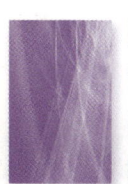

Practical Guide to the Care of the Gynecologic/Obstetric Patient

Series Editor
Fred F. Ferri, MD, FACP
Clinical Professor
The Warren Alpert Medical School of Brown University
Providence, Rhode Island

OTHER VOLUMES IN THE "PRACTICAL GUIDE SERIES"
Goldberg: *Practical Guide to the Care of the Psychiatric Patient*
Alario & Birnkrant: *Practical Guide to the Care of the Pediatric Patient*
Wachtel & Fretwell: *Practical Guide to the Care of the Geriatric Patient*
Ferri: *Practical Guide to the Care of the Medical Patient*

Practical Guide to the Care of the Gynecologic/Obstetric Patient

2nd Edition

George T. Danakas, MD, FACOG
Clinical Assistant Professor
Department of Gynecology/Obstetrics
University at Buffalo School of Medicine
 and Biomedical Sciences
Buffalo, New York

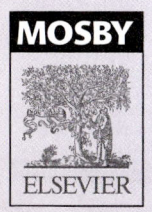

MOSBY
ELSEVIER

MOSBY
ELSEVIER

1600 John F. Kennedy Blvd.
Suite 1800
Philadelphia, PA 19103-2899

PRACTICAL GUIDE TO THE CARE
OF THE GYNECOLOGIC/OBSTETRIC
PATIENT, SECOND EDITION

ISBN: 978-0-323-04708-1

Copyright © 2007, 1997 by Mosby, Inc., an affiliate of Elsevier Inc.

All rights reserved. No part of this publication may be reproduced or transmitted in any form or by any means, electronic or mechanical, including photocopying, recording, or any information storage and retrieval system, without permission in writing from the publisher. Permissions may be sought directly from Elsevier's Rights Department: phone: (+1) 215 239 3804 (US) or (+44) 1865 843830 (UK); fax: (+44) 1865 853333; e-mail: healthpermissions@elsevier.com. You may also complete your request on-line via the Elsevier website at http://www.elsevier.com/permissions.

Notice

Knowledge and best practice in this field are constantly changing. As new research and experience broaden our knowledge, changes in practice, treatment, and drug therapy may become necessary or appropriate. Readers are advised to check the most current information provided (i) on procedures featured or (ii) by the manufacturer of each product to be administered to verify the recommended dose or formula, the method and duration of administration, and contraindications. It is the responsibility of the practitioner, relying on their own experience and knowledge of the patient, to make diagnoses, to determine dosages and the best treatment for each individual patient, and to take all appropriate safety precautions. To the fullest extent of the law, neither the Publisher nor the Editor assumes any liability for any injury and/or damage to persons or property arising out of or related to any use of the material contained in this book.

The Publisher

Library of Congress Cataloging-in-Publication Data
Practical guide to the care of the gynecologic/obstetric patient / [edited by] George T. Danakas. — 2nd ed.
  p. ; cm.
  Includes bibliographical references and index.
  ISBN 978-0-323-04708-1
  1. Gynecology—Handbooks, manuals, etc. 2. Obstetrics—Handbooks, manuals, etc. I. Danakas, George T.
  [DNLM: 1. Gynecology—methods—Handbooks. 2. Obstetrics—methods—Handbooks. WP 39 P8947 2007]
  RG110.P73 2007
  618—dc22
                                                                    2007023050

Acquisitions Editor: Jim Merritt
Developmental Editor: Andrea Deis
Project Manager: Mary Stermel
Design Direction: Ellen Zanolle
Marketing Manager: Alyson Sherby

Working together to grow
libraries in developing countries

www.elsevier.com | www.bookaid.org | www.sabre.org

ELSEVIER   BOOK AID International   Sabre Foundation

Printed in the United States of America

Last digit is the print number: 9 8 7 6 5 4 3 2 1

This book is dedicated to my wonderful wife, Maria, who has given me so much love and support throughout the years. I also want to dedicate this book to my two beautiful daughters, Rose and Alexandra, who have inspired me to be a better person in all areas of my life.

Contributors

Philip J. Aliotta, MD, MSHA, FACS, CPI
Clinical Instructor
Department of Urology and Neurology
State University of New York at Buffalo
Attending Urologist
Sisters of Charity Hospital
Director, Bladder and Pelvic Floor Disorders
Department of Neurology
Jacobs Neurological Institute of Buffalo General Hospital
Medical Director
Center for Urologic Research of Western New York
Main Urology
Buffalo, New York

Brad Angle, MD
Associate Professor of Pediatrics
Northwestern University Feinberg School of Medicine
Attending Physician, Genetics
Division of Birth Defects and Metabolism
Children's Memorial Hospital
Chicago, Illinois

Farkad Balaya, MD
Clinical Assistant Professor
Department of Gynecology/Obstetrics
School of Medicine and Biomedical Sciences
State University of New York at Buffalo
Clinical Assistant Professor
Department of Gynecology/Obstetrics
Women and Children's Hospital
Clinical Assistant Professor
Department of Gynecology/Obstetrics
Sisters of Charity Hospital
Buffalo, New York

John R. Barton, MD
Volunteer Professor of Obstetrics and Gynecology
Department of Obstetrics and Gynecology
University of Cincinnati
Cincinnati, Ohio
Director, Maternal-Fetal Medicine
Central Baptist Hospital
Lexington, Kentucky

Ronald E. Batt, MD, MA
Professor of Clinical Gynecology
Department of Gynecology/Obstetrics
State University of New York at Buffalo
Women and Children's Hospital of Buffalo
Buffalo, New York

Harold E. Bays MD, FACP
Medical Director/President
Louisville Metabolic and Atherosclerosis Research Center
Louisville, Kentucky

Beth Buehler, MS, CGC
Director, Genetic Counseling
The Prenatal Center
Palm Beach Gardens, Florida

S. J. Carlan, MD
Program Director, Residency Program
Director, Maternal-Fetal Medicine
Department of Obstetrics and Gynecology
Orlando Regional Healthcare
Orlando, Florida

Vernon Cook, MD
Assistant Professor
Department of Obstetrics and Gynecology
University of Louisville School of Medicine
Louisville, Kentucky

Maria A. Corigliano, MD, FACOG
Clinical Assistant Professor
Department of Obstetrics and Gynecology
Kaleida Health
Clinical Assistant Professor
Department of Obstetrics and Gynecology
Sisters of Charity Hospital
Buffalo, New York

George T. Danakas, MD, FACOG
Clinical Assistant Professor
Department of Gynecology/Obstetrics
University at Buffalo School of Medicine and Biomedical Sciences
Buffalo, New York

Carolyn Maud Doherty, MD
Assistant Professor
Department of Obstetrics and Gynecology
Creighton University
Director, Assisted Reproductive Lab
Department of Obstetrics and Gynecology
Methodist Hospital
Omaha, Nebraska

Ivan D'Souza, MD, FRCS, FACOG
Clinical Assistant Professor
Department of Obstetrics and Gynecology
State University of New York at Buffalo School of Medicine
Buffalo, New York

J. Kevin Fitzpatrick, MD
Clinical Instructor
Department of Obstetrics and Gynecology
State University of New York at Buffalo
Buffalo, New York

Stanley A. Gall, MD
Professor
Department of Obstetrics, Gynecology, and Women's Health
University of Louisville
Department of Obstetrics, Gynecology, and Women's Health
University of Louisville Hospital
Louisville, Kentucky

Lawrence J. Gugino, MD
Clinical Associate Professor
Department of Obstetrics and Gynecology
State University of New York at Buffalo School of Medicine
Children's Hospital of Buffalo
Buffalo, New York

Patricia D. Harris, RD, LD, CDE
Senior Nutritionist
Department of Obstetrics, Gynecology, and Women's Health
University of Louisville
Louisville, Kentucky

Joseph Hersh, MD
Professor
Department of Pediatrics
Child Evaluation Center
University of Louisville School of Medicine
Louisville, Kentucky

Karen Houck, MD
Carol G. Simon Cancer Center
Morristown Memorial Hospital
Morristown, New Jersey

Helen Y. How, MD
Assistant Professor
Department of Obstetrics and Gynecology
Marshall University School of Medicine
Department of Obstetrics and Gynecology
Cabell Huntington Hospital
Huntington, West Virginia

Ibrahim Joulak, MD
Clinical Assistant Instructor
Department of Gynecology and Obstetrics
State University of New York at Buffalo
Buffalo, New York

Luanne Lettieri, MD
Assistant Professor
Director of Maternal-Fetal Medicine
Department of Obstetrics and Gynecology
Texas Tech University Health Sciences Center
Odessa, Texas

Germaine M. Louis, PhD, MS
Chief and Senior Investigator
Epidemiology Branch
National Institute of Child Health and Human Development
Rockville, Maryland

David L. Marchetti, MD
Clinical Associate Professor
Department of Gynecology/Obstetrics
State University of New York at Buffalo
Department of Gynecology/Obstetrics
Sisters of Charity Hospital
Department of Gynecology/Obstetrics
Roswell Park Cancer Institute
Buffalo, New York
Department of Gynecology/Obstetrics
Kaleida Health Systems
Williamsville, New York

Michael P. Marcotte, MD
Member, Division of Maternal-Fetal Medicine
Department of Obstetrics and Gynecology
Good Samaritan Hospital
Cincinnati, Ohio

John M. O'Brien, MD
Director, Perinatal Diagnostic Center
Maternal-Fetal Medicine
Central Baptist Hospital
Lexington, Kentucky

Alexander B. Olawaiye, MD, MRCOG, FACOG
Division of Gynecologic Oncology
Department of Obstetrics, Gynecology, and
 Reproductive Biology
Massachusetts General Hospital/Harvard Medical School
Boston, Massachusetts

Michael Parsons, MD
Associate Professor
Department of Obstetrics and Gynecology
University of South Florida
Tampa General Hospital
Tampa, Florida

Marcello Pietrantoni, MD
Associate Professor
Department of Obstetrics and Gynecology
Division of Maternal-Fetal Medicine
University of Louisville School of Medicine
Louisville, Kentucky

Arundathi G. Prasad, MD
Faculty Physician
Department of Obstetrics and Gynecology
Health Net, Inc.
Indianapolis, Indiana

Bruce D. Rodgers, MD
Associate Professor of Clinical Obstetrics and Gynecology
Director, Maternal-Fetal Medicine
State University of New York at Buffalo School of Medicine and
 Biomedical Sciences
Director, Maternal-Fetal Medicine
Women and Children's Hospital of Buffalo
Buffalo, New York

Mary Self, MD

Baha M. Sibai, MD
Professor
Department of Obstetrics and Gynecology
University of Cincinnati College of Medicine
Cincinnati, Ohio

Avi Sklar, MD, FACOG, FACS, FRCSC
Clinical Associate Professor
Department of Obstetrics and Gynecology
Stanford University
Palo Alto, California
Co-Chief, Gynecology
Santa Clara Valley Medical Center
San Jose, California

D. Michael Slate II, MD, FACS
Clinical Assistant Professor
Department of Pathology and Anatomical Sciences
State University of New York at Buffalo
Medical Director, Clinical Microbiology
Kaleida Health
Buffalo, New York
Medical Director, Essential Services Laboratory
Kaleida Health Millard Fillmore Suburban Hospital
Williamsville, New York

Diane J. Sutter, MD, FACOG
Attending Physician
Department of Obstetrics and Gynecology
Kaleida Health Millard Fillmore Suburban Hospital
Williamsville, New York
Attending Physician
Department of Obstetrics and Gynecology
Mercy Hospital at Buffalo
Buffalo, New York

Salvador M. Udagawa, MD, FACS
Attending Surgeon, Colon and Rectal Surgery
Sisters of Charity Hospital
Buffalo, New York

Louis Weinstein, MD
Bowers Professor and Chairperson
Department of Obstetrics and Gynecology
Thomas Jefferson University
Chairperson
Department of Obstetrics and Gynecology
Thomas Jefferson University Hospital
Philadelphia, Pennsylvania

Dennis M. Weppner, MD, FACOG
Associate Professor of Clinical Gynecology
Department of Obstetrics/Gynecology
State University of New York at Buffalo School of Medicine
Clinical Chief
Department of Obstetrics/Gynecology
Millard Fillmore Suburban Hospital
Buffalo, New York

Mark Williams, MD
Assistant Professor
Department of Obstetrics and Gynecology
University of South Florida
Tampa General Hospital
Tampa, Florida

P. Gail Williams, MD
Associate Professor, Pediatrics
University of Louisville
Louisville, Kentucky

Scott J. Zuccala, DO, FACOG
Staff Physician
Department of Obstetrics and Gynecology
Mercy Hospital at Buffalo
Buffalo, New York
Managing Partner
Hamburg Obstetrics/Gynecology Group, PC
Blasdell, New York

Preface

Practical Guide to the Care of the Gynecologic/Obstetric Patient, second edition, is a concise and portable source to aid third-year medical students, physician assistants, and nurse practitioners. The book is divided into two sections: first gynecology and then obstetrics.

The book follows an outline format, and although complete, it is not meant to be used as a replacement for standard textbooks in the fields of obstetrics and gynecology. References have been included for readers who desire more information.

I would like to acknowledge all the contributors to this text and Dr. Donald Schmidt for reviewing the chapter on high-risk obstetrics.

I am grateful for the help of my editors at Elsevier, James Merritt, Andrea Deis, and Leah Bross, and their assistants, artists, and copy editors.

And special thanks to my good friend and colleague, Dr. Fred Ferri, for his guidance and encouragement, which made a dream reality.

George T. Danakas

Contents

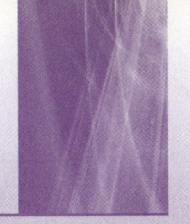

1 Charting, 1
George T. Danakas

- 1.1 History and Physical Examinations, 1
- 1.2 Progress Notes, 4
- 1.3 Admission Orders, 4
- 1.4 Preoperative Evaluation, 5
- 1.5 Preoperative Note, 6
- 1.6 Postoperative Orders, 6
- 1.7 Discharge Summary, 7

2 Gynecologic Anatomy, 8
David L. Marchetti

- 2.1 Anterior Lateral Abdominal Wall, 8
- 2.2 Muscles and Fascia of the Anterior Lateral Abdominal Wall, 9
- 2.3 External Genitalia, 13
- 2.4 The Perineum, 13
- 2.5 Pelvic Diaphragm, Obturator, and Piriformis Muscles, 20
- 2.6 The Pelvic Viscera, 23
- 2.7 Spaces, 24
- 2.8 Pelvic Peritoneum, 28
- 2.9 Cardinal and Uterosacral Ligaments, 28
- 2.10 The Vagina, 28
- 2.11 The Urinary Tract, 28
- 2.12 Blood Supply of the Pelvis, 30
- 2.13 Lymphatic Drainage of the Pelvis, 34
- 2.14 Pelvic Joints, 34
- 2.15 Ligaments, 35
- 2.16 Nerves of the Lesser Pelvis, 35
- 2.17 The Autonomic Nervous System, 40

3 Abdominal Surgical Approaches, 46
J. Kevin Fitzpatrick

- 3.1 Anatomy of the Anterior Abdominal Wall, 46
- 3.2 Abdominal Incisions, 50
- 3.3 Closing the Abdomen, 65

4 Diagnostic Studies, 69

- 4.1 Papanicolaou Smear, 69
  George T. Danakas
- 4.2 Colposcopy, 70
  George T. Danakas and Karen Houck
- 4.3 Hysteroscopy, 71
  Scott J. Zuccala
- 4.4 Abdominal–Pelvic Diagnostic Laparoscopy, 72
  Scott J. Zuccala
- 4.5 Bowel Injury, 77
  Salvador M. Udagawa, Germaine M. Louis, and Ronald E. Batt
- 4.6 Ureteral Dissection, 80
  Ronald E. Batt and Germaine M. Louis
- 4.7 Urodynamic Studies, 83
  Philip J. Aliotta

5 Contraception, 100
Maria A. Corigliano

- 5.1 Oral Contraceptives, 101
- 5.2 Progestin-Only Contraception, 107
- 5.3 Postcoital Contraception, 113
- 5.4 Barrier Methods, 118
- 5.5 Lactation Amenorrhea Method, 123
- 5.6 Abstinence, 123
- 5.7 Withdrawal, 124
- 5.8 Rhythm Method—Natural Family Planning, 124
- 5.9 Sterilization, 125

6 Infertility Evaluation, 137

- 6.1 Female Infertility, 137
  Carolyn Maud Doherty
- 6.2 Male Infertility, 150
  Philip J. Aliotta

7 Amenorrhea, 167
Ivan D'Souza

- 7.1 Classification, 167
- 7.2 Clinical Assessment, 171
- 7.3 Secondary Amenorrhea, 173

8 Abnormal Uterine Bleeding, 179
George T. Danakas and Diane J. Sutter

- 8.1 Etiology, 179
- 8.2 Definitions of Abnormal Bleeding, 179

- 8.3 Diagnosis, 180
- 8.4 Management, 182

9 Endometriosis, 184
Ronald E. Batt and Germaine M. Louis

- 9.1 Definition, 184
- 9.2 Epidemiology, 184
- 9.3 Theories of Histogenesis, 185
- 9.4 Clinical Manifestations, 185
- 9.5 Physical Examination, 186
- 9.6 Tools for Assessment, 187
- 9.7 Findings at Laparoscopy, 187
- 9.8 Host Responses to Endometriosis, 188
- 9.9 Disease Patterns, 189
- 9.10 Complications of Treatment of Complex Disease Patterns, 189
- 9.11 Options for Treatment, 190
- 9.12 Physician–Patient Follow-Up from Diagnosis Until Postmenopause, 192
- 9.13 Overview of Management, 192

10 Gynecologic Infections, 194
D. Michael Slate II and Lawrence J. Gugino

- 10.1 Gonorrhea, 194
- 10.2 Chlamydia, 197
- 10.3 Lymphogranuloma Venereum, 199
- 10.4 Syphilis, 200
- 10.5 Chancroid, 203
- 10.6 Donovanosis (Granuloma Inguinale), 204
- 10.7 Genital Herpes Simplex Virus, 205
- 10.8 Pelvic Inflammatory Disease, 208
- 10.9 Bacterial Vaginosis, 213
- 10.10 Vulvovaginal Candidiasis, 215
- 10.11 Trichomoniasis, 218

11 HIV Infection in Women, 222
D. Michael Slate II and Lawrence J. Gugino

- 11.1 Background, 222
- 11.2 Epidemiology, 222
- 11.3 Major Routes of Transmission of HIV-1, 222
- 11.4 Pathophysiology, 223
- 11.5 HIV Testing and Counseling in Women, 223
- 11.6 Clinical Manifestations and Diagnosis, 224
- 11.7 HIV Infection in Pregnancy, 228

12 Evaluation of Lower Abdominal and Pelvic Pain, 233
Avi Sklar and Farkad Balaya

12.1 Anatomy and Physiology, 233
12.2 Assessment, 234
12.3 Early Pregnancy Complications, 238
12.4 Ectopic Pregnancy, 239
12.5 Hemorrhagic Corpus Luteum of Pregnancy, 243
12.6 Gestational Trophoblastic Disease, 243
12.7 Pregnant Uterine Incarceration, 243
12.8 Pelvic Infections, 244
12.9 Pain of Adnexal Origin, 244
12.10 Ovarian Hyperstimulation Syndrome, 245
12.11 Leiomyomas, 246
12.12 Intestinal Sources of Pain, 246
12.13 Urinary Tract Sources of Pain, 249
12.14 Vascular Sources of Pain, 250
12.15 Systemic Causes of Abdominal Pain, 251
12.16 Dysmenorrhea, 251
12.17 Endometriosis, 252
12.18 Adenomyosis, 253
12.19 Adhesions, 253
12.20 Ovulatory Pain (Mittelschmerz), 254
12.21 Ovarian Remnant Syndrome, 254
12.22 Pelvic Congestion Syndrome, 254
12.23 "Trigger Point" Abdominal Wall Pain, 255
12.24 Functional Bowel Disorders, 255
12.25 Chronic Pelvic Pain, 256

13 Differential Diagnosis of Benign Gynecologic Conditions, 258
Dennis M. Weppner

13.1 Abnormal Genital Tract Bleeding, 258
13.2 Amenorrhea, 261
13.3 Ascites, 263
13.4 Breast Inflammatory Lesion, 263
13.5 Breast Mass, 264
13.6 Endocrinopathies, 265
13.7 Female Reproductive Tract Abnormalities, 268
13.8 Genital Discharge, 269
13.9 Infertility, 270
13.10 Lower Reproductive Tract Infection, 272
13.11 Ovarian Failure, 273
13.12 Pelvic Mass—Gynecologic Causes, 274
13.13 Pelvic Mass—Nongynecologic Causes, 280
13.14 Pelvic Pain, 281
13.15 Premenstrual Syndrome, 283

13.16 Sexual Dysfunction, 284
13.17 Upper Genital Tract Infection, 285
13.18 Urinary Incontinence, 286
13.19 Vulvar Lesions, 287

14 Gynecologic Oncology, 290
Alexander B. Olawaiye

14.1 Cervical Cancer, 290
14.2 Uterine Cancer, 291
14.3 Vaginal Cancer, 295
14.4 Vulvar Cancer, 297
14.5 Ovarian Cancer, 299

15 Hirsutism, 304
Arundathi G. Prasad

15.1 Definitions, 304
15.2 Physiology of Hair Growth, 304
15.3 Androgen Production, 305
15.4 Etiology of Hirsutism, 305
15.5 Evaluation, 308
15.6 Treatment, 308

16 Premenstrual Syndrome, 310
George T. Danakas and Ibrahim Joulak

16.1 Definition, 310
16.2 Epidemiology, 310
16.3 Diagnostic Criteria, 310
16.4 Etiology, 310
16.5 Symptoms, 311
16.6 Diagnosis, 311
16.7 Management, 311

17 Menopause, 320
Diane J. Sutter

17.1 Menopause, 320
17.2 Osteoporosis, 323
17.3 Cardiovascular Disease, 325
17.4 Hormone Replacement Therapy, 327

18 Labor, Delivery, and Obstetrics Pain Management, 329
Farkad Balaya

18.1 Normal Labor and Delivery, 329
18.2 Abnormal Labor, 340
18.3 Analgesia and Anesthetics in Obstetrics, 347

19 High-Risk Obstetrics, 362

- 19.1 Diabetes in Pregnancy, 362
  Bruce D. Rodgers
- 19.2 Insulin Treatment in Pregnancy, 383
  Harold E. Bays and Mary Self
- 19.3 Intrauterine Growth Retardation, 395
  Mark Williams
- 19.4 Genetic Counseling, 414
  Beth Buehler
- 19.5 Hypertension in Pregnancy, 426
  John R. Barton and Baha M. Sibai
- 19.6 HIV in Pregnancy, 444
  Stanley A. Gall
- 19.7 Group B *Streptococcus* and Bacterial Vaginosis, 451
  Michael P. Marcotte and Louis Weinstein
- 19.8 Pulmonary Disease, 464
  Michael Parsons
- 19.9 Renal Disease, 480
  Helen Y. How

20 Antenatal Assessment, 492

- 20.1 Antenatal Assessment, 492
  S. J. Carlan
- 20.2 Ultrasound and Fetal Aneuploidy, 508
  Luanne Lettieri
- 20.3 Nutrition in Pregnancy, 515
  Patricia D. Harris and Marcello Pietrantoni
- 20.4 Assessment of Fetal Pulmonary Maturity, 525
  George T. Danakas
- 20.5 Genetics, 525
  Brad Angle, P. Gail Williams, and Joseph Hersh
- 20.6 Amniocentesis and Chorionic Villus Sampling, 556
  Vernon Cook

21 Postpartum Hemorrhage, 565
John M. O'Brien

- 21.1 Importance and Perspective, 565
- 21.2 Etiologies, 565
- 21.3 Treatments, 567
- 21.4 Algorithm for Management, 572

22 Physiology in Pregnancy, 573
Arundathi G. Prasad

- 22.1 Maternal Nutrition, 573

22.2 Maternal Skin Changes, 574
22.3 Maternal Blood Volume, 575
22.4 Maternal Vascular Changes, 576
22.5 Fetal and Placental Physiology, 577
22.6 Maternal Respiratory System, 581
22.7 Maternal Urinary System, 583
22.8 Maternal Gastrointestinal System, 587
22.9 Maternal Reproductive System, 588
22.10 Common Discomforts of Pregnancy: Causes and Relief, 589
22.11 Endocrinology and Physiologic Changes, 596

Index, 603

Charting

George T. Danakas

1.1 History and Physical Examinations

1. **Chief complaint:** Reason patient has come to see you; should be in her own words (Why have you come in to see me today?)
2. **Present illness:** The patient describes each presenting problem in detail. When did the problem begin (onset)? Is this a new problem or a recurrence?
3. **Past medical history:**
4. **Past surgical history:**
   a. Transfusions:
   b. Current medications:
   c. Allergies:
   d. Habits (drugs, alcohol, tobacco, exercise, diet):
5. **Family history:**
6. **Systems review:**
   a. General: weakness, fatigue, change in weight, appetite, sleeping habits, chills, fever, night sweats
   b. Integument: color changes, pruritus, nevus, infections, tumor (benign or malignant), dermatosis, hair changes, nail changes
   c. Hematopoietic: anemia, abnormal bleeding, adenopathy, excessive bruising
   d. Central nervous system:
      (1) General: syncope, loss of consciousness, convulsions, meningitis, encephalitis, stroke
      (2) Mentative: speech disorders, emotional status, orientation, memory disorders, change in sleep pattern, history of nervous breakdown
      (3) Motor: tremor, weakness, paralysis, clumsiness of movement
      (4) Sensory: radicular or neuralgic pain (head, neck, trunk, extremities), paresthesias, anesthesias
   e. Eyes: vision, glasses or contact lenses, date of last eye examination, scotomata, pain, excessive tearing
   f. Ears: tinnitus, deafness, other
   g. Nose, throat, and sinuses: epistaxis, discharge, sinusitis, hoarseness
   h. Dentition: caries, pyorrhea, dentures
   i. Breasts: masses, discharge, pain, family history of breast cancer, any past problems, monthly breast self-examination: yes or no

j. Respiratory: cough (productive or nonproductive), change in cough, amount and characteristic of sputum, duration of sputum production, smoking, number of packs a day, years of tobacco use, wheezing, hemoptysis, recurrent respiratory tract infections, positive tuberculin test
k. Cardiovascular: chest pain, typical angina pectoris, dyspnea on exertion, orthopnea, paroxysmal nocturnal dyspnea, peripheral edema, murmur, palpitation, varicosities, thrombophlebitis, claudication, Raynaud's phenomenon, syncope, near syncope
l. Gastrointestinal (GI): nausea, vomiting, diarrhea, constipation, melena, hematemesis, rectal bleeding, change in bowel habits, hemorrhoids, dysphagia, food intolerance, excessive gas or indigestion, abdominal pain, jaundice, use of antacids, use of laxatives
m. Urinary tract: renal colic, frequency of urination, nocturia, polyuria, dysuria, micturition (retention, hesitancy, urgency, dysuria, narrowing of stream, dribbling incontinence), hematuria, albuminuria, pyuria, kidney disease, renal stones, cystoscopy
n. Genitoreproductive system:
   (1) Gynecologic history: age of menarche, last menstrual period, age at menopause, postmenopausal bleeding, abnormal menses, amount of bleeding, intermenstrual bleeding, postcoital bleeding, leukorrhea, pruritus, history of venereal disease, serology, last Papanicolaou smear and results, menopausal symptoms, hormone replacement therapy history
      (a) Dysmenorrhea (onset, duration, severity)
      (b) Cycle interval, amount of flow (light, moderate, heavy)
      (c) Vaginal discharge (onset, color, odor, itching, burning, or pain)
      (d) Methods of contraception (past and present)
   (2) Obstetric history:
      (a) **G** Gravida—number of pregnancies
          P Parity—full term, preterm, abortion, living children
      (b) Description of each pregnancy
          (i) Date
          (ii) Vaginal; spontaneous or operative (forceps or vacuum); Cesarean
          (iii) Weight and sex
          (iv) Complications (antepartum, intrapartum, postpartum)
      (c) Complications of pregnancies, infertility (Has the patient ever had difficulty becoming pregnant? Was she ever evaluated or treated for this problem? If yes, describe in detail.)
   (3) Sexual history: age of first coitus, consensual?; number of partners, orgasmic?; dyspareunia; libido
o. Musculoskeletal system:
   (1) Joints: pain, edema, heat, rubor, stiffness, deformity
   (2) Muscles: myalgias
p. Endocrine system: goiter, heat intolerance, cold intolerance, change in voice, polyuria, polydipsia, polyphagia

q. Psychiatric: hyperventilation, nervousness, depression, insomnia, nightmares, memory loss

7. **Physical examination:**
   a. Vital signs: blood pressure, pulse, respirations, temperature
   b. Height and weight
   c. Integument: turgor, texture, pigmentation, cyanosis, telangiectasis, petechiae, purpura, ecchymosis, infection, lesions, hair, nails, mucous membranes
   d. Lymph nodes: cervical, postauricular, supraclavicular, axillary, inguinal, epitrochlear
   e. Skull: trauma, bruits, other
   f. Eyes: lacrimal glands, cornea, lids, sclerae, conjunctivae, exophthalmos, lid lag
   g. Fundi: discs, arteries, veins, hemorrhages, exudates, microaneurysm
   h. Ears: tophi, tympanic membranes, external canal, hearing
   i. Mouth, nose, and throat: dentition, gingiva, tongue, tonsils, pharynx, nasal mucosa, nasal septum, sinuses
   j. Neck: mobility, scars, masses, thyroid, bruit, salivary glands, tracheal shift
   k. Breasts: masses, discharge, nipples, asymmetry, skin retraction, axillary adenopathy
   l. Chest: respiratory rate: /min; amplitude: shallow/deep/normal; clear, rales, rhonci, wheezes
   m. Cardiovascular system: S1, S2, gallops, systolic murmur, diastolic murmur
   n. Peripheral pulses: carotid, brachial, radial, aorta, femoral, popliteal, dorsalis pedis
   o. Extremities: edema, cyanosis, stasis, ulceration, hair distribution, clubbing
   p. Abdomen: obesity, contour, scars, tenderness, cerebrovascular accident, tenderness, masses, rebound, rigidity, fluid wave, shifting dullness, frank ascites, bruits, hernia, venous collaterals
      (1) Bowel sounds: normal, absent, hyperactive, hypoactive, obstructive
      (2) Organomegaly: liver, spleen, kidneys, bladder, gallbladder
   q. Genitoreproductive system:
      (1) External genitalia: labia, clitoris, introitus, urethra, perineum; document any lesions.
      (2) Internal genitalia: vagina, cervix, adnexa, cul-de-sac, discharge.
      (3) Papanicolaou smear: done, omitted.
      (4) Rectal: hemorrhoids, sphincter tone, bleeding, masses.
      (5) Stool for occult blood.
      (6) External genitalia: hair pattern, labia majora and minora, clitoris, urethral Bartholin, periurethral and Skene's glands.
      (7) Speculum examination: Choose the appropriate-size speculum (either a medium Graves, a Smith-Anderson, or a pediatric) and insert it into the vagina. The speculum may be moistened with warm water, if necessary, but no other kinds of lubrication

should be used because they can affect cultures and cytology. Spread the labia and insert the speculum vertically through the introitus and then rotate horizontally. Note any lesions on the cervix, if present. Obtain a Papanicolaou smear. Next obtain cervical cultures for chlamydia, gonorrhea, and human papillomavirus (HPV) if clinically warranted.
- (8) Bimanual examination: Palpate vagina, cervix, uterus, adnexa, and cul-de-sac. Insert the index and middle fingers of the examining hand into the vagina. The abdominal hand brings down the organs to the examining hand in the vagina. Specifically note the following:
  - (a) Cervix: position, consistency, pain with cervical motion
  - (b) Uterus: size, shape (normal, globular, irregular), position (anterior, posterior, midline), tenderness on motion
  - (c) Adnexa: masses or tenderness
- (9) Rectovaginal examination: With the index finger in the vagina and the middle figure in the rectum, palpate rectovaginal septum, uterosacral ligaments, cardinal ligaments, cul-de-sac, looking for masses or tenderness.
r. Joints: deformity, rubor, calor, tenderness, edema
  - (1) Range of motion: fingers, wrists, elbow, shoulder, hips, knees, ankles
  - (2) Spine: deformity (kyphosis, lordosis, scoliosis), thoracic excursion
s. Neurologic system: reflexes; cerebral function: alert wakefulness, lethargic, obtunded, stuporous, semicomatose, comatose

1.2 Progress Notes

Use the mnemonic "SOAP":

- **S** Subjective patient complaints
- **O** Objective—physical exam and testing results
- **A** Assessment
- **P** Plan

1.3 Admission Orders

Use the mnemonic "ABC-DAVID":

- **A** Admit
- **B** Because—diagnosis
- **C** Condition
- **D** Diet—nothing by month (NPO), clear liquids, regular house diet, diabetic diet
- **A** Allergies and activity
- **V** Vital signs—frequency
- **I** Intravenous (IV) fluids—solution and rate
- **D** Diagnostic tests; laboratory studies; x-rays; drugs/medications: dose, frequency, rate of administration (e.g., Motrin 800 mg q8h orally [PO] prn for pain)

Practical Guide to the Care of the Gynecologic/Obstetric Patient 5

1.4 Preoperative Evaluation

1. Medical history and physical examination
   a. Significant medical history or illnesses that may complicate anesthesia or recovery
   b. Current medications: prescription and nonprescription
   c. Allergies
   d. Previous surgery: Review operative reports from previous pelvic surgery especially if patient has had surgery for pelvic inflammatory disease (PID), endometriosis, pelvic abscess, or malignancy.
   e. Family history: excessive bleeding, malignant hyperthermia
   f. General review of systems, especially GI and genitourinary
2. Laboratory evaluation
   a. Complete blood count (CBC)
   b. Serum chemistry with liver function tests (LFTs)
   c. Chest x-ray (CXR), electrocardiogram (ECG) if over 40 (if under 40 only if medical history warrants these studies)
   d. Intravenous pyelogram (IVP), barium enema, upper GI with small bowel follow-through, computed tomography (CT) if felt necessary
3. Obtaining informed consent is not merely getting the patient to sign the hospital consent form. A detailed discussion with the patient, her significant other, and any other family member she thinks necessary should be undertaken before surgery. The discussion should include the following:
   a. Risks and complications of proposed surgery: blood loss, infection, anesthesia, injury to bowel, bladder, ureter, venous thrombosis, return to surgery, and death
   b. Benefits of surgery
   c. Postoperative recovery period—length of time unable to perform usual activities
   d. Long-term effects of the surgery (e.g., menopausal symptoms and consequences after bilateral salpingo-oophorectomy [BSO]) or if surgery not done
   e. The nature and extent of the disease process
   f. Alternative methods of therapy along with the risks and benefits of these other methods of therapy
   g. Failure rates of procedure (e.g., sterilization)
   h. Type of anesthesia planned: Questions should be addressed to the anesthesiologist. If the patient has preexisting medical condition that could complicate anesthesia, a presurgical consult with the anesthesia department would be a good idea.
   i. Expected length of surgery
   j. Description of the surgical procedure: Use pictures if felt necessary; is procedure only diagnostic or is it therapeutic?
   k. Time for the patient and family members to ask questions
4. Bowel preparation should be performed in patients with pelvic mass, endometriosis, cancer, multiple previous abdominal surgeries, or previous bowel surgery.

5. Antibiotic prophylaxis
   a. It is generally accepted to use preoperative antibiotics 30 minutes before initial incision.
   b. Prophylactic antibiotics should not be used for more than 24 hours. I prefer only a single dose because there is no definitive proof that continuing antibiotics over 24 hours is any more effective. First-generation cephalosporin is adequate.
6. Thromboembolic prophylaxis needs to be considered in patients at risk for thromboembolic event after surgery (i.e., previous thromboembolic disease, venous insufficiency, obesity, anticipation of prolonged immobility). Low-dose heparin 5000 units subcutaneously (SC) 2 hours preoperative, followed by 5000 units q12h until ambulatory well, pneumatic stockings.

1.5 Preoperative Note

1. Brief summary of history and physical (only significant facts listed)
2. Proposed surgery
3. Indication for proposed surgery
4. Consent reviewed and signed
5. Lab results, x-ray reports, ECG (if done)
6. Patient allergies
7. If major surgery, whether or not blood typed and crossed
8. Operating room (OR) note
   a. Preoperative diagnosis:
   b. Postoperative diagnosis:
   c. Procedure:
   d. Anesthesia:
   e. Surgeon:
   f. Assistants:
   g. Findings:
   h. Transferred to recovery room in (satisfactory) condition

1.6 Postoperative Orders

1. Admit: to recovery room and then to floor
2. Diagnosis: status post (S/P) total abdominal hysterectomy (TAH) for endometrial carcinoma
3. Condition:
4. Diet:
5. Activity:
6. Fluids:
7. Graphics: vitals, weights, urine output, etc.
8. Allergies:
9. Nursing instructions: Foley, nasogastric, spirometry, drains
10. Labs:
11. Medication: pain, antibiotics, sleeper
12. Call house officer for:

1.7 Discharge Summary

1. Patient name:
2. Discharge date:
3. Medical records number:
4. Admitting diagnosis:
5. Statement of history and physical findings:
6. Significant findings (x-ray film, laboratory results, consults, etc.):
7. Course in hospital (complications, progress of patient, etc.):
8. Condition on discharge:
9. Instructions to patient and family:
    a. Diet
    b. Level of activity
    c. Medications
    d. Follow-up instructions
10. Principal diagnosis:
11. Secondary diagnosis:
12. Procedures:

Gynecologic Anatomy

David L. Marchetti

The anatomic study of the female reproductive tract and related anatomy is a necessary adjunct to proper diagnosis and treatment of gynecologic disease. Such knowledge is a prerequisite of advanced surgical technique. This chapter presents this information from both a surgical and an anatomic perspective.

2.1 Anterior Lateral Abdominal Wall

Anatomic study of the abdomen includes the abdomen proper and the pelvis. The perineum is continuous with the anterior abdominal wall and is located at the outlet of the pelvis. For descriptive purposes, the abdomen can be divided into nine regions by three horizontal and two vertical planes (Fig. 2-1).

SUPERFICIAL FASCIA
The superficial fascia of the anterior abdominal wall is composed of Camper's fascia, which is the superficial fatty layer (Fig. 2-2). It is continuous over the inguinal ligament with the similar corresponding layer of the thigh and medially continues into the labia majora.

DEEP LAYER
The deep layer of the membranous subcutaneous fascia is identified as Scarpa's fascia and is a membranous sheath containing little or no adipose tissue (see Fig. 2-2). It forms a continuous sheath across the midline, where it attaches to the linea alba. Inferiorly it passes over the inguinal ligament and is securely attached to either the ligament itself or to the fascia lata just beyond it. Inferior to the ligament, the corresponding layer is called the fascia cribrosa as it covers and fills the fossa ovalis. At the medial end of the inguinal ligament, it passes over the external inguinal ring without attachment and continues along the groove between the labia majora and thigh into the perineum, where it is called the fascia of Colles. These attachments of Scarpa's fascia form a gutter that empties into the superficial perineal pouch. The abdomen and perineum communicate through the abdominal labial opening posterior to the fascia of Scarpa and Colles. Hemorrhage of the anterior abdominal wall may be associated with extravasation into the perineum.

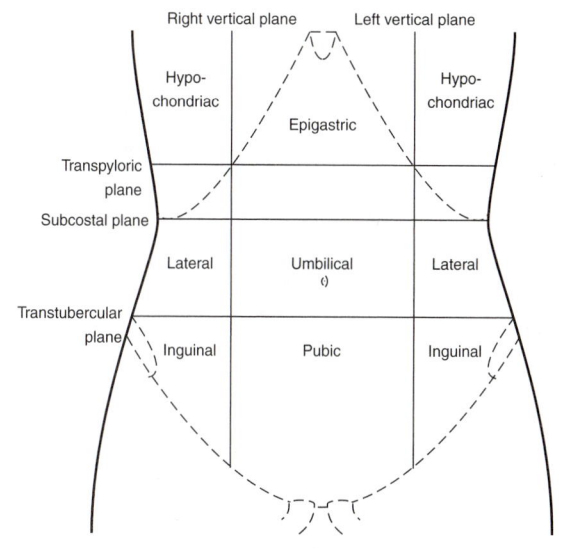

Practical Guide to the Care of the Gynecologic/Obstetric Patient

Figure 2-1 Anatomical subdivisions of the anterior abdominal wall.

DEEP FASCIA

The deep fascia (Gallaudet's fascia) is identified easily in the lateral portion of the anterior abdominal wall, where it covers the fleshy fibers of the external oblique muscle. It is continuous with the fascia of the latissimus dorsi and the pectoralis major. More medially, it is indistinguishable from the muscular fascia of the external abdominal oblique muscle, and it is thickened in the midline to form the suspensory ligament of the clitoris.

In the superficial fascia of Camper, the superficial circumflex iliac artery, the superficial epigastric artery, and the superficial external pudendal artery are seen as inguinal branches of the femoral artery, whereas the corresponding venous tributaries drain into the great saphenous vein.

2.2 Muscles and Fascia of the Anterior Lateral Abdominal Wall

At each side of the abdomen there are three flat muscles: the external oblique, the internal oblique, and the transversus abdominis. There is one vertical muscle, the rectus abdominis.

EXTERNAL OBLIQUE MUSCLE

The external oblique muscle arises from the lower eight ribs to insert at the outer lip of the anterior half of the iliac crest. The fibers of the muscle continue anteriorly as a thin but dense aponeurosis to decussate with

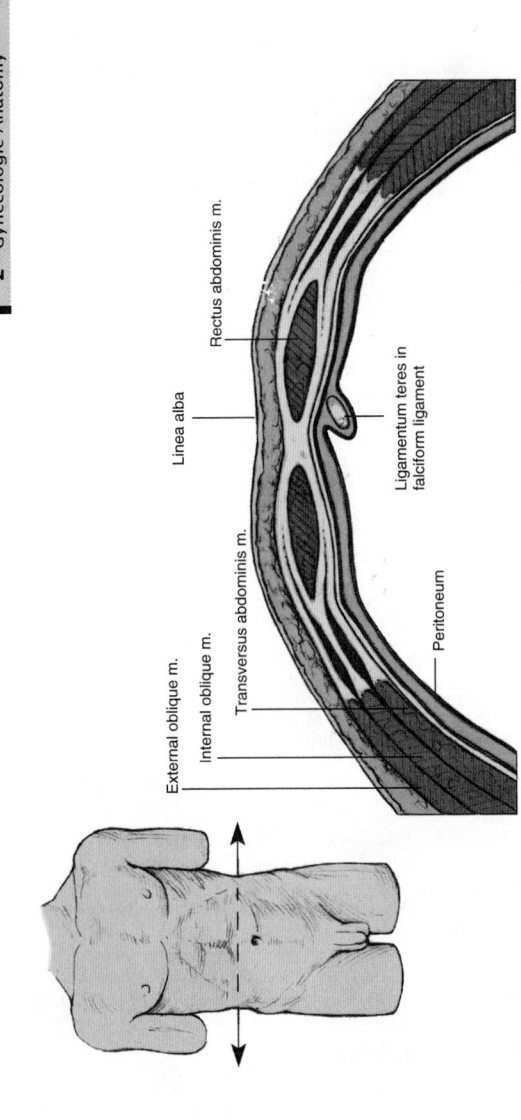

10   Practical Guide to the Care of the Gynecologic/Obstetric Patient

Figure 2-2 Fascial and muscular layers of the anterior abdominal wall and the inguinal and subinguinal regions. (From Mathers L, Chase R: *Clinical anatomy principles*, St. Louis, 1995, Mosby.)

those of the opposite side at the linea alba (Fig. 2-3). The linea alba represents the insertion of the muscles of the anterior abdominal wall at the midline. Below, it attaches with the pubic tubercle medially and the anterior superior iliac spine laterally, with the free lower border of the aponeurosis folding inward to become the inguinal ligament. Short of the pubic tubercle, the fibers form the triangular lacunar ligament, whereas those fibers that extend along the pectineal line form the pectineal ligament of Cooper. Fibers attaching to the pubic tubercle constitute the lateral crus of the superficial inguinal ring, whereas the fibers extending to the front of the pubis form its medial crus.

INTERNAL OBLIQUE MUSCLE

The internal abdominal oblique arises from the anterior two thirds of the intermediate lip of the iliac crest and the lateral two thirds of the inguinal ligament. Most of the fibers are directed upward and forward at a right angle to those of the external oblique muscle and continue as the aponeurosis. Posterior fibers ascend vertically to insert in the lower four ribs, whereas the lowest fibers run horizontally and inferiorly.

LINEA ARCUATA

The linea arcuata is a tendinous band in the posterior rectus sheath located at the approximate midpoint between the umbilicus and the pubic symphysis. Above the arcuate line, the aponeurosis of the internal oblique splits at the lateral border of the rectus muscle (linea semilunares) into anterior and posterior layers. These participate in the formation of the rectus sheath and decussate with the opposite muscle at the linea alba. Below the arcuate line, the aponeurosis does not split but joins totally the anterior lamina of the rectus sheath.

TRANSVERSUS ABDOMINUS MUSCLE

The transversus abdominus muscle arises from the thoracolumbar fascia, the inner surface of the lower six costal cartilages, the inner lip of the anterior two thirds of the iliac crest, and the lateral one third of the inguinal ligament. Its fibers course transversely forward and continue as the aponeurosis, joining the posterior lamina of the rectus sheath above the arcuate line and the anterior lamina below the arcuate line.

FASCIA TRANSVERSALIS

The fascia transversalis is thin and is part of the endoabdominal fascia and forms the posterior wall of the rectus sheath below the arcuate line. When fat is absent, the fascia transversalis adheres to the peritoneum as a single layer.

THORACOLUMBAR FASCIA

The thoracolumbar fascia consists of three layers arising from the vertebral spines, the tips of the transverse processes, and the anterior portion of the transverse processes, respectively. Layers join laterally to provide origin for the internal oblique and transversus muscles.

RECTUS SHEATH

The rectus sheath contains the rectus abdominus muscle, which arises by a tendon from the pubic bone medial to the tubercle. The muscle

2—Gynecologic Anatomy

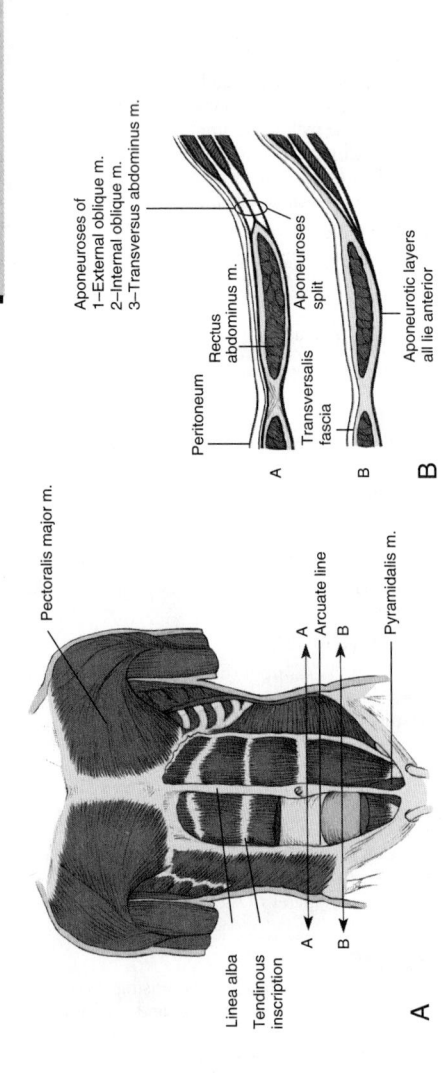

12 Practical Guide to the Care of the Gynecologic/Obstetric Patient

Figure 2-3 The rectus abdominis muscle. **A,** The anterior abdominal wall is made up on each side of three layers of flattened muscle and a pair of elongated vertical muscles, each known as rectus abdominis. The rectus muscle has two or three transverse whitish bands, the tendinous inscriptions, between the level of the umbilicus and the xiphoid. In cross-section A-A, just inferior to the umbilicus, the external oblique aponeurosis lies anterior to the rectus; the aponeurosis of the internal oblique muscle split passes both in front of and behind the rectus; and the aponeurosis of the transversus abdominus muscle passes posterior to the rectus. In cross-section B-B, all three of these aponeurotic layers lie anterior to the rectus; only the transversalis fascia and peritoneum lie posterior. **B,** A portion of the rectus muscle has been removed to reveal the arrangement of aponeuroses derived from the more lateral abdominal muscles. The gently curved aponeurotic edge, the arcuate line, represents the point at which all the aponeurotic layers first lie anterior to the rectus. Viewed from the interior, the arcuate line marks the point at which the inferior epigastric vessels enter and lie in the transversalis fascia posterior to the rectus. The small pyramidalis muscle lies anterior to the lower end of the rectus abdominis muscle.

inserts into the fifth and seventh costal cartilages and the xiphoid process. The pyramidalis muscle is present in front of the lower part of the rectus muscle, rising from the pubis below the origin of the rectus, and inserts into the linea alba. In addition to these two muscular structures, the rectus sheath contains the anterior cutaneous branches of the seventh through twelfth thoracic nerves and the superior and inferior epigastric vessels, which lie posterior to the muscle bed. The superior epigastric artery is a terminal branch of the internal thoracic, whereas the inferior is a branch of the external iliac artery. As described previously, the rectus sheath is formed by the aponeuroses of the external oblique, internal oblique, and transversus muscles. Fibers of the right and left sheaths decussate at the midline to form the linea alba. The anterior lamina of the sheath (see Fig. 2-3) is composed of all the aponeuroses below the level of the arcuate line but only of the external oblique and anterior layer of the internal oblique above the arcuate line. The posterior lamina above the arcuate line is formed by the aponeurosis of the transversus muscle and the posterior lamina of the internal oblique aponeurosis.

GROUP ACTIONS

Group actions of the abdominal wall muscles include constriction of the cavity, assisting in the noble function of parturition and the more servile functions of defecation, urination, and emesis. They also assist in flexion of the thorax or pelvis as well as in rotation of the trunk. They can also assist in expiration.

2.3 External Genitalia

The female urogenital triangle (Fig. 2-4) is separated into right and left halves by the pudendal cleft, which is bounded by the two labia majora. The labia majora emerge in front of the pubic symphysis and form the mons pubis. Inside the pudendal cleft are skin folds identified as the labia minora, which are devoid of hair and subcutaneous fat. The labia minora join to form the prepuce of the clitoris superiorly and the frenulum of the clitoris inferiorly. The clitoris, which consists of the glans, a body, and two crura, is connected to the pubic symphysis by the suspensory ligament of the clitoris. The space between the two labia minora is designated the vestibule and opens into the vagina posteriorly and the urethra anteriorly. The ostia of the major vestibular glands (of Bartholin) are located between the vaginal orifice and labia minora. The opening of the vagina is partially closed by the hymen.

2.4 The Perineum

Boundaries of the perineum (Fig. 2-5) are anteriorly, the pubic symphysis; posteriorly, the coccyx; anterolaterally, the pubic arch and ischiotuberosity; and posterolaterally, the sacrotuberous ligament. The floor of the perineum is the skin and the roof is the pelvic diaphragm (levator ani and coccygeus muscles). The perineum can be divided into a posterior anal triangle and an anterior urogenital triangle.

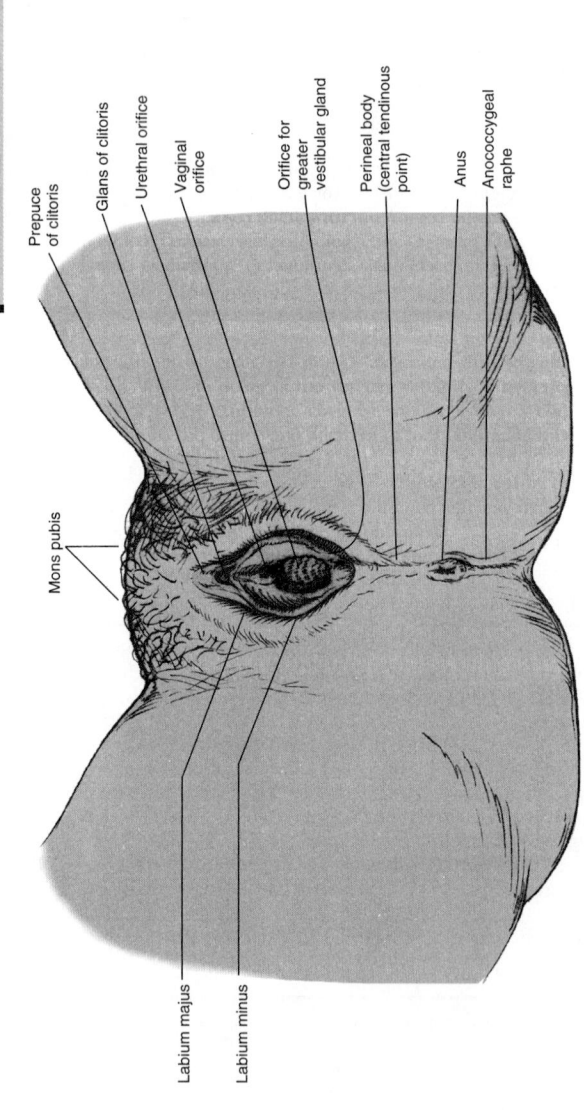

14 Practical Guide to the Care of the Gynecologic/Obstetric Patient

Figure 2-4 External genitalia of the female. The labia majora flank the labia minora, and the urethral and vaginal orifices are seen between the labia minora. (From Mathers L, Chase R: *Clinical anatomy principles*, St. Louis, 1995, Mosby.)

Practical Guide to the Care of the Gynecologic/Obstetric Patient 15

2—Gynecologic Anatomy

Figure 2-5 Urogenital and anal triangles. The perineum is a diamond-shaped region. It is bordered by the two ischiopubic rami and the two sacrotuberous ligaments. (Some authors define the posterior margins of this region to be imaginary lines on each side extending from the ischial tuberosity to the coccyx.) A horizontal line connecting the two ischial tuberosities divides the perineum into the anterior urogenital triangle and the posterior anal triangle. At the midpoint of this line is found the perineal body, just anterior to the anal canal. (From Mathers L, Chase R: *Clinical anatomy principles*, St. Louis, 1995, Mosby.)

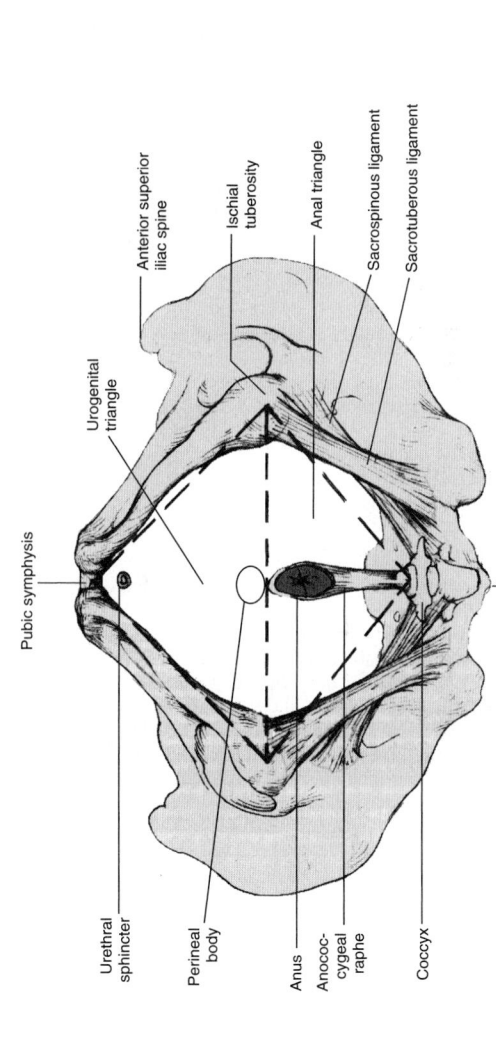

ANAL TRIANGLE

The anal triangle consists of a central anal canal and the lateral ischiorectal fossae. The sphincter ani externus muscle has three parts: subcutaneous, superficial, and deep. Muscle fibers are attached to the perineal body anteriorly and to the anococcygeal ligament posteriorly. The muscle is supplied by the inferior rectal nerve and vessels.

The ischiorectal fossae occupy the lateral portion of the anal triangle. The medial boundaries are the sphincter ani externus muscle and anal canal, the levator ani and coccygeus muscles, and their fasciae. The obturator internus muscle identifies the lateral wall. The posterior wall is the sacrotuberous ligament, covered by the gluteus maximus muscle. The anterior wall is the superficial and deep spaces of the urogenital triangle. The superior roof of the fossa is formed by the obturator internus and levator ani muscles. The skin and superficial fascia form the base of the fossa.

The contents of the ischiorectal fossae include the inferior rectal nerve, which is a branch of the pudendal nerve, supplying the levator ani and sphincter ani externus muscles; the inferior rectal artery, which is a branch of the internal pudendal artery; and the inferior rectal vein, which drains to the internal pudendal vein. All these structures then communicate with the pudendal nerve and internal pudendal artery and vein, which are located in the pudendal canal. The canal is formed by the obturator internus fascia and is located in the lateral wall of the ischiorectal fossa.

UROGENITAL TRIANGLE

The urogenital triangle consists of three layers of fasciae that separate the superficial and deep perineal spaces (Figs. 2-6 and 2-7). They consist of the superficial fascia, which is attached laterally to the pubic arch and posterosuperiorly to the perineal membrane. As in the abdomen, there are two layers. There is a superficial fatty layer and a deeper membranous layer, referred to as the fascia of Colles instead of Scarpa. Anteriorly, the deep layer of the superficial fascia is continuous with Scarpa's fascia in the abdomen. The fusion of this superficial perineal fascia and the perineal membrane forms the posterior boundary of the superficial perineal space. The middle fascial layer is the perineal membrane (inferior fascia of the urogenital diaphragm), which is also attached laterally to the pubic arch. In the middle of the line of fusion between the anus and the vagina is the central perineal tendon or perineum. The perineal membrane is fused posteriorly with the deeper superior fascia of the urogenital diaphragm to form the deep perineal space.

Superficial Perineal Pouch

The contents of the superficial perineal pouch are as follows:

1. The posterior labial nerve is a branch of the pudendal nerve.
2. The posterior labial artery is a branch of the internal pudendal artery.
3. The superficial transverse perineal muscles form the posterior boundary of the superficial pouch. These muscles arise from the ischiotuberosities and insert into the perineal body. Their function is to stabilize the perineum.

Practical Guide to the Care of the Gynecologic/Obstetric Patient   17

Figure 2-6 Female perineum, superficial dissection. Here the female perineum is partially dissected to show the inferior layer of the fascia of the urogenital diaphragm, otherwise known as the perineal membrane, and on the opposite side the course and distribution of pudendal vessels and nerves in the perineal region. (From Mathers L, Chase R: *Clinical anatomy principles*, St. Louis, 1995, Mosby.)

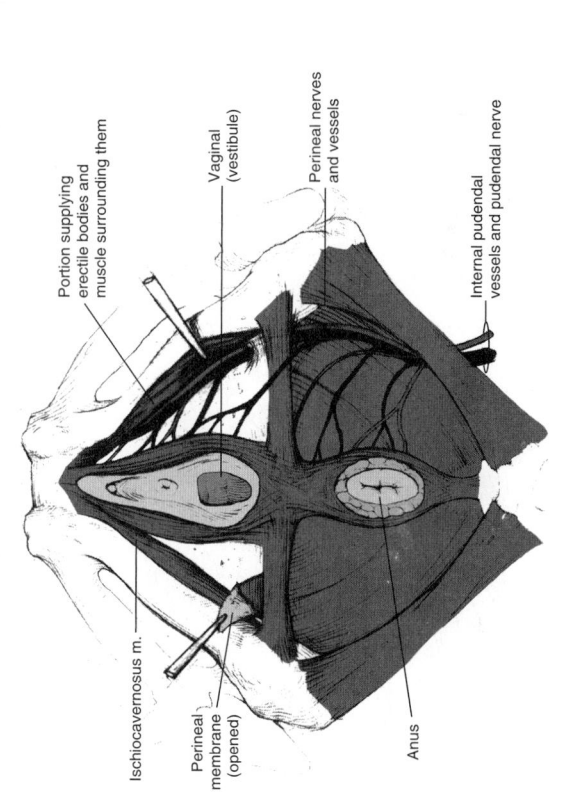

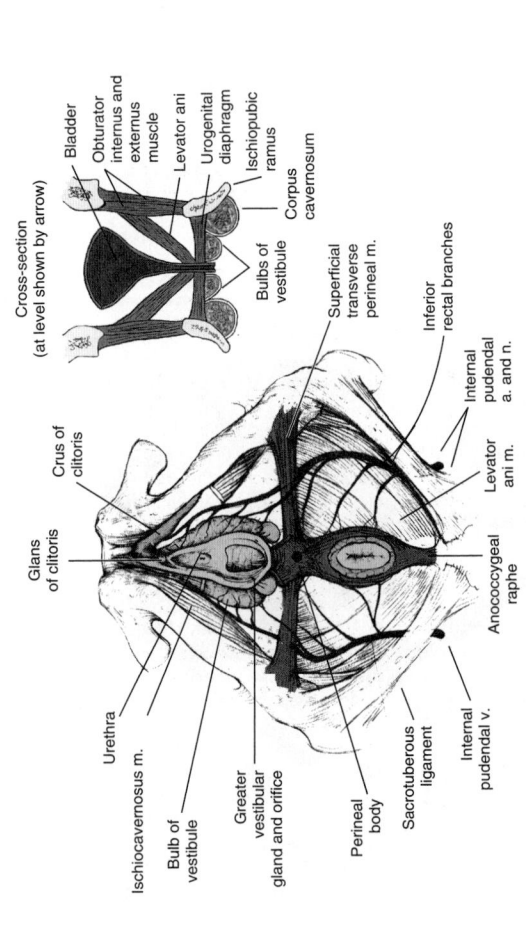

Figure 2-7 Female perineum, deeper dissection. Erectile bodies are present in the superficial pouch. The pudendal arteries and veins are shown, each on one side of the perineum. The glans and frenulum of the clitoris are also shown here. The striated ischiocavernosus muscle surrounds the proximal part of each corpora cavernosa, where they are attached firmly to the medial sides of the ischiopubic rami. (From Mathers L, Chase R: *Clinical anatomy principles*, St. Louis, 1995, Mosby.)

4. The bulbospongiosis muscles are exposed by cutting away the labia minora, and they cover the bulb of the vestibule. They arise from the perineal body and insert into the dorsum of the clitoris. Their function is to close the vaginal orifice.
5. The vestibular bulbs consist of erectile tissue that lies on each side of the vaginal orifice and are attached to the perineal membrane overlapping the greater vestibular glands (of Bartholin) posteriorly. The bulbs are united anteriorly by a plexus of veins (the commissure) between the urethra and the clitoris. The commissure is attached to the glans of the clitoris by a thin strip of erectile tissue.
6. The ischiocavernosus muscles cover the two crura of the clitoris and arise from the ischial ramus and insert into the crura of the clitoris. They cause erection of the clitoris. The clitoris itself has a free glans and a fixed body composed of two corpora cavernosa, which attach to the ischial pubic rami by two crura.

Deep Perineal Pouch

The deep perineal pouch is bounded by the perineal membrane inferiorly and the superior fascia of the urogenital diaphragm superiorly (Figs. 2-7 and 2-8). The perineal membrane or inferior fascia of the urogenital diaphragm is a layer of dense fibrous tissue. The membrane separates the superficial and deep perineal pouches. Its attachments laterally are the pubic arch, whereas anteriorly it is thickened to form the transverse perineal ligament. Between this ligament and the inferior pubic ligament, the deep dorsal vein of the clitoris passes. The contents of the deep perineal pouch include the following:

1. The urethra.
2. The vagina.
3. The sphincter urethrae muscle is thin and divisible into a central and a peripheral portion. The central circular fibers surround the urethra, whereas the peripheral, transverse fibers attach to the pubic arch and the perineal membrane. These fibers run anterior and posterior to the urethra. This muscle functions to constrict the urethra and is supplied by the deep perineal nerve. The posterior fibers of the sphincter urethrae muscle are continuous with the deep transverse perineal muscle, which together form the urogenital diaphragm.
4. The deep transverse perineal muscles arise from the ischial rami and perineal membrane. They insert into the perineal body. Their function is to stabilize the perineum, and their nerve supply arises from the deep perineal nerve. The muscles of the urogenital diaphragm also function to constrict the urethra.
5. The internal pudendal artery enters the deep perineal pouch posteriorly after leaving the pudendal canal and courses along the pubic arch, terminating as the deep and dorsal arteries of the clitoris. There is also a branch distributed to the bulbocavernosus.
6. The pudendal nerve terminates as the dorsal nerve of the clitoris, entering the deep perineal pouch on the lateral sides of the internal

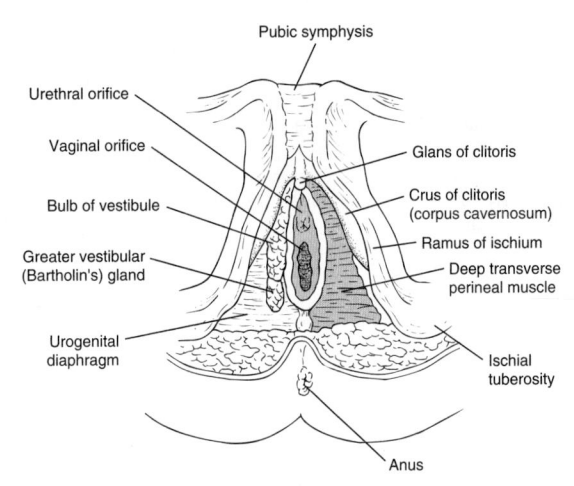

Figure 2-8 The female urogenital diaphragm seen from below. Also illustrated are the swelling bodies or cavernosus bodies. On the right side, the urogenital diaphragm is cut to show the major vestibular gland. (From Hafferl A: *Lehrbuch der topographischen anatomie*, Berlin, 1957, Springer-Verlag.)

pudendal artery, which is medial to the pubic arch. It functions as a sensory nerve supplying the erectile tissue of the clitoris. The deep perineal nerve, representing a second terminal branch of the pudendal nerve, gives off the posterior labial nerve from the anterior part of the pudendal canal along with several muscular branches to supply all the muscles of the superficial and deep perineal pouches.

LYMPHATIC DRAINAGE

Lymphatic drainage from the inferior perineal structures, which include the inferior anal canal, lower vagina, and distal urethra, drains to the medial superficial inguinal lymph nodes. Superiorly, lymphatic flow is directed to the pelvic lymph nodes.

2.5 Pelvic Diaphragm, Obturator, and Piriformis Muscles

Muscles of the pelvic diaphragm are the levator ani and coccygeus muscles. These muscles are both the roof of the perineum and the floor of the pelvis (Figs. 2-9 and 2-10).

LEVATOR ANI MUSCLE

The levator ani muscle originates anteriorly from the body of the pubis, the tendinous arch, and the ischial spine. The four components of this muscle are listed in Table 2-1.

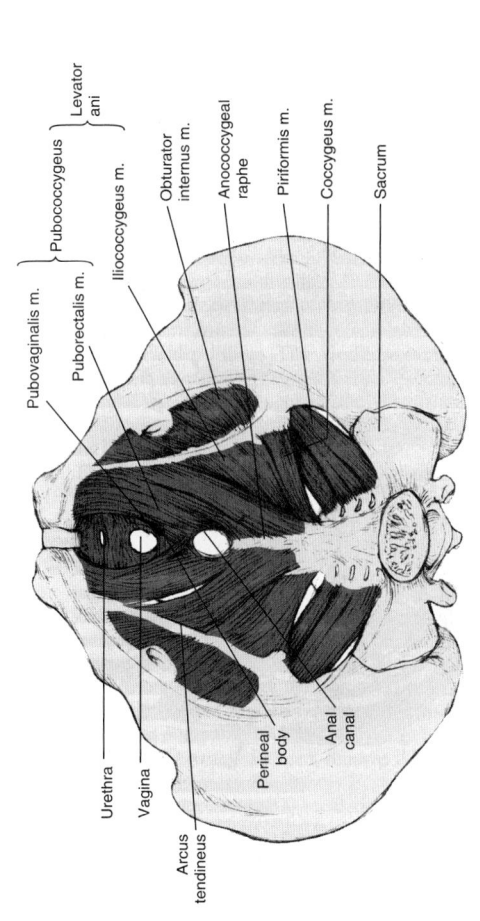

Practical Guide to the Care of the Gynecologic/Obstetric Patient 21

Figure 2-9 Pelvic diaphragm, superior view, female. All of the viscera have been removed to reveal the muscles forming the pelvic floor, with apertures for the rectum/anus, vagina, and urethra. The most medial and largest muscle in this area is the pubococcygeus, with its subdivisions puborectalis and pubovaginalis shown as well. Further posterior, on each side, is the iliococcygeus muscle. The posterior margin of this muscle is at the level of the sacrospinous ligament, with which the coccygeus muscle is often blended. The iliococcygeus muscle is also unique in originating from the ischial spine and along the fibrous arcus tendineus, on the medial surface of the obturator internus muscle. The piriformis muscle appears to "fill in" the gap between the posterior edge of the coccygeus and the sacrum but is not a true pelvic floor muscle. (From Mathers L, Chase R: *Clinical anatomy principles*, St. Louis, 1995, Mosby.)

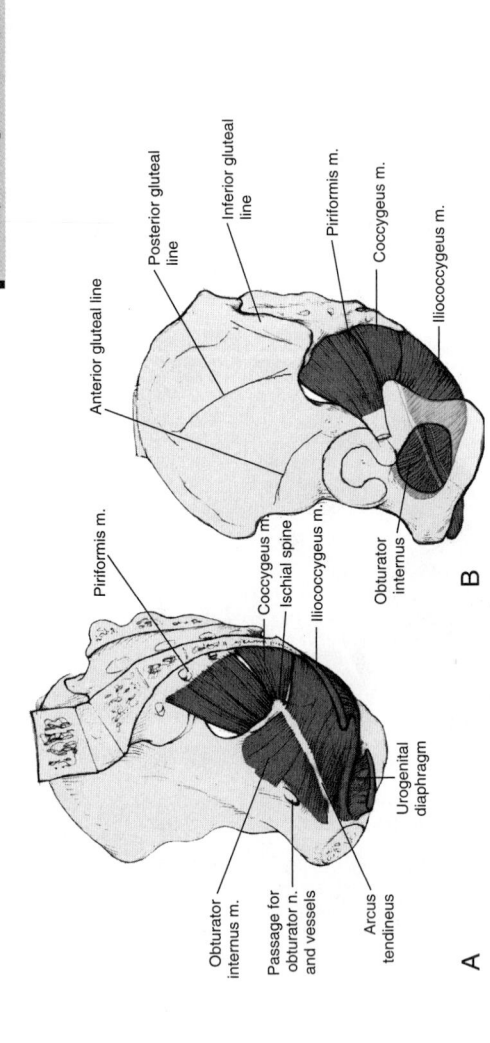

22 Practical Guide to the Care of the Gynecologic/Obstetric Patient

2—Gynecologic Anatomy

Figure 2-10 Pelvic and urogenital diaphragms. Internal view of the right hemipelvis and an external view of the left hemipelvis. It is as though the intact pelvis had been split in the midsagittal plane and the two halves separated. **A**, In the internal view, the piriformis, obturator internus, and obturator foramen are labeled. Note the arcus tendineus, extending from the inner surface of the pubic symphysis anteriorly to the ischial spine posteriorly. Anteriorly, note the deep transverse perineal muscle, and the anterior recess of the ischiorectal fossa that lies between it and the iliococcygeus. **B**, On the lateral or external view, the posterior half of the bony ring surrounding the obturator foramen has been removed. The portion of the obturator internus inferior to the arcus tendineus has also been removed to reveal the inferior surface of the iliococcygeus muscle. (From Mathers L, Chase R: *Clinical anatomy principles*, St. Louis, 1995, Mosby.)

Practical Guide to the Care of the Gynecologic/Obstetric Patient

Table 2-1 Components of the Levator Ani Muscle

Muscle	Origin	Insertion	Function
Pubovaginalis	Pubic bone	Perineal body	Constriction of the vagina
Puborectalis	Pubic bone	Posterior rectum	Sphincter of anal canal
Pubococcygeus	Tendon of obturator fascia	Anococcygeal ligament	Constriction of the anal canal
Iliococcygeus	Tendon of obturator fascia	Anococcygeal ligament	Constriction of the anal canal

The nerve supply includes branches of the third, fourth, and fifth sacral nerves, and the inferior rectal nerves. The function is to elevate the pelvic floor, increase intraabdominal pressure during forced respiration, and assist in defecation and vomiting.

COCCYGEUS

The coccygeus originates from the ischial spine and inserts into the lower border of the sacrum and coccyx. This muscle tends to be fibrous and is incorporated in the sacrospinous ligament. It is supplied by the fifth sacral nerve and has no significant function.

OBTURATOR INTERNUS

The obturator internus arises from the medial, inferior, and lateral margins of the obturator foramen and inserts into the medial side of the greater trochanter of the femur. It is covered by the obturator fascia, which is thickened to form the tendinous arch for the attachment of the levator ani muscle. The fascia, as previously mentioned, forms the pudendal canal. Its function is the same as that of the piriformis muscle.

PIRIFORMIS

The piriformis originates from the second, third, and fourth segments of the sacrum, leaving the pelvis through the greater sciatic foramen, and is inserted into the upper border of the greater trochanter of the femur. It laterally rotates and abducts the hip.

2.6 The Pelvic Viscera

The ovaries are intraperitoneal structures measuring approximately 3 × 1.5 × 1 cm. The ovary lies in the lateral wall of the pelvic cavity between the ureter, medially, and the external iliac vein, laterally. The uterine tube lies anteriorly. The distal portion of the tube curves around the lateral end of the ovary and is attached by one or more fimbriae. The ovary is attached to the superior surface of the broad ligament by the mesovarium and is attached to the uterus by the ligament of the ovary. The ovarian artery arises from the aorta below the renal artery and ascends along the posterior abdominal wall, crossing the external iliac artery, and entering the lateral part of the broad ligament via the suspensory ligament of the ovary or infidulopelvic ligament. The peritoneum covering the uterine tube forms the broad ligament that extends from both sides of the uterus to the lateral walls of the pelvis. The broad ligament can be divided into the mesovarium, mesosalpinx, and mesometrium (Fig. 2-11). The ovarian ligament proper connects the ovary to the uterus. The round ligament extends from the uterus to the labia majora. The uterine tube has three parts: the medial isthmus, middle ampula, and distal infundibulum, leading to the internal ostia and outer fimbria of the tube, respectively. The uterus is a fibromuscular organ, the dimensions of which vary considerably in premenopausal and postmenopausal women. This is a function of estrogenic stimulation and parturition. The uterus is composed of the upper muscular corpus and the lower cervix. The portion of the corpus above the fallopian tubes is identified as the fundus. The isthmus of the uterus is located between the body and the cervix. The uterine corpus is lined by the endometrium, which is composed of epithelium, forming glands, and also contains a specialized stroma. The portion of the cervix protruding into the vagina is identified as the portio vaginalis. The cervix consists of predominant fibrous connective tissue with a small amount of smooth muscle. The border of the cervical canal, where the canal widens into the endometrial cavity, is termed the internal os. The lower portion of the canal is the external os (Fig. 2-12). The uterine artery, which is a branch of the internal iliac artery, joins the uterus above the junction of the cervix and isthmus, where it communicates with the marginal artery along the lateral wall of the uterus. The marginal artery also communicates with the ovarian artery.

2.7 Spaces

PARAVESICAL SPACE

The anterior leaf of the broad ligament forms the roof of the paravesical space, blending with the bladder peritoneum medially and the parietal peritoneum laterally. The space is composed of connective tissue and fat. The bladder occupies the medial border, and the obturator internus muscle forms the lateral border. The posterior limit of the space is formed by the cardinal ligament, and the floor is composed of the levator ani muscle. The anterior leaf of the broad ligament should be opened at the midportion of the round ligament (Fig. 2-13). The incision extends laterally to expose the pelvic vessels and medially to reflect the bladder peritoneum. The space is entered on the lateral side of the obliterated hypogastric artery, and blunt dissection is carried to the level of the levator ani muscle.

PARARECTAL SPACE

The pararectal space lies beneath the pelvic peritoneum. Its borders include the cardinal ligament anterolaterally and the uterosacral ligament medially. The sacrum forms the posteromedial margin of the space and the ureter is attached to the peritoneum, forming the roof of the space.

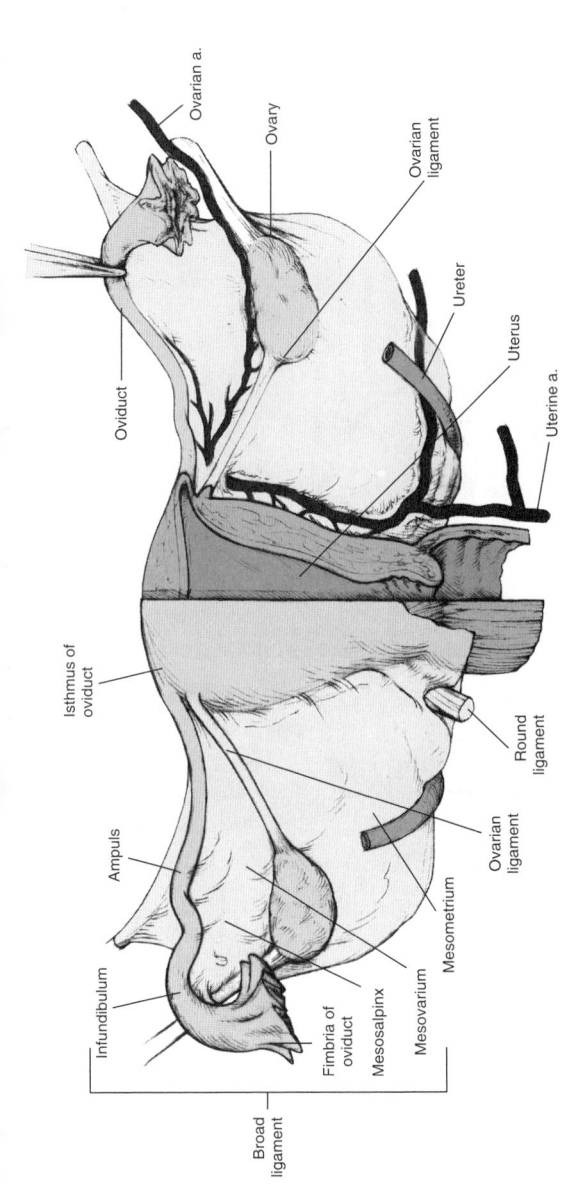

Practical Guide to the Care of the Gynecologic/Obstetric Patient   25

Figure 2-11 Female internal genitalia. Viewing the ovaries and uterus from the posterior aspect, the structures that lie lateral to the uterus can be seen enclosed within the two layers of the broad ligament. The structures are shown intact on the left side and are revealed by removing the posterior leaflet of the broad ligament on the right. (From Mathers L, Chase R: *Clinical anatomy principles*, St. Louis, 1995, Mosby.)

2—Gynecologic Anatomy

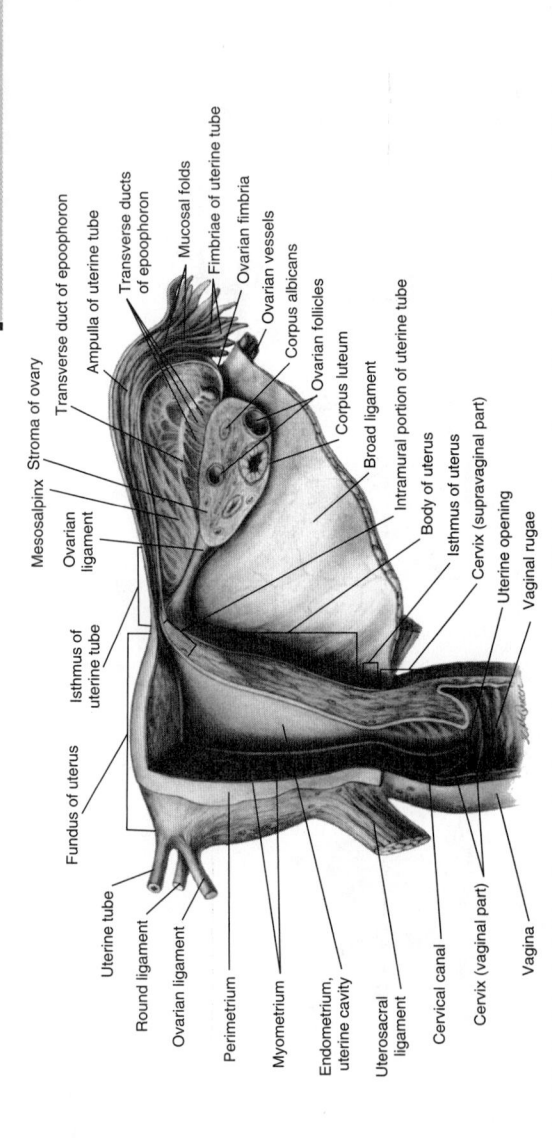

26 Practical Guide to the Care of the Gynecologic/Obstetric Patient

Figure 2-12 A schematic drawing of a posterior view of the cervix, uterus, fallopian tube, and ovary. Note that the cervix is divided by the vaginal attachment into an external portio segment and a supravaginal segment. Note that the uterus is composed of the dome-shaped fundus, the muscular body, and the narrow isthmus. Note the fimbria ovarica, or ovarian fimbria, attaching the oviduct to the ovary. (From Droegemueller W: *Comprehensive gynecology*, ed 2, St. Louis, 1987, Mosby.)

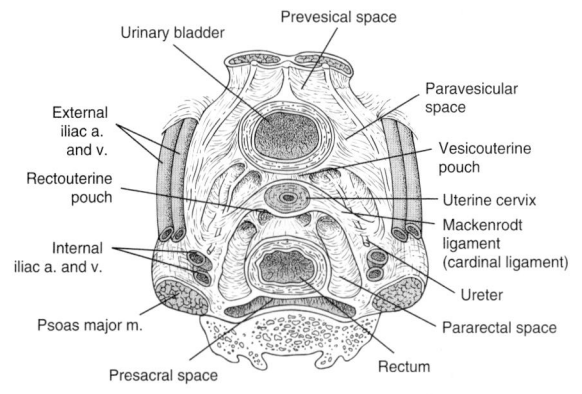

Figure 2-13 Schematic sectional drawing of the pelvis shows the firm connective tissue and the paraspaces (Amreich). The bladder, cervix, and rectum are surrounded by a connective tissue covering. The Mackenrodt ligament extends from the lateral cervix to the lateral abdominal pelvic wall. The vesicouterine ligament originating from the anterior edge of the Mackenrodt ligament leads to the covering of the bladder on the posterior side. The sagittal rectum column spreads both to the connective tissue of the rectum and to the sacral vertebrae closely nestled against the back of the Mackenrodt ligament and lateral pelvic wall. Between the firm connective tissue bundles there is loose connective tissue (paraspaces). (From Von Peham H, Amreich JA: *Gynaekologische operationslehre*, Berlin, 1930, S Karger.)

The hypogastric artery and vein are located in the pararectal space, and entry should be cautious, with medial displacement of the ureter and its attached peritoneum. Surgical entry is accomplished by cephalad extension of the previous incision for the paravesical space along the lateral border of the infundibulopelvic ligament.

RETROPUBIC SPACE

The retropubic space is developed anterior to the peritoneum and bladder by posteriorly retracting the bladder to expose the retropubic space. The space is filled with loose fatty tissue and is bordered anteriorly by the pubic symphysis and superiorly by the anterior abdominal wall between the two obliterated umbilical arteries. The posterior border is the rectovesical fascia, which encloses the ureter and blood vessels of the posterolateral border of the bladder. The lateral structures include the pubic bone, the obturator internis and levator ani muscles, the obliterated umbilical artery, and the obturator nerve. The inferolateral surface of the bladder is the medial border. The floor of the space includes two thickened fascial cords that represent the pubovesical ligament. This ligament extends from the neck of the bladder to the inferior border of the pubic symphysis.

2.8 Pelvic Peritoneum

The structure of the pelvic floor forms the sigmoid mesocolon and pararectal and paravesical fossa. The uterus divides the peritoneal cavity into a rectouterine fossa (pouch of Douglas) bounded laterally by the rectouterine folds and an anterior vesicouterine fossa. The peritoneum covering the folds also forms the broad ligament. The pelvic viscera are connected to the pelvic wall by their adventitial layers. Between these attachments are cleavage planes separating one organ from the other. These planes include the vesicovaginal space, the rectovaginal space, the retrorectal space, and the pararectal and paravesical spaces previously mentioned.

2.9 Cardinal and Uterosacral Ligaments

The cardinal ligaments are fibromuscular bands embedded in the adipose tissue of the lower portion of the broad ligaments. These bands extend from the lower portion of the cervix and upper portion of the vagina across the pelvic floor as a deeper continuation of the broad ligament. As the ligaments reach the lateral pelvic diaphragm, their ventral and dorsal extensions attach to the deep fascia on the inner surface of the levator ani, coccygeus, and piriformis muscles. This forms a white line 2 cm below the arcus tendineus of the levator ani, which is called the arcus tendineus of the pelvic fascia. Ventral extension is continuous with the supporting tissue of the bladder, whereas the dorsal extension blends with the uterosacral ligaments.

The uterosacral ligaments are the prominent fibrous bands extending from the cervix to the sacrum. They are attached to the periosteum and fascia of the sacrum. The peritoneum surrounding the ligaments creates the rectouterine folds that enclose the pouch of Douglas.

2.10 The Vagina

The vagina is approximately 9 cm long posteriorly and approximately 7 cm long anteriorly. It forms an angle with the uterus that is greater than 90 degrees (Fig. 2-14). The recess posterior to the cervix is the posterior fornix, and there are similar but smaller recesses anteriorly and laterally. The posterior surface of the vagina is separated from the upper rectum by the rectouterine fossa. The middle portion of the rectum is separated from the vagina by the rectovaginal fascia (of Denonvillier), and the lower fourth is separated from the anal canal by the perineal body.

2.11 The Urinary Tract

The abdominal ureter is a muscular tube, approximately 25 cm long and 5 mm wide, extending from a slight constriction at its junction with the pelvis of the kidney and descending vertically in a line parallel with the tips of the lumbar transverse processes to the

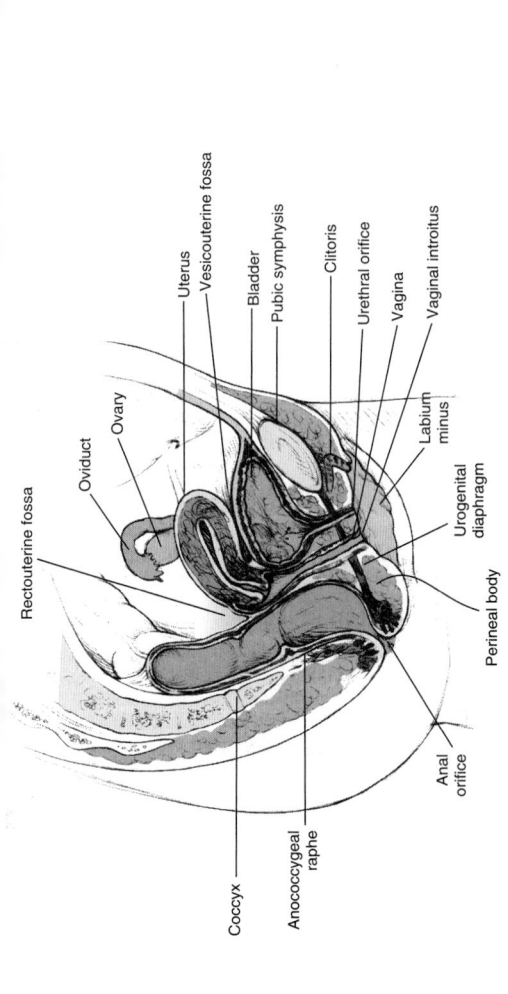

Practical Guide to the Care of the Gynecologic/Obstetric Patient 29

Figure 2-14 Female pelvic floor, midsagittal view. The anterior limit of the perineal area is the pubic symphysis, and the posterior limit the coccyx. Just anterior to the anal canal is the perineal body, an important landmark and point of attachment for several perineal muscles, ligaments, and organs. The anterior parts of the two corpora cavernosa are seen as the clitoris, lying just inferior to the pubic symphysis. Note that the urethral orifice is about halfway between the clitoris and the vaginal opening. The peritoneal membrane, covering the superior surfaces of the organs located in the pelvis, forms two special areas, the vesicouterine fossa and the rectouterine fossa (or pouch of Douglas). (From Mathers L, Chase R: *Clinical anatomy principles*, St. Louis, 1995, Mosby.)

midpoint of the ureter. This midpoint lies at the origin of the external iliac artery, where the ureter then enters the lesser pelvis. The blood supply of the ureter includes small branches from the renal and ovarian arteries, as well as the aorta and the common, internal iliac, uterine, and superior vesical arteries. These branches form longitudinal anastomoses that lie on the surface of the ureter. Because of this anastomotic network, branches can be divided without interfering with the blood supply.

The pelvic ureter runs posteroinferiorly anterior to the internal iliac artery and deep to the peritoneum of the lateral wall of the pelvis (Fig. 2-15). It travels along the lateral fornix of the vagina inferior to the broad ligament and uterine artery turning superiorly into the broad ligament. It enters the bladder wall to open into the superolateral angle of the trigone of the bladder.

The internal surface of the bladder is ridged by folds of mucous membrane, whereas on the posterior wall there is a smooth triangular area previously mentioned as the trigone of the bladder. The median internal urethral orifice is located at the inferior angle of the triangle. Fibrous bundles between the anteroinferior part of the pubic symphysis and the urethra represent the pubourethral ligament, which stabilizes the urethra and forms the inferior boundary of the retropubic space.

2.12 Blood Supply of the Pelvis
(Figs. 2-16 and 2-17)

OVARIAN ARTERIES

The ovarian arteries arise from the aorta just below the renal arteries. They pass distally under the peritoneum, resting on the psoas major muscle. On entering the pelvis, the arteries are enclosed in the layers of the suspensory ligament of the ovary.

SUPERIOR RECTAL ARTERY

The superior rectal artery is the continuation of the inferior mesenteric artery and descends between the layers of the mesentery of the sigmoid colon crossing the left common iliac artery. Opposite the distal portion of the sacrum the artery divides into two branches that descend on either side of the rectum.

MIDDLE SACRAL ARTERY

The middle sacral artery arises from the distal portion of the aorta posteriorly, descending behind the left common iliac vein and anterior to the fifth lumbar vertebra and the sacrum. The corresponding vein drains into the left common iliac vein.

COMMON ILIAC ARTERIES

The common iliac arteries descend obliquely from the fourth lumbar vertebra to the pelvic brim. The vessels bifurcate into the external and internal iliac arteries opposite the lumbosacral joint. There are accompanying common iliac veins that unite to form the inferior

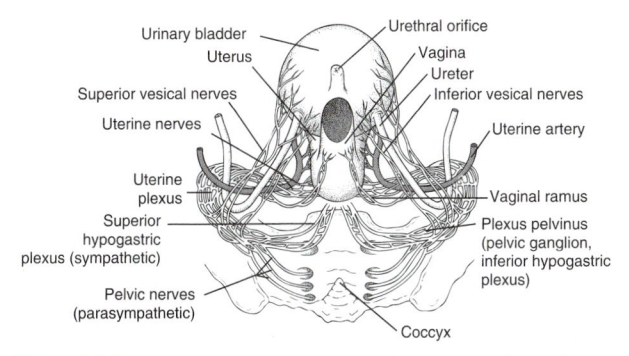

Practical Guide to the Care of the Gynecologic/Obstetric Patient

Figure 2-15 Innervation of uterus, bladder, and vagina, viewed from the perineum. *1*, Inferior vesical nerves; *2*, superior vesical nerves; *3*, uterine artery; *4*, uterine plexus (uterovaginal); *5*, plexus pelvinus (pelvic ganglion, inferior hypogastric plexus); *6*, pelvic nerves (parasympathetic); *7*, superior hypogastric plexus (sympathetic); *8*, vaginal ramus; *9*, uterine nerves; *10*, vagina; *11*, uterus; *12*, ureter; *13*, urinary bladder. (From Reiffenstuhl G, Platzer W: *Die vaginalen operationen. Chirug anatomie u operationslehre*, Berlin, 1974, Urban-Schwarzenberg.)

vena cava. These vessels are slightly posterior and a portion of the right common iliac vein is lateral to the right common iliac artery, whereas the left common iliac is always medial. Each common iliac vein receives the iliolumbar and sometimes the lateral sacral veins. As stated previously, the left common iliac vein receives the middle sacral vein as well.

EXTERNAL ILIAC ARTERY

The external iliac artery passes laterally along the medial border of the psoas major muscle to a midpoint beneath the inguinal ligament between the anterior superior iliac spine and the pubic symphysis. It enters the thigh and becomes the femoral artery.

INTERNAL ILIAC ARTERY

The internal iliac artery is the main arterial supply of the pelvis. It enters the pelvis behind the ureter and anterior to the internal iliac vein in the sacroiliac joint. The artery divides into anterior and posterior trunks at the upper border of the greater sciatic foramen. The anterior trunk has three somatic branches and four visceral branches.

Anterior Trunk

1. The umbilical artery is the intrapelvic portion of the fetal umbilical artery. It retains its lumen for a short distance from the internal iliac and gives off the superior vesical artery. Distally it forms a fibrous cord running beside the bladder to the umbilicus as the lateral umbilical ligament or the obliterated hypogastric artery.

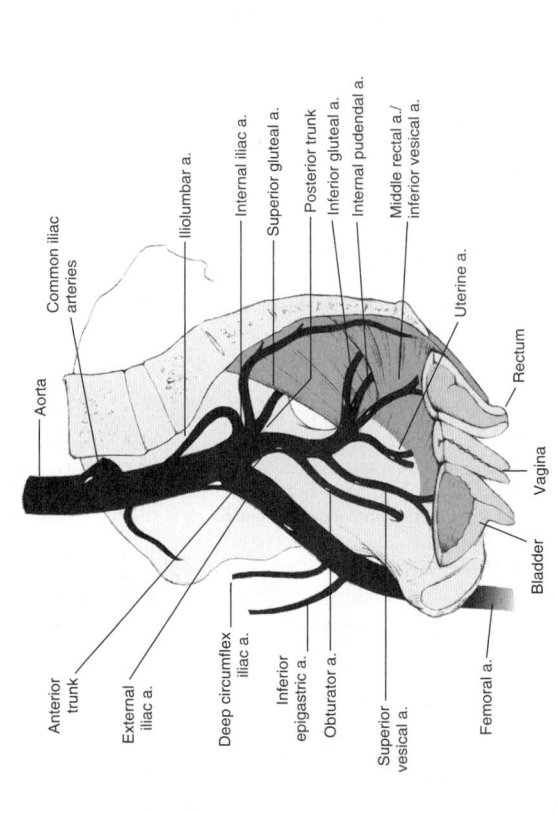

32   Practical Guide to the Care of the Gynecologic/Obstetric Patient

2—Gynecologic Anatomy

Figure 2-16 Branches of the common iliac artery. The common iliac artery divides into an internal and an external branch. The internal iliac artery supplies the gluteal and internal pelvic structures, whereas the external iliac artery continues inferiorly as the femoral artery, the major blood supply to the entire lower limb. (From Mathers L, Chase R: *Clinical anatomy principles*, St. Louis, 1995, Mosby.)

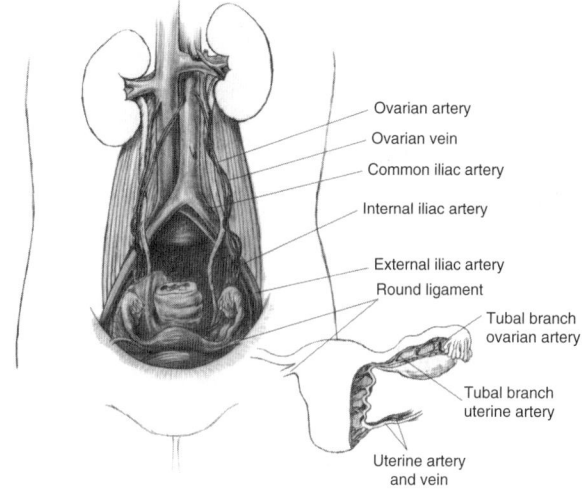

Practical Guide to the Care of the Gynecologic/Obstetric Patient 33

Figure 2-17 Pelvic blood supply. (From Davis JH et al, editors: *Surgery*, ed 2, St. Louis, 1995, Mosby.)

2. The obturator artery courses along the lateral wall of the pelvis to the obturator canal. Superior to the artery is the obturator nerve, and the vein is inferior. There is a pubic branch communicating with the pelvic surface of the pubic bone and anastomosing with a similar branch from the inferior epigastric artery. This anastomosis may replace the more common course of the obturator artery originating from the internal iliac and is called the abnormal obturator artery.
3. The uterine artery runs forward to the base of the broad ligament, where it crosses the ureter anteriorly and ascends along the lateral border of the uterus. It forms an anastomosis with the ovarian and vaginal arteries.
4. The vaginal artery corresponds to the inferior vesical artery in the male; it supplies the vagina, the uterus, and the inferior portion of the bladder.
5. The middle rectal artery arises from a common trunk with the vaginal artery. It communicates with the superior and inferior rectal arteries.
6. The internal pudendal artery leaves the pelvis through the greater sciatic foramen and reenters at the lesser sciatic foramen, where it goes forward to the pudendal canal.
7. The inferior gluteal artery also leaves the pelvis through the greater sciatic foramen and passes to the gluteal region. It is located posterior to the internal pudendal artery.

Posterior Trunk

1. The iliolumbar artery passes posteriorly and laterally between the fourth and fifth lumbar nerves, passing behind the psoas major muscle and proximal portion of the obturator nerve. Its vein terminates in the common iliac vein.
2. The lateral sacral artery has a superior and an inferior branch that may have separate or common origins. The superior branch enters the vertebral canal between the upper two anterior sacral foramina, and the inferior branch is directed to the lower two foramina and the coccyx.
3. The superior gluteal artery runs posteriorly between the fourth and fifth lumbar nerves or between the lumbosacral trunk and the first sacral nerve. It travels through the greater sciatic foramen to the gluteal region.

COLLATERAL CIRCULATION

Collateral circulation between the branches of the internal iliac artery and the systemic circulation is clinically significant. The lumbar branch of the iliolumbar artery communicates with the lumbar arteries of the systemic circulation. The lateral sacral artery communicates with the median sacral artery. The middle rectal artery communicates with the inferior and superior rectal arteries.

2.13 Lymphatic Drainage of the Pelvis

1. **External iliac lymph nodes:** The external iliac lymph nodes receive lymphatic drainage from the bladder, the isthmus of the uterus, and deep inguinal nodes.
2. **Internal iliac lymph nodes:** The internal iliac lymph nodes receive drainage from the pelvic viscera, the gluteal region, and the deep perineum. They do not receive drainage from the ovaries or uterine tubes.
3. **Sacral group:** The sacral group is located along the median and lateral sacral arteries, and these nodes receive drainage from the posterior pelvic wall, the rectum, and the isthmus of the uterus.
4. **Lower paraaortic nodes:** The lower paraaortic nodes communicate with lymphatics from the ovaries and uterine tubes.

2.14 Pelvic Joints

1. **Lumbosacral:** The lumbosacral is located between the fifth lumbar vertebra and the upper end of the sacrum.
2. **Sacroiliac:** The sacroiliac connects the auricular surfaces of the sacrum and the ilium.
3. **Pubic symphysis:** The pubic symphysis is joined by the interpubic disc of fibrocartilage, which is strengthened by the anterior, posterior, superior, and inferior (arcuate) ligaments.
4. **Sacrococcygeal and coccygeal joints:** The sacrococcygeal and coccygeal joints are miniatures of intervertebral joints.

2.15 Ligaments

SACROTUBEROUS LIGAMENT

The sacrotuberous ligament (Fig. 2-18) originates from the dorsal surface of the sacrum and coccyx and from the posterior and inferior iliac spine, passing inferiorly and laterally to the medial surface of the ischiotuberosity. It helps form the medial margin of the greater and lesser sciatic foramen.

SACROSPINOUS LIGAMENT

The sacrospinous ligament (see Fig. 2-18) originates from the lateral margin of the coccyx and the lowermost portion of the sacrum and attaches to the ischial spine. The greater and lesser sciatic foramina are located superiorly and inferiorly to the sacrospinous ligament. The greater sciatic foramen is superior to the pelvic diaphragm, whereas the lesser is located inferiorly. As a result, structures passing to the perineum and ischiorectal fossa initially travel through the greater sciatic foramen and reemerge through the lesser. The pudendal nerve and artery are dorsal and posterior to the sacrospinous ligament and are seen just medial to the ischial spine. The sciatic nerve is similarly located but is lateral to the ischial spine. It is for this reason that surgical fixation of the vagina to the sacrospinous ligament is performed approximately 2 to 3 cm medial to the ischial spine. The coccygeus muscle is located anterior to the sacrospinous ligament and the fibers of both structures are intimately adherent.

2.16 Nerves of the Lesser Pelvis (Fig. 2-19)

LUMBOSACRAL TRUNK

The lumbosacral trunk (L4, L5) is a thick nerve formed from the entire ventral ramus of the fifth lumbar nerve and the descending portion of the fourth. It descends distally anterior to the sacral ala posterior to the pelvic fascia and joins the ventral rami of the sacral nerves anterior to the piriformis muscle.

SACRAL PLEXUS

The sacral plexus (L4, L5, and S1 to S4) is formed by the ventral rami of the fifth lumbar vertebra, the first three sacral rami, and a portion of the fourth lumbar and fourth sacral rami. The lumbosacral trunk unites with the first sacroventral ramus and, together with the second, third, and part of the fourth sacral ramus, forms the solid triangular sacral plexus. The plexus is located between the piriformis and the pelvic fascia.

SCIATIC NERVE

The sciatic nerve (L4, L5, S1, S2, and S3), as a terminal branch of the sacral plexus, is composed of fibers from the fourth and fifth lumbar nerves and the first through third sacral nerves. The sciatic nerve later splits into the common peroneal and tibial nerves.

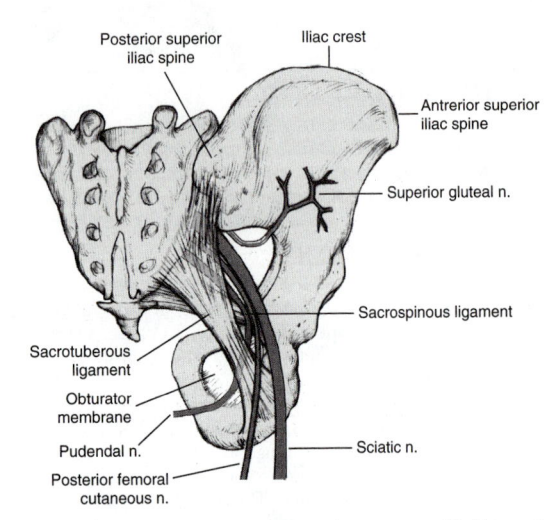

Figure 2-18 Pelvic ligaments, external view from posterior. Visible are the sacrotuberous and sacrospinous ligaments, as well as the sciatic, superior gluteal, posterior femoral cutaneous, and pudendal nerves. (From Mathers L, Chase R: *Clinical anatomy principles*, St. Louis, 1995, Mosby.)

PUDENDAL NERVE

The pudendal nerve (S2, S3, S4) is composed of sacral branches from the second, third, and fourth sacral nerves and leaves the pelvis through the greater sciatic foramen and, as mentioned previously, reenters through the lesser sciatic foramen to enter the pudendal canal.

COCCYGEAL PLEXUS

The coccygeal plexus (S4, S5) is formed from ventral rami of the fourth and fifth sacral nerves, as well as the coccygeal nerve, innervating the pelvic diaphragm and the skin posterior to the coccyx.

LUMBAR PLEXUS

The lumbar plexus is formed by the ventral rami of the first three and the greater part of the fourth lumbar nerves. It is located dorsal to or within the fasciculi of the psoas major muscle. Although these fibers emerge from the posterior abdominal wall, many traverse the pelvis en route to their site of innervation. The branches of the lumbar plexus are listed in Table 2-2.

Iliohypogastric Nerve

The iliohypogastric nerve emerges from the upper part of the lateral border of the psoas major muscle, penetrates the posterior part of the

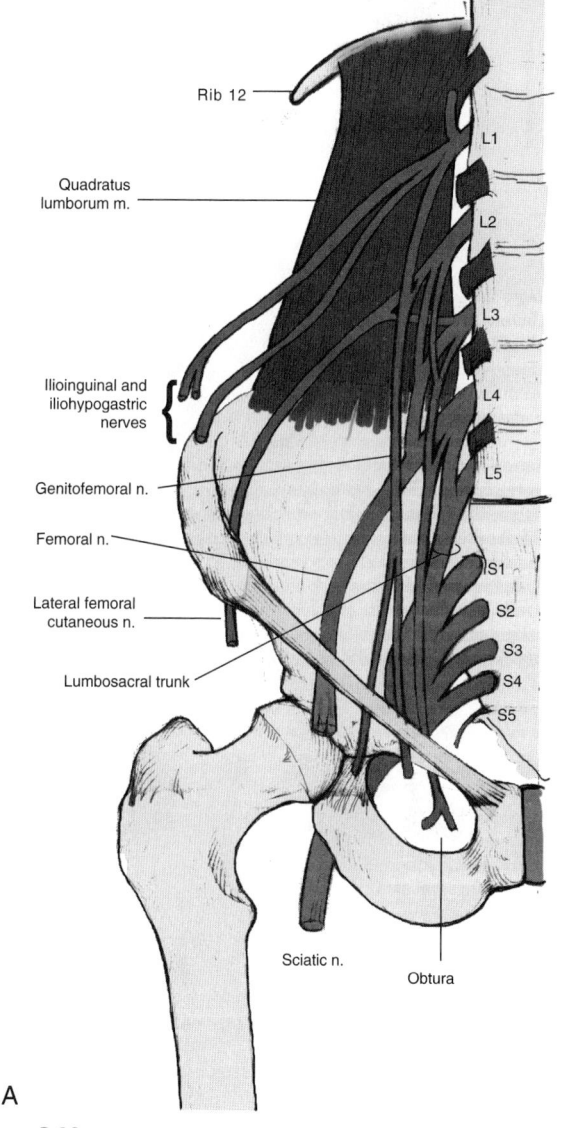

Figure 2-19 Lumbosacral plexus. **A,** The lumbar and sacral plexuses are shown here as a continuum of nerve fibers emerging from vertebral levels L1 to S5. The lumbar plexus is directed at innervation of the lower anterolateral abdominal wall and the inguinal canal. The sacral plexus innervates pelvic organs and continues outside the pelvis to supply the posterior thigh and nearly all of the lower limb below the knee. *(continued)*

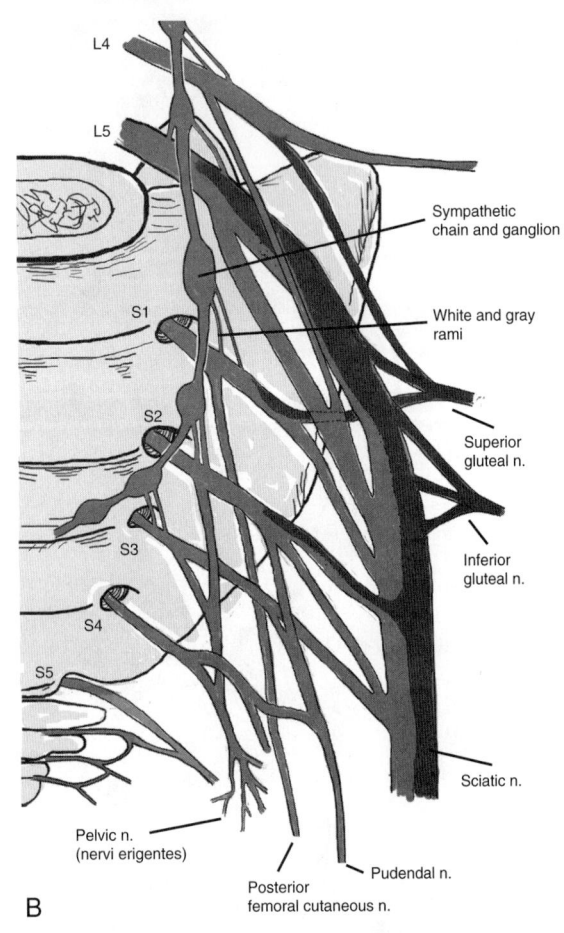

Figure 2-19, cont'd **B,** This schematic drawing of the sacral plexus illustrates formation of its major branches and the distribution of anterior and posterior division branches in them. (From Mathers L, Chase R: *Clinical anatomy principles*, St. Louis, 1995, Mosby.)

transversus abdominus muscle near the crest of the ilium, and divides into a lateral and an anterior cutaneous branch.

1. The lateral cutaneous branch is distributed to the skin of the gluteal region.
2. The anterior cutaneous branch continues on a course between the internal oblique and transversus muscles and penetrates the

Table 2-2 Branches of the Lumbar Plexus

Branch	Level
Iliohypogastric	L1, T12
Ilioinguinal	L1
Genitofemoral	L1, L2
Lateral femoral cutaneous	L2, L3
Obturator	L2, L3, L4
Femoral	L2, L3, L4

aponeurosis of the external oblique 2 cm above the external inguinal ring, where it is distributed to the skin of the hypogastric region.

Ilioinguinal Nerve

The ilioinguinal nerve arises just caudal to the iliohypogastric nerve, traversing posteriorly to the crest of the ilium. It penetrates the internal oblique muscle, travels through the external inguinal ring, and is distributed to the skin of the mons pubis and labia majora.

Genitofemoral Nerve

The genitofemoral nerve passes distally through the substance of the psoas major muscle, emerging at the level of the fourth lumbar vertebra, where it is covered by peritoneum.

1. The genital branch progresses to the inguinal ligament, where it accompanies the round ligament of the uterus. It provides sensory fibers to the round ligament and the labia majora.
2. The femoral branch, which is lateral to the genital branch, passes under the inguinal ligament with the external iliac artery and enters the femoral sheath, penetrating the fascia lata to supply the skin of the proximal anterior thigh.

Lateral Femoral Cutaneous Nerve

The lateral femoral cutaneous nerve emerges from the lateral portion of the psoas major, where it passes under the inguinal ligament and over the sartorius muscle, dividing into an anterior and posterior branch.

1. The anterior branch innervates the skin of the lateral and anterior thigh as far distally as the knee.
2. The posterior branch innervates the lateral and posterior surfaces of the thigh. This innervation extends from the level of the greater trochanter to the midportion of the thigh.

Obturator Nerve

The obturator nerve provides motor innervation to the adductor muscles of the thigh. It emerges from the medial border of the psoas near the pelvic brim posterior to the common iliac vessels. It continues distally lateral to the internal iliac vessels and the ureter, then runs along the lateral wall of the pelvis to enter the obturator foramen with the obturator artery and vein.

Femoral Nerve

The femoral nerve represents the largest branch of the lumbar plexus and is the principal motor innervation of the anterior thigh. It originates in the pelvis within the fibers of the psoas major, emerging from the psoas below the iliac crest. It descends between the psoas and iliacus muscles covered by the fascia. It passes underneath the inguinal ligament and remains lateral to the femoral sheath. Besides its motor function, it has sensory cutaneous function. The cutaneous branches penetrate the fascia lata of the thigh approximately 7 to 8 cm distal to the inguinal ligament, dividing into an anterior and a medial branch.

2.17 The Autonomic Nervous System

The autonomic nervous system (Figs. 2-20 and 2-21) affecting the pelvic viscera can by divided into a sympathetic (thoracolumbar) system and a parasympathetic (craniosacral) system. The neurotransmitter for the sympathetic nervous system is adrenergic, whereas the parasympathetic is cholinergic. In general, adrenergic stimulation favors storage and cholinergic stimulation favors evacuation.

SYMPATHETIC PATHWAY

The sympathetic pathway from the spinal cord to the viscera always involves two neurons. The synapse occurs either in the paravertebral ganglia of the sympathetic trunk or in prevertebral ganglia (i.e., the inferior mesenteric ganglion). Preganglionic sympathetic fibers supplying the pelvic organs originate from the white rami of the upper two lumbar nerves and from the lowest thoracic nerve. These fibers pass through the corresponding ganglia of the sympathetic trunk (paravertebral ganglia) terminating in the inferior mesenteric ganglia (prevertebral). Postganglionic fibers or axons are then sent by way of the superior hypogastric and inferior hypogastric plexi to the pelvic viscera. Each spinal nerve receives gray rami communicantes from the sympathetic trunk. The gray ramus consists of postganglionic sympathetic fibers, which innervate blood vessels, hair, and glands of the body wall. The four pairs of ganglia of the sympathetic trunk anterior to the sacrum contribute branches from the first two ganglia to the inferior hypogastric plexus, whereas the last two supply the rectum directly.

PARASYMPATHETIC SYSTEM

The parasympathetic system consists of preganglionic fibers that originate from the second, third, and fourth sacral nerves forming the pelvic nerve (also termed nervi erigentes) and terminate in the ganglia of the pelvic plexi. Postganglionic fibers from these plexi supply the effectors of the pelvic organs, including the urinary bladder, the descending colon, the rectum, and the reproductive organs.

Anatomically (Fig. 2-22), the two sympathetic trunks descend into the pelvis along the medial side of the anterior sacral foramina and end as a single ganglion impar anterior to the coccyx. Each trunk usually has four ganglia, which send gray rami to the sacral and the coccygeal nerves. The superior hypogastric plexus lies in front of the fifth lumbar vertebra,

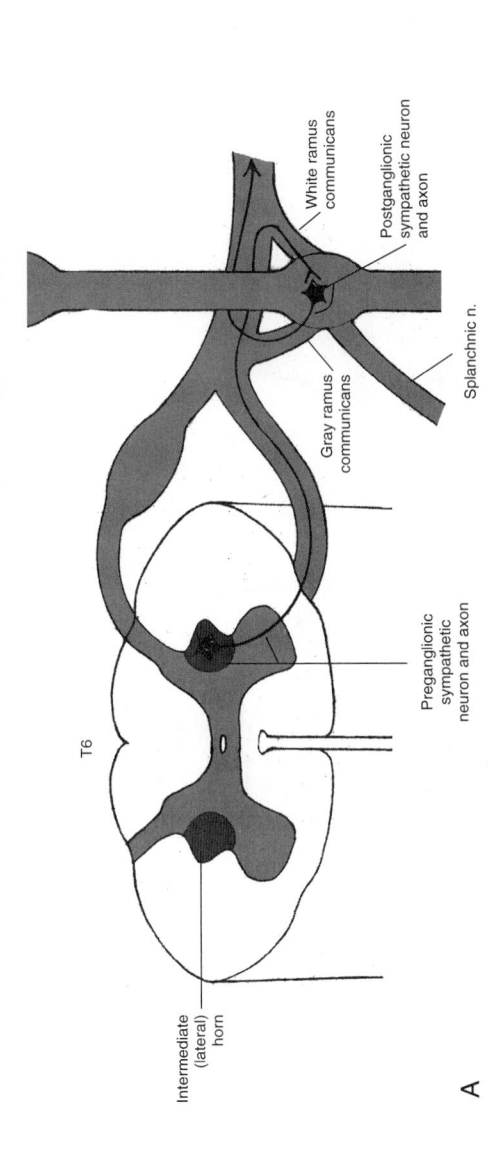

Practical Guide to the Care of the Gynecologic/Obstetric Patient 41

Figure 2-20 Sympathetic nerves at different vertebral levels. **A,** At vertebral levels T1 to L2, preganglionic sympathetic neuron cell bodies are located in the intermediate horn, and their axons travel in the ventral root to reach the sympathetic chain. The axons then traverse the white ramus communicans to enter the sympathetic ganglion and, as shown here, synapse in a neuron in that ganglion (other options would be to enter the splanchnic nerve or to ascend or descend in the sympathetic chain). When they synapse in the sympathetic ganglion, the postganglionic axon then traverse the gray ramus communicans to reenter the spinal nerve. *(continued)*

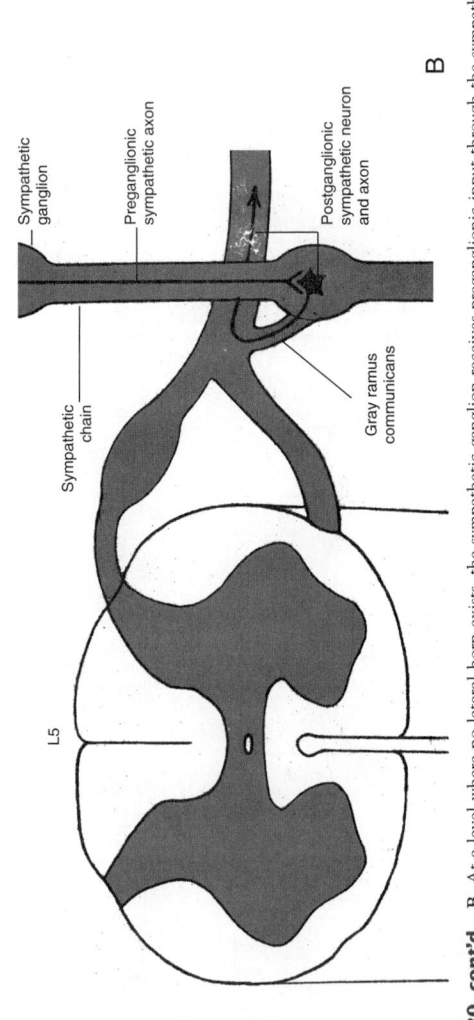

42 Practical Guide to the Care of the Gynecologic/Obstetric Patient

2—Gynecologic Anatomy

Figure 2-20, cont'd B, At a level where no lateral horn exists, the sympathetic ganglion receives preganglionic input through the sympathetic chain. The postganglionic axons traverse the gray ramus to enter the spinal nerve for that level. (From Mathers L, Chase R: *Clinical anatomy principles*, St. Louis, 1995, Mosby.)

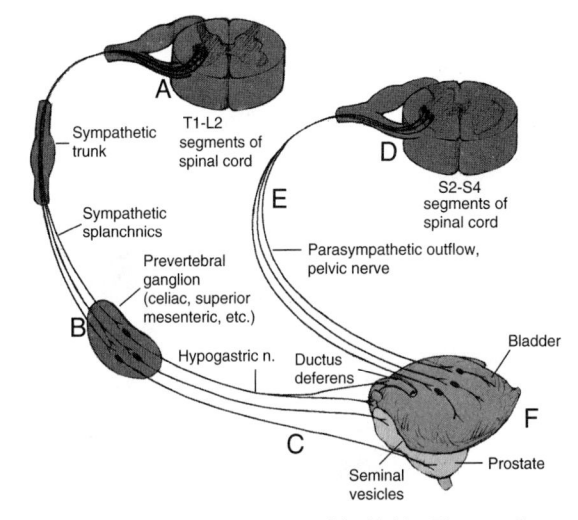

Figure 2-21 Autonomic innervation of the bladder. The sympathetic innervation begins with preganglionic axons arising in the lower thoracic spinal cord (A) in the intermediolateral cell column. These axons must synapse in a peripheral ganglion, and it is from the neurons of those ganglia that the axons actually innervating the intended target tissues arise. For pelvic viscera, preganglionic axons travel as part of the group of splanchnic nerves (greater, lesser, and least) that separate from the segmental thoracic nerves and descend along the posterior thoracic wall to enter the abdomen. Here they synapse in one of the large prevertebral ganglia (B) along the aorta (e.g., the celiac, superior mesenteric, renal, etc.). Postganglionic axons arising in these ganglia distribute themselves along the arterial branches of the abdominal aorta, and, in addition, a portion of them continues inferiorly to descend from the bifurcation of the aorta into the pelvis and the hypogastric nerve (or plexus) (C). Parasympathetic innervation begins with preganglionic axons arising in spinal cord segments S2 to S4 (D). These axons travel in the pelvic nerve (E) to small groups of neurons embedded in the walls of target organs. Here the preganglionic axons synapse, and the small neurons give rise to postganglionic axons (F), which actually innervate the muscle or glands in that organ. (From Mathers L, Chase R: *Clinical anatomy principles,* St. Louis, 1995, Mosby.)

the sacral promontory, and the ventral surface of the lower aorta. This plexus also receives important pain fibers from the pelvic viscera. From the superior hypogastric plexus descend two hypogastric nerves along the course of the internal iliac vessels. These nerves terminate as the inferior hypogastric plexus.

The inferior hypogastric plexus consists of the uterovaginal plexus along the medial surface of the uterine vessels lateral to the uterosacral ligament. In addition, extensions of the inferior hypogastric plexi are located on the walls of the pelvic viscera. This includes the rectal plexus and the vesical plexus.

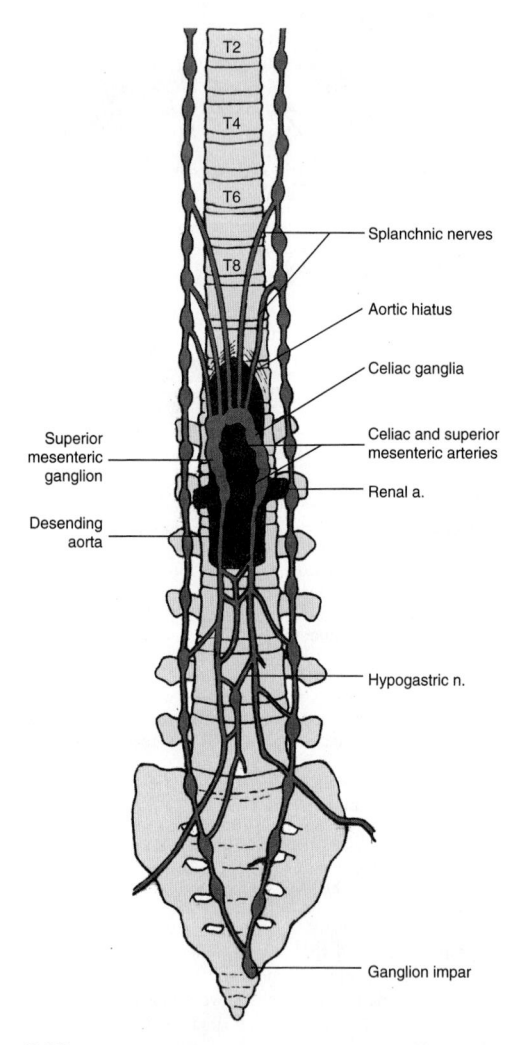

Figure 2-22 Sympathetic chains and splanchnic nerves. The sympathetic chains emit medial branches from the T6 to T12 levels (the splanchnic nerves). These synapse in ganglia positioned at the origin of branches of the abdominal aorta, especially the celiac ganglion. The sympathetic chains continue inferiorly in the abdomen and eventually meet in the midline, anterior to the coccyx (the ganglion impar). (From Mathers L, Chase R: *Clinical anatomy principles,* St. Louis, 1995, Mosby.)

SUGGESTED READINGS

Anderson J: *Grant's atlas of anatomy*, ed 8, Baltimore, 1983, Williams & Wilkins.
Standring S: *Gray's anatomy*, ed 39, New York, 2005, Churchill Livingstone.
Mathers LH et al: *Clinical anatomy principles*, St. Louis, 1996, Mosby.
Nichols DH: *Gynecologic and obstetric surgery*, St. Louis, 1993, Mosby.
Romanes G: *Cunningham's manual of practical anatomy, vol 1, Upper and lower limbs*, New York, 1993, Oxford University Press.
Romanes G: *Cunningham's manual of practical anatomy, vol 2, Thorax and abdomen*, New York, 1992, Oxford University Press.

Abdominal Surgical Approaches

J. Kevin Fitzpatrick

3.1 Anatomy of the Anterior Abdominal Wall

SKIN AND SUBCUTANEOUS TISSUE
1. The skin is composed of epidermis and dermis.
2. It is traversed by lines of cleavage called Langer's lines. First described by Langer in 1861, these lines represent parallel rows of collagen bundles present in the dermal tissue. When these lines are transected the skin edges are pulled apart.
3. Skin incisions following these lines generally heal with a thinner scar.
4. The Langer's lines on the abdomen run in a transverse fashion (Fig. 3-1).

FASCIAL LAYERS (Fig. 3-2)
1. Camper's fascia: Superficial fatty layer that can be several centimeters thick in an obese patient
2. Scarpa's fascia
   a. A membranous layer lying beneath Camper's fascia
   b. Continuous with Colle's fascia of the perineum and joins the deep fascia lata of the anterior thigh 2 cm inferior to the inguinal ligament
3. Rectus fascia
   a. The rectus fascia is a tough band of connective tissue that is composed of the aponeuroses of the external oblique, internal oblique, and transversus abdominis muscles and their point of insertion at the midline in the avascular linea alba.
   b. Superior to the arcuate line, a landmark found in the midline at the level of the anterior superior iliac spine, the aponeuroses form an anterior and posterior sheath to the rectus abdominis muscles.
      (1) The anterior rectus sheath consists of the aponeuroses of the external oblique and the split aponeurosis of the internal oblique.
      (2) The posterior rectus sheath consists of the remaining portion of the internal oblique coupled with the aponeurosis of the transversus abdominis muscle.
   c. Inferior to the arcuate line, the posterior rectus sheath disappears.
   d. The transversus abdominus and the entire internal oblique aponeurosis is found anterior to the rectus abdominus muscle.

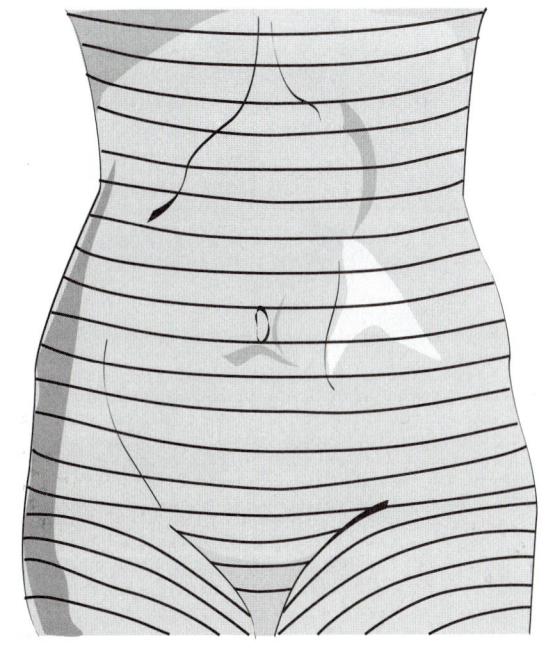

Figure 3-1 Langer's lines of the abdomen.

- e. Therefore, below the arcuate line, the anterior rectus sheath consists of the aponeuroses of the external and the entire internal oblique and transversus abdominus.
- f. In this region the anterior abdominal wall is weaker and there is an increased incidence of incisional hernias.
- g. Tendinous insertions between the rectus abdominus muscles and the anterior rectus sheath exist in several horizontal bands along the course of the muscle.
4. Transversalis fascia: a membranous layer that lies deep to the rectus muscles and superficial to the peritoneum

MUSCLE LAYERS (Fig. 3-3)

1. Rectus abdominis
    a. The rectus abdominis is a paired group of longitudinal muscles found in the midline.
    b. They are separated by the linea alba and held in the rectus sheath as described above.
    c. Their origin is on the symphysis pubis and the pubic crest and the rectus abdominis runs to the xiphoid process and lower costal cartilage.

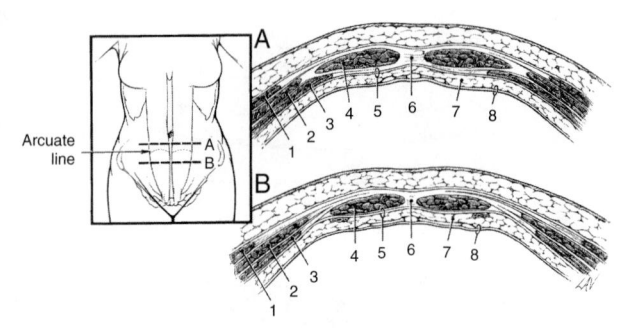

Figure 3-2 **A,** Transverse section of the anterior abdominal wall above the arcuate line. The posterior leaf of the aponeurosis of the internal oblique muscle and the aponeurosis of the transversus abdominis muscle unite to form the posterior wall of the rectus sheath. **B,** A transverse section through the anterior abdominal wall. Below the arcuate line, the posterior wall of the rectus sheath is formed only by the transversalis fascia. *1,* External oblique; *2,* internal oblique; *3,* transversus abdominis; *4,* rectus abdominis; *5A,* posterior rectus sheath; *5B,* transversales fascia; *6,* linea alba; *7,* perperitioneal fat; *8,* peritoneum. (From Nichols DH, editor: *Gynecologic and obstetric surgery,* St. Louis, 1993, Mosby.)

    d. There are also tendinous insertions between the muscle and the anterior rectus sheath found mainly above the arcuate line. These function to anchor the muscle to the anterior sheath.
    e. Function of the rectus abdominis is in locomotion and increasing intraabdominal pressure.
    f. The inferior epigastric artery supplies the lower portion of the muscle and enters the rectus sheath posteriorly at the arcuate line. This vessel anastomoses with the superior epigastric artery, which supplies the upper portion of the muscle.
    g. Nerve supply to the rectus abdominis is derived from the intercostal and lumbar nerves, which enter the rectus sheath laterally.
2. External oblique muscle
    a. The most superficial of the lateral abdominal muscles.
    b. It runs from its origin on the lower eight ribs to its insertion on the pubic crest, pubic tubercle, linea alba, and xiphoid process.
    c. This muscle functions mainly to assist respirations and increasing abdominal pressure. It has a minor role in locomotion.
    d. Its aponeurosis forms part of the anterior rectus sheath.
3. Internal oblique muscle
    a. This muscle is found deep to the external oblique.
    b. Its origin is on the lumbar fascia, iliac crest, and inguinal ligament.
    c. It inserts on the symphysis pubis, linea alba, lower ribs, and xiphoid process.
    d. The rectus sheath is partially formed by its aponeurosis, as mentioned previously.
    e. Its fibers run perpendicular to the external oblique's fibers.

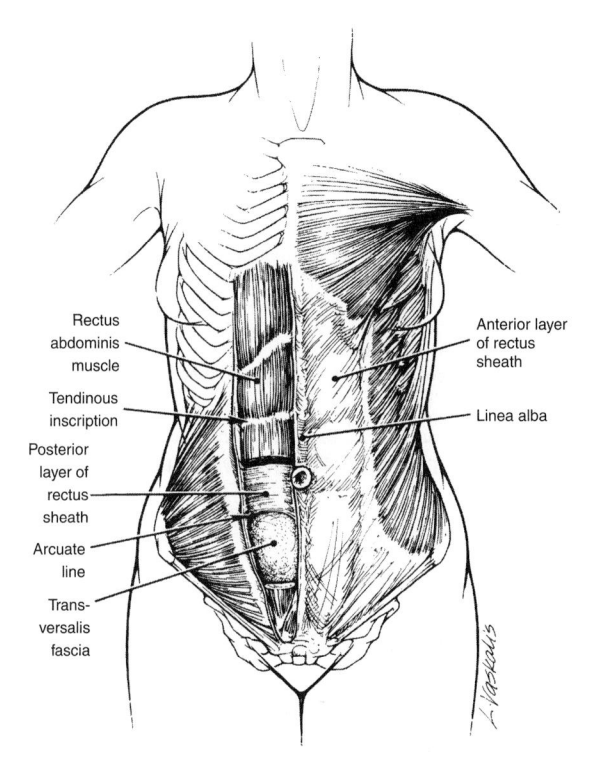

Practical Guide to the Care of the Gynecologic/Obstetric Patient 49

Figure 3-3 A composite of the muscles of the anterior abdominal wall of the adult female. The superficial muscles are shown in the left side of the drawing, and the rectus abdominis and external and internal oblique muscles have been removed in the right side of the drawing. (From Nichols DH, editor: *Gynecologic and obstetric surgery*, St. Louis, 1993, Mosby.)

    f. It, too, functions mainly in respiration, increasing abdominal pressure, and locomotion.
4. Transversus abdominis
    a. This muscle lies deep to the internal oblique.
    b. It arises from the lower costal cartilages, lumbar fascia, iliac crest, and inguinal ligament.
    c. Its insertion is found on the symphysis pubis, linea alba, and xiphoid process.
    d. Functions include respiration, increasing abdominal pressure, and locomotion.
    e. Its aponeurosis is part of the anterior and posterior rectus sheath, as mentioned.

BLOOD SUPPLY (see Fig. 2-16)

1. The blood supply for the anterior abdominal wall arises mainly from the inferior and superior epigastrics near the midline.
2. Laterally, the blood supply is derived from the intercostal, lumbar, and deep circumflex iliac arteries.

NERVE SUPPLY (Fig. 3-4)

1. The intercostal and lumbar nerves run between the internal oblique and transversus muscles.
2. These enter the rectus sheath at various points laterally and innervate the rectus abdominis.
3. The skin over the symphysis pubis and upper lateral thigh is innervated by branches of the iliohypogastric and ilioinguinal nerves.
4. This is important in transverse incisions, in which numbness over the abdomen and upper thigh may result from transection of these branches.

3.2 Abdominal Incisions

SELECTION OF THE APPROPRIATE INCISION
(Fig. 3-5)

There are several considerations when selecting an abdominal approach. The main factor is exposure. It is absurd to select a limited incision that will not grant adequate exposure to perform the necessary surgery.

1. Midline incisions
   a. Midline incisions provide excellent exposure.
   b. They can be extended cranially without compromising the strength of the abdominal wall.
   c. These incisions, however, do not heal as well as the transverse incision and are less cosmetically appealing.
   d. The midline incision is generally reserved for cases in which a transverse incision would not allow for adequate exposure.
   e. Another factor is the speed of entry in an emergency situation. In this regard, the low midline incision is again generally considered the incision of choice.
2. Transverse incisions
   a. The transverse incisions usually provide adequate exposure, are stronger, and are more cosmetically appealing than the midline incisions.
   b. The transverse incisions are the most common abdominal incisions in gynecologic and obstetric surgery.

TRANSVERSE INCISIONS

There are several types of transverse incisions. As mentioned previously, these incisions are used preferentially, provided adequate exposure can be achieved. This is because they heal better, with lower incidence of incisional hernias than the midline incision. Also, because they follow Langer's lines, they heal with a thinner scar. They do, however, have a higher incidence of skin numbness inferior to the incision and damage to

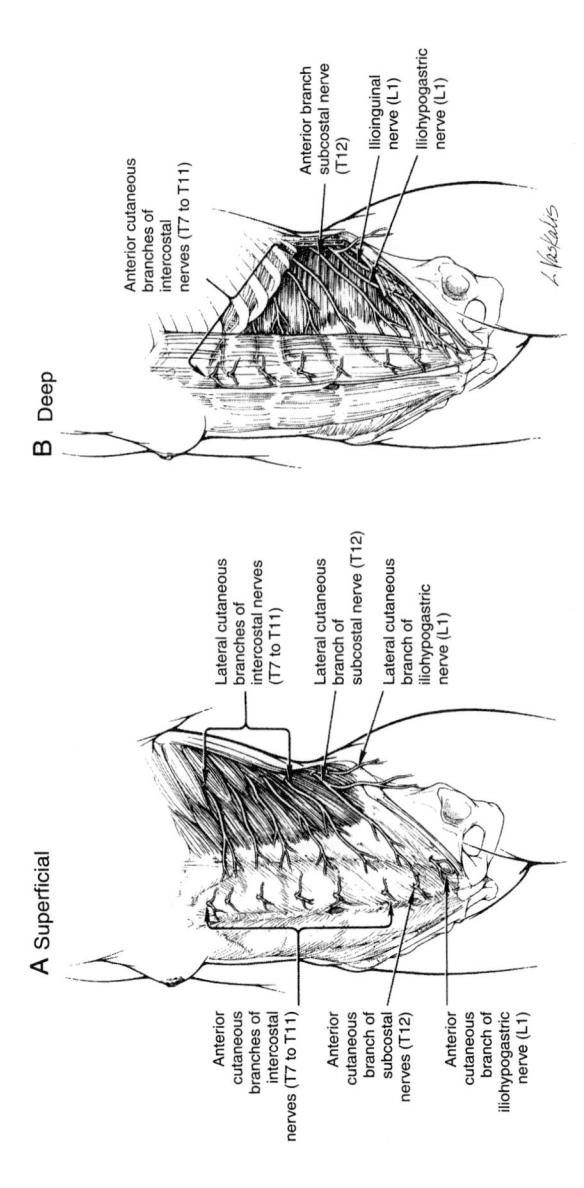

Practical Guide to the Care of the Gynecologic/Obstetric Patient 51

Figure 3-4 **A,** Superficial nerves of the anterior abdominal wall. **B,** Deep nerves of the anterior abdominal wall. (From Nichols DH, editor: *Gynecologic and obstetric surgery*, St. Louis, 1993, Mosby.)

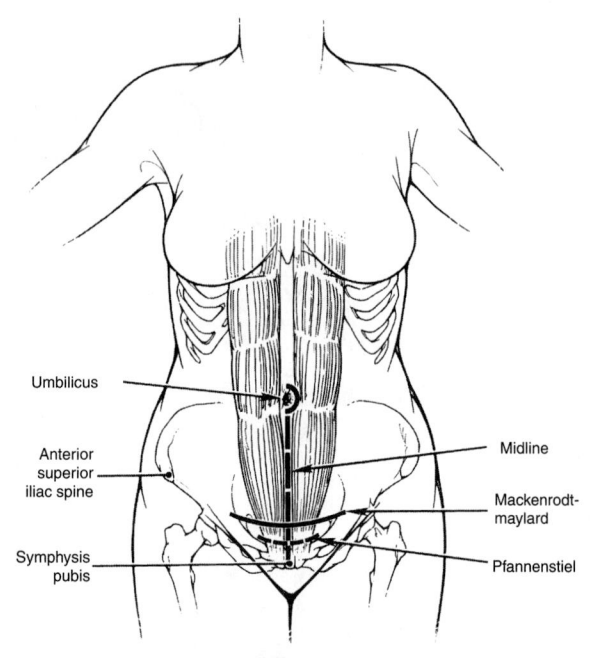

52 Practical Guide to the Care of the Gynecologic/Obstetric Patient

Figure 3-5 The frequent incisions of the anterior abdominal wall are shown in relation to the anterior superior iliac spines. (From Nichols DH, editor: *Gynecologic and obstetric surgery*, St. Louis, 1993, Mosby.)

the femoral nerve by crushing it to the psoas with the deep blades of retractors.

1. Pfannenstiel incision (Fig. 3-6)
    a. This is a transverse incision that is generally considered to have the best postoperative strength.
    b. However, it offers probably the least exposure of any abdominal incision.
    c. To perform this incision, the following is done:
        (1) The skin is incised approximately 2 cm above the symphysis pubis in a transverse fashion.
        (2) This incision is carried down through Camper's and Scarpa's fascia to the rectus fascia with either the scalpel or electrocautery.
        (3) The rectus fascia is then nicked in the midline, again in a transverse fashion.
        (4) This incision is then carried laterally through the rectus fascia with either Mayo scissors, scalpel, or cautery.

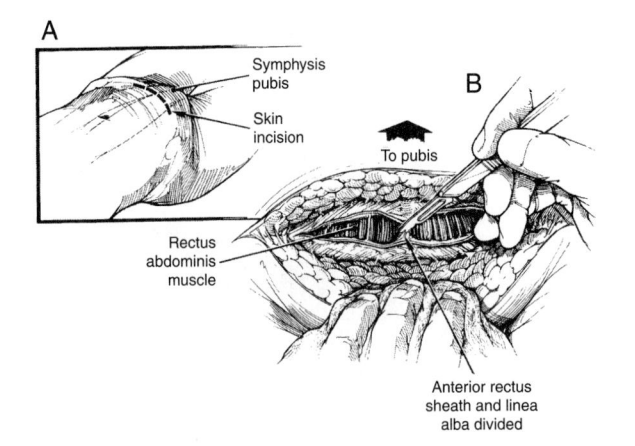

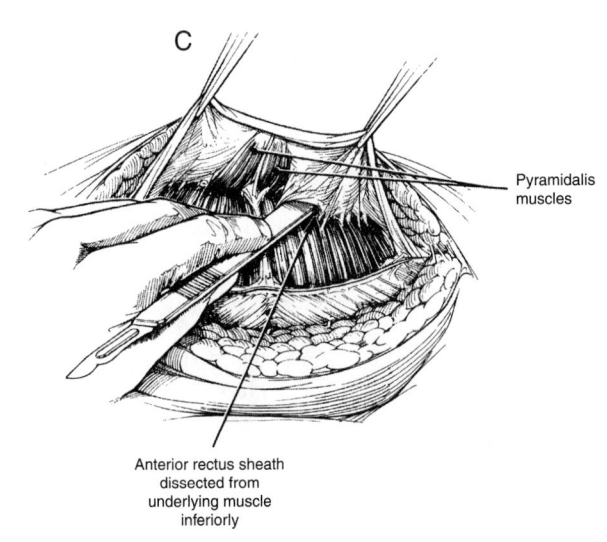

Practical Guide to the Care of the Gynecologic/Obstetric Patient 53

Figure 3-6 Pfannenstiel's incision. **A,** A transverse elliptical skin incision is made in the suprapubic area. **B,** Subcutaneous tissue is incised, exposing the anterior rectus sheath, which is incised to expose the underlying rectus abdominis muscle. The anterior sheath is separated from the muscle by sharp and blunt dissection **(C)**, first in the caudal portion of the incision, *(continued)*

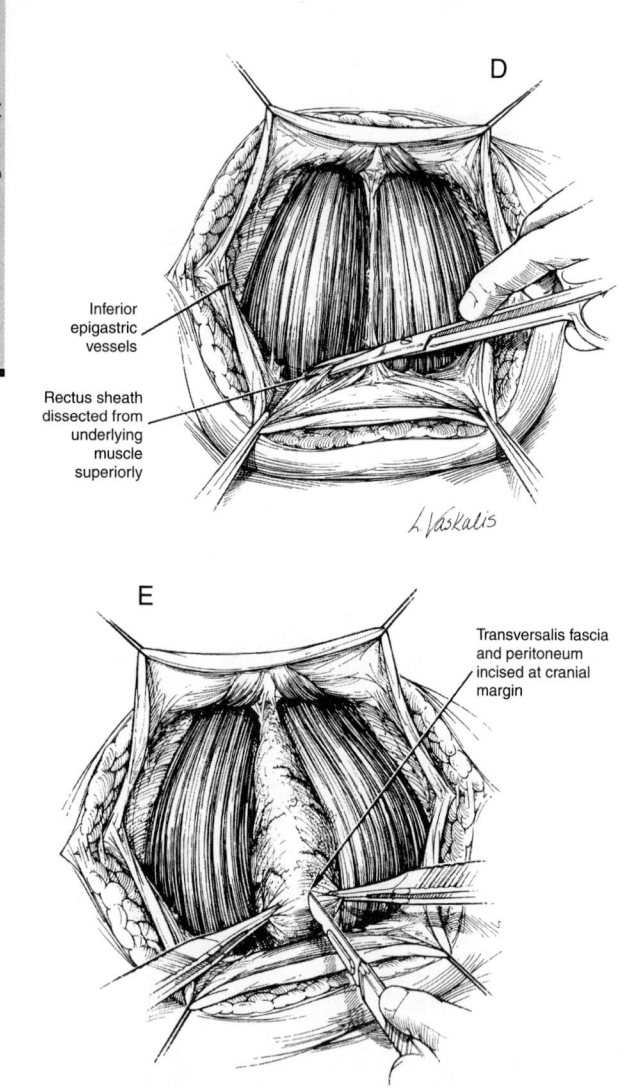

Figure 3-6, cont'd and then beneath the cranial portion of the anterior rectus sheath **(D)**. The peritoneum is identified between the bellies of the rectus muscles, and the transversalis fascia and peritoneum are grasped with forceps and incised in the midline at the cranial margin of the exposure **(E)**.

Peitoneal incision extended caudally

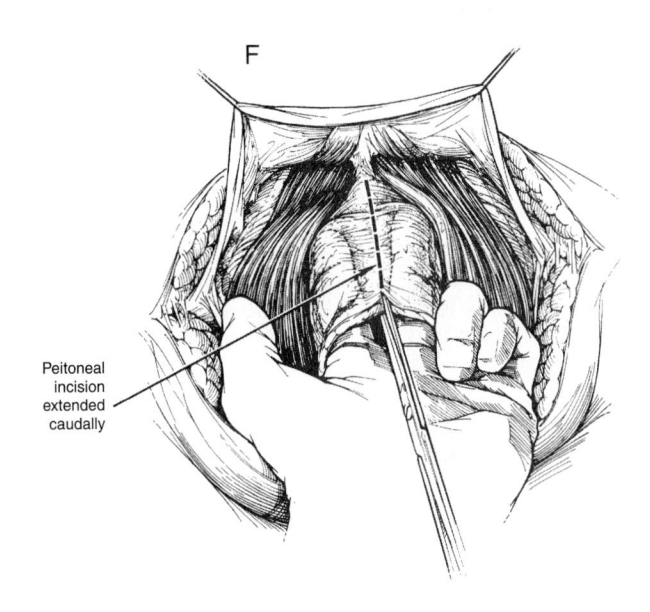

Figure 3-6, cont'd **F,** The surgeon's fingertips are inserted caudally beneath the peritoneum, and the incision is extended downward between the surgeon's fingers, with care being taken to recognize and avoid the cranial margin of the apex of the bladder at the inferior pole of the incision. At the completion of surgery, it is optional whether the parietal peritoneum and transversalis fascia are closed. (From Nichols DH, editor: *Gynecologic and obstetric surgery,* St. Louis, 1993, Mosby.)

- (5) Often, the fascia can be elevated with a Rochester clamp to allow incision without extension into the deeper tissues.
- (6) Once the rectus fascia has been incised, Kocher clamps are used to grasp the superior leaf of the fascia.
- (7) This is then dissected off the rectus abdominis and pyramidalis muscles using either blunt or sharp dissection.
- (8) While dissecting the fascia off the muscle, it is important to be aware of perforating vessels that come through the rectus muscle, mainly lateral to the midline, to give a blood supply to the anterior rectus sheath. These can be controlled with either cautery or fine free ties.
- (9) After dissection of the superior leaf of the fascia is complete, attention is given to the inferior leaf of the incised fascia.
  - (a) This too is grasped with two Kocher clamps and dissected off the pyramidalis muscle using either blunt or sharp dissection.
  - (b) The dissection should be carried down to the level of the pubic symphysis.

(10) Following this, the rectus muscles are separated in the midline and retracted laterally, exposing the transversalis fascia and peritoneum.
(11) This layer is then grasped with two clamps and elevated.
  (a) It is important at this point to make sure that the peritoneum is grasped sufficiently cranially to ensure the bladder is not included in the clamp.
  (b) The possibility of picking up adherent bowel or omentum in the clamp should also be considered, particularly in a patient with previous abdominal surgery, endometriosis, or intraabdominal infection.
(12) Once the presence of bowel or omentum in the clamp has been ruled out by palpation, Metzenbaum scissors can be used to sharply enter the peritoneum.
d. This incision can be extended cranially using the Metzenbaum scissors.
e. When extending the incision caudally, the transversalis fascia can be dissected sharply off the peritoneum and incised.
  (1) Care must be taken at this point not to enter the bladder.
  (2) Transillumination should be used while extending the peritoneal incision to ensure this does not occur.
  (3) It may also be necessary to split the pyramidalis muscle in the midline to provide adequate exposure.
f. This completes the steps necessary to enter the abdomen through a Pfannenstiel incision.
g. As mentioned previously, this incision is limited by the amount of exposure it provides. If a Pfannenstiel incision is done and exposure is suboptimal, it can be converted to a Cherney incision. It is important that this incision not be converted to a Maylard, because once the fascia has been dissected off the rectus muscles, as in the Pfannenstiel, transecting the rectus abdominis muscle corpus, as is done in the Maylard, may cause the rectus muscle to retract and, without its insertions to the anterior sheath, it may not heal well.

2. Maylard incision (Fig. 3-7)
a. This incision allows for greater exposure than the Pfannenstiel as the rectus abdominis muscle is transected and retracted superiorly and inferiorly.
b. Through this incision, pelvic and paraaortic node dissections can be done, as well as the removal of large pelvic tumors.
c. When compared with the midline incision, the Maylard has less postoperative pain, stronger healing, and fewer adhesions, although accessibility to the upper abdomen through this incision is limited.
d. To perform the Maylard incision, the following is done:
  (1) An incision is made 2 to 3 cm above the pubic symphysis and carried down to the rectus fascia, as is done in the Pfannenstiel incision.
  (2) Once the rectus fascia has been identified, it is nicked using the scalpel and extended bilaterally using sharp dissection.
  (3) At this point, the incision differs from the Pfannenstiel in that the rectus fascia is not dissected off the rectus abdominis

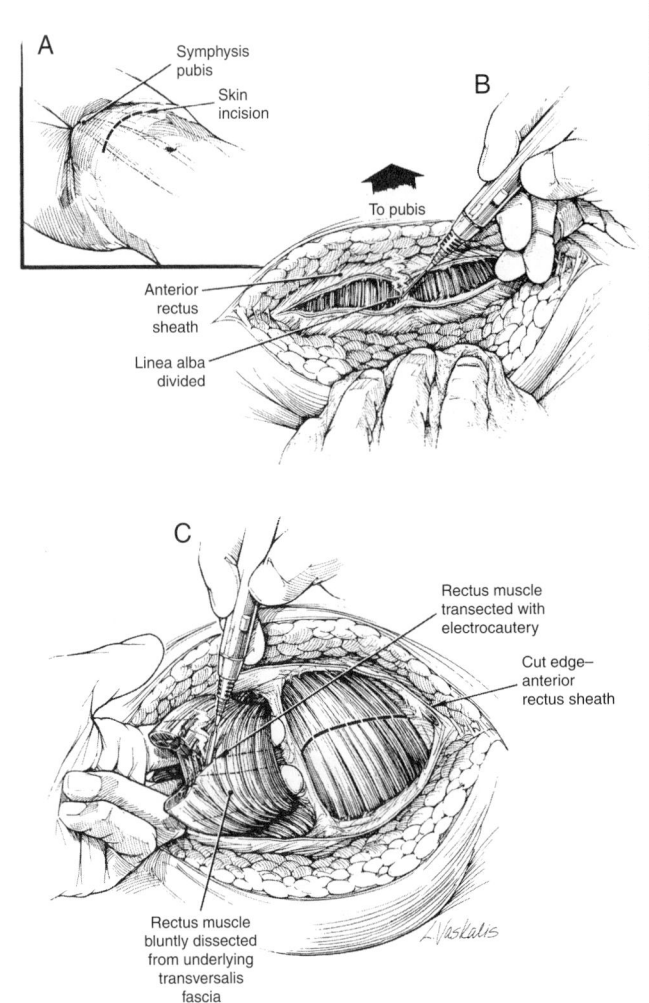

Practical Guide to the Care of the Gynecologic/Obstetric Patient 57

Figure 3-7 The Maylard incision. **A,** A transverse skin incision is made 5 cm above the superior border of the pubis. **B,** The anterior rectus sheath is incised in the same line, exposing the bellies of the rectus abdominis muscles. The muscle is bluntly dissected from the underlying transversalis fascia and incised transversely on each side, along the path of the broken side, using the electrosurgical scalpel **(C).** *(continued)*

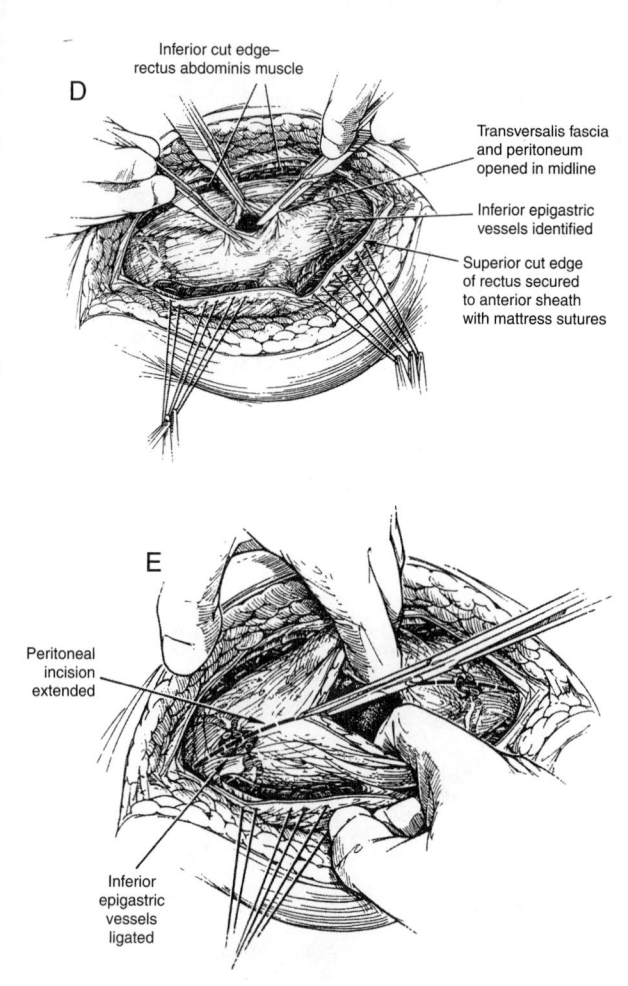

Figure 3-7, cont'd D, The transversalis fascia and peritoneum are opened, and the superior cut edge of the rectus abdominis is secured to the anterior sheath with mattress sutures. E, The peritoneal incision is extended laterally, and the inferior epigastric vessels must usually be ligated and cut. (From Nichols DH, editor: *Gynecologic and obstetric surgery,* St. Louis, 1993, Mosby.)

muscles. Instead, the inferior epigastric arteries are isolated in the connective tissue lying at the lateral border of the rectus muscles.
- (a) These can be identified by palpation and dissected out using blunt dissection with a clamp.
- (b) Once identified, they should be ligated by passing a free 2-0 Vicryl tie around the vessel on a right-angle clamp.
- (c) They should be doubly ligated and incised in between the ligatures.
- (4) After the epigastrics are ligated, attention can be turned to the rectus abdominis muscles. These can be transected, about 3 to 5 cm above their origin on the pubic symphysis, using electrocautery, and proceeding across the muscle in a zigzagging motion to achieve adequate hemostasis.
- (5) Often, a Penrose drain can be passed beneath each rectus muscle, allowing elevation of the muscle while the incision is made.
- (6) This also serves to protect the underlying tissues from extending beyond the limits of the muscle with the electrocautery.
- (7) Once the rectus muscle has been transected, it can be retracted superiorly and inferiorly and the transversalis fascia and peritoneum can be entered using the technique mentioned previously, with the only difference being that the peritoneum is opened in a transverse fashion parallel to the skin incision.
- (8) When closing this incision, it is not necessary to reapproximate the rectus muscles because these will spontaneously heal provided their tendinous insertions to the anterior rectus sheath remain intact.

3. Cherney incision (Fig. 3-8)
  a. This incision differs from the Maylard in that the rectus muscle is not transected through its corpus; instead, it is cut across its tendinous origin on the pubic symphysis.
  b. The muscle is then reflected cranially.
  c. Following the surgery, the tendinous insertion is reattached to the pubic symphysis.
  d. This incision is strong and allows adequate exposure to the pelvis.
  e. Like the Maylard it is limited in its exposure of the upper abdomen.
   (1) A Cherney incision begins like the Maylard and Pfannenstiel in that the skin and superficial fascia are cut down to the level of the rectus fascia.
   (2) The rectus fascia is then nicked in the midline and the incision is extended transversely with sharp dissection as described.
      (a) At this point, the Cherney differs from the Maylard in that the inferior leaf of the split fascia is grasped with two Kocher clamps, is elevated, and is dissected off the rectus abdominis and pyramidalis muscles using either sharp or blunt dissection.

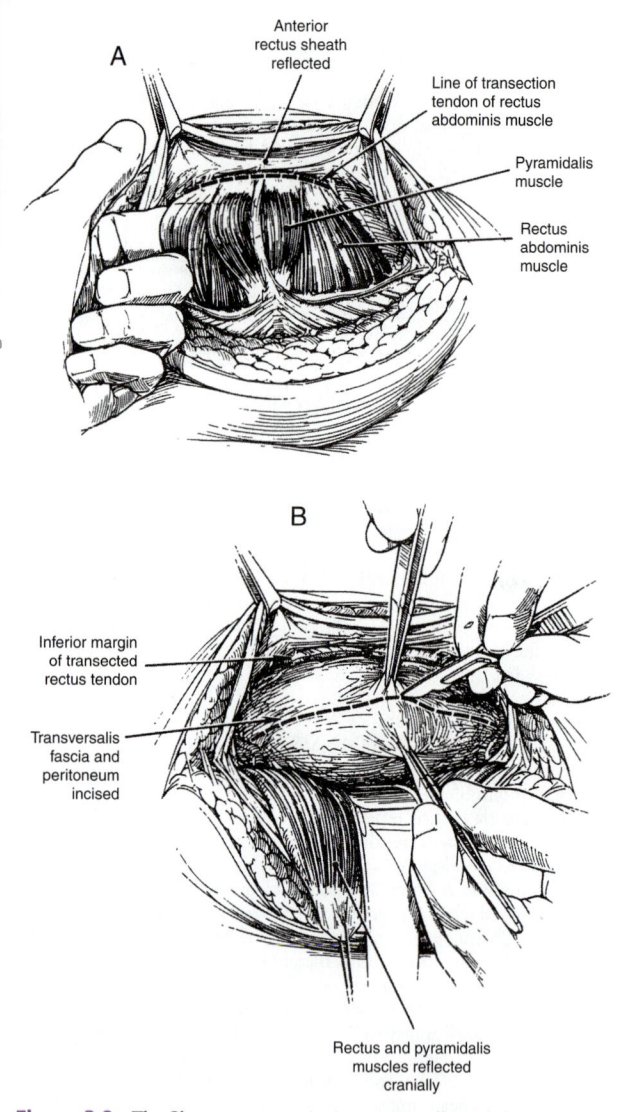

Figure 3-8 The Cherney incision. **A,** A transverse elliptical skin incision is made through the skin and subcutaneous tissue. The tendon of the rectus abdominis muscle and pyramidalis is transsected on each side as shown by the broken line. **B,** The muscles are reflected cranially, and the peritoneum and transversalis fascia are picked up between forceps and incised transversely.

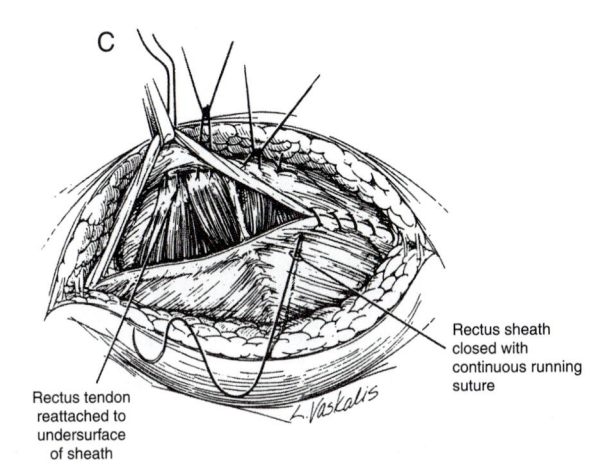

Figure 3-8, cont'd C, At the conclusion of surgery, the tendon of the rectus muscle is attached to the undersurface of the rectus sheath by several interrupted stitches, and the original incision in the rectus aponeurosis is closed with a continuous running suture. The skin incision is closed with staples or a subcuticular closure. (From Nichols DH, editor: *Gynecologic and obstetric surgery*, St Louis, 1993, Mosby.)

- (b) This dissection is carried down to the level of the pubic symphysis, where the aponeurosis of the rectus and pyramidalis muscles are identified.
- (3) The tendon is then incised with Mayo scissors, releasing the muscles from their origin on the pubic symphysis.
- (4) This allows the muscles to be retracted superiorly, and out of the operative field.
- (5) Once retracted, the transversalis fascia and peritoneum can be entered as described.
- (6) Following the operation, the tendon of the rectus and pyramidalis muscles should be reattached to the pubic symphysis using interrupted permanent suture.
- (7) Because this incision reattaches the muscle to the pubic symphysis, the rectus muscle cannot retract cranially into the rectus sheath. Therefore, a Pfannenstiel incision, if found to be inadequate intraoperatively, can be converted to a Cherney without compromising the integrity of the midline musculature.

VERTICAL INCISIONS

As mentioned, the vertical incisions allow for unparalleled exposure to both the pelvis and upper abdomen and can be extended from xiphoid to pubis if need be. They are, however, not as strong as the transverse incisions and, because Langer's lines are transected, heal with a larger, less cosmetically appealing scar.

1. Median incision (Fig. 3-9)
    a. In this procedure, the following is done:
        (1) An incision is made between the umbilicus and pubic symphysis.
        (2) This is carried down through the superficial fascia to the level of the rectus fascia, using either the scalpel or cautery.
        (3) The fascia is then nicked in a vertical direction and a Rochester clamp is placed beneath the fascia to elevate it and allow it to be incised without extension into the deeper tissues.
        (4) A scalpel or cautery can then be used to incise the fascia, opening it to the limits of the skin incision.
        (5) The rectus muscles are then split in the midline along the linea alba and retracted laterally.
        (6) Using clamps, the deeper tissues are then bluntly dissected and the transversalis fascia and peritoneum are identified and elevated between two clamps. As described previously, the

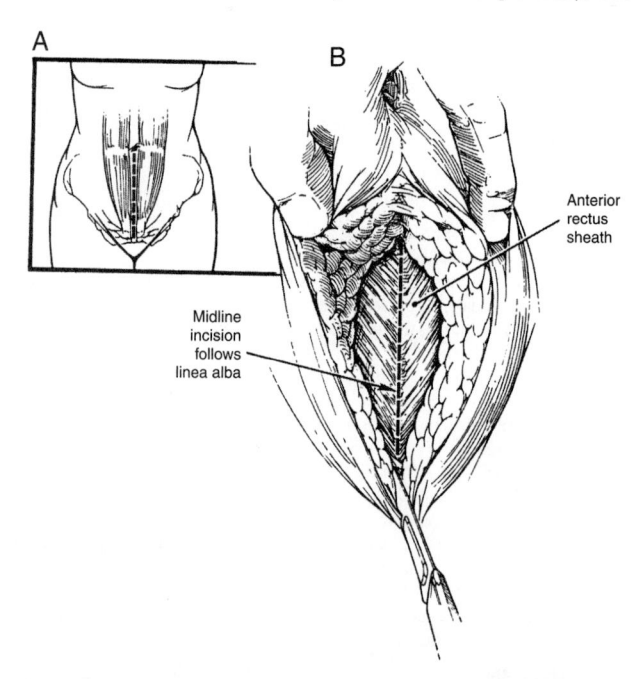

Figure 3-9 The technique of a midline incision in the lower abdomen. **A,** Site of the incision between the umbilicus and the pubis. **B,** The midline incision continues through the subcutaneous tissue to expose the linea alba of the anterior rectus sheath.

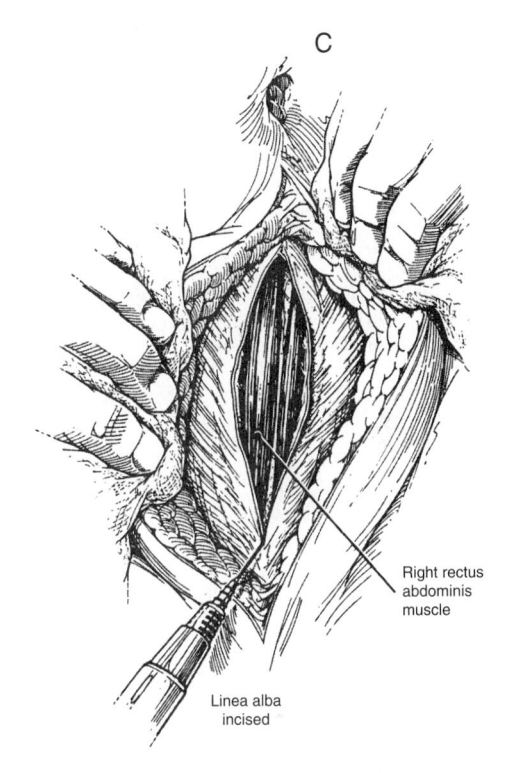

Practical Guide to the Care of the Gynecologic/Obstetric Patient   63

[Illustration labeled C showing: Right rectus abdominis muscle, Linea alba incised]

Figure 3-9, cont'd C, This sheath is incised. *(continued)*

   peritoneum is palpated to ensure no bowel or omentum is adherent to the posterior surface of the peritoneum.
(7) The peritoneum is then entered sharply using Metzenbaum scissors.
(8) This incision is then carried cranially using Mayo scissors and transecting the posterior rectus sheath, transversalis fascia, and peritoneum in the midline. While making this portion of the incision, the posterior surface of the peritoneum should be explored intermittently to ensure that no bowel or omentum is adherent to the posterior surface.
(9) Once the incision has been extended to the length of the skin incision, the peritoneum can be incised in a caudal direction.
   (a) Again, the position of the bladder should be demonstrated by transillumination to avoid entering it with extension of the incision.

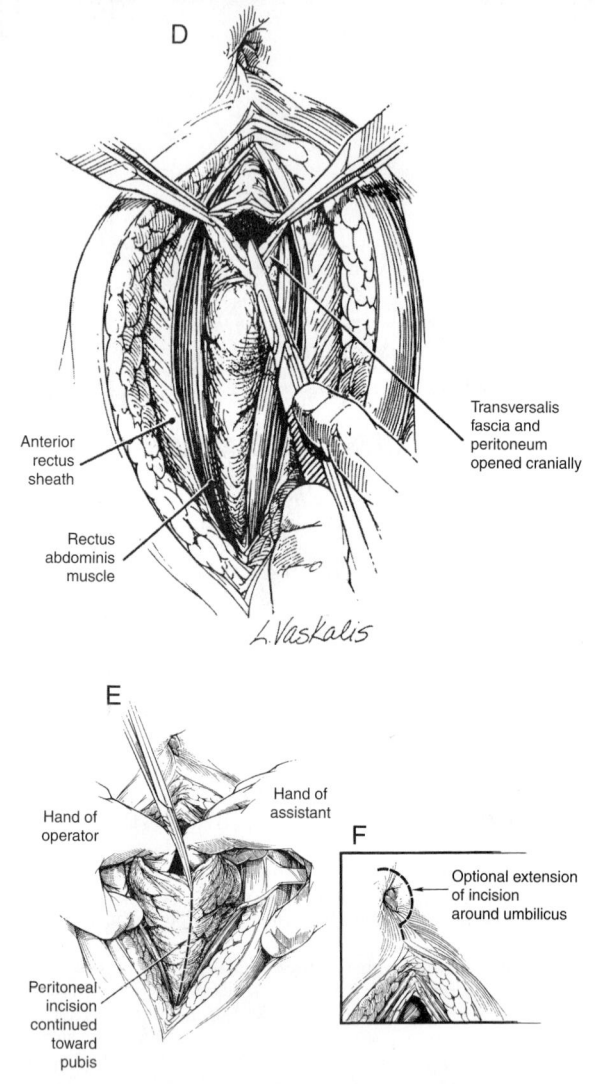

Figure 3-9, cont'd D, The peritoneum and transversalis fascia are grasped between forceps and opened at the cranial end of the incision. Transillumination of this flap by looking through its peritoneal side discloses the outline of the apex of the bladder, marking the caudal limit of the pubic peritoneal dissection (**E**). When it is necessary to extend the midline incision cranially to obtain additional exposure, it should be performed around the left side of the umbilicus to avoid the ligamentus teres (**F**). (From Nichols DH, editor: *Gynecologic and obstetric surgery*, St. Louis, 1993, Mosby.)

(b) Once complete, this incision will allow adequate exposure for pelvic surgery and exploration of the upper abdomen and paraaortic lymphatics.

(c) Should the need arise, the incision can be carried around the umbilicus and as far cranially as the xiphoid process, allowing exposure to the entire upper abdomen.

2. Paramedian incision (Fig. 3-10)
   a. This incision is made to one side of the midline, usually on the side of the expected pathology.
      (1) Instead of entering the peritoneal cavity through the linea alba, the rectus muscle is split longitudinally and reflected laterally.
      (2) Or the abdomen is entered lateral to the rectus muscle following ligature of the inferior epigastric artery.
   b. This incision is reported to be stronger than the median incision, as the avascular linea alba is left intact.
   c. Denervation of the rectus muscle can occur if the incision is extended too far along the lateral border of the muscle. This can result in muscle atrophy.

3.3 Closing the Abdomen

TRANSVERSE INCISIONS

1. Peritoneum
   a. It is currently controversial whether to close the peritoneum following laparotomy or leave it to heal spontaneously.
   b. Several recent studies have shown no benefit in closing the peritoneal membrane; however, surgeons are still concerned that failure to close this layer will result in pelvic and abdominal organs becoming adherent to the anterior abdominal wall.
   c. One exception is with the Maylard incision; in this case, the peritoneum should be closed to keep the split ends of the rectus muscles outside the peritoneal cavity.
   d. To close the peritoneum, the following is done:
      (1) The entire length of the defect can be grasped with clamps. This allows definition of the membrane and its elevation to aid in suturing.
      (2) Using an absorbable or delayed absorbable suture, this layer can be closed in a running stitch, which generally begins at the cranial apex of the incision and extends to the inferior apex.
      (3) When suturing near the caudal aspect of the incision, more superficial stitches should be used to avoid including the bladder.
      (4) A malleable ribbon can be used to protect the bowel from inadvertent needle punctures.
   e. Manipulation of this layer in patients under regional anesthesia, as at cesarean section, can result in discomfort, nausea, and vomiting.

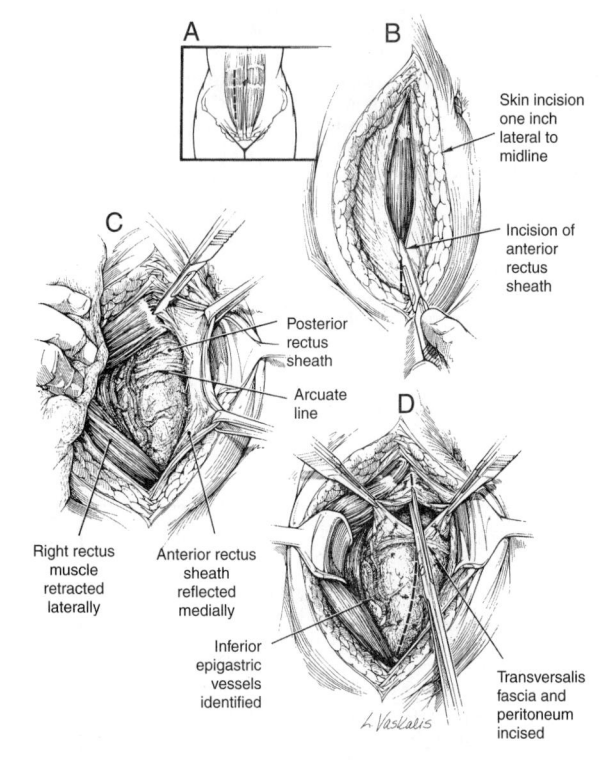

Figure 3-10 Paramedian incision. The skin incision is made on either the right or the left side of the abdomen along the path of the dashed line as shown in **A,** 1 inch lateral to the midline. The anterior rectus sheath is incised over the midportion of the underlying rectus muscle **(B)** and retracted laterally. The anterior rectus sheath is reflected immediately **(C).** The posterior rectus sheath, transversalis fascia, and peritoneum are incised in the bed temporarily vacated by the muscle **(D).** (From Nichols DH, editor: *Gynecologic and obstetric surgery*, St. Louis, 1993, Mosby.)

2. Muscle
   a. Closing the muscle defect in the Maylard incision is not useful in providing extra strength for the incision because the rectus will be reapproximated when the rectus fascia is closed and will heal spontaneously.
   b. Reapproximation of the rectus muscles in the Pfannenstiel incision is also of little value.

c. In the Cherney incision, it is necessary to reattach the aponeurosis of the rectus and pyramidalis muscles to their origin on the pubic symphysis using a permanent suture.
d. Should one choose to close the muscle layer in a Pfannenstiel incision, wide bites of a delayed absorbable or absorbable suture should be used and these should be loosely tied, just allowing for gentle reapproximation of the musculature.

3. Rectus fascia: This layer should be closed using a delayed absorbable or permanent suture of sufficient strength.
   a. The apex of the defect should be identified and the initial suture placed behind the apex, through both leaves of the fascia.
   b. Care should be taken not to include the corpus of the oblique or transverse musculature because ligature of these could result in damage to the ilioinguinal and iliohypogastric nerves, causing numbness inferior to the incision and over the upper thigh.
   c. The sutures should be placed at 1-cm to 2-cm intervals and at least 1.5 cm away from the cut edge. This avoids strangulation of the fascia and weakening the incision.
   d. Again, the fascia should be approximated with gentle pressure and not pulled taut. This too avoids strangulation of the tissues and postoperative pain.

4. Superficial fascia
   a. Recent reports have shown that closure of the superficial fascia in patients with greater than 3 cm of tissue in this plane results in a decreased incidence of wound separation.
   b. When dealing with an obese patient, it is often prudent to leave this layer and the skin open to heal by secondary intention or by a delayed primary closure.
   c. Other cases in which leaving this layer open is desirable include infected or contaminated cases.
   d. Leaving the skin and superficial fascia open with aggressive wound care allows the area to remain clean and for good granulation tissue to accumulate before closure.
      (1) Closure of this layer can be achieved by using a fine absorbable or delayed absorbable suture that can be run from apex to apex of the incision.
      (2) Again, it is only necessary to approximate the edges of the tissue gently.
      (3) Apart from allowing fewer wound separations, this stitch serves to support the skin and allows better anatomical reapproximation at skin closure.

5. Skin
   a. There are multiple methods for closing the skin; these include the following:
      (1) Skin clips
      (2) A running subcuticular stitch
      (3) Mattress stitches
      (4) Interrupted through-and-through stitches

b. An important consideration when closing the skin is potential compromise of the microvasculature.
c. This can be avoided with any of the above techniques, provided that the tissue is not strangulated at closure.
d. An advantage to the skin clips is their ease of removal to allow opening and drainage of the wound should a hematoma, seroma, or wound infection develop.
e. Another consideration when closing the skin is whether it should be closed at all. As mentioned previously, in certain cases (such as infected cases, contaminated cases, and in obese patients) leaving the skin open has certain advantages.
f. In these cases, permanent mattress sutures can be placed in the skin and subcuticular tissues and not tied. These can be left loose until adequate granulation tissue has developed in the wound and then tied at the bedside, giving a delayed primary wound closure.

VERTICAL INCISIONS

1. A running mass closure is an excellent means of closing a midline incision.
2. With this technique, a permanent, thick suture is used to grasp the peritoneum, the posterior and anterior rectus sheath, and the superficial fascia.
3. This is carried in a running fashion from apex to apex, avoiding the inclusion of muscle in the suture.
4. Stitches should be taken at 1-cm to 2-cm intervals and at least 1.5 cm from the fascial edge.
5. This allows the microcirculation to remain intact and results in a decreased incidence of wound eviscerations.

Diagnostic Studies

4.1 Papanicolaou Smear

George T. Danakas

PATIENT PREPARATION

The patient should be instructed to avoid douching or using vaginal creams for at least 24 hours before her examination. Also, Papanicolaou smears should not be obtained during menstruation because the red blood cells may obscure the sample. Sampling should be done before a bimanual pelvic examination, and the use of lubrication should be avoided if possible. However, water used to warm the speculum will not affect the sample. After the patient is positioned in the dorsal lithotomy position, choose a speculum that allows visualization of the entire cervix. Note any abnormalities of the cervix at this time.

SAMPLING

Liquid-based screening systems have been approved by the Food and Drug Administration and were developed to improve the transfer of cells from the collection device to the slide, provide uniformity of the cell population in each sample, and thus decrease interpretational errors. The two systems currently available are ThinPrep and SurePath. Liquid-based cytology has been shown to result in an increased detection rate of both low-grade and high-grade cervical dysplasia, as well as a decrease in the ambiguous diagnosis of atypical squamous cells of undetermined significance (ASCUS). An added benefit of liquid-based cytology systems is the ability to perform "reflex" human papillomavirus (HPV) testing, if desired. For this and other reasons, many health care providers have made liquid-based cytology their test system of choice despite higher cost.

In the ThinPrep test kit, cervical specimens are collected in the usual fashion with either a broom-type device or a spatula and endocervical brush, and cells are collected directly in the methanol-based fixation liquid.

GRADING OF THE SMEAR

Table 4-1 lists the classification of Papanicolaou smears.

Table 4-1 Classification of Papanicolaou Smears

Bethesda System	WHO System	CIN System	Class
Within normal limits	Normal	Normal	I
Infection/reactive and reparative changes	Inflammatory atypia		II
Squamous cell abnormalities: atypical squamous cells of undetermined significance (ASCUS)	Squamous atypia	CIN	
Squamous intraepithelial lesion	Dysplasia		III
Low-grade SIL: HPV	Mild	CIN I	
High-grade SIL	Moderate	CIN II	
	Severe	CIN III	IV
	Carcinoma in situ	CIN IV	
Squamous cell cancer	Squamous cell cancer	Squamous cell cancer	V

SIL, Squamous intraepithelial lesion; *HPV*, human papillomavirus; *CIN*, cervical intraepithelial neoplasia.

4.2 Colposcopy

George T. Danakas and Karen Houck

1. A colposcope is a binocular microscope with magnification from 6× to 40× and a variable intensity light source to allow visualization of the lower genital tract. Box 4-1 lists the common terms in colposcopy.
2. **Patient preparation and procedure**
   a. The patient is placed in the lithotomy position, and the largest speculum that can comfortably be inserted is used to visualize the cervix and upper vagina.
   b. Any excess mucus is gently removed with a cotton swab.
   c. The entire cervix and transition zone must be clearly visualized. Inability to visualize the entire squamocolumnar junction results in an unsatisfactory colposcopy.
   d. A green filter and high magnification may be used to allow improved visualization of the subepithelial angioarchitecture and to help identify abnormal vasculature.
   e. Acetic acid (3% to 5%) is gently applied to the cervix with a cotton swab. Acetic acid reacts with nuclear protein, causing the tissue to swell, which prevents light from passing through it. Abnormal or dysplastic lesions have a large amount of nuclear protein; they therefore have a strong reaction to acetic acid and appear white (acetowhite).

> **BOX 4-1 Colposcopic Terminology**
>
> 1. Acetowhite epithelium (modification of epithelium after application of 5% acetic acid solution).
>   Grade 1: pale, pinkish appearance of underlying stroma still visible
>   Grade 2: whiter epithelium, increased thickness
>   Grade 3: very opaque, irregular surface
> 2. Punctation: set of vascular red dots disseminated in acetowhite lesion. Regularity and coarseness vary with severity of lesion.
> 3. Mosaic: surface vessels arranged in a mosaic pattern. Density and irregularity of epithelial paving vary with grade of lesion.
> 4. Hyperkeratosis: white epithelial lesion present before acetic acid application representing surface keratin.
> 5. Abnormal vessels: abnormal forms of surface vessels described as commas, corkscrews, or spaghetti like. These vessels are signs of invasive disease.

From Alexander Meisels, Carol Morin: *Cytopathology of the uterine cervix*, p. 196. © 1991 by the American Society of Clinical Pathologists.

    f. Once abnormal tissue has been identified, colposcopic biopsy can be performed using a cervical biopsy punch. If needed, multiple biopsies can be obtained. Each biopsy should be sent separately and labeled as to its location of origin. Any bleeding from the biopsy site can be controlled with Monsel's solution or a silver nitrate stick.

    g. An endocervical curettage (ECC) allows sampling of the endocervical canal above the squamocolumnar junction.

    h. It is necessary to make a carefully diagrammed picture of the findings in the chart as well as to document plans for follow-up.

4.3 Hysteroscopy

Scott J. Zuccala

This is the gold standard for evaluation of suspected intrauterine pathology, providing both diagnostic as well as therapeutic intervention. Effectively replaces dilation and curettage (D&C).

INDICATIONS
1. Abnormal uterine bleeding, whether premenopausal or postmenopausal
2. Infertility
3. Retained or lost intrauterine device (IUD)
4. Abnormal radiologic studies, i.e., hysterosalpingogram or sonogram

CONTRAINDICATIONS

1. Infection of cervix or vagina
2. Known cervical or uterine malignancy
3. Suspected pregnancy
4. Hemodynamically unstable patient (hemorrhage)

EQUIPMENT

1. Hysteroscope (0.12 degree or 30 degree)
2. Uterine distention media
   a. Carbon dioxide (CO_2): diagnostic procedures
   b. Solutions: diagnostic as well as therapeutic advantage. Hyskon (32% dextran), nonelectrolyte (3% sorbitol or glycine), electrolyte (saline or Lactated Ringer's)
3. Equipment to monitor inflow and outflow of distention media
4. May be done in office or hospital-based setting

PROCEDURE

1. Ascertain position of uterus.
2. Dilate cervix to accommodate hysteroscope; if 5-mm diagnostic scope is used, may not need to dilate.
3. Pass scope to fundus under *direct visualization*.
4. Observe shape of cavity, ostia, thickness of endometrium, presence or absence of septa, adhesions, myomas, polyps, and irregular surface contour.
5. Observe cervical canal as scope is slowly withdrawn.
6. Avoid intrauterine pressure greater than 100 mm Hg (uterine distension is achieved at 75 mm Hg) by gauge if using CO_2 or by hanging fluids 1.5 m above patient.

BENEFITS

1. Diagnosis and treatment of polyps, myomas, septa, adhesions, adenomyosis, polypoid endometrial hyperplasia, carcinoma, and IUDs
2. Directed tissue sampling

COMPLICATIONS

1. Infection
2. Bleeding
3. Uterine perforation
4. Malabsorption of fluid distention media
5. Cervical laceration (by tenaculum or dilator)
6. Note: D&C has the same complications but also results in a missed diagnosis 10% to 35% of the time.

4.4 Abdominal–Pelvic Diagnostic Laparoscopy

Scott J. Zuccala

PREADMISSION PREPARATION

1. Dictate a problem-oriented preoperative note summarizing all previous operative reports, consultations, history, and physical and laboratory

findings. Read this note 5 minutes before surgery to focus on the patient's problems.
2. Obtain an operative consent in the office as part of the process of informed consent. Discuss risks, benefits, and alternatives to the procedure.
3. Advise the patient not to take any nonsteroidal antiinflammatory drugs (NSAIDs) for 2 weeks before surgery.
4. Order mechanical cleansing of bowel and betadine douche the night before surgery.

OPERATING ROOM PREPARATION

1. Lower genital tract instruments
   a. Straight catheter in urinary bladder
   b. Uterine dilator in uterus for manipulation
   c. Rectal probe available for manipulation
2. Instruments for open laparoscopy
   a. Toothed forceps
   b. No. 15 scalpel
   c. (2) Narrow S retractors
   d. (2) Short, straight Kocher clamps
   e. (2) Tonsil clamps (Varco clamps)
   f. Metzenbaum scissors
   g. 2-0 Vicryl suture on urology needle for fascia
   h. Hasson laparoscopic cannula
   i. 10-mm 180-degree laparoscope
   j. Video camera
   k. (2) Video monitors, one with photographic printer
   l. (2) Short, screw-type 5-mm trocars
   m. Suction irrigator with Lactated Ringer's solution
   n. Calibrated probe
   o. Ovarian biopsy forceps to grasp and palpate lesions
   p. Bipolar forceps
   q. 10-mm 30-degree laparoscope (available)
   r. 5-mm laparoscope (available)
3. Instruments for laparoscopic surgery
   a. 10-mm laser-operating laparoscope with coupler
   b. Hot water, to warm laparoscope to body temperature
   c. Harmonic
   d. Sharp scissors (available)
   e. (2) Atraumatic grasping forceps
   f. Monopolar dissecting needle and generator
4. Allen stirrups: While awake, the patient is placed in the low thigh dorsal lithotomy position to ensure comfort to back, hips, and lower extremities.
5. Left arm: The left armboard should be avoided. The patient's left arm should be tucked across the chest to increase the right-handed surgeon's access to the operative field. Comfort reduces fatigue.
6. Right arm: The right arm is extended on an armboard to receive the intravenous (IV) fluids.

7. General anesthesia: The patient is anesthetized with an intratracheal tube and a warming unit for the upper half of the body to prevent hypothermia during surgery.
8. Examination under anesthesia: Betadine preparation and sterile draping; bladder emptied by straight metal catheter. Examine the pelvis thoroughly. Determine the position of the uterus. Insert and fix an intrauterine dilator or HUMI catheter to control uterine movement during the operation. Place straight catheter to drainage in anticipation of an operative laparoscopic surgery.
9. Height of operating table for laparoscopy: Height should be adjusted to the comfort of the tallest surgeon; shorter members of the operating team should stand on stools as needed for comfort.
10. One surgeon controls the operation: Both diagnostic and operative laparoscopy should be performed by one surgeon. The assistant should assist, not attempt to perform the surgery. The assistant should be still, maintain surgical exposure, and hold the video camera for the surgeon if requested.

EXAMINATION PROCEDURE

1. Placement of Hasson cannula
   Note: The patient should remain supine with no degree of Trendelenburg before the insertion of all trocars to prevent injury to the aorta, the vena cava, and the iliac vessels.
   a. Umbilicus: The depths of the umbilicus must be thoroughly cleaned with cotton swabs and betadine to remove all lint and powder.
   b. Vertical infraumbilical skin incision: The surgeon elevates the skin of umbilicus at 6 o'clock with a toothed forceps, while the assistant spreads the umbilicus open with a tonsil clamp. The surgeon makes a vertical incision through the skin starting near the base of the umbilicus. The surgeon spreads the subcutaneous tissues with tonsil clamps to identify the white anterior fascia.
   c. Vertical fascial incision: Using two S clamps, the assistant separates the subcutaneous tissue and exposes the fascia. The surgeon identifies, grasps, and elevates the white anterior fascia with two straight Kocher clamps and incises in the midline with scalpel. The surgeon spreads the incision with the tonsil clamp. The rectus muscles should be visible. The surgeon places two stay sutures through the fascia for later fixation of the Hasson cannula.
   d. Vertical incision in posterior sheath: Using two S clamps, the assistant separates the areolar tissue to expose the posterior sheath. The surgeon identifies, grasps, and elevates the white posterior sheath with two tonsil clamps. The surgeon carefully incises the posterior sheath with scissors. (Occasionally the peritoneum is incised at the same time.)
   e. Vertical incision in peritoneum: Using two S clamps, the assistant separates the areolar tissue to expose the peritoneum. The surgeon identifies, grasps, and elevates the white peritoneum with two tonsil clamps, being observant for underlying bowel adhesions.

The surgeon incises the peritoneum vertically with scissors. In obese patients, the peritoneum may be entered bluntly with the index finger. Neither technique guarantees prevention of bowel injury.

    f. Insertion of Hasson cannula: With confirmation of intraabdominal entry, an S retractor is placed thorough the opening and the Hasson cannula is inserted using the retractor as a guide. Insufflate the abdomen with CO_2 to a pressure of 18 mm Hg, not to exceed 20 mm Hg. Insert the laparoscope and check for bleeding.

    g. Depth adjustment of Hasson cannula: Withdraw the laparoscope into the cannula. Loosen the screw and, holding the acorn tip snugly against the abdomen, withdraw the cannula until the edge of the peritoneum comes into view; then insert the cannula inward 0.5 cm, tighten the screw, and fix the stay sutures.

2. Placement of trocars lateral to deep epigastric vessels

    a. Identify deep epigastric vessels: On the video screen, the surgeon identifies the right, deep epigastric vessels. The deep epigastric vessels are marked with the surgeon's left hand, and the anterior superior iliac spine is marked with the index finger of the surgeon's left hand. The abdominal wall is transilluminated between the deep epigastric vessels and the anterior superior iliac spine to identify superficial blood vessels. The skin is incised in a clear area.

    b. The surgeon inserts the 5-mm trocar through the fascia and peritoneum, keeping the sharp point under constant visual control. The trocar is directed toward the uterus. The trocar is never directed laterally or inferiorly toward the iliac vessels. The sharp stylet is removed, and the calibrated probe is inserted.

    c. The procedure is repeated for the left lower quadrant trocar with the deep epigastric vessels marked with the index finger of the surgeon's left hand and the left anterior superior iliac spine marked with the thumb of the surgeon's left hand. The suction irrigator is inserted.

3. Bipolar forceps test: The surgeon identifies a fine, superficial blood vessel on the bladder peritoneum and tests the bipolar forceps.

4. Three-step laparoscopic examination

    a. Step 1: abdominal examination in supine position

        (1) The gall bladder, liver, diaphragms, stomach, omentum, spleen, splenic flexure, transverse colon, hepatic flexure, ascending colon, cecum, and vermiform appendix are examined. Endometriosis, adhesions, malrotation of the bowel, or inflammatory disease are looked for.

        (2) A calibrated probe is placed through the right lower quadrant portal to elevate the liver for examination of the gall bladder. The suction irrigator is placed through the left lower quadrant portal to lift the liver to examine the stomach. The omentum is moved to examine the spleen, splenic flexure of the colon, transverse colon, and hepatic flexure of the colon. The left

lower quadrant suction irrigator is lain in the right colic gutter, and the cecum is gently lifted and rotated medially. The mobility of the right colon and the status of the vermiform appendix are ascertained.
   (3) Where detailed examination of the transverse colon and jejunum is required, the surgeon should stand between the patient's legs and use two atraumatic instruments to run the bowel.
 b. Step 2: examination of small bowel and left colon
   (1) With the patient in the steep Trendelenberg position, the surgeon examines the distal 150 cm of ileum, descending colon, sigmoid colon, rectum, rectovaginal pouch of Douglas, and uterosacral ligaments. The ileum is checked for endometriosis, Crohn's disease, adhesions, and Meckel's diverticulum. The surgeon examines the descending colon, sigmoid colon, and rectum for endometriosis, malignancy, diverticulitis, and adhesive disease, and the rectovaginal pouch and uterosacral ligaments for endometriosis.
   (2) Starting at the ileal–cecal junction, the surgeon uses two instruments to gently elevate the loops of small bowel out of the pelvis to a position above the sacral promontory.
   (3) With the uterus anteverted, the surgeon uses two instruments to elevate the sigmoid colon out of the pelvis and put the rectum on stretch for examination. The rectum points like an arrow to any deep rectal endometriosis adherent to the uterosacral ligaments or uterus.
   (4) The surgeon examines the rectovaginal pouch for endometriosis. The rectal probe may be used with advantage to differentiate between an open, partially obliterated, and obliterated rectovaginal pouch, and between rectal and pararectal endometriosis. Rectal lesions can be palpated between the rectal and abdominal probes. Deep peritoneal endometriosis can be grasped with a pair of toothed ovarian biopsy forceps, elevated and evaluated for size and depth of invasion.
 c. Step 3: alpha sequence examination of the pelvis
   (1) Alpha sequence: The surgeon examines the anterior abdominal wall, round ligaments, bladder, anterior uterus, posterior uterus, and uterosacral ligaments; then the left anterior broad ligament, fallopian tube, ovary, ureter, and posterior broad ligament; and last, the right anterior broad ligament, fallopian tube, ovary, ureter, and posterior broad ligament.
   (2) The surgeon examines for endometriosis, malignancy, fibroids, salpingitis isthmica nodosa, hydrosalpinx, pelvic adhesions, and congenital anomalies: inguinal hernias, peritoneal pockets, deep recesses in the lateral pelvic wall(s), medial displacement of the ureter(s), and pelvic kidney.
   (3) With the uterus retroverted into the rectovaginal pouch, the surgeon examines the anterior abdominal wall, round ligaments, bladder, anterior uterus, and uterine fundus.

(4) With the uterus anteverted, the surgeon examines the posterior uterus, the uterosacral ligaments, and the rectovaginal pouch for a second time.
(5) Then the surgeon examines the left fallopian tube from the cornual angle laterally. The left ovary is examined on all surfaces, elevating it with the contralateral instrument and holding it with the ipsilateral instrument. Still holding the ovary and tube, the surgeon lifts the sigmoid colon medially with the right lower quadrant instrument and examines the left pelvic wall and posterior broad ligament. The surgeon locates the pulsations of the hypogastric artery. Usually the ureter runs lateral to the hypogastric artery in the posterior pelvis. The relation of the ureter to the hypogastric artery, the infundibulopelvic ligament, and the uterosacral ligament should be noted.
(6) The surgeon examines the right fallopian tube, the right ovary, the right pelvic wall and broad ligament, the right hypogastric artery, and the ureter in same sequence.

5. Proceed to laparoscopic surgery.

HEMOSTASIS

The surgeon checks for complete hemostasis; all trocars are withdrawn under direct visualization and the pneumoperitoneum is decompressed. Fascial sutures are tied on all 10-mm incisions. The skin is closed with inverted 5-0 Vicryl subcuticular sutures or with interrupted nylon skin sutures.

OPERATIVE REPORT

The laparoscopic photographs, preadmission note, and the American Fertility Society Revised Classification form are assembled. The surgeon dictates the operative report immediately in the same sequence as the three-step abdominal–pelvic laparoscopic examination.

SUGGESTED READINGS

Batt RE, Wheeler JM: Endometriosis: advanced diagnostic laparoscopy. In Hunt RB, editor: *Atlas of female infertility surgery*, ed 2, St. Louis, 1992, Mosby, pp. 422-435.

Batt RE, Wheeler JM: Endometriosis: advanced laparoscopic surgery. In Hunt RB, editor: *Atlas of female infertility surgery*, ed 2, St. Louis, 1992, Mosby, pp. 436-453.

Hasson HM: Open techniques for equipment insertion. In Martin DC, editor: *Manual of endoscopy*, Santa Fe Springs, Calif., 1990, American Association of Gynecologic Laparoscopists, pp. 23-29.

Hulka JF, Reich H: *Textbook of laparoscopy*, ed 2, Philadelphia, 1994, WB Saunders.

Soderstom RM: *Operative laparoscopy: the masters' techniques*, New York, 1993, Raven Press.

4.5 Bowel Injury

Salvador M. Udagawa, Germaine M. Louis, and Ronald E. Batt

SMALL INTESTINE

Injury to the small intestine may occur during difficult operations; this is especially true of operations in the pelvis for neoplastic or inflammatory diseases, in endometriosis, or when there have been previous multiple surgeries. Injuries vary from partial to through-and-through small or large lacerations, perforations, monopolar or bipolar burn injuries, and avulsion injuries to the mesentery and hemorrhages. Success in management of these complications depends on their immediate recognition and treatment. Failure or delay in identifying these injuries may lead to other more serious complications.[1,2]

1. Laceration injury to small bowel
    a. After proper local hemostasis, irrigation, and debridement, the bowel may be closed safely with interrupted nonabsorbable sutures. It is closed transversely according to the Heineke-Mikulicz principle.
    b. Large lacerations or multiple small lacerations in the same segment are treated with a limited resection and an end-to-end anastomosis.
    c. Lacerations to the mesenteric border, unless they are quite small, are difficult to repair and may be associated with vascular impairment. When in doubt of the vascular integrity, a resection should be undertaken. Antibiotic coverage should be used accordingly in relation to the degree and duration of local contamination.
2. Perforation injury to small bowel
    a. Sharp and small perforations, such as those inflicted by the Veress needle used in laparoscopy, are self-limited and may require a small purse-string closure if leakage is confirmed.
    b. Sharp and large perforations such as those inflicted by primary and secondary laparoscopic trocars need a careful local assessment and immediate primary closure using interrupted, nonabsorbable suture material. As in all penetrating or stab wounds of the bowel, ideally the trocar or sleeve should not be removed to facilitate location and repair of single, through-and-through and multiple puncture injuries to the bowel.
3. Thermal injury to small bowel
    a. The most serious injury is the one caused by monopolar energy with necrosis of the bowel wall beyond the area of actual perforation. If a persistent blanched area or a blanched area around a perforation is found, resect at least 5 cm of bowel on either side of the injury.[5] Examine minutely for active bleeding from the wound edges after debridement or resection before local repair or bowel anastomosis is done. Active bleeding from the wound edges indicates healthy blood supply that is necessary for optimal healing.
    b. Wound resection adequate to reach viable tissue is less extensive after a bipolar or a laser energy burn to the bowel. Nevertheless, the surgeon is encouraged to resect and debride the injury until there is active bleeding from the wound edges before proceeding to local repair or bowel anastomosis as needed.
4. Avulsion injury to mesentery: Avulsion injuries usually occur from undue traction exerted on the mesentery. Copious bleeding is the most troublesome. Safe control of the hemorrhage requires adequate exposure and visualization. The surgeon can confidently and deliberately control the exact bleeding point without resorting to the use of

mass suture ligatures or thermocoagulation. It is better to provide local tamponage, for a few minutes, with steady finger pressure to the bleeding area or by means of a small pack. The bleeding will have ceased and individual ligation of lacerated blood vessels can be done. Repair of large and important veins may be necessary.

COLON AND RECTUM

1. The morbidity and mortality from injuries to the colon have been significantly reduced by an aggressive surgical approach. Sepsis is the most formidable added risk when dealing with colonic injury.
2. Specific care should be directed by the type, location, and extent of injury as well as the condition of the colon, whether or not it is obstructed and distended or is simply filled with fecal content. Also, the anatomic location of the injury is important; whereas injuries to the intraperitoneal right, transverse, and sigmoid colon do not require drainage, injuries to the retroperitoneal descending colon and rectum require that the suture line be protected by retroperitoneal drainage and/or fecal diversion by colostomy.
3. It is important that the time from injury to definitive operation be as short as possible. It is similarly important to avoid, by all means, fecal soilage or contamination. Antimicrobials are not a substitute for surgical technique. However, antibiotics should be used judiciously preoperatively and postoperatively.
4. Diagnosis
   a. A sudden smell of fecal odor during an abdominal or laparoscopic procedure, even in the absence of visible extravasation of stool, indicates an entrance into the colon or rectum. Careful inspection leads to the recognition of the injury and a complete repair.
   b. Plain film of the abdomen should be employed if there is a perforated colon with leakage of air into the free peritoneal cavity following laparotomy. This examination is of limited value after laparoscopic procedures. Sigmoidoscopy or colonoscopy can be used in the examination of patients suspected of colonic perforation after surgery. Computed tomography (CT) scan of the abdomen and pelvis may be helpful in selected cases. Barium contrast material should not be used because of the high morbidity and mortality associated with leakage of barium and feces into the free peritoneal cavity. Aqueous opaque media such as Gastrografin are preferable when penetration of the colon is suspected.
5. Treatment
   a. An incision capable of an easy extension is used because operation on the colon often requires wide mobilization of at least two flexures. Incisional infections are discouraged by protecting the wound with moist pads or 7-in. ring plastic wound protectors (Vidrape, 3M Corporation).
   b. First the peritoneal cavity should be carefully explored and close examination of the lesion itself reserved for last. The strategy of the operation is planned, and the procedure is conducted with the avoidance of contamination or bleeding.

REFERENCES

1. Levy BS, Soderstrom RM, Dail DH: Bowel injuries during laparoscopy: gross anatomy and histology. *J Reprod Med* 30:168-179, 1985.
2. Soderstrom RM: Bowel injury litigation after laparoscopy. *J Am Assoc Gynecol Laparoscopists* 1:74-77, 1993.
3. Soderstom RM: *Operative laparoscopy: the masters' techniques*, New York, 1993, Raven Press, pp. 195.

4.6 Ureteral Dissection

Ronald E. Batt and Germaine M. Louis

Precise localization of the ureters is recommended before all operative interventions. Ureteral dissection and displacement from harm is recommended whenever the possibility of ureteral injury exists. Placement of ureteral catheters preoperatively is recommended in patients with extensive pelvic disease that distorts the pelvic anatomy.

INDICATION FOR URETERAL DISSECTION

1. When operating near the ureter, it is safer and faster to dissect and expose the ureter to clear view than to stop repeatedly and check its position or perform the dissection under emergency circumstances.
2. Ureteral dissection is recommended in the following instances:
   a. Obliteration of rectovaginal pouch by deep fibrotic endometriosis
   b. Medial displacement of ureter near uterosacral ligaments
   c. Excision of deep fibrotic endometriosis from vaginal cuff and uterosacral ligaments, status posthysterectomy
   d. Deep endometriosis adherent to or partially obstructing the ureter
   e. Left-frozen-pelvis from endometriosis
   f. Ovary, oviduct, or sigmoid colon adherent to ureter
   g. Extensive chronic salpingo-oophoritis
   h. Laparoscopically assisted vaginal hysterectomy (LAVH) for endometriosis
   i. Extraperitoneal lymphadenectomy for malignancy
   j. To isolate and ligate retracted bleeding uterine artery
   k. Salpingo-oophorectomy

TOPOGRAPOHICAL ANATOMY

1 Anatomic divisions of the ureter
   a. The iliopectineal line divides the ureter into abdominal and pelvic portions. The pelvic ureter is divided into the following three parts:
      (1) The pars posterior, which runs from the sacroiliac joint along the lateral pelvic wall to the entrance of the preformed tunnel in the cardinal ligament
      (2) The pars intermedia, which runs within the broad ligament to the vesicouterine ligament
      (3) The pars anterior, which runs from the entrance into the vesicouterine ligament to the ureteral orifice of the bladder
   b. The left ureter may be identified above the iliopectineal line at the apex of the intersigmoid fossa by displacing the left adnexa

anterolaterally and the sigmoid colon medially and cephalad. In difficult cases, the ureter may be located near the pelvic brim, lateral to the pulsations of the hypogastric artery. Normal peristalsis should be observed. When the ureter lies close to the infundibulopelvic ligament, the infundibulopelvic ligament must be displaced laterally. This maneuver compresses the peritoneum over the ureter and facilitates identification.
   c. The right ureter crosses the iliac vessels at the bifurcation of the common iliac artery and is easier to locate than the left ureter. Near the pelvic brim, it lies lateral to the pulsations of the hypogastric artery.
2. Congenital anomalies: medial displacement of one or both ureters occurs in the following ways[1]:
   a. As an isolated congenital anomaly
   b. In association with peritoneal pockets in the posterior pelvis
   c. As the medial border of a large broad ligament recess
3. The sigmoid colon traps menstrual detritis against the left ureter, increasing the risk of endometriosis. It may also envelop the left tube and ovary in dense obliterative adhesions in response to repeated ruptures of an ovarian endometrioma.

OPERATIVE PROCEDURES FOR URETERAL DISSECTION

1. Preoperative preparation
   a. The surgeon examines old operative reports.
   b. An intravenous pyelogram (IVP) is recommended when there is severe and extensive endometriosis and selectively in other situations.
   c. Cleansing enemas or a formal bowel preparation are recommended the day before surgery.
2. Excision of endometriosis at the level of the left ovary[2]: Endometriotic plaques overlying or invading the ureter are often associated with endometriomas of the ovary.
   a. The course of the left ureter must be explored and defined before adhesiolysis is attempted.
   b. The surgeon elevates the peritoneum lateral to the ureter with a toothed forceps and incises (with scissors or CO_2 laser) for a distance of 2 cm to expose the ureter and the endometriosis.
   c. The surgeon separates the ureter from surrounding tissues, using blunt aquadissection and perpendicular and parallel spreading with a blunt dissecting forceps.
   d. With the ureter exposed, the ovarian adhesions are placed on tension and the initial incision is made with scissors or a CO_2 laser. Gentle blunt aquadissection with the suction irrigator usually completes the ovariolysis.
   e. The ovarian endometrioma(s) is excised to improve surgical exposure.
   f. The peritoneal incision is extended lateral to the endometriotic plaque.

g. The surgeon grasps the lateral margin of the endometriotic plaque with a pair of toothed forceps and reflects it medially.
h. The endometriotic plaque is dissected with aquadissection and blunt spreading forceps, cutting the peritoneum and dense adhesion bands to the muscularis of the ureter with scissors or a harmonic scalpel.
i. Caution must be exercised so that the dense adhesion bands do not tent the ureter. This dissection may be tedious and time consuming. The surgeon should be gentle and persistent, avoiding impulsive moves and rough dissection.
j. Hemoclips or fine bipolar forceps can be used for hemostasis. The surgeon excises the endometriosis.
k. The surgeon examines the ureter. Additional ureterolysis is performed if needed.
l. The peritoneal wounds are left open to heal.

3. Excision of endometriosis at level of the left uterosacral ligaments[2]: Medial displacement of the ureter adjacent to the uterosacral ligament may occur as a congenital anomaly or from contraction of deep fibrotic endometriosis in the uterosacral or broad ligament. Dissection of the ureter must be performed very carefully to avoid brisk bleeding from the extensive venous network in the cardinal ligament and from the uterine artery. The retroperitoneal approach is recommended.[3]
   a. The peritoneum is incised lateral to the ureter 2 cm from the cardinal ligament, and the incision is extended caudally.
   b. The ureter is dissected free with aquadissection and perpendicular and parallel spreading with a blunt dissecting forceps, until it can be displaced laterally with a blunt probe.
   c. Hemostasis is applied with clips or bipolar coagulation. If bipolar coagulation is necessary to control bleeding, the power density must be kept low to prevent the lateral spread of thermal energy, but it must be sufficient for hemostasis.
   d. With the ureter displaced laterally, the surgeon grasps the endometriosis with a pair of toothed forceps and maintains constant medial traction.
   e. Excision with hemostasis is facilitated by use of the harmonic scalpel. Scissors dissection may require hemostasis with hemoclips or bipolar electrocoagulation.
   f. To prevent or control bleeding or hematoma formation in the broad ligament, the uterine artery must be ligated. The paravesical and pararectal spaces must be opened and developed. The surgeon identifies the external iliac vein and artery, the internal iliac artery, the uterine artery, and the ureter. The surgeon displaces the ureter medially out of harm's way and ligates the uterine artery with clips, bipolar electrocoagulation, or ligature.[4]

4. Dissection of left-frozen-pelvis: In some cases of extensive endometriosis (greater than RAFS stage IV-70), the left tube and ovary are irrecoverably damaged, trapped by obliterative, adhesive disease between the sigmoid colon and the pelvic wall. The left-frozen-pelvis may be a complication of previous conservative surgery. The ureter is particularly at risk for ligation or transection. The experienced pelvic endosurgeon may attempt retroperitoneal dissection and left

salpingo-oophorectomy; however, the prudent course in most cases is to gain access to the pelvis by laparotomy.[5]

5. Dissection of frozen pelvis and frozen ureter: When the pelvic anatomy is totally distorted by obliterative endometriotic disease and the ureters are firmly embedded in endometriosis, laparotomy is recommended as the only mode of access. The surgical team (gynecologist, colorectal surgeon, and urologist) should be prepared for bowel resection as well as resection of the ureter(s) and implantation into the bladder.

PREOPERATIVE URETERAL CATHETERS

Surgery for severe and extensive endometriosis is often more challenging than surgery for malignancy. Deeply invasive disease combined with dense, obliterative adhesions so distort pelvic anatomy that dissection is long, tedious, and bloody. Ureteral catheters facilitate identification of the ureters and should be used in such cases. This gives the urologist an opportunity to meet the patient, read the detailed preoperative note, and perform a cystoscopy and insert the ureteral catheters. If a urologic problem arises, the urologist comes to the operating table prepared.

URETERAL INJURIES

A detailed discussion of detection and intraoperative repair of ureteral injuries, as well as the diagnosis and treatment of unrecognized ureteral injuries and unsuccessful ureteral repairs, is beyond the scope of this chapter. Detailed information is readily available.[5]

REFERENCES

1. Batt RE, et al: A case-series study of peritoneal pockets and endometriosis: rudimentary duplications of the mullerian system. *Adolesc Pediatr Gynecol* 2:47, 1989.
2. Batt RE, Wheeler JM: Endometriosis: advanced laparoscopic surgery. In Hunt RB, editor: *Atlas of female infertility surgery*, ed 2, St. Louis, 1992, Mosby, pp. 436-453.
3. Kadar N: An operative technique for laparoscopic hysterectomy using a retroperitoneal approach. *J Am Assoc Gynecol Laparoscopists* 1:365-377, 1994.
4. Batt RE, Udagawa SM, Wheeler JM: Endometriosis: microconservative surgery. In Hunt RB, editor: *Atlas of female infertility surgery*, ed 2, 1992, Mosby, pp. 454-481.
5. Gynecologic and obstetric surgery. *Intraoperative ureteral injuries and urinary diversion*, St. Louis, 1993, Mosby, pp. 900-910.

4.7 Urodynamic Studies

Philip J. Aliotta

DEFINITION

Urodynamics is the study of the changing parameters of bladder filling, storage, and emptying, dealing with the interaction of the bladder with its urethra.[1]

STEPS IN THE MICTURITION PROCESS

1. Voluntary relaxation of the external sphincter
2. Reduced sympathetic nervous system outflow
3. Smooth muscle relaxation with resultant funneling of the bladder neck and opening of urethra
4. Bladder contraction with evacuation of the bladder's contents

URODYNAMIC EVALUATION OF THE FEMALE PATIENT

1. History, focusing on the following:
   a. Existing systemic disorders
   b. Congenital disorders
   c. Psychosocial factors
   d. Existing neurologic disorders
   e. Disorders specific to the urologic tract
2. Physical examination
   a. General examination
   b. Evaluation of estrogen status
   c. Examination of the vagina and periurethral area for signs of fistula, abscess, and diverticula
   d. Examination for cystocele, rectocele, and enterocele
   e. Rectal examination to assess sphincter tone and the bulbocavernosus reflex
   f. Neurologic examination
      (1) Mental status assessment
      (2) Assessment of cranial nerves II through XII
      (3) Cerebellar testing for truncal ataxia, gait ataxia, finger–nose test, heel–shin test
         (a) Clinically, cerebellar lesions produce spontaneous, high-amplitude detrusor reflex contractions
         (b) Poor hand coordination makes clean intermittent catheterization impractical
      (4) Deep tendon reflexes
         (a) Supranuclear lesions: hyperreflexia
         (b) Cauda equina lesions: diminished or absent reflex
         (c) Peripheral neuropathy: diminished or absent reflex
      (5) Sensory assessment
         (a) Pain and temperature awareness
         (b) Position, vibration, light, and crude touch
3. Frequency/volume voiding diary: an investigational record of fluid intake, output, and other voiding characteristics occurring in a 24-hour period that includes the following:
   a. Daily intake and output
   b. Frequency of micturition
   c. Time interval between voidings
   d. Volume voided
   e. Urgency
   f. Incontinence
   g. Number of continence pads used per day
4. Urinalysis and culture
   a. Treatment for existing infections
   b. Hematuria workup
5. Radiographic evaluation
   a. Plain film of abdomen: to rule out bony abnormalities of the vertebral column and pelvis
   b. IVP to assess the following:

(1) Upper tract anatomy and anomalies
(2) Ureters: ureteral ectopy and duplication
(3) Bladder configuration and abnormalities of contour and position
(4) Postvoid residual
(5) Vesicovaginal fistula

c. Video cystourethrography combines voiding cystourethrography (VCUG), fluroscopy, and pressure recordings of the bladder and abdomen along with urinary flow rates

6. Urethroscopy
   a. Under direct visualization, the urethra is examined using a 0-degree, 5-degree, or 30-degree lens.
   b. Gas urethroscopy allows measurement of urethral opening pressure, which in a normal patient is between 70 and 90 cm of water.[2]
   c. Water urethroscopy does not allow for urethral opening pressures.
   d. The interior of the urethra is examined for any obstructing lesions, discharge from periurethral glands, diverticuli, or an ectopic ureter. The normal urethra has a pink epithelium.
   e. The bladder is entered, and the urethrovesical junction is examined during bladder filling. The urethrovesical junction is normally described as round and symmetric. The trigone, located on the floor of the bladder, is pale pink. The ureteral orifices appear as slitlike openings on the floor of the bladder and should be observed for expulsion of urine.
   f. The following changes are seen with bladder filling[2]:
      (1) The urethrovesical junction closes.
      (2) The periurethral striated muscles tighten (Table 4-2).

7. Residual urine
   a. Integrates the activity of the bladder and outlet during the emptying phase of micturition[3]
   b. Defined as the volume of fluid remaining in the bladder immediately following the completion of micturition[4]
   c. Estimated by using the following:
      (1) Catheter
      (2) Cystoscopy
      (3) IVP
      (4) VCUG
      (5) Radioisotope studies
   d. Findings
      (1) Increased residual (>100 cc): failure to empty. Possible causes include the following:
         (a) Anxiety (if suspected, repeat test)
         (b) Increased outlet resistance
         (c) Decreased bladder contractility
         (d) Combination of all of the above
      (2) No residual of significance (<100 cc). Possible causes include the following:
         (a) Normal function
         (b) Increased bladder contractility
         (c) Incompetent sphincter

Table 4-2 Urethroscopy of Normal and Abnormal Patients

Dynamic Function of the Urethrovesical Junction	Normal	Genuine Stress Incontinence	Unstable Bladder
Empty bladder	Closed	Closed	Closed
Partially filled bladder	Closed	Slowly opens	Closed if no vesical contraction
Full bladder	Closed	Slowly opens	Closed if no vesical contraction
Holding	Closes	Sluggish closure	Closes
Straining	Remains closed	Opens	Remains closed if no vesical contraction
Coughing	Remains closed	Opens	Remains closed if no vesical contraction
Vesical contraction	Opens, then closes, with suppression		Opens and remains open due to inability to suppress
Ability to suppress a vesical contraction	Present	Present	Absent

Modified from Robertson JR: Dynamic urethroscopy. In Ostergard DR, Bent AE, editors: *Urogynecology and urodynamics—theory and practice*, Baltimore, 1991, Williams & Wilkins.

Practical Guide to the Care of the Gynecologic/Obstetric Patient 87

> BOX 4-2 Urine Flow Rate Parameters
>
> Flow time: time over which measurable flow occurs
> Time to maximum flow: time elapsed from the onset of flow to maximum rate
> Maximum flow rate: the maximal rate of flow
> Voided volume: the total volume expelled by way of the urethra
> Average flow rate: the voided volume divided by flow time
> Voiding time: the total duration of micturition, including interruptions
> Flow pattern: may be continuous, interrupted, or specifically described

8. Uroflow studies: defined as the volume of fluid expelled from the urethra per unit time expressed in mL/s.[3] It expresses the combined activity of the detrusor and urethra. Box 4-2 lists the terminology of the International Continence Society relating to the urodynamic description of urinary flow. The flow pattern in Figure 4-1 is normal. Minimum acceptable urine flow rates are listed in Table 4-3. Volumes under 150 cc should be interpreted with caution.[5]
9. Urethral pressure profile
   a. Allows for the measurement of the active and passive tone of the urethra.[1]
   b. Measures urethral pressure with the patient lying down, the bladder at rest, and the urethra closed.

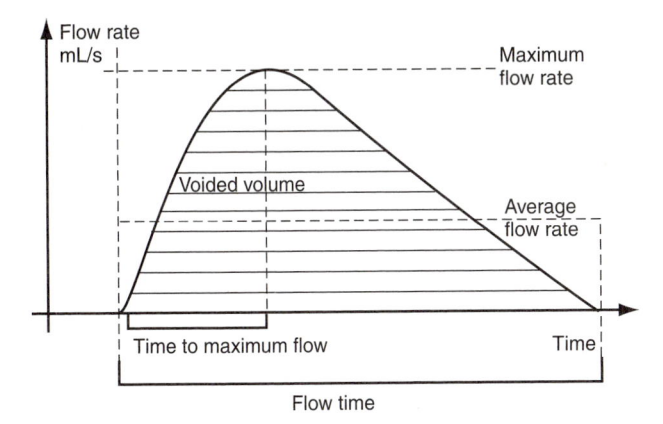

Figure 4-1 Terminology of the International Continence Society as it applies to a normal flow pattern (see also Box 4-2). (From Wein AJ, English WS, Whitmore KE: *Urol Clin North Am* 15:621, 1988.)

Table 4-3 Minimum Acceptable Urine Flow Rates

Age (yr)	Minimum Voided Volume (Ml)	Flow Rates (mL/s) Males	Flow Rates (mL/s) Females
4-7	100	10	10
8-13	100	12	15
14-45	200	21	18
46-55	200	22	15
56-80	200	9	10

Data from Abrams P: The urethral pressure profile measurement. In Mundy AR et al, editors: *Urodynamics: principles, practice, and application*, Edinburgh, 1984, Churchill Livingstone.

    c. Uses a specially designed catheter with multiple side holes and an occluded tip. (Fluid infused along the catheter escapes through the side holes and the urethral pressure profile measures the resistance of the urethral walls to distension by the escaping fluid.)

    d. Nomenclature for the urethral pressure profile.
      (1) Maximum urethral pressure: the maximum pressure of the profile
      (2) Maximum urethral closing pressure: the difference between the maximum urethral pressure and bladder pressure
      (3) Functional profile length: the length of the urethra along which the pressure exceeds bladder pressure
      (4) Total urethral length: functional length plus the additional length to reach atmospheric pressure

    e. Types of urethral pressure profile.
      (1) Static: measures urethral pressure with the patient lying down, the bladder at rest, and the urethra closed.
      (2) Perfusion: using saline or gas perfusion through a motorized syringe pump.
      (3) Stress: while the catheter is withdrawn from the bladder through the urethra at a rate of 0.1 cm/s, the patient is asked to cough. In patients with genuine stress urinary incontinence, there is a failure of pressure transmission to the proximal two thirds of the urethra. Normal patients demonstrate intraabdominal pressure transmission to the proximal two thirds of the urethra.
      (4) Dynamic: shows variation in sphincteric closure pressure under various physiologic events, various stresses, and various commands (Table 4-4). It uses the membrane catheter or microtransducer technique.

    f. Figure 4-2 shows a normal perfusion urethral pressure profile.

10. Cystometrogram (Fig. 4-3)
    a. Measures changes in bladder pressure with increases in bladder volume; evaluates the bladder's ability to fill uniformly and store

Practical Guide to the Care of the Gynecologic/Obstetric Patient 89

Table 4-4 **Dynamic Changes Seen with Urethral Pressure Profiles: Dynamic Function of the Urethral Sphincteric Mechanism in Normal Women and in Patients with Genuine Stress Incontinence**

Changes with Urethral Closure Pressure Profile in Response to the Following	*Closure Pressure Response*	
	Normal Patient	**Stress Incontinent Patient**
Cough	Increased	Minimal to none
Valsalva	Increased	Minimal to none
Holding urine	Increased	Minimal to none
Contraction of perineal muscles	Increased	Minimal to none
Bladder distension*		
Empty	—	—
Partially full	Increase	Minimal to none
Full distension	Further increase	Minimal to none
Position*		
Supine	—	—
Sitting	Increase	Minimal to none
Standing	Further increase	Minimal to none

Data from Tanagho EA, Stoller ML: Urodynamics: cystometry and urethral closure pressure profile. In Ostergard DR, Bent AE, editors: *Urogynecology and urodynamics theory and practice*, Baltimore, 1991, Williams & Wilkins.
*Response in pressure, length, or both.

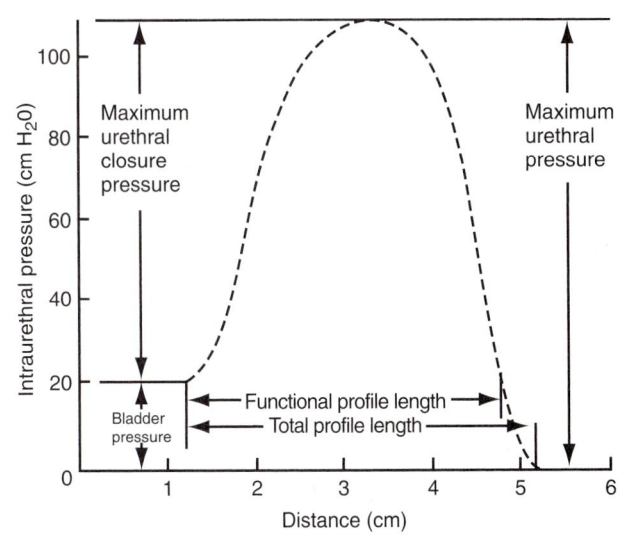

Figure 4-2 Normal perfusion urethral pressure profile.

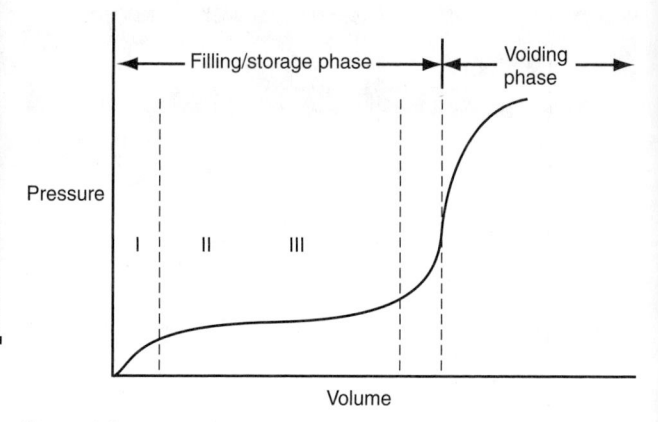

Figure 4-3 Normal adult cystometrogram. *I*, The compliance phase; *II*, the contraction phase; *III*, the voiding phase.

urine, by assessing detrusor activity, sensation, capacity, and compliance
  b. Definitions[4]
    (1) Intravesical pressure: the pressure within the bladder
    (2) Abdominal pressure: the pressure surrounding the bladder
    (3) Detrusor pressure: a measure of the passive and active forces within the bladder wall, obtained by subtracting abdominal pressure from intravesical pressure
    (4) Bladder sensation: subjective; involves the following:
      (a) First desire to void
      (b) Normal desire to void: feeling that leads the patient to pass urine at the next convenient moment (can be delayed or postponed)
      (c) Strong desire to void: persistent desire to void without fear of leakage or pain
      (d) Urgency: the strong desire to void accompanied by fear of leakage and pain
11. Three phases of bladder filling[6] (Fig. 4-4)
  a. The compliance phase is composed of the following:
    (1) An initial rise in pressure to achieve resting bladder pressure
    (2) A tonus limb that reflects the bladder's viscoelastic response to accommodating filling
      (a) Bladder compliance: the change in detrusor pressure that accompanies an increase in bladder volume during filling; not to exceed 15 cm of water. Compliance depends on the following:
        (i) Rate of filling
        (ii) The volume interval over which compliance is calculated

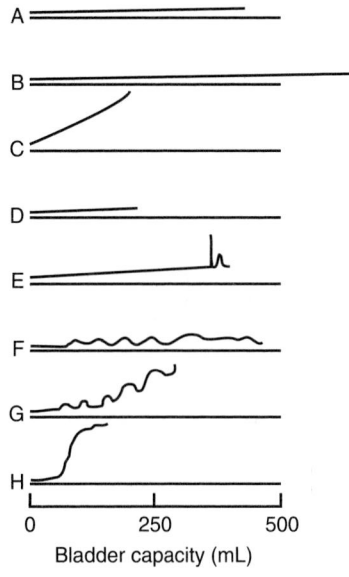

Practical Guide to the Care of the Gynecologic/Obstetric Patient 91

Figure 4-4 Various representative adult cystometrograms. **A,** Normal filling curve in a patient with a bladder capacity of 450 mL, normal compliance, and no involuntary bladder contractions. Nothing can be said about bladder activity during the emptying phase of micturition from this tracing. **B,** Large-capacity bladder with increased compliance at medium fill rate. This type of curve is characteristic of an individual with decreased sensation and bladder decompensation. Although most individuals will in fact have no or poor detrusor contraction, that conclusion cannot be made on the basis of this curve. **C,** Decreased compliance. **D,** Small-capacity bladder secondary to hypersensitivity without decreased compliance or involuntary bladder contraction. **E,** Bladder contraction provoked by cough. This particular tracing represents total bladder pressure. To make this diagnosis from just this tracing would require either a very astute examiner or separate recordings of intravesical pressure and intraabdominal pressure (intrarectal pressure). **F,** Low-amplitude detrusor contractions. This is a subtracted bladder pressure, and this type of recording may be seen most characteristically in a patient with suprasacral neurologic disease or idiopathic detrusor instability. **G,** Decreased compliance and involuntary bladder contractions. **H,** High-amplitude early involuntary bladder contraction. (Redrawn from Wein AJ, English NS, Whitmore KE: *Urol Clin North Am* 15:609, 1988.)

        (iii) Bladder wall thickness
        (iv) Mechanical bladder wall properties
        (v) Shape of the bladder
        (vi) Contractile and relaxant properties of the bladder wall
  b. The contraction phase characterizations
    (1) A rapid rise in intravesical pressure
    (2) Ability of patient to suppress voluntary voiding contractions

c. The voiding phase
   (1) Requires an intact neural pathway to the brainstem micturition center
   (2) Coordination of the detrusor contraction with concomitant relaxation of the sphincter results in voiding
d. Gas cystometry[1]
   (1) Clean and efficient
   (2) Allows rapid filling of the bladder
   (3) Impairs accommodation, producing a low-volume total capacity
   (4) Irritating to the urothelium, producing discomfort and dysuria
   (5) Gas compressibility may mask low-amplitude phasic contractions and blunt high-pressure contractions
   (6) Gas can leak
e. Other terminology
   (1) Involuntary detrusor contraction: a phasic rise, uninhibited, in bladder pressure, generally provoked by a stimulus, which signifies a lack of accommodation on the part of the bladder during filling; pressures exceed 15 cm of water
   (2) Two phases of voluntary control
      (a) The ability to initiate a bladder contraction
      (b) The ability to inhibit the bladder contraction
   (3) Maximum functional capacity: the largest amount voided at any one time over a 24-hour observation period
   (4) Maximal cystometric capacity: the volume at which the patient feels micturition can no longer be delayed
12. Electromyography (EMG) (Fig. 4-5): defined as the study of electrical potentials generated by depolarization of muscle[4]
   a. Motor unit: functional unit in EMG
   b. Motor unit: described as a single motor neuron and the muscle fibers it innervates; comprises a single motor neuron and the muscle fibers it innervates
   c. Motor unit action potential: the recorded depolarization of muscle fibers that results from activation of a single anterior horn cell; muscle action potentials are detected by the following:
      (1) Surface electrode
         (a) Noninvasive
         (b) Comfortable
         (c) Determines gross motor activity
         (d) Cannot detect individual EMG potentials
         (e) Represents a total net record of anal or urethral sphincteric activity
      (2) Needle electrode
         (a) Monopolar/concentric
         (b) Invasive and uncomfortable
         (c) Produces an "injury potential"
         (d) Must be placed directly into the striated sphincter
         (e) Simultaneously records urethral, bladder, and rectal pressure changes and flow

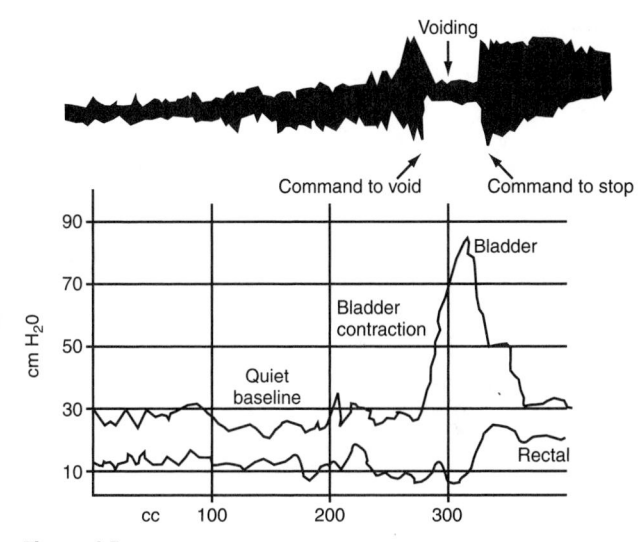

Figure 4-5 Normal pressure EMG tracing. (From Wein AJ, English WJ, Whitmore KE: *Urol Clin North Am* 15:609, 1988.)

    d. In a normal EMG tracing, with the bladder empty and at rest, there is a flat "quiet" baseline of activity with few random potentials.
    e. As bladder volume increases to 150 to 350 mL, more muscles depolarize and contract to maintain continence.
    f. As the bladder capacity is reached, maximal activation of perineal floor muscles occurs, producing a full interference pattern. With voiding there is silence.
    g. The progression from minimal activity to maximal activity with bladder filling is called the guarding reflex.
    h. Abnormal findings can be subdivided into the following categories[7]:
      (1) Upper motor neuron lesions
        (a) Loss of ability to contract or relax the sphincter voluntarily
        (b) Example: detrusor sphincter dyssynergia
      (2) Lower motor neuron lesions
        (a) Complete lesion: lesions of the spinal cord or cauda equina; total denervation of the striated sphincter
        (b) Incomplete lesion: partial denervation of the striated sphincter with consequent sphincteric contractions of poor magnitude
      (3) Mixed neuron lesions
        (a) Demonstrate features of both upper and lower motor neuron lesions
        (b) Examples: myelodysplasia and multiple sclerosis

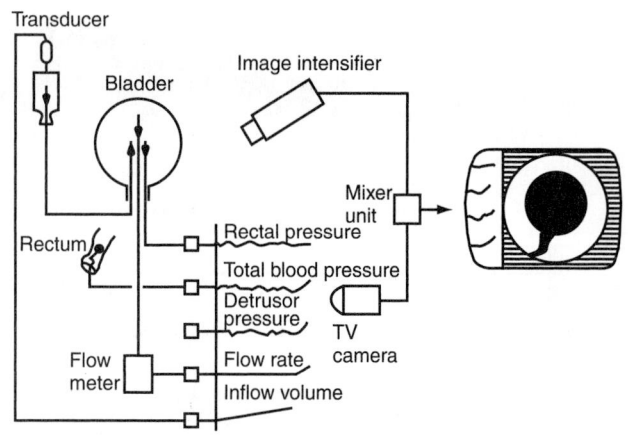

Figure 4-6 Typical videourodynamic system.

13. Videourodynamics (Fig. 4-6): Combines measurement of intravesical intraabdominal and striated urethral sphincter pressures with bladder filling, bladder emptying, and flow rate, all done simultaneously with fluoroscopy
14. Sacral evoked responses[8]
    a. This test quantitates the integrity of the innervation of the striated pelvic floor and perineal muscles along with the supraspinal pathways involved in lower urologic tract function.
    b. The nerve conduction time (latency) and the stimulation threshold are the two parameters most commonly measured.
    c. Bulbocavernosus reflex latency is clinically measured. Normal is 30 to 40 msec.
    d. Any neurologic process that interferes with the integrity of the reflex arc will result in a prolonged latency.
    e. The following are common disorders associated with prolonged latency:
       (1) Diabetes mellitus
       (2) Alcoholic neuropathy
       (3) Disc disease
15. Abdominal-valsalva leak point pressures[9,10]
    a. This measures the amount of abdominal pressure required to induce urinary leakage. A normal patient should remain continent regardless of the amount of abdominal pressure exerted on the lower urinary tract.
    b. This is used to document type III incontinence, associated with an incompetent sphincter.
       (1) These patients leak at low to moderate abdominal pressures.
       (2) Patients with types I and II incontinence require higher abdominal pressures to leak.

c. The abdominal-valsalva leak point pressure is the change in intravesical pressure documented before the valsalva maneuver to the pressure at which incontinence occurs.
d. Abdominal-valsalva leak point pressures.
    (1) Greater than 120 cm H_2O: Type I incontinence is characterized by the bladder neck gradually opening with heavy exercise or exertion. There is support for the pelvic floor and no movement of the bladder neck. Treatment: medication.
    (2) 60 to 100 cm H_2O: Type II incontinence is characterized by bladder neck hypermobility with herniation through the pelvic floor with straining, disrupting the ability of the bladder to remain closed. Treatment: bladder neck suspension.
    (3) Less than 60 cm H_2O: Type III, or intrinsic sphincter deficiency, is characterized by a dysfunctional bladder neck and proximal urethra. Treatment: pubovaginal sling, an injectable agent, or an artificial sphincter.
16. Detrusor leak point pressure[9,10]
    a. This is the pressure obtained by filling the bladder until intravesical pressure overcomes urethral resistance and incontinence occurs. Detrusor pressure can force the sphincter open, whereas the abdominal pressure cannot.
    b. It is an indirect measure of bladder storage.
    c. It is an assessment of intravesical pressure, useful in the patient with a neuropathic bladder to determine if urine is being stored at pressures that will not cause upper urinary tract deterioration.
    d. Normal detrusor leak point pressure is below 40 cm H_2O. Pressures above this can over time cause upper tract damage.
17. Specialized testing
    a. Rapid fill cystometry[11]
        (1) Used to rule out detrusor areflexia
        (2) Rapid filling of the bladder at rates of flow up to 300 cc/min
    b. Bethanechol supersensitivity test[12]
        (1) Bethanechol chloride.
            (a) Parasympathomimetic
            (b) Selective for bladder and gut
            (c) Cholinesterase resistant
            (d) Causes bladder muscle to contract (spares ganglia and cardiovascular)
            (e) Minimal effects on the normal bladder
                (i) Decreases capacity slightly
                (ii) Increases detrusor tone
                (iii) Increases voluntary micturition pressure
                (iv) Does not cause detrusor instability
        (2) Basis for test: Cannon's law of denervation; when an organ is deprived of its nerve supply, it will develop hypersensitivity to its own neurotransmitter substance.[5]
        (3) Method: Subcutaneous injection of 2.5 mg of bethanechol chloride followed in 15 to 30 minutes by repeat cystometrogram study.

(a) A rise of at least 15 cm of water after 100-cc infusion at a medium rate of between 100 and 200 cc/min in excess of the pretreated cystometrogram pressure is indicative of parasympathetic dysfunction (denervation). It is seen with lower motor neuron lesions (also called decentralized bladder).
(b) This test is contraindicated in patients with cardiac disease, asthma, hyperthyroidism, peptic ulcer disease, enteritis bowel obstruction, and bladder outlet obstruction.
(c) Blaivas reported a false-negative rate of 24%, attributing such testing factors as repeated overdistension of the bladder, bethanechol absorption, emotional stress, time, and bladder volume to the high false-negative rate.[13]
(d) False-positive test results occur in the presence of active urinary tract infections, azotemia, emotional stress, and detrusor hypertrophy.[8]
(e) Studies by Mattiason[14] and Malkowicz[15] suggest that end organ supersensitivity is not an end organ response to denervation but may measure supersensitivity at the pelvic reflex arc or demonstrates another aspect of vesical pressure generation such as detrusor muscle hypertrophy.
c. Phentolamine testing[15,16]
  (1) Premise: Inappropriate smooth muscle or striated muscle activity with bladder outlet obstruction has been associated with the neurologically impaired bladder. Smooth muscle components are under the control of the autonomic nervous system. The striated muscle is under peripheral nervous system control. When symptoms are caused by the smooth muscle component, the pharmacologic manipulation of the sympathetic nervous system has been shown to be of benefit.
  (2) The phentolamine test is used to select patients most likely to benefit from the use of adrenergic blocking agents. See relaxation of the urethral smooth muscle component of bladder neck.
  (3) This test compares the urethral closure pressure profile before and after injection of phentolamine.
  (4) An IV bolus of phentolamine mesylate, 0.1 mg/kg, is given, after which blood pressure and pulse are recorded every minute until a tachycardia of at least 10 beats per minute occurs. The urethral pressure profile is then repeated and the patient is observed for 30 minutes for any untoward effects from the drug.
  (5) A positive test: A decrease of 30% or more occurs in the maximum urethral closure pressure after injection of phentolamine.
  (6) These patients can be offered a trial of alpha-1 blockers.
d. Glycopyrrolate test[3,8] (formerly pro-banthine stimulation test)
  (1) Glycopyrrolate is an anticholinergic test.
  (2) IV glycopyrrolate, 0.4 mg, is given.

(3) A cystometrogram is done before and 10 to 25 minutes after injection.
(4) The disappearance or decrease in the amplitude or the frequency of uninhibited contractions indicates that the patient may respond to outpatient therapy.
(5) Note: This test is almost never performed in clinical practice. The efficacy of newer anticholinergic medications, their rapid absorption (sublingual forms), and their different concentrations makes it far easier to use them than to expose a patient to IV glycopyrrolate.
(6) Glaucoma and obstructive gastrointestinal disease are contraindicated.
e. Urethral denervation sensitivity testing[1] (also listed as noradrenaline supersensitivity test of the urethra)
(1) The primary innervation of the urethra is through sympathetic alpha fibers.
(2) Baseline maximum urthral closure pressure is determined.
(3) Four mg IV ethylphenylephrine is given.
(4) Five minutes later, a repeat maximum closure pressure is obtained.
(5) Chronic urethral denervation is present when there is a rise of 15 cm or greater of water in the closure pressure from control.
f. Marshall-Marchetti-Bonney stress test[16] (also called the cough-stress test)
(1) The patient coughs with a full bladder while the examiner observes the urethra for urine loss.
(2) The examiner manipulates the urethrovesical angle either by placing Allis clamps on the anterior vaginal wall, lateral to the urethrovesical angle, or more commonly by inserting two fingers into the lateral fornices of the vagina, pushing the bladder base up and anteriorly without compressing the urethra closed. The patient coughs and bears down again. The practitioner observes leak with cough but no leak with bladder base elevation: true stress urinary incontinence.
(3) Controversy: This test presumes to simulate the results of the planned surgical procedure by elevation and stabilization of the urethra and vesical neck. Evidence by Bergman[16] has demonstrated that this test restores continence by occlusion of the urethra and vesical neck. Regardless, it remains a mainstay of tests in the evaluation of female incontinence.
g. Q-tip test
(1) Using an orthopedic goniometer
    (a) Normal: with straining, 0-degree to 20-degree deflection
    (b) Urethral hypermobility (associated with genuine stress incontinence); greater than 25-degree deflection
(2) Note: Recent evidence indicates that the Q-tip test is not specific for stress urinary incontinence because a positive result reflects anterior vaginal muscle relaxation rather than sphincteric incompetence. In addition, this test is thought to

have a false-negative rate for the diagnosis of stress urinary incontinence of 30%, especially in elderly females.[6]

h. Pessary test[17]
   (1) Premise: The vaginal pessary may increase urethral closure and urethral functional length in women with a mild to moderate cystocele. The pessary restores continence by stabilization of the bladder base, allowing proper pressure transmission to the urethra, and by active enhancement of urethral resistance, by increasing urethral functional length and closure pressure.
      (a) Positive: surgical correction
      (b) Negative: urodynamic evaluation
   (2) Note: This test is thought to be unpredictable in the elderly.

REFERENCES

1. Snyder JA, editor: Urologic perspectives: urinary incontinence. *Special Supplement to Urology Grand Rounds*, Number 27, Chicago, McCann Healthcare Advertising.
2. Robertson JR: Dynamic urethroscopy. In Ostergard DR, editor: *Urogynecology and urodynamics theory and practice*, Baltimore, 1991, Williams & Wilkins.
3. Wein AJ, Barrett DM, editors: *Voiding function and dysfunction: a logical and practical approach*, Chicago, 1988, Yearbook Medical Publishers.
4. Ostergard DR, Bent AE, editors: *Appendix I: the standardisation of terminology of lower urinary tract function*, Baltimore, 1991, Williams & Wilkins.
5. Cannon WB, Rosenbleuth A: *The supersensitivity of denervated structures*, New York, 1949, McMillan, pp. 96-105.
6. DuBeau CE, Resnick NM: Evaluation of the causes and severity of geriatric incontinence: a critical appraisal. *Urol Clin North Am* 18:243, 1991.
7. Bhatia NN: Urogynecology and urodynamics theory and practice. *Neurourology and urodynamics: sphincter electromyography and electrophysiological testing*, Baltimore, 1991, Williams & Wilkins.
8. Wein AJ: Voiding dysfunction: neurogenic or non neurogenic? AUA Update Series, vol VII, Lesson 23, Houston, 1988, American Urological Association, Inc., Office of Education.
9. McGuire EJ, et al: Clinical assessment of urethral sphincter function. *J Urol* 150:1452-1454, 1993.
10. Montella JM, Ostergard DR: Specialized testing procedures. *Urogynecology and urodynamics theory and practice*, Baltimore, 1991, Williams & Wilkins.
11. Wein AJ, English WS, Whitmore KE: Office urodynamics. *Urol Clin North Am* 15:609, 1988.
12. Wan J, et al: Stress leak point pressure: a diagnostic tool for incontinent children. *J Urol* 150:700-702, 1993.
13. Blaivas J, et al: Failure of bethanechol denervation supersensitivity as a diagnostic aid. *J Urol* 123:199, 1980.
14. Mattiason A, et al: Supersensitivity to carbachol in the parasympathetically decentralized feline urinary bladder. *J Urol* 131:562, 1984.
15. Malkowicz SB, et al: The effect of parasympathetic decentralization on the feline urinary bladder. *J Urol* 133:521, 1985.

16. Bergman A: Invalidity of the Marshall Marchetti and Bonney stress tests. In Ostergard DR, Bent AE, editors: *Urogynecology and urodynamics theory and practice*, Baltimore, 1991, Williams & Wilkins.
17. Bergman A: Nonsurgical treatment for stress urinary incontinence. In Ostergard DR, Bent AE, editors: *Urogynecology and urodynamics theory and practice*, Baltimore, 1991, Williams & Wilkins.

Contraception

Maria A. Corigliano

Contraception is an integral and very important aspect of a general obstetric and gynecologic practice. Not only should the effectiveness of a method be considered but also what is best for each individual patient in regard to probable compliance with the method, medical history, and desire or lack of desire for future fertility. Emotional and social issues at the time of decision should also be discussed and evaluated.

Each patient should be informed of all options that are appropriate for her. Many times misconceptions about safety, fertility after use, and positive benefits of the different forms of contraception are very freely volunteered by the patient during a consultation. Many patients are pleasantly surprised by the fact that they are candidates for certain contraceptive methods that they never thought they would be eligible for because of misinformation given to them by friends. The clinician's job is not only to inform patients of their options and the risks of certain methods but also to stress the benefits of using them. The reason a particular method is not recommended for an individual patient may also be discussed at this time.

A full history and physical examination should be completed before a method is prescribed. History should include the usual data as follows:

1. Medical history.
2. Surgical history.
3. Obstetric history: Establish whether patient could be already pregnant; desire for future fertility.
4. Gynecologic history.
5. History of sexually transmitted diseases.
6. Number of partners.
7. Previous difficulties with contraception use.
8. Frequency of intercourse.
9. Family history: Include family members with history of vascular events or female cancers. Workup for thrombophilia is indicated if family history reflects risk. Risk of vascular events are increased fivefold to tenfold in the groups that are homozygous and heterozygous for factor V leiden, prothrombin gene mutation, antithrombin III deficiency, protein S&C deficiency, and methylene tetrahydrofolate reductase (MTHFR) deficiency.
10. A full physical examination: Papanicolaou smear and cultures of the cervix should be obtained.

5.1 Oral Contraceptives

1. Oral contraceptive types.
    a. Monophasic: Contain a constant dose of estrogen and progesterone in each of the 21 contraceptively active pills (e.g., Orthonova 1/35, ovcon 35, and yasmin).
    b. Biphasic: Contain a constant dose of estrogen progestin over 21 days. The last 7 days contain estrogen only in a lower dose (e.g., mircette).
    c. Triphasic: Contain a varying dose of progestin. In some types the estrogen dose in the 21 contraceptively active pills is varied. The purpose of this manipulation is to keep the patient on the lowest dose possible throughout the cycle, while preventing pregnancy at the same rate (e.g., Estrostep, trilevelen, and orthotricyclen).
    d. Progestin-only pill: Contains even lower doses of progestin in 28 contraceptively active pills (e.g., Micronor and ovrette).
    e. Ring therapy: A nonbiodegradeable vaginal ring that contains a progestin etonogestrel and ethinyl estradiol. The patient receives an average of 0.015 mg/day of the estrogen and 0.120 mg/day of progestin. The ring is inserted into the vagina for 3 weeks and is removed for 1 week to provoke a menstrual cycle. Indications and contraindications are the same as oral contraceptives (e.g., Nuvaring).
    f. The contraceptive patch: It is a transdermal trilayer patch. The inner layer carries the active compounds norelgestromin, progestin, and 20 µg of ethinyl estradiol. Currently the patch is being reevaluated concerning steady-state blood levels. It is applied weekly to the abdomen, buttocks, upper back, and upper outer arm. The patch is changed weekly for 3 weeks and rotated each time to a different site. Indications and contraindications are equal to other hormonal combined contraceptives (e.g., Orthoevra).
2. The most commonly used estrogen is ethinyl estradiol in a dose containing less than 35 µg of estrogen.
3. Mestranol is the estrogen used in the higher-dosed pills. Pills with estrogen levels greater than 50 µg are no longer available.
4. Most commonly used progestins are norethindrone, levonorgestrel, norgestrel, norethindrone acetate, or ethynodiol diacetate.
5. Less androgenic progestins are norgestimate and destogestrel. Gestodene is another new progestin along with norelgestromin, drosperidone, and etongetrel.
6. Mechanism of action: Suppression of pituitary follicle-stimulating hormone (FSH) and luteinizing hormone (LH) secretion, which suppresses ovulation. The progestin portion of the pill causes changes in cervical mucus and endometrium, which afford birth control because ovulation may occur on oral contraceptives.
7. Effectiveness rate: If taken correctly, only 1 in 1000 women is expected to get pregnant within the first year on combined oral contraceptives. The typical failure rate of combined oral contraceptives is

about 3%. Progestin-only pills have about the same effectiveness rate as the combined pills.
8. Administration of combination oral contraceptives.
   a. A daily ritual should be associated with oral contraceptive use. Many women are more likely to remember to take the pills at night before bedtime. This may prevent nausea because the patient will be sleeping. A woman should begin taking oral contraceptives either on the Sunday following the first day of her period or on the first day of her period.
   b. It should be stressed that taking the pills daily at the same time is necessary for optimum effectiveness.
   c. If one or two pills are missed, have the patient double up on the pills until she catches up.
   d. If two or more pills are missed, backup birth control should be used and the pack should be completed.
9. Antibiotic use and the Pill: The only antibiotic proven to decrease the effectiveness rate of the Pill is rifampin. The dermatologic literature has produced a guideline to follow regarding contraceptive pill and antibiotic mixing (Box 5-1).

BOX 5-1 Categories of Antibiotics

Category A: Antibiotic That Likely Reduces Birth Control Pill Effectiveness

Rifampicin

Category B: Antibiotics Associated with Oral Contraceptive Failure in Three or More Case Reports

Ampicillin
Amoxicillin
Metronidazole
Tetracycline

Category C: Antibiotics Associated with Oral Contraceptive Failure in at Least One Case Report

Cephalexin
Clindamycin
Dapsone
Erythromycin
Griseofulvin
Isoniazid
Phenoxymethylpenicillin
Telampicillin
Trimethoprim

From Miller DM et al: *J Am Acad Derm* 30:1009, 1994.

10. Benefits of hormonal contraception.
    a. Menstruation becomes more regular; there is a 63% reduction in dysmenorrhea and a 29% reduction of premenstrual syndrome [PMS]).
    b. There is decrease in the amount and duration of menstrual flow.
    c. The Pill corrects iron-deficiency anemia.
11. Preventions.
    a. Benign breast disease: An Oxford study showed a 30% reduction in fibrocystic breast disease (FCBD) and 60% fewer fibroadenomas. An American study showed a 30% reduction with 13 to 24 months' use, and a 65% reduction when used for 25 months or more.
    b. Hospitalization: The chance of hospitalization resulting from pelvic inflammatory disease (PID) is decreased secondary to thicker impenetrable cervical mucus. Menstrual blood flow is reduced by 50% to 60%. Smaller cervical openings, which do not prevent cervical *Chlamydia*, do decrease upper tract disease.
    c. Epithelial ovarian cancer: There is 40% to 50% reduction in occurrence if oral contraceptives are used for 5 years; an 80% to 90% reduction in occurrence if used for 10 years. Protection from cancer lasts up to 15 years after discontinuation. There is also a decrease in endometrial cancer (50% reduction, lasts for 15 years).
    d. Ectopic pregnancy: A tenfold decrease in ectopic pregnancy is seen, compared with nonusers.
    e. Acne: Decreasing serum testosterone improves acne.
    f. Estrogen deficiency: Symptoms are improved.
    g. Fear of pregnancy: The fear of pregnancy decreases, therefore sexual enjoyment is heightened.
    h. Fibroid size: An Oxford study showed a 30% reduction in size over 10 years.
12. Possible benefits.
    a. Prevention of rheumatoid arthritis: The onset may be postponed, but estrogen dose does not decrease the pain of rheumatoid arthritis.
    b. Prevention of ovarian cysts: The rate of recurrent hemorrhagic cysts is decreased.
    c. Increased bone density: not as beneficial as endogenous estrogen.
    d. Decreased endometriosis and atherosclerosis with low-dose oral contraceptives.
13. Disadvantages or side effects that prompt discontinuation.
    a. Nausea: Usually disappears after first month.
    b. Breast tenderness.
    c. Breakthrough bleeding (initial months).
    d. Amenorrhea (prolonged use): May add estrogen or change pills.
    e. Depression.
    f. Decreased libido: May result from decreased free testosterone circulation.
    g. Expense (pharmacy dependent).
    h. Headaches.
        (1) Only classical migraine types should prompt stopping the Pill. Progestin-only pills may be tried in this case.

(2) Often the headaches are experienced during the pill-free interval. This may be remedied through the use of continuous oral contraceptives (eliminate pill-free interval).
  i. *Chlamydia* infection: *Chlamydia* cervicitis (not PID) is more common in contraceptive pill users secondary to the increased ectropion caused by the pill than in nonusers (Box 5-2).
14. Major risks to health (Box 5-3 and Tables 5-1 and 5-2).
  a. Cardiovascular disease.
    (1) Cardiovascular disease includes thrombophlebitis, pulmonary embolus, and stroke. All of these may occur in women who are at risk for these events (i.e., women who are smokers, sedentary, overweight, over 50 years old, and who have increased low-density lipoprotein/high-density lipoprotein [LDL/HDL] cholesterol ratio). History of hypertension, history of diabetes, a family history of cardiovascular events, and diabetes in a premenopausal women also indicate a higher risk level.
    (2) Estrogen and progesterone doses have decreased by fourfold and tenfold, respectively, from the original birth control pills, which were studied in the 1960s and 1970s. The use of low-dose oral contraceptives markedly decreases the risk of cardiovascular side effects. For select outpatients who are at increased risk for cardiovascular events, it is wise to suggest alternate forms of birth control.
    (3) Smokers: Smoking increases dangerous cardiovascular side effects. Smoking fewer than 15 cigarettes per day increases the risk of myocardial infarction threefold. Smoking more than 15 cigarettes a day increases the risk of myocardial infarction to twenty-one-fold. After age 35, smokers should not use the Pill.
  b. Cancer: A major concern of women and the most common reason for women to decline use of oral contraceptives.
    (1) Breast cancer: The final word on the Pill's influence on breast cancer is not in. There is no convincing evidence in the literature that birth control pill use increases the rate of breast cancer.
    (2) A recent study done in Canada shows a 50% reduction in breast cancer risk for women who used combination oral contraceptives for 5 years.
    (3) Cervical cancer: Five out of thirteen studies have shown a significant increase in cervical cancer in women who use oral contraceptives. Seven studies showed no significant increase. One study showed a relationship between the Pill and dysplasia and carcinomas of the cervix, especially in women who were on oral contraceptives for prolonged periods of time. However, this may be because Pill users generally have multiple sexual partners and are screened more frequently by Papanicolaou smears than non–Pill users. Human papillomavirus (HPV) plays a large role in cervical cancer, and oral contraception users are less likely to use barrier methods than non–Pill users.

BOX 5-2 Relation of Side Effects to Hormone Content

Reproductive System

ESTROGEN EXCESS
Breast cystic changes
Cervical extrophy
Dysmenorrhea
Hypermenorrhea, menorrhagia, and clotting
  Increase in breast size
  Mucorrhea
  Uterine enlargement
  Uterine fibroid growth

ESTROGEN DEFICIENCY
Absence of withdrawal bleeding
Bleeding and spotting during pill days 1 to 9
Continuous bleeding and spotting
Flow decrease, hypomenorrhea
Pelvic relaxation symptoms
Vaginitis atrophic

PROGESTIN EXCESS
Cervicitis
Flow length decrease
Moniliasis

PROGESTIN DEFICIENCY
Breakthrough bleeding and spotting during pill days 10 to 21
Delayed withdrawal bleeding
Dysmenorrhea (also estrogen excess)
Heavy flow and clots (also estrogen excess), hypermenorrhea, menorrhagia

Premenstrual Syndrome

ESTROGEN EXCESS OR PROGESTERONE DEFICIENCY
Bloating
Dizziness, syncope
Edema
Headache (cyclic)
Irritability
Leg cramps
Nausea, vomiting
Visual changes (cyclic)
Weight gain (cyclic)

Box continued on following page

> **BOX 5-2 Relation of Side Effects to Hormone Content** *(Continued)*

General

ESTROGEN EXCESS
Chloasma
Chronic nasal pharyngitis
Gastric influenza and varicella
Hay fever and allergic rhinitis
Urinary tract infection

ESTROGEN DEFICIENCY
Nervousness
Vasomotor symptoms

PROGESTIN EXCESS
Appetite increase
Depression
Fatigue
Hypoglycemia symptoms
Libido decrease
Neurodermatitis
Weight gain (noncyclic)

ANDROGEN EXCESS
Acne
Cholestatic jaundice
Hirsutism
Libido increase
Oily skin and scalp
Rash and pruritus
Edema

Cardiovascular System

PROGESTIN EXCESS
Hypertension
Leg vein dilation

ESTROGEN EXCESS
Capillary fragility
Cerebrovascular accident
Deep vein thrombosis hemiparesis (unilateral weakness and numbness)
Telangiectasias
Thromboembolic disease

From Dickey R: *Managing contraceptive pill patients*, ed 8, Durant, OK, 1994, Essential Medical Information Systems.

> BOX 5-3 **Contraindications to Using Oral Contraceptives**
>
> Present or past history of thrombophlebitis
> Stroke
> Coronary artery disease
> Breast cancer
> Estrogen-dependent neoplasia
> Hepatic disease, benign or malignant
> Smokers over 35 years old
> Women who smoke more than 15 cigarettes per day
> Migraine headaches that started after oral contraception use
> Hypertension
> Pregnancy
> Major surgery that involves immobilization
> Lactation
> Sickle cell disease (theoretical increase risk for thrombosis)
> Active gallbladder disease
> Undiagnosed vaginal bleeding
> Gilbert's disease (congenital hyperbilirubinemia)
> Women over 50 years old
> Immediate postpartum period (up to 14 days still in hypercoagulable state)
> Cardiac and renal disease (severe)
> Mental illness, substance abusers (less likely to take pills correctly)
> Family history of hyperlipidemia
> Family history of female sibling or parents who died from myocardial infarction before menopause

(4) Ovarian and endometrial cancer: Many studies show a decreased risk of ovarian epithelial cancers and endometrial cancers for women on oral contraceptives. The longer the use, the more long term the protection.

(5) Hepatocellular carcinomas: Benign hepatic adenomas occur with oral contraceptive use. However, increased risk of hepatocellular cancer has not been proved in women using oral contraceptives.

(6) Adolescents: The Pill is not contraindicated; however, compliance and sexually transmitted disease (non–condom users) become issues.

5.2 Progestin-Only Contraception

1. Hormonal implants (Norplant) have the most use experience and clinical trials. Norplant is no longer marketed in the United States. Implanon is approved by the Food and Drug Administration (FDA).

Table 5-1 Symptoms of a Serious or Potentially Serious Nature

Symptom	Possible Cause
Serious: Pills Should Be Stopped Immediately	
Loss of vision, proptosis, diplopia, papilledema	Retinal artery thrombosis
Unilateral numbness, weakness, or tingling	Hemorrhagic or thrombotic stroke
Severe pains in chest, left arm, or neck	Myocardial infarction
Hemoptysis	Pulmonary embolism
Severe pains, tenderness or swelling, warmth, or palpable cord in legs	Thrombophlebitis
Slurring of speech	Hemorrhagic or thrombotic stroke
Hepatic mass or tenderness	Liver neoplasm
Potentially Serious: Pills May Be Continued with Caution While Patient Is Being Evaluated	
Absence of menses	Pregnancy
Spotting or breakthrough bleeding	Cervical, endometrial, or vaginal cancer
Breast mass, pain, or swelling	Breast cancer
Right upper quadrant pain	Cholecystitis, cholelithiasis, or liver neoplasm
Midepigastric pain	Thrombosis of abdominal artery or vein, myocardial infarction, or pulmonary embolism
Migraine (vascular or throbbing) headache	Vascular spasm, which may precede thrombosis
Severe nonvascular headache	Hypertension, vascular spasm
Galactorrhea	Pituitary adenoma
Jaundice, pruritus	Cholestatic jaundice
Depression	B_6 deficiency
Uterine size increase	Leiomyomata, adenomyosis, pregnancy

From Dickey R: *Managing contraceptive pill patients*, ed 8, Durant, OK, 1984, Essential Medical Information Systems.

Implanon has two advantages over Norplant: Implanon is one implant, and the effectiveness rate is not affected by obesity.
  a. Composition and mode of action: Norplant consists of six soft plastic implants, each filled with 36 mg of levonorgestrel daily. Levonorgestrel suppresses the LH surge responsible for ovulation. Ovulation occurs in about two thirds of all cycles with Norplant. Levonorgestrel thickens and decreases the amount of cervical mucus and blocks sperm penetration. It suppresses estrogenic maturation of the endometrial lining.
  b. Effectiveness rate.

Table 5-2 Choosing Oral Contraceptives (OCs)

Step 1	Step 2	Step 3	Step 4
Can this individual be prescribed a pill with estrogen? Definitely refrain from prescribing a pill with estrogen to women with a history of a cerebrovascular accident, ischemic heart disease, uncontrolled hypertension, insulin-dependent diabetes with vascular disease, classic migraine with neurologic impairment that has increased with estrogen, breast cancer, estrogen-dependent neoplasia, active hepatic disease with impaired liver function at the present time, benign or malignant liver tumor, or deep vein thrombosis. Some clinicians would make an exception and provide combined OCs to women following postpartum pelvic vein thrombosis or women	YES, she can use an estrogen. NO, it would be best if she did not use an estrogen. Therefore, you can consider: **A.** Progestin-only pills, such as: Micronor (0.35 mg norethindrone daily) NOR QD (0.35 mg norethindrone daily) Ovrette (0.075 mg norgestrel daily) Norplant (5-year levonorgestrel implants) Depo-Provera (150 mg medroxyprogesterone acetate injection every 3 months) **B.** Intrauterine device Copper T 380-A Progestasert System	Therefore, you may choose between any of the following OCs based on: Number of micrograms of ethinyl estradiol Availability of pill Ease of remaining on schedule because of pills Price of pills to clinic* Price of pills to client* Prior experience of this individual woman or the clinician caring for this woman with a special pill	Other clinical considerations that may help in OC choice: **A.** To minimize the risk potential for thrombosis caused by estrogen in a woman 40 to 50 years of age or a woman at increased risk for thrombosis from another cause (e.g., diabetic or heavy smoker), prescribe: Loestrin 1/20 **B.** To minimize nausea, breast tenderness, vascular headaches, and estrogen-mediated side effects, prescribe: Loestrin 1/20 Or a 30-μg pill, such as: Desogen Levlen Loestrin 1.5-30 Lo-Ovral Nordette Ortho-Cept **C.** To minimize spotting and/or breakthrough bleeding, prescribe: Lo-Ovral, Nordette, or Levlen

Table continued on following page

Table 5-2 Choosing Oral Contraceptives (OCs) (Continued)

Step 1	Step 2	Step 3	Step 4
whose thrombophlebitis has resulted from trauma or IV. Also, in most instances refrain from providing combined pills to women over 35 who smoke. Breast-feeding women, in general, should avoid estrogen.	**C.** Condoms (male or female) **D.** Diaphragm, cervical cap **E.** Foam, vaginal contraceptive film, suppository **F.** Sponge		A new progestin pill: Desogen, Ortho-Cept, Ortho-Cyclen, or Ortho Tri-Cyclen **D.** To minimize androgen effects such as *acne, hirsutism, oily skin, sebaceous cysts, pilonidal cysts, or weight gain*, prescribe: Desogen, Ortho-Cept Ortho Tri-Cyclen Ortho Cyclen Ovcon-35, Brevicon, or Modicon (of norethindrone pills) Demulen-35 (of ethnodiol diacetate pills) **E.** To produce the most *favorable lipid profile*, prescribe: Ortho Cyclen or Ortho Tri-Cyclen Desogen or Ortho-Cept Ovcon-35, Brevicon, or Modicon (of norethindrone pills)

Modified from Hatcher RH, et al: *Contraceptive technology*, ed 16, New York, 1994, Irvington Publishers.
*On December 11, 1992, *The Medical Letter* published the cost to pharmacists for a 1-month cycle of OCs based on "Average Wholesale Price Listing in Drug Topics Red Book 1992" and its November Update.

Table 5-3 **Rates of Ectopic Pregnancy per 1000 Women-Years by Contraceptive Method and for All U.S. Women**

Method	Rate
Norplant	0.28*
TCu380A	0.20[†]
Noncontraceptors	3.00[‡]
All U.S. women	1.50[§]

Data from Darney PD: *Am J Obstet Gynecol* 170:1536-1543, 1994.
*Sivin I: *Stud Fam Plann* 19:81, 1988.
[†]Sivin I: *Contraception* 19:151, 1979.
[‡]Franks AL et al: *Am J Obstet Gynecol* 163:1120, 1990.
[§]Centers for Disease Control and Prevention: *MMWR* 38:1, 1989.

(1) About 1% of women are pregnant within the first 5 years of using Norplant. The rate goes up to 2% in the sixth year. Therefore removal and reinsertion is advised after 5 years. Implanon is reinserted after 3 years (Tables 5-3 and 5-4).

(2) If fertilization does occur, it is more likely to be an ectopic pregnancy. Table 5-3 shows ectopic pregnancy rates per 1000 women-years with different types of birth control. The failure rate is increased by carbamazepine, phenytoin, phenobarbital, primidone, phenylbutazone, and rifampin.

c. Side effects most commonly occur in the first few months and can include irregular menses, headaches, weight change, breast tenderness, acne, hirsutism, depression, mood swings, galactorrhea, amenorrhea, and hair loss. Menstrual irregularities are the most common reason for discontinuation.

d. Fertility returns quickly after discontinuation. Plasma levels of levonogestrel are subcontraceptive level within 24 hours of removal.

e. Indications: Women who breast-feed: The implant may be inserted in noncompliant patients while in hospital. However, most studies do not start the method before 4 weeks postpartum. Biodegradable systems, such as capronor and norethindrone pellets, will eliminate removal. Undesirable side effects will be eliminated by the use of

Table 5-4 **Norplant Capsules: Gross Cumulative Pregnancy Rates at 5 Years of Use by Weight and Type of Tubing**

Weight at Insertion (kg)	N	Total	Pliable Tubing	Rigid Tubing
<50	532	0.2	0.0	0.3
50-59	1041	3.5	2.0	4.3
60-69	585	3.5	1.5	4.5
>70	309	7.6	2.4	9.3
Total	2496	3.5	1.6	4.9

Data from Darney PD: *Am J Obstet Gynecol* 170:1536-1543, 1994; Sivin IL: *Stud Fam Plann* 19:86, 1988.

less androgenic progestins such as desogestrel, gestodene, norgestimate, or ST 14356.
2. Depo-Provera.
    a. Depo-medroxy progesterone acetate (Depo-Provera) is the most commonly used injectable progestin in the world. It was finally approved for use in the United States in 1992. It is excellent for use in women who breast-feed or for short-term use where estrogen is contraindicated.
    b. Composition and mode of action.
        (1) Depo-medroxy progesterone acetate is given by deep intramuscular injections. A dosage of 150 mg must be given every 3 months.
        (2) Its action is to shut down the LH surge and suppress LH and FSH levels. It also causes an atrophic endometrium and thick impenetrable cervical mucus. Depo-Provera is so effective that long-time users may be as much as 2 weeks late for their next injections.
    c. Efficacy: Only 0.3% of women will experience accidental pregnancy within the first year of use. Giving 400 mg of Depo-Provera in the more concentrated form every 6 months decreases the effectiveness rate throughout the 6-month period.
    d. Indications: Women who may not use estrogen, women who breast-feed, older women, women who need short-term but effective contraception may use Depo-Provera.
    e. Advantages.
        (1) Risk of endometrial and ovarian cancer and PID is decreased.
        (2) There is less menstrual blood loss, and therefore anemia is decreased.
        (3) A decrease in dysmenorrhea and mittelschmerz is seen.
        (4) Depo-Provera is a reversible form of birth control, although the return of fertility is slower than it is for other types of hormonal contraception.
        (5) Risk of ectopic pregnancies decreases to 1.3/1000 women-years as compared with 6.5/1000 women-years in women who use no contraception.
        (6) Amenorrhea is of advantage in certain women because as many as 80% of women are amenorrheic after 3 years of use.
        (7) Use with antibiotics is safe. The only drug known to decrease the effectiveness of Depo-Provera is cytodren. Because it is given parenterally, it is not dependent on the gastrointestinal tract. Improvement of seizure disorder results from the sedating effects of progestins.
    f. Side effects.
        (1) The menstrual cycle changes (increased days of light bleeding but not increased blood loss).
        (2) Amenorrhea develops with time.
        (3) Weight gain: The patient may gain up to 14 pounds with 4 years of use.
        (4) Breast tenderness may occur.
        (5) Depression may occur.

(6) Bone density decreases, which is reversible after discontinuation.
(7) The return of fertility is delayed for 6 months to 1 year after discontinuing use.
3. Minipill: The progestin-only pill has many of the advantages of the Norplant and Depo-Provera injection. It is used very infrequently. It is known to be less effective than combination oral contraceptives, Norplant, and Depo-Provera. However, it is a viable alternative in women who breast-feed and are unable to use estrogen. It has the advantage of being stopped easily. Its effectiveness rate is intensified if it causes anovulation, menstrual irregularities, and amenorrhea.
   a. Efficacy: The failure rate of the Minipill in the first year of typical use is 1.1% to 13.2%. If used perfectly, only 5 in 1000 women become pregnant in the first year. It is nearly 100% effective in lactating women and does not affect milk production.
   b. Indications.
      (1) Women for whom estrogen is contraindicated
      (2) Decreases blood loss during menses, therefore decreasing anemia, dysmenorrhea, and mittelschmerz
      (3) Decrease in endometrial and ovarian cancer and PID
      (4) Immediate reversibility
      (5) Indicated for women who develop headache and hypertension on combination oral contraceptives
   c. Side effects.
      (1) There are changes in menstrual cycles (more spotting and irregularity). These changes are sometimes unacceptable to women.
      (2) Interaction with anticonvulsants makes the Minipill less effective.
      (3) The risk of pregnancy is greater unless the cycles are disturbed.
      (4) The Minipill must be taken with exact regularity.
      (5) The Minipill is less available.
      (6) Practitioners have less experience with the Minipill.
      (7) Ovarian cysts (functional) are increased with use of the Minipill.
      (8) Ectopic pregnancy is more common with failures.
4. Delivery systems: Delivery systems for progestin-only contraceptives and combined pills are outlined in Table 5-5.

5.3 Postcoital Contraception

Postcoital contraception is used when condoms break, when combination oral contraceptives have been forgotten, or in cases of rape or misuse of present contraceptive method.

1. Contraceptive pills: The so-called morning after pill is highly effective in preventing pregnancy if it is used within 12 to 24 hours after coitus. The most commonly used regimen is 100 µg ethinyl estradiol and 1 mg of norgestrel or 0.5 mg levonorgestrel given immediately and then repeated 12 hours later. Antiemetics are sometimes needed with this

Table 5-5 Delivery Systems for Progestin-Only Contraceptives and Combined Pills

Administration	Injectable Depo-Provera	Implant Norplant	Oral Progestin-Only Pill	Oral Combined OC
Frequency	Every 3 months	5 years	Daily	Daily
Progestin dose	High	Ultra low	Ultra low	Low
Blood levels	Initial peak, then decline	Constant	Rapidly fluctuating	Rapidly fluctuating
First pass through liver	No	No	Yes	Yes
Major Mechanisms of Action				
Ovary: decreases ovulation*	+++	++	+	+++
Cervical mucus: decreases sperm penetrability	Yes	Yes	Yes	Yes
Endometrium: decreases receptivity to bastocyst	Yes	Yes	Yes	Yes
First-year failure rate (perfect use)	0.3	0.09	0.5	0.1
Menstrual pattern	Very irregular	Very irregular	Often irregular	Regular
Amenorrhea during use	Very common	Common	Occasional	Rare
Reversibility				
Immediate termination possible	No	Yes	Yes	Yes
By woman herself at any time	No	No	Yes	Yes
Median time to conception from first omitted dose, removal	6 months	About 1 month	<3 months	3 months

Data from Hatcher R: *Contraceptive technology*, ed 16, New York, 1994, Irvington Publishers.
*By several mechanisms—LH and FSH surges suppressed; preovulatory follicles suppressed.

regimen. For example, Ovral, 2 double doses are given 12 hours apart totaling 4; Loovral/Nordette/Levelen/Triphasil, 4 tablets are given every 12 hours, totaling 8 pills; or Danazol, 400 mg given every 12 hours, two to three times, totaling 800 to 1200 mg, are effective alternatives for women who are not able to use estrogen. For Plan B (Preven), 2 tablets containing 50 μg per tablet are taken 12 hours apart. Also available is levonorgestrel, 0.75 mg, 1 tablet every 12 hours or 1.5 mg stat.

2. Intrauterine device (IUD): Insertion of a copper IUD within 7 days of coitus is very effective in preventing pregnancy. However, use in women who are at high risk for PID is discouraged. Also it is not to be used in rape situations or nulliparous women. An IUD is an excellent option for properly selected patients such as multiparous women who do not desire surgery for birth control. The IUD is indicated in monogamous women.

   a. Fewer than 2% of the women in the United States are IUD users. In the 1970s, before many IUDs were taken off the market, about 10% of American women were IUD users. There are presently two IUDs available. The Mirena IUD, approved for 5 years, is produced by Berlex. The copper 380A (Paragard) is a desirable IUD option because it has been recently approved for 10 years of use. It is produced by Gynopharma and is the most commonly used IUD.

   b. Composition and mode of action.

   (1) The CU T 380A (Paragard) is shaped like a T. The polyethylene T is wrapped with a fine copper wire on all three arms of the T. A single-filament white string projects from the base of the T. The Mirena IUD is a polyethylene T wrapped with levonorgestrel on the vertical arm. Two blue single-filament strings project from the base of the T. The advantage of the Mirena is that it drastically decreases menstrual flow and therefore has a therapeutic indication.

   (2) Gyneflex, developed in Belgium, is a new IUD being trialed in Europe. It consists of a monofilament polypropylene thread that dangles six copper bands in the uterus. It is fixed to the fundus by an anchoring loop in the uterus. It is approved for 5 years. Special training for users is required.

   (3) The mechanism of action of the IUD includes sperm immobilization and increased speed of ovum transport through the fallopian tubes. It was once thought that IUDs caused abortion of the fertilized egg by preventing implantation. However, it is now known that the device prohibits the sperm from meeting the egg in the fallopian tube.

   c. Considerations before insertion of the IUD.

   (1) A detailed history must be completed and a thorough physical must be done. Cervical cultures for *Chlamydia* and gonorrhea must be negative. All abnormal Papanicolaou smears should be diagnosed and treated first.

   (2) Discussion of risks and benefits for this form of birth control should be thorough. Patients with the following history should

not be considered candidates for IUD insertion: Known or possible pregnancy, acute PID, or current behavior that suggests the patient is high risk for PID, recent postpartum endometritis, postabortion infection. The IUD should be used with caution in the following patient populations:
- (a) Those at risk for sexually transmitted diseases and PID.
- (b) Those with impaired immune response: human immunodeficiency virus (HIV) positive, diabetics, leukemics, or patients on steroids.
- (c) Patients with menorrhagia, undiagnosed irregular vaginal bleeding (i.e., known or suspected uterine or cervical malignancies).
- (d) Those who have had previous complications associated with IUDs, such as pregnancies, expulsion, or perforation.
- (e) Women with anatomic uterine abnormalities that make insertion difficult (e.g., leiomyoma, cervical stenosis).
- (f) Genital actinomycosis.
- (g) Mucopurulent cervicitis.
- (h) Those with valvular heart disease (women with cardiac lesions are more susceptible to subacute bacterial endocarditis).
- (i) History of a previous ectopic pregnancy is no longer a contraindication because IUDs actually decrease the risk of ectopic pregnancies.
- (j) Mitral valve prolapse is not a contraindication to IUD use.

d. IUD insertion.
  (1) An IUD may be inserted any time in a menstrual cycle as long as pregnancy has been ruled out.
  (2) The patient should be educated thoroughly before insertion. Gynopharma and Berlex provide a very complete patient education pamphlet that reviews everything from composition to side effects, effectiveness rate, and how to check the IUD postinsertion. The patient should read this material carefully before the device is inserted. The more informed the patient is, the better selected the patient will be. For insertion instructions see package inserts and other written sources (Fig. 5-1).
  (3) Prophylactic antibiotics: Two published studies differ on whether the use of antibiotics is necessary at the time of insertion. I prefer to use them. At this time it is well established that antibiotics should be used after insertion due to the fact that at insertion time bacteria from the vagina is introduced and may cause infection.
    (a) Giving 200 mg of doxycycline at the time of insertion and 100 mg 12 hours after insertion is appropriate in women who are not breast-feeding.
    (b) In women who are breast-feeding erythromycin 500 mg orally (PO) 1 hour before insertion and 500 mg 6 hours after is appropriate. Azithromax also may be used.

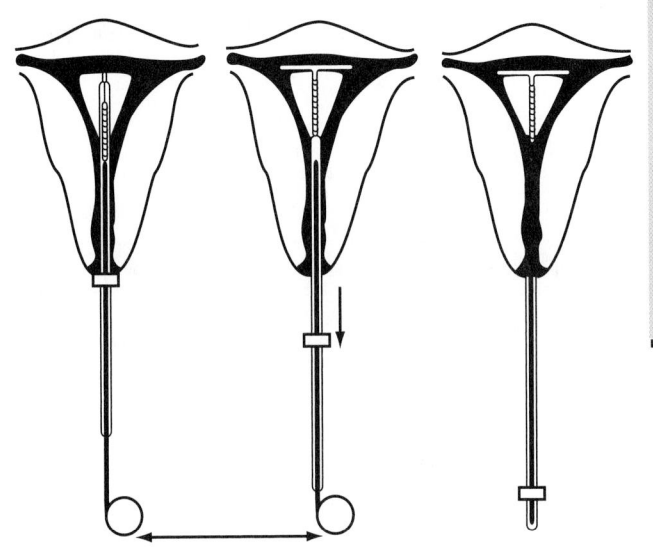

Figure 5-1 Withdrawal technique for an intrauterine device.

- e. IUD removal: Paragard CU T 380A is now approved for 10 years of use; Mirena for 5 years. Removal should be done gently with ring forceps or any type of long grasping forceps.

    Difficult removals may require cervical dilation with dilators or laminaria. An IUD hook or Novak's curette may be used to grasp an IUD in which strings are not visible.
- f. Pregnancy with an IUD.
    (1) Ectopic pregnancy must be ruled out.
    (2) The patient must be informed of signs and symptoms of infection and perforation if IUD strings are not seen.
    (3) If IUD strings are seen, remove IUD gently.
- g. Perforation.
    (1) There is a 1 in 1000 incidence.
    (2) The most common sites include fundus, body of the uterus, and cervical wall.
    (3) If IUD partially perforates it can be removed as a simple IUD removal.
    (4) If total perforation is diagnosed by ultrasound and x-ray film, PID or bowel obstruction may occur. In this case antibiotics and removal by laparoscopy is suggested. If no PID or obstruction occurs, then patient has option of leaving the IUD and watching for signs or symptoms of PID or obstruction.
- h. If PID develops, treatment should be instituted, the IUD removed, and hospitalization with intravenous (IV) antibiotics started.

A simple mnemonic device* to remind patients of symptoms that indicate a problem with the IUD is:

P Period late (pregnancy), abnormal bleeding
A Abdominal pain
I Infection exposure, abnormal discharges
N Not feeling well, fever, chills
S String missing, shorter, or longer

5.4 Barrier Methods

1. Diaphragms and cervical cap: These have about the same rate of effectiveness.
   a. Composition and use of diaphragm.
      (1) The diaphragm is a dome-shaped rubber cup with a flexible rim.
      (2) It fits in the vagina between the symphysis pubis and the posterior fornix of the vagina, covering the cervix.
      (3) It must be used with contraceptive gel.
      (4) It is effective for 6 hours.
      (5) The diaphragm is not to be worn more than 24 hours (risk of toxic shock syndrome).
      (6) The size is 50 to 95 mm.
      (7) Disposable diaphragms packaged with spermicide are being developed for single use.
      (8) Types (Fig. 5-2).
         (a) Flat spring rim: good for women with good vaginal muscle tone
         (b) Coil spring: good for women with average muscle tone and average pubic arch depth
         (c) Arcing spring: good for poor vaginal muscle tone
         (d) Wide seal: arcing or coil spring
   b. Cervical cap (Fig. 5-3).
      (1) A deep rubber cup, smaller than the diaphragm and fits snugly over the cervix only (Prentif cavity rim cervical cap)
      (2) Must be one-third filled with contraceptive gel, effective continuously for 48 hours
      (3) May repeat intercourse without additional spermicide
      (4) Not to be left in more than 48 hours, may cause toxic shock syndrome
   c. Fitting a diaphragm.
      (1) Domed and fitting rings are available.
      (2) The average size is 70 to 75 mm.
      (3) Vaginal depth is estimated by inserting the middle and index finger into the posterior fornix of the vagina; the thumb will mark the pubic bone.
      (4) Several rings or dome sizes should be used to get the best fit, which is the tighter but comfortable fit.

---

*From *Contraceptional Tech*, p. 375.

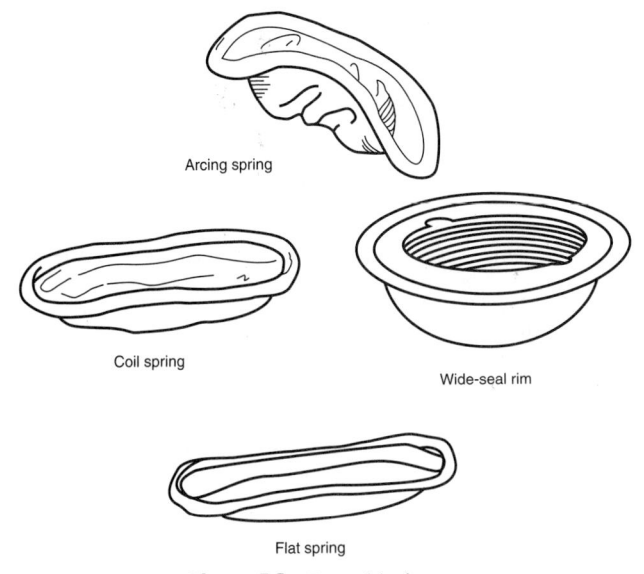

Practical Guide to the Care of the Gynecologic/Obstetric Patient   119

Figure 5-2 Types of diaphragms.

d. Fitting a cervical cap (the Femcap and Lea shield are now marketed).
   (1) The cervical cap is available in sizes 22, 25, 28, and 31 mm.
   (2) Six percent to ten percent of patients are unable to be fitted.
   (3) When the cap is fitted, it should be the exact diameter (within a few millimeters only) of the base of the cervix.
   (4) The dome should not be tight to the cervix.
   (5) If the cap is too tight, it will cause cervical trauma.
   (6) The rim of the cap forms suction around the cervix.

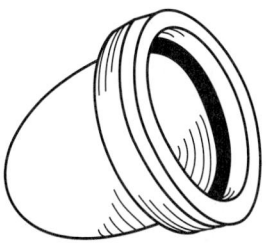

Figure 5-3 Cervical cap.

e. Efficacy of female barriers.
   (1) All types of barriers have a failure rate of 5% to 9% in nulliparous and 5% to 26% in multiparous users in the first year of use.
   (2) Failures are also more likely to occur in women who have intercourse three or more times weekly or are less than 25 years old.
   (3) Increased failures result from use with oil-based lubricants such as mineral oil, baby oil, suntan oil, butter, vaginal medications, yeast preparations, estrogen creams, and Vagisil. Latex will break down.
f. The vaginal sponge is again available. It releases nonoxynol 9, soaks up sperm, and is a physical barrier. The sponge was discontinued in the United States in 1995, but the Protectaid Sponge is available on the Internet.
g. Advantages of female barrier methods.
   (1) No systemic side effects
   (2) Efficacy equal to condoms
   (3) Good for women who are much less sexually active
   (4) Protection against sexually transmitted diseases such as gonorrhea, *Chlamydia*, cervical intraepithelial neoplasia
h. Side effects and contraindications.
   (1) Allergy to spermicide, rubber, latex, or polyurethane
   (2) Abnormalities in anatomy (may affect the fit)
   (3) Patient insertion error
   (4) May cause recurrent urinary tract infections
   (5) History of toxic shock syndrome
   (6) Lack of experience in fitting cap/diaphragm
   (7) Vaginal bleeding
   (8) Should not be used before 6 weeks postpartum
   (9) Known malignancy (cervix, uterus)
   (10) Unresolved Papanicolaou smears or infections of the genital tract

2. Female condoms.
   a. Female condoms look like a combination of a diaphragm and a condom.
   b. The condoms are composed of soft polyurethane, with one end closed, one end open.
   c. They come with extra lubricant.
   d. Insertion: The closed ring is inserted into the vagina and covers the cervix. The open end covers the labia and base of penis (Fig. 5-4).
   e. Removal: The open end is twisted to contain semen and the condom is discarded; it should never be reused.
   f. Efficacy: There is a 5.1% pregnancy failure rate with perfect use; failure is 12.4% with average use. The FDA labeling states a 25% failure rate.
   g. Advantages.
      (1) Highly effective protection against HIV (94% protection) and all other sexually transmitted diseases
      (2) May be used if male partner refuses to use a condom

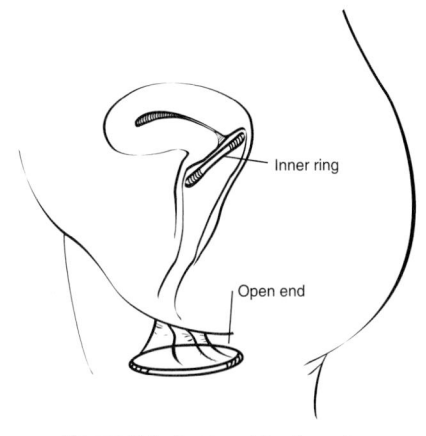

Figure 5-4 Position of female condom.

3. Male condom.
   a. Composition: Ninety-five percent are latex (rubber) condoms. Five percent are skin or natural membrane.
      (1) Most condoms are 7 inches long (170 mm) and 2 inches (50 mm) wide.
      (2) Most condoms are 0.001 to 0.004 inches (0.03 to 0.10 mm) thick.
   b. Proper use of male condom (Fig. 5-5).
      (1) The condom should be placed on the erect penis before genital contact.
      (2) The condom is unrolled to the base of the penis; the rolled portion should remain on the outside of the condom.
      (3) One-half inch of empty space is left at the tip of the condom.
      (4) The condom must be lubricated; if it is dry it may tear.
      (5) Oil-based lubricants should not be used.
      (6) To prevent spillage, the condom is held to the base of penis while withdrawing.
   c. Efficacy.
      (1) Perfect use has a 3% failure rate. Typical use has a 12% failure rate.
      (2) Breakage rate is 1 or 2 per 100 condoms used.
   d. Advantages.
      (1) Accessibility
      (2) Hygienic
      (3) Erection enhancement
      (4) Prevention of sperm allergies
      (5) Prevention of sexually transmitted diseases: effective barrier against HIV, HPV, gonorrhea, herpes simplex, *Chlamydia*

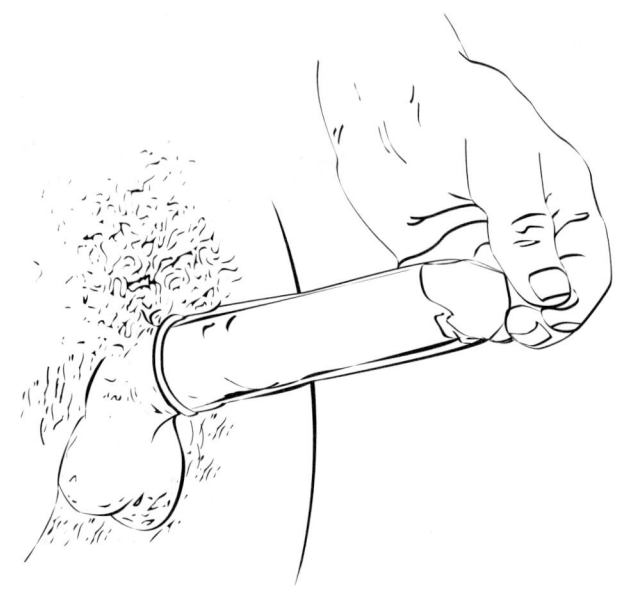

Figure 5-5 Placement of male condom.

  e. Disadvantages.
    (1) Interruption of foreplay
    (2) Decreased sexual pleasure for the female
    (3) Latex allergies (1% to 3% of the U.S. population)
    (4) Breakage of condoms
    (5) Sheepskin condoms do not act as a barrier to viruses
4. Spermicides.
  a. Chemical methods of contraception are used alone or with other barriers.
  b. Types: There are nonoxynol and octoxynol forms; jellies, creams, foams, suppositories, tablets, and soluble films kill sperm.
  c. Effectiveness depends on correct use. Perfect use has a 3% failure rate, typical use a 36% failure rate.
  d. Use.
    (1) Films and suppositories should be inserted into the vagina about 15 minutes before intercourse so they may dissolve.
    (2) They should be inserted deeply into the vagina.
    (3) Spermicide should be reapplied for each episode of intercourse.
    (4) Spermicide should be left in place for 6 to 8 hours after intercourse.
    (5) Users should not douche after intercourse.

(6) Spermicides should be stored in a cool, dry place.
e. Advantages.
  (1) Sold over the counter
  (2) Inexpensive
  (3) Easy to use
  (4) Can also be used as a lubricant with other barriers
  (5) May help prevent sexually transmitted diseases
f. Disadvantages.
  (1) Irritation in either partner
  (2) May not prevent HIV transmission because of irritation
  (3) Needs to be used after every act of intercourse
  (4) Messy

5.5 Lactation Amenorrhea Method

1. The lactation amenorrhea method can provide contraception in the early postpartum months.
2. Mechanism of action.
   a. There are decreased progesterone and estrogen levels after delivery.
   b. Ovulation suppression lasts 70 to 100 days after delivery.
   c. Nipple stimulation sends nerve impulses to the hypothalamus that cause release of beta-endorphin, which decreases gonadotropin-releasing hormone (GNRH) secretion; there is no follicle development.
   d. Increased levels of prolactin make ovaries unresponsive to LH, suppressing positive feedback effects of estrogen on the midcycle rise of GNRH or directly interfering with ovarian steroid production.
   e. The sucking mechanism is crucial for effectiveness. A woman who is fully or nearly fully breast-feeding and remains amenorrheic for 6 months postpartum is protected against pregnancy.
   f. Breast-feeding is effective as birth control for 6 months if 15 or more feedings lasting 10 minutes are accomplished daily.
   g. This method depends on the intensity of breast-feeding and rate of menses return.
   h. Most of the women in the United States do not practice full, on-demand breast-feeding, which is the basis of the lactation amenorrhea method; they need to use complementary contraceptive methods.

5.6 Abstinence

1. Abstinence is defined as refraining from intercourse.
2. Abstainers outnumber people choosing to have intercourse in the United States until age 15.
3. In all, 13% of women 30 to 34 years old have never had sex.
4. The goal of abstinence is to avoid sexually transmitted diseases.
5. Abstinence should be seriously discussed with adolescents.
6. Adolescents should plan on how to say "No" to intercourse.

7. High-pressure sexual situations should be avoided. "No" should be said clearly.

5.7 Withdrawal

1. Mechanism: withdrawal of the penis from the vagina before ejaculation
2. Effectiveness: 4% failure rate for perfect use; 19% failure in typical use
3. Advantages
   a. There are no costs, devices, or chemicals.
   b. This is a backup method that is always available.
   c. Only 2% of women use this method.
4. Disadvantages
   a. The excitement is interrupted.
   b. The method relies on self-control.
   c. The partners are not protected from transmission of sexually transmitted diseases before ejaculation.

5.8 Rhythm Method—Natural Family Planning

1. Mechanism of action.
   a. This method depends on the awareness of the physiology of the male and female reproductive tracts.
   b. Sperm and ovum life spans are as follows:
      (1) Sperm viability averages 3 days; however, the range is 2 to 7 days.
      (2) Ovum life span is about 24 hours.
   c. The unsafe period is considered to be up to 7 days before ovulation and 3 days after ovulation.
   d. Avoid intercourse at these unsafe times or use other methods such as barriers for backup.
2. Effectiveness rate.
   a. There is a 20% failure rate for typical use in the first year.
   b. Perfect use has a failure rate of 1% to 9%.
   c. The most effective version is the postovulation method.
   d. If used perfectly, the symptothermal and ovulation method is very effective.
   e. The calendar method is the least effective.
3. Types include the postovulation method, the symptothermal method, the ovulation method, and the calendar method.
   a. Symptothermal
      (1) Cervical mucus basal body temperature (thermal) is measured.
      (2) Lower abdominal pain with ovulation is experienced (symptom).
      (3) Perfect use: Intercourse can be resumed only on the fourth day peak mucus and the third day after thermal rise.
   b. Ovulation method (Billings method)
      (1) Mucus is checked from the vagina before urination.
      (2) Mucus is checked for lubrication, elasticity, wetness, and tackiness (it ferns midcycle).

- (3) Ovulation occurs 1 day before, after, or during the last day of the most slippery and abundant mucus.
- (4) The fertile period is any time mucus is noted before ovulation.
- (5) Note: Some women have very insignificant mucus discharges at ovulation time.

c. Basal body temperature (BBT) charting (temperature method)
- (1) Body temperature is taken every morning.
- (2) The temperature is charted on a BBT chart.
- (3) Look for a biphasic temperature chart (Fig. 5-6).
- (4) However, 6 out of 30 women ovulate but do not have biphasic changes on a temperature chart.

4. Advantages.
   a. There are no side effects.
   b. Some couples like to be totally involved in fertility prevention.
5. Disadvantages.
   a. There is no protection against sexually transmitted diseases.
   b. The male partner sometimes objects to participating.
   c. It is not as reliable a method of contraception with women who have irregular cycles, recent menarche, approaching menopause, or who are unable to keep records.

5.9 Sterilization

1. Male vasectomy
   a. Vasectomy interrupts the vas deferentia. This prevents the passage of sperm into the seminal ejaculate. It is about half as common as female sterilization in the United States.
   b. The failure rate of this method is about 0.1% in the first year. This does not include pregnancies that occur secondary to a couple's failure to wait for sperm to be cleared from the distal vas deferentia.
   c. Techniques: Sterilization is done under aseptic conditions with 1% lidocaine injection.
      (1) Scalpel technique
         (a) The vas deferentia are divided through an open skin incision (Fig. 5-7).
         (b) The divided ends are either fulgurated (more effective) or tied. A portion of the vas may be removed (not necessary).
         (c) The fascia may be sutured over one end of the divided vas; this may increase the effectiveness.
      (2) No-scalpel technique
         (a) The vas is grasped through the closed skin of the scrotum by a ring forceps (Fig. 5-8).
         (b) A sharp tipped forceps punctures the skin.
         (c) The vas is drawn out.
         (d) The same occlusion technique is used as for the scalpel technique.
         (e) The no-scalpel technique avoids skin incisions, decreases the rate of hematoma formation, affords bloodless surgery, and may be more acceptable in societies where skin scrotum incisions are not acceptable.

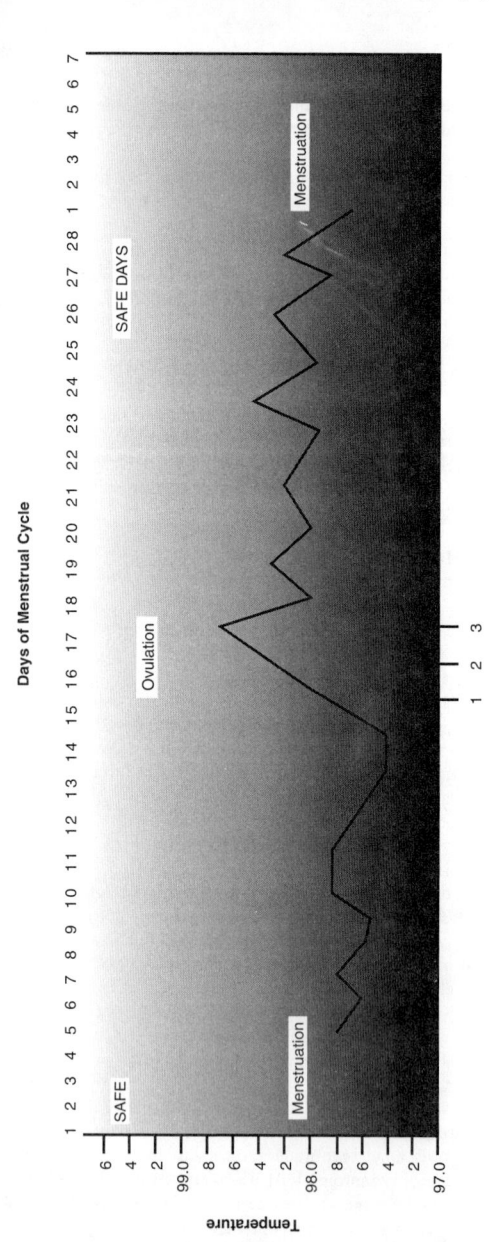

Figure 5-6 Basal body temperature variations during a model menstrual cycle.

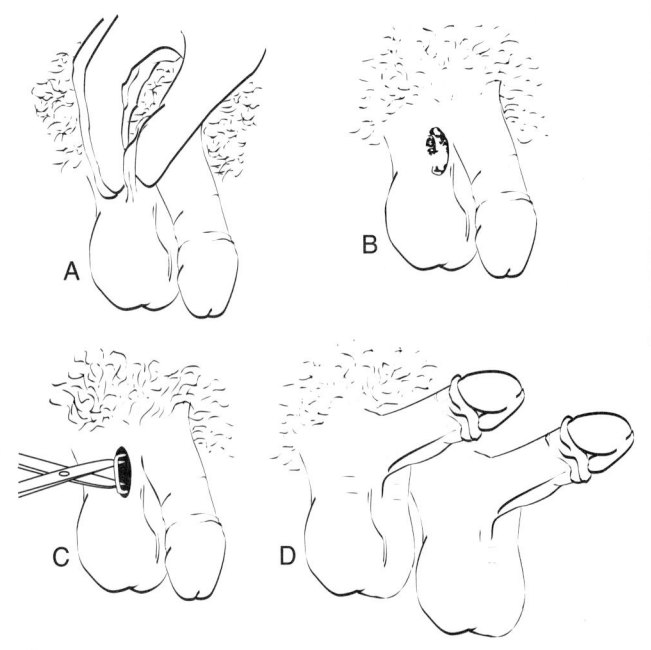

Figure 5-7 Scalpel vasectomy. Vas deferens is located (**A**) and an incision made (**B**). The vas is isolated (**C**) and fulgurated or tied. Either one or two incisions can be used (**D**).

    d. Advantages: vasectomy versus female sterilization.
      (1) Safer procedure than female sterilization
      (2) More easily performed
      (3) Less expensive than female sterilization
      (4) Does not require general anesthesia
    e. Disadvantages.
      (1) There is no protection against sexually transmitted diseases.
      (2) The procedure is permanent. Reversal cannot always be accomplished.
      (3) This is a "male only" form of birth control.
      (4) Five percent to ten percent of men regret having the procedure.
      (5) One third to two thirds of men develop sperm antibodies postvasectomy.
    f. Safety of vasectomy: continually studied.
      (1) Fears of increased risk of cardiovascular disease have been allayed by the Sichuan study, 1983-1986.
      (2) Also, studies have shown that there is no increased risk of developing prostate cancer postvasectomy.

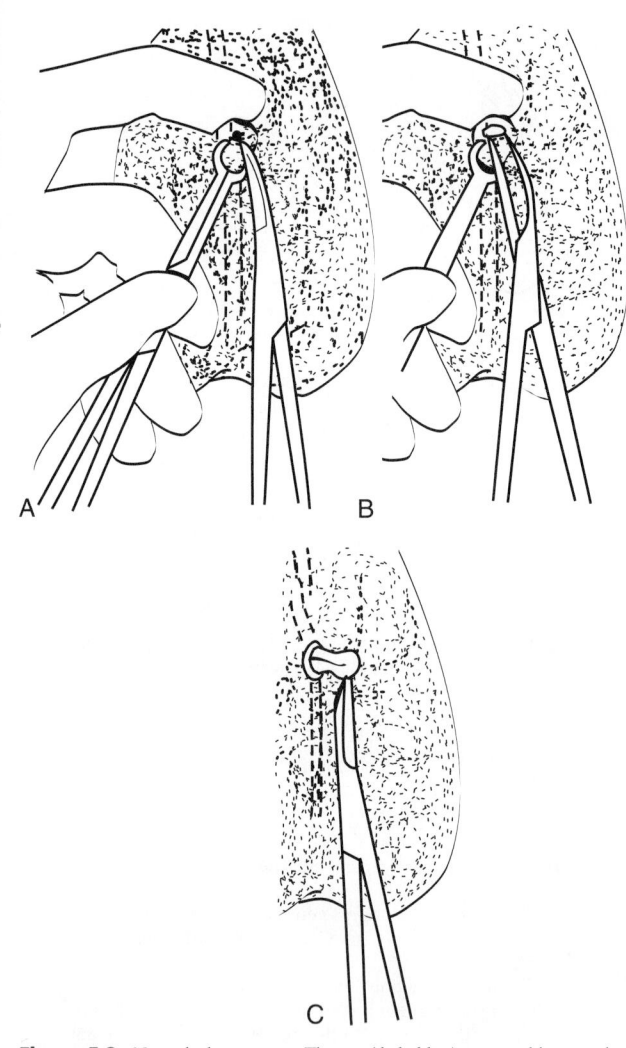

Figure 5-8 No-scalpel vasectomy. The vas (*dashed line*) is grasped by special ring forceps, and the skin and the vas sheath are pierced by sharp-tipped dissecting forceps **(A).** The forceps stretch the opening **(B),** and the vas is lifted out **(C).**

2. Female sterilization
   a. Female sterilization is the leading popular method of fertility control in the United States, especially in women over 30 years old.
   b. Fifty percent are done at the time of delivery; 50% are done outside of pregnancy (interval).
   c. Women should be carefully counseled before they make such a permanent decision.
   d. All possible future situations should be discussed (i.e., divorce, remarriage, death of a spouse or child, future improvement of economic situation).
   e. Women younger than 30 years old have a greater tendency to regret the decision and seek reversal. Between 5% and 15% regret it. Only 1% to 2% seek reversal.
   f. Only the partner who has made the decision to end the possibility for child bearing should have the permanent procedure done.
   g. All other birth control options should be reviewed with the patient because she may not realize the benefits connected with other birth control options and the importance of keeping the option to have children in the future open.
   h. Also, it must be made very clear to the patient that this procedure should be viewed as permanent even though it has a failure rate.
   i. Types.
      (1) Pomeroy technique
         (a) The technique was published in 1930; it's considered "the gold standard."
         (b) A loop of fallopian tube is grasped with a babcock clamp. An absorbable, plain, catgut suture is tied around the loop; the loop is excised and is sent to pathology.
      (2) Irving technique
         (a) Described in 1924.
         (b) Destroys no tube, is highly effective, and is highly reversible.
         (c) The tube is divided at the isthmus. The proximal end is buried in the myometrium, and the distal end is buried in the broad ligament.
         (d) There is no known failure rate.
         (e) The morbidity is higher than for other tubal ligation methods.
      (3) Fimbriectomy
         (a) The procedure is not reversible; it is permanent.
         (b) Fimbria is totally excised, including the fimbria ovarica (portion of the tube connected to the ovary).
         (c) Failures are secondary to not excising the fimbria ovarica.
      (4) Postpartum tubal
         (a) It is done 1 day postpartum.
         (b) The incision is a small infraumbilical incision and may be done transversely very close to the umbilicus. Often the incision is hidden within the umbilicus and is no larger than a laparoscopic incision.

j. Techniques.
   (1) Uchida technique
      (a) A saline epinephrine solution is injected into tubal musculature to separate the serosa from the inner circular muscle of the tube.
      (b) The edematous tube is incised on its antimesenteric side.
      (c) The inner circular muscle of the tube is excised.
      (d) The proximal stump is buried beneath the edematous serosa and the distal stump outside the serosa.
      (e) The excised portions are sent to pathology.
   (2) Clip application technique (Fig. 5-9)
      (a) Spring loaded clips are used (same as for laparoscopy).
      (b) The isthmus of the tube is stretched between two babcock clamps.
      (c) The clip is put on by hand by holding the jaws of the clip between the thumb and the third finger. The index finger pushes the spring into locked position.
3. Interval sterilization
   a. Original unipolar technique was described by Steptoe.
   b. The introduction of laparoscopy made it a popular procedure not associated with pregnancy.
   c. Vaginal sterilization by fimbriectomy was the only interval form of tubal ligation before laparoscopy.
   d. Types (all done through the laparoscopy).
      (1) Unipolar coagulation
         (a) The tube was grasped and burned until blanching.
         (b) Scissors were used to excise the blanched portion, which was sent to pathology.
         (c) A current ran through patient's body. Morbidity is secondary to bowel and skin burn.
         (d) No longer used because morbidity, secondary to extensive tissue destruction, is too high.
      (2) Bipolar technique: developed independently in the 1970s by Kleppinger (United States), Rioux (Canada), and Hirsh (Germany)
         (a) This is the most common laparoscopic tubal ligation.
         (b) This technique is the easiest to perform.
         (c) The bipolar technique works by concentrating the electricity between two paddles; therefore, the patient does not carry the current.
         (d) Kleppinger recommends that the tube be burned in three places so there is at least a 3-cm gap between healthy portions of tube.
         (e) It is recommended that the cauterization begin 2 to 3 cm from the cornual angles, preventing uteroperitoneal fistulization and ectopic pregnancy formation.
      (3) Falope Ring (silastic band)
         (a) The Falope Ring is safer than cautery.

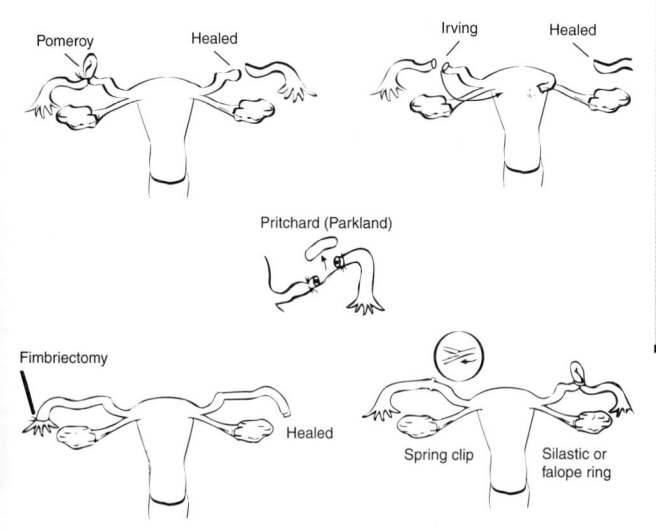

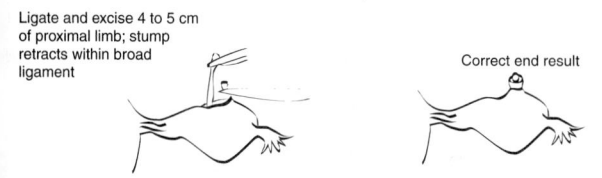

Practical Guide to the Care of the Gynecologic/Obstetric Patient   131

Figure 5-9 Techniques for tubal sterilization.

- (b) It was developed in the 1970s.
- (c) The fallopian tube is grasped into a metal cylinder with grasping prongs.
- (d) The silastic ring occludes the base of a 3-cm portion of tube, which necroses.
- (e) It is associated with a 2.5% incidence of hemorrhage secondary to stretching of vessels beneath the tube or tearing of the tube.
- (f) The patient has pain from 48 to 96 hours from tubal hypoxia.
- (4) Spring clip
  - (a) Of the laparoscopic methods, it is the most difficult technically.

- (b) The clip must go across the whole tube.
- (c) The spring clip is applied across the isthmus of the tube.
- (d) Most procedures are reversible; destroys only 5 mm of the tube.
- (e) This is the best method for women under 30 years.
  - (5) Minilaparotomy tubal
    - (a) Minilaparotomy tubal may be used if there is a contraindication to laparoscopy.
    - (b) It is described as a technique using local anesthesia and intravenous sedation. General anesthesia also may be used.
    - (c) A 2-cm to 5-cm suprapubic incision is made. The Pomeroy technique, clips, or silastic rings may be used on the tubes.
    - (d) A dilator is placed in the uterus before the technique is done for manipulation and uterine elevation.
- e. Failure rates of sterilization: All laparoscopic tubal ligations have a failure rate of between 2 and 10 pregnancies per 1000 operations (Tables 5-6 and 5-7).
- f. Posttubal syndrome: an irregular cycle and dysmenorrhea post–tubual ligation.
  - (1) Studies have been done, but none have been conclusive.
  - (2) Menstrual irregularities and dysmenorrhea are probably not caused by tubal ligation.
  - (3) It is more likely that the woman's own cycles are surfacing.
  - (4) Complication rate (Table 5-8).
    - (a) Defined as those requiring laparotomy for repair.
    - (b) Has stayed below 2 in 1000 for the past decade.
    - (c) Mortality has not been reported since 1982.
    - (d) Major vessel laceration from trocar needle insertion in 1/1000 to 1/10,000 cases.
    - (e) Thermal bowel injury in 1/1000 cases.
- g. Essure: Hysteroscopic placement of tubal plugs inserted at the uterotubal junction. Another form of birth control must be used for 3 months while the coil scars over. Long-term sterilization is quoted at 85% to 90%. Advantage is that it is quick, and may be done without anesthesia.

Table 5-6 Technical Difficulties

Author	Electrocoagulation	Ring	Hulka Clip	Filshie Clip
Bhiwandiwal	3.03%	4.03%	6.06%	—
Khandwal	—	4.24%	8.50%	—
Parikh	—	—	—	10.72%

Data from Khandwala S: *J Reprod Med* 5:465, 1988.

Table 5-7 **Technical Failures**

Author	Bipolar Coagulation	Endocoagulation	Ring	Hulka Clip	Filshie Clip
Hirsch	0.08%	—	—	—	—
Kleppinger	0%	—	—	—	—
Reidel	—	0.1%	—	—	—
Bhiwandiwala	—	—	0.93%	0.74%	—
Khandwala	—	—	0.17%	0.3%	—
Chi	—	—	3.8%	—	—
Hulka	—	—	—	0.4%	—
Parika	—	—	—	—	0%

Data from Khandwala S: *J Reprod Med* 5:465, 1988.

Table 5-8 Effectiveness and Mortality of Contraceptive Methods

Method	Pregnancies per 100 Women-Years (All Ages)		Estimated Annual Deaths Resulting from Contraceptive Method and/or Pregnancy per 100,000 Women-Years (by Age)						
	Lowest Expected	Typical	15-19	20-24	25-29	30-34	35-39	40-44	
No Contraception	85	85	6	5	7	14	19	22	
Surgical Sterilization									
Tubal ligation	0.2	0.4	4	4	4	4	4	4	
Combination Oral Contraceptives									
Nonsmokers	0.1	3	1	1	1	2	4	3	
Smokers	0.1	3	2	2	2	11	13	59	
Progestin-Only Oral Contraceptives	0.5	3	1	1	1	1	1	1	
Progestin Injections									
Medroxyprogesterone acetate (MPA)	0.3	0.3	1	1	1	1	1	1	
Norethindrone enanthanate (NET)	0.4	0.4	1	1	1	1	1	1	
Progestin Implants									
Levonorgestrel (LNG)	0.3	0.3	1	1	1	1	1	1	
Intrauterine Devices									
Progestasert	2.0	3	1	1	1	1	2	1	
Copper T 380A	0.8	3	1	1	1	1	1	1	
Barrier Methods*									
Diaphragm, cap	6	18	1-2	1-2	1-2	1-4	1-6	1-7	

Condoms	2	1-3	1-3	1-4	1-7	1-12
Aerosol foam, jelly, cream, tablets	3	1-3	1-3	1-4	1-7	1-12
Sponge						
Parous women	9	1-2	1-2	1-3	1-6	1-10
Nulliparous women	6	1-2	1-2	1-2	1-4	1-7
Periodic Abstinence (Rhythm)	1-9	1-2	1-2	1-2	1-4	1-16

From Dickey R: *Managing contraceptive pill patients*, ed 8, Durant, OK, 1994, Essential Medical Information Systems.
*In a comparative study of 1437 women using the sponge versus diaphragm and a study of 1394 women using the cervical cap versus diaphragm, the 12 months failure rate was diaphragm, 5.2% and 6.9%; cervical cap 11.4%; sponge 11.7%. Failure rates increased to 26.4% for the cap and 20% for the sponge among parous users. The failure rate for condoms was estimated at 2.7%. J. Trussel, Office of Population Research, Princeton University, 1993.

SUGGESTED READINGS

The use of hormonal contraception in women with coexisting medical conditions, *ACOG Practice Bulletin*, Number 18, July 2000.

Giannouris T: Contraception for your challenging patient and the evolving role of intrauterine contraception. Supplement to *The Female Patient Ob/Gyn*, 2005.

Guillebaud J: *Your questions answered contraception*, ed 4, 2004, Churchill Livingstone.

Gynopharma Inc: Patient package insert, Paragard T 380A, May 1994.

Speroff L, Darney P: *A clinical guide for contraception*, 2005, Lippincott, Williams & Wilkins.

Physician desk reference, ed 59, 2005, Thomson.

University of Illinois Urbana/Champaign, Carle Cancer Center: Hematology Resource Page, Patient resources: Prothrombin gene mutation 20210A.

Infertility Evaluation

6.1 Female Infertility

Carolyn Maud Doherty

HISTORY AND EVALUATION

1. Definition: Infertility is generally defined as the inability to achieve a conception after 1 year of unprotected intercourse.
2. Prevalence.
   a. Infertility affects 13% to 15% of married couples in the United States.
   b. An episode of infertility will be experienced by 25% of women during their reproductive years.
3. Evaluation of the infertile female.
   a. History: A detailed patient history is important.
      (1) Age of patient: fertility decreases with increasing age
      (2) Exposure to chemicals, toxins, or radiation in the work environment
      (3) Smokers: three to four times more likely to experience longer than a 1-year delay to conception when compared with nonsmokers; a relative risk of 3:1 for an ectopic pregnancy when compared with control pregnant patients
      (4) Caffeine: may be associated with an increased risk of miscarriage
      (5) Alcohol use
      (6) Current drugs or medications
         (a) Antihistamines: can decrease mucus production and also diminish vaginal lubrication
         (b) Nonsteroidal antiinflammatory drugs: can inhibit the luteinizing hormone (LH) surge
         (c) Barbiturates: can decrease or inhibit gonadotropin-releasing hormone (GnRH) release
      (7) Excessive physical activity: can lead to anovulatory cycles
      (8) Marital history
         (a) Number of years
         (b) Contraception used
      (9) Sexual intercourse
         (a) Frequency: times per month
         (b) Adequate penetration
         (c) Ejaculation: retrograde, normal

(d) Difficulties: impotence
(e) Coital positions
(f) Use of lubricants: type
(g) Pain or discomfort: either partner
(h) Orgasm
(i) Masturbation: frequency, especially by the male partner
(10) Pregnancy history
   (a) All pregnancies: term, preterm, abortions
   (b) Dates
   (c) Outcome
   (d) Weight
   (e) Sex
   (f) Complications
   (g) Abortions: date, length of pregnancy, complications
   (h) Number of natural children
(11) Previous marriages: all partners
   (a) Number of years
   (b) Contraception use: number of years, type
   (c) Children
   (d) Miscarriages
(12) Past workup
   (a) Tests performed: repeating same tests should be avoided
   (b) Dates, results, physician's name
(13) Menstrual history
   (a) Age at onset of menses
   (b) Age of sexual development
   (c) Present menstrual cycle
      (i) Length: start to start
      (ii) Duration of flow
      (iii) Date of last menstrual period
   (d) Dysmenorrhea
      (i) What was the age of onset?
      (ii) Does it occur with each cycle?
   (e) Vaginal discharge
      (i) Color: Green or bright yellow is abnormal.
      (ii) Odor: If odor present, it should be cultured.
      (iii) Irritation: Wet mount and culture are probably required.
(14) Medical history
   (a) Allergies
   (b) Surgeries
   (c) Medications
   (d) Blood transfusion
   (e) Pelvic infection: syphilis, gonorrhea, *Chlamydia*
   (f) Thyroid disease
   (g) Other chronic medical problems
b. Physical examination.
   (1) Head, ears, eyes, nose, and throat.
      (a) Clinicians should be alert for exophthalmos (Graves' disease).
      (b) The thyroid should be palpated to check for enlargement or nodules.

(2) Breast.
   (a) A complete breast examination is necessary.
   (b) Clinicians should be alert for galactorrhea; if present, prolactin and thyroid-stimulating hormone (TSH) should be checked.
   (c) Of patients with polycystic ovaries (PCO), 25% will have hyperprolactinemia.
(3) Abdomen.
   (a) Clinicians should palpate to check for masses.
   (b) Often, myomas can be palpated abdominally.
(4) External genitalia: The size of the clitoris should be carefully examined. Enlargement is a sign of excessive androgens.
(5) Cervix.
   (a) A yearly Papanicolaou smear should be performed.
   (b) Clinicians should observe for scarring secondary to cones, cryotherapy, and Loop electrosurgical excision procedure (LEEP).
   (c) Observe the canal for signs of stenosis.
(6) Uterus, ovaries.
   (a) Size
   (b) Position
   (c) Fixed vs. mobile
   (d) Contour: smooth versus nodular
   (e) Pain

COMMON CAUSES OF INFERTILITY

1. Endometriosis.
   a. Endometriosis is a condition characterized by ectopic endometrial glands and stroma.
   b. The etiology of endometriosis is unknown. Possible etiologies are as follows:
      (1) Retrograde menstruation
      (2) Vascular or lymphatic transport
      (3) Transformation of coelomic epithelium into endometrial type glands (coelomic metaplasia)
      (4) Immunologic alteration leading to a decreased cellular immunity to endometrial tissue
   c. Symptoms.
      (1) Dysmenorrhea
      (2) Dyspareunia, especially with deep penetration
      (3) Low back pain
      (4) Infertility
   d. Examination: Certain findings should raise a physician's index of suspicion.
      (1) Retroverted uterus
      (2) Enlarged ovaries
      (3) Fixed uterus or ovaries
      (4) Tender, nodular uterosacral ligaments

e. Diagnosis.
   (1) Laparoscopy should be performed.
   (2) Suspicious lesions on the cervix should be biopsied.
f. Treatment.
   (1) Surgical
      (a) Operative laparoscopy to ablate all visible lesions and debulk ovarian endometriomas
      (b) Laparotomy: debulking procedure
   (2) Medical
      (a) GnRH agonist (Depo-Lupron, Zoladex)
      (b) Oral contraceptives: decidualize endometrial tissue
      (c) Danazol: should be used only in cases of persistent pain
      (d) Progestational agents (Depo-Provera, Provera)
2. Cervical factor.
   a. Scarring: previous cone, LEEP, or cryotherapy
   b. Diethylstilbesterol (DES) exposure
   c. Clomiphene citrate: antiestrogenic mechanism of action leads to thick cervical mucus
3. Uterine factor.
   a. Müllerian anomalies
   b. Anatomic abnormalities
      (1) Myomas
      (2) Asherman's syndrome
      (3) Adenomyosis: presence of endometriosis within the myometrium; these patients have chronic pelvic pain
   c. Diagnosis
      (1) Hysterosalpingogram (HSG): needed by all infertility patients
      (2) Ultrasound
      (3) Magnetic resonance imaging (MRI): especially for Müllerian anomalies and myomas
   d. Treatment
      (1) Surgical: See Surgical Therapy for Infertility, p. 146.
      (2) Medical: See Medical Management of Infertility, p. 144.
4. Male factor infertility.
   a. Semen analysis: Physicians should never make a diagnosis based on a single semen analysis.
      (1) Normal semen parameters[2]
         (a) Volume: 2.0 mL or greater
         (b) pH: 7.2 to 8.0
         (c) Concentration: 20×10^6 spermatozoa per mL or greater
         (d) Motility: 50% or greater
         (e) Morphology: 30% or greater normal forms
         (f) White blood cells: 1×10^6 per mL or fewer
      (2) Specimen collection rules
         (a) Three days of abstinence is optimal.
         (b) Specimens should be produced via masturbation.
         (c) No lubricants may be used.
         (d) Specimens should be collected in a sterile specimen container.
         (e) Extremes of temperature should be avoided while transporting to the laboratory.

b. See Section 6.2 for further information on male factor infertility.
5. Hormonal dysfunction.
    a. Disorders of ovulation
        (1) Polycystic ovarian syndrome: LH/follicle-stimulating hormone (FSH) ratio of 3:1 or greater
        (2) Hypothyroidism: high TSH
        (3) Oligo-ovulation: etiology unknown
    b. Luteal phase defect: Defined as a lag of more than 2 days in the histologic development of the endometrium as compared with the actual day of the cycle. It is diagnosed by an appropriately timed endometrial biopsy. It is best to time the biopsy by the LH surge rather than the start of the menses. Luteal phase defects have one of the following etiologies:
        (1) Lack of adequate progesterone production
        (2) Inability of the endometrium to respond to the progesterone that is present
6. Pelvic adhesions.
    a. Diagnosis
        (1) HSG: look for tubal occlusion or contrast loculation
        (2) Laparoscopy: direct evaluation of pelvic anatomy
    b. Therapy
        (1) Surgical lysis
        (2) Assisted reproductive technology (ART)
7. Ovarian failure.
    a. Diagnosis: serum FSH
        (1) Less than 15: There is a good chance for successful ART.
        (2) Greater than 15 to less than 25: There is a diminished chance for success. Oocyte donation should be discussed with the patient.
        (3) Greater than 25: Estrogen replacement should be started and oocyte donation discussed.
8. Unexplained infertility: This is a diagnosis of exclusion. A complete workup should be done before this diagnosis is made.

DIAGNOSTIC STUDIES

1. Complete history and physical examination: as previously outlined.
2. HSG.
    a. An HSG is a fluoroscopic examination used to demonstrate uterotubal disease.
    b. An HSG should be performed early in the workup of the infertile female. Laparoscopy and HSG are complementary procedures. Chromotubation at the time of laparoscopy does not replace the HSG. Valuable information about the uterine cavity, such as intrauterine filling defects and the status of the fallopian tubes (i.e., the location of tubal occlusion), can be delineated by HSG.
    c. HSG should be done before laparoscopy to verify and treat (if possible) at the time of surgery.
    d. The timing of HSG should be just after the patient finishes her menses and well before the time of ovulation.

e. Indications for HSG.
   (1) Infertility
   (2) Abnormal uterine bleeding
   (3) Repetitive pregnancy loss
   (4) Confirmation of uterine myomas
f. Contraindications.
   (1) Current or suspected pelvic infection: HSG can lead to salpingitis or endometritis if performed during an active infection. Patients with a history of pelvic inflammatory disease (PID) have a 1% to 3% risk of recurrent infection after an HSG and therefore should be treated with antibiotics (doxcycline 100 mg, bid) beginning 24 hours before the examination.
   (2) Active bleeding: Active bleeding at the time of HSG can lead to contrast extravasation; passage of blood into the peritoneal cavity, possibly leading to endometriosis; and an inaccurate diagnosis of an intrauterine filling defect because of the presence of blood clots in the cavity.
   (3) Pregnancy: When HSG is inadvertently done during an early pregnancy, it is usually an "all-or-none phenomenon." If the fetus survives (which is usually the case), it will not be affected by the exposure.
g. Procedure technique.
   (1) The physician inquires as to allergies to shellfish or iodine.
   (2) The physician inserts speculum and cleans cervix with betadine.
   (3) The physician places a single-tooth tenaculum on the anterior lip of the cervix and introduces the Kahn cannula into the os.
   (4) The speculum is removed slowly to avoid disrupting the cannula.
   (5) Contrast is injected slowly while always visualizing the uterine cavity for filling defects and the tubes for abnormal contour.
   (6) The physician should attempt to demonstrate tubal patency. However, the patient should not be tortured in the attempt.
3. Semen analysis.
4. Hormonal development: The menstrual cycle consists of three distinct phases.
   a. Follicular phase (time during which the follicle develops): This phase is characterized by a rising estradiol.
      (1) The estradiol should peak at the time of ovulation at approximately 300 pg/mL.
      (2) Progesterone in the follicular phase is always less than 1.
      (3) It should be remembered that actual ovulation occurs 36 hours after the onset of the LH surge.
      (4) An easy way to determine the day of ovulation is to subtract 14 days from the total cycle length to give the day of ovulation.
   b. Luteal phase (begins after ovulation, which is brought about by the LH surge).
      (1) Any time the LH level rises two to four times above the baseline level, it is considered to be the ovulatory surge.

(2) This phase is characterized by rising progesterone levels (>2 ng/mL) and also by a secondary peak of the estradiol level on day 21.
(3) If a pregnancy occurs, then the hormone levels remain elevated.
(4) If no pregnancy occurs, then the hormone levels drop and menses begin.
(5) The basal body temperature (BBT) will rise 0.3° to 0.5° during the luteal phase and is associated with progesterone levels greater than 4 ng/mL.
(6) Care must be taken because BBT charts can be misleading.
   c. Menstrual phase: A drop in hormones leads to the onset of menses.
5. Follicular development.
   a. The follicle is a fluid-filled sac that contains the oocyte. It should be 18 to 25 mm at the time of ovulation.
   b. The development of the follicle can easily be followed by transvaginal ultrasound.
   c. An easy way to determine whether follicles of the correct size are being produced is to scan the patient 15 days before her expected menses. This should be just before ovulation.
6. Cervical mucus or postcoital testing.
   a. Cervical mucus is estrogen dependent. There should be an increase in production at the time of ovulation.
   b. Mucus is evaluated for the following:
      (1) Consistency: should be thin, clear
      (2) Spinnbarkeit: thready stretchability
      (3) Ferning: product of estrogen influence
      (4) Cellularity
      (5) Volume: should be abundant
      (6) pH: 6.4 to 8.0
   c. A postcoital test (PCT) should be done 6 to 10 hours after intercourse. The endocervical specimen should contain 25 sperm per high-power field (HPF). Ten or more sperm with progressive motility should be considered an adequate PCT.
7. Endometrial biopsy.
   a. The endometrial biopsy is used to diagnose a luteal phase defect (LFD). LFD is defined in one of the two following ways:
      (1) An inadequate amount of progesterone being secreted by the corpus luteum
      (2) The inability of the endometrium to respond to adequate progesterone concentrations
   b. The diagnosis of LFD is made by two endometrial biopsies greater than 2 days out of phase.
   c. Endometrial biopsy should be done 12 days after the LH surge.
   d. Samples should be removed via a small pipette (Pipelle) from the anterior uterine wall to avoid possibly disrupting an early implantation, because the posterior surface is the most common site of implantation.
   e. Pretreatment of patients with acetaminophen or Naprosyn is advised.

8. Laparoscopy/hysteroscopy.
   a. Surgery should be the last step in the workup.
   b. Laparoscopy.
      (1) Laparoscopy can be both diagnostic and therapeutic.
      (2) Visualization of the pelvis must be done to make the diagnosis of endometriosis or pelvic adhesions.
      (3) Laparoscopy can be done in the follicular or the luteal phase of the cycle. If chromotubation is planned, it should not be done during the menstrual cycle.
   c. Hysteroscopy.
      (1) Hysteroscopy should be done when there is a suspected or known intrauterine defect. This is why hysterosalpingography is so important.
      (2) Tubal cannulation of proximal obstruction of the fallopian tubes can be accomplished hysteroscopically.
      (3) Intraoperative HSG can be done to assess the uterine cavity during an operative hysteroscopic procedure.

MEDICAL MANAGEMENT OF INFERTILITY

The approach in this section is to take the most common causes of infertility as outlined in the first two sections of this chapter and discuss medical management options.

1. Endometriosis: Endometriosis lesions have estrogen, androgen, and progesterone receptors. The concentration of these receptors is lower than that of eutopic endometrium. However, estradiol is the critical hormone regulating growth and development of endometriosis. Androgens and progestins produce atrophy in endometriosis lesions. Treatment options:
   a. Danazol
      (1) Derivative of 17-ethinyltestosterone.
      (2) Produces a high-androgen, low-estrogen environment.
      (3) Should no longer be used as first-line treatment for endometriosis.
      (4) Dose greater than 100 mg/day leads to pain relief in most patients.
      (5) Doses of 100 to 800 mg/day are most effective for treatment purposes.
   b. GnRH analogs
      (1) The mechanism of action is effectively to shut down GnRH stimulation of FSH and LH, leading to a hypoestrogenic state.
      (2) The first 8 to 10 days after administration, the effects are stimulatory until downregulation occurs. Therefore, Depo-Lupron should be administered 8 to 10 days before expected menses (day 20) and then every 28 days after this for 6 months.
      (3) Most patients can be started on 3.75 mg of Depo-Lupron. Two weeks after the second shot, a serum estradiol level should be checked to make sure the patient is suppressed (E2 < 20 pg/mL). If the level is greater than 20 pg/mL, the next injection should be 7.5 mg.

(4) Most patients require 6 months of therapy.
  c. Progestins
    (1) These agents produce a hypoestrogenic state by suppressing FSH and LH.
    (2) Good choices are Provera (10 to 30 mg day) and Depo-Provera 150 mg every 3 months.
  d. Oral contraceptives
    (1) There is a dual mechanism of action (i.e., suppression of LH and FSH as well as decidualization of the endometrium).
    (2) The most effective regime is a continuous regimen, but cyclic administration can also provide relief.
    (3) This is not a "treatment" for endometriosis; it is suppressive therapy.
    (4) Lo-Ovral is a good choice for this therapy.
2. Cervical factor.
  a. The medical treatment of choice for cervical factor infertility is intrauterine insemination.
  b. The oral administration of estrogen does not improve cervical mucus or enhance pregnancy rates and should not be done.
3. Uterine factor.
  a. Myomas
    (1) Indications for medical therapy of myomas
      (a) Bleeding
      (b) Pain
      (c) Preoperative therapy: to improve hemoglobin and decrease the risk of blood transfusion
    (2) GnRH agonists
      (a) They are the only real medical therapy.
      (b) They must suppress estradiol levels to less than 45 pg/mL.
      (c) Optimal therapeutic benefit comes after 3 months of therapy (Depo-Lupron, 3.75 mg, every 28 days).
      (d) Myomas will undergo rapid regrowth upon cessation of therapy.
  b. Adenomyosis
    (1) Adenomyosis is a condition in which endometriosis is found within the myometrium.
    (2) It is characterized by chronic pelvic pain.
    (3) It is found in approximately one of every six patients at the time of hysterectomy (most are multiparous).
    (4) Its effect on fertility is unknown.
    (5) Medical therapy is the same as that for pelvic endometriosis.
4. Male factor. (See Section 6.2.)
5. Hormonal dysfunction.
  a. Disorders of ovulation (usually require ovulation induction)
    (1) Clomid.
      (a) Clomid works by blocking estrogen receptor binding or replenishment at hypothalamic or pituitary level, thus blocking estrogen feedback, leading to increased serum gonadotropins.
      (b) It is administered orally day 3 to day 7 or day 5 to day 9.

(c) Dosage can be increased if ovulation does not occur. Recommended doses are 50 to 150 mg.
(d) Human chorionic gonadotropin (HCG) (Profasi) can be added to increase ovulation rates. Administer IM 5000 or 10,000 IU when follicles are greater than 20 mm.
(2) Humegon/Pergonal.
  (a) These are injectable gonadotropins consisting of 75 IU of FSH and 75 IU of LH or HCG.
  (b) They act by directly stimulating the ovaries to produce follicles. Ovulation is accomplished by using HCG (Profasi).
  (c) Monitoring is by serum estradiol and LH. There should be a serum E2 level of approximately 250 pg/mL for each follicle.
  (d) Patients are also monitored by ultrasound.
  (e) Each follicle should be 18 to 20 mm at the time of ovulation.
(3) Metrodin: partially purified FSH. It is the drug of choice in the treatment of patients with PCO.
(4) GnRH pump (Factrel or Lutrepulse).
  (a) It is administered via an automatic portable infusion pump with a pulsatile mechanism.
  (b) It is a good choice for hypothalamic amenorrhea.
b. Lymphoproliferative disease (LPD)
(1) The correction of a LPD is usually directed at enhancing the follicular phase, thus leading to an improved luteal phase with Clomid or Pergonal/Humegon.
(2) Progesterone supplementation can benefit those patients with a LPD who produce inadequate amounts of progesterone.
6. Pelvic adhesions: The treatment of pelvic adhesions is surgical.
7. Ovarian failure: The current therapy for infertility associated with ovarian failure is egg donation.
8. Unexplained infertility.
  a. Unexplained infertility is a diagnosis of exclusion.
  b. Therapy is usually ovulation induction with intrauterine insemination or an assisted reproductive procedure.

SURGICAL THERAPY FOR INFERTILITY

1. Endometriosis.
  a. Basic tenets
    (1) The definitive diagnosis of endometriosis is by direct visualization and biopsy via laparoscopy.
    (2) Lesions can have a variety of appearances, including the following:
      (a) Clear: most likely early lesions
      (b) Red: histologically active
      (c) White: scarring
      (d) Brown-black: inactive endometrial glands and stroma
    (3) All patients found to have endometriosis should be surgically staged via the American Fertility Society Classification.
  b. Indications for surgery
    (1) Pain is present in 50% of patients with endometriosis.

(2) Adnexal masses are unexplained ovarian enlargements that necessitate ultrasound and surgery.
(3) Infertility: Endometriosis can lead to adhesions, ovarian dysfunction, tubal abnormalities, LPDs, and decreased fertilization.
c. Surgical procedures
  (1) Conservative surgery by laparoscopy, the goal of which is to ablate and resect lesions and lyse adhesions with minimal disruption to normal surrounding tissue.
    (a) Electrosurgery
      (i) This procedure is most commonly used.
      (ii) Electrosurgery may be unipolar or bipolar.
      (iii) A variety of instruments are available to operate with. A point coagulator is especially useful for small, individual lesions.
    (b) Thermocoagulator: causes tissue desiccation by increasing the temperature to 100° to 120° F and not by electric current
    (c) Laser
      (i) This procedure offers precise tissue destruction.
      (ii) CO_2 laser is best for vaporization.
      (iii) Nd:YAG is best for coagulation.
  (2) Conservative surgery by laparotomy: The goal of this surgery is also to ablate and resect lesions and to lyse adhesions with minimal disruption to normal surrounding tissue.
    (a) Microsurgical technique: Tissues must be handled carefully to avoid trauma.
    (b) Ablation and resection of lesions: Uses the previously mentioned modalities to achieve the best results.
    (c) Preoperative suppression: Successful surgery can be more easily accomplished in certain cases with preoperation suppression with GnRH agonist. Some argue that this makes the lesions more difficult to resect, but in most cases this is not the case.
    (d) Laparoscopy versus laparotomy.
      (i) Laparoscopy is probably most dependent on the surgeon's skills.
      (ii) Current data supports the less costly, probably more effective laparoscopic approach.
  (3) Definitive surgical therapy.
    (a) Hysterectomy with bilateral salpingoophorectomy is the definitive surgical therapy.
    (b) Estrogen replacement should be instituted after surgery is completed with little risk of disease recurrence.
2. Cervical factor.
  a. Stenosis: The surgical therapy for cervical stenosis is dilation.
  b. Myomas: Removal is via hysteroscope resectoscope.
  c. Polyps: Removal is via hysteroscope resectoscope.
3. Uterine factor.
  a. Leiomyomata: They should be removed only if they impinge on the cavity or are thought to be causing repeated losses.
    (1) Hysteroscopic resection

(2) Abdominal myomectomy
    (a) Abdominal myomectomy causes adhesions.
    (b) A second-look laparoscopy 7 days after the myomectomy should be considered to lyse early adhesions.
 b. Polyps should be removed hysteroscopically.
 c. Intrauterine adhesions.
    (1) Hysteroscopic resection with scissors
        (a) An intraoperative HSG should be performed to confirm complete lysis of the adhesions.
        (b) An 8-French, 3-cc pediatric Foley catheter should be placed in the endometrial cavity at the end of the procedure to prevent reformation of adhesions. The Foley should be left in place for 5 to 7 days, during which time the patient is on antibiotics and estrogen (Premarin 2.5 mg bid or Estrace 4 mg bid). The estrogen is continued for 25 days with 10 mg of Provera administered on days 16 to 25. Menses should occur 48 to 72 hours after the estrogen and Provera are discontinued.
 d. Congenital uterine anomalies.
    (1) Unicornuate: No surgery is necessary unless a rudimentary horn is present and requires removal.
    (2) Bicornuate versus septate uterus: This diagnosis can be made only by laparoscopy. A septum can be resected hysteroscopically. A bicornuate uterus requires a metroplasty if it is associated with repeated losses.
    (3) Uterine didelphys: Surgery is not generally required.
4. Male factor. (See Section 6.2.)
5. Hormonal dysfunction: This is usually corrected via controlled ovarian hyperstimulation, with or without insemination or assisted reproductive technology. (See 6.b.)
6. Pelvic adhesions.
   a. Surgical lysis of adhesions
      (1) Laparoscopy
      (2) Laparotomy
   b. Assisted reproduction
      (1) In vitro fertilization (IVF)
         (a) Indications
             (i) Poor prognosis tubal factor
             (ii) Endometriosis
             (iii) Male factor
             (iv) Immunologic infertility
             (v) DES exposure
             (vi) Unexplained infertility
         (b) Process
             (i) Ovarian hyperstimulation
             (ii) Oocyte retrieval
             (iii) Oocyte insemination fertilization
             (iv) Transcervical embryo transfer
         (c) Outcome
             (i) Approximately 20% ongoing pregnancy rate

(ii) Multiple pregnancy rate of 30%
(iii) May need embryo manipulation, such as assisted hatching, to facilitate implantation
(2) Gamete intrafallopian transfer (GIFT)
(a) Indications
(i) Cervical factor
(ii) Mild to moderate male factor infertility
(iii) Pelvic adhesions: need one healthy tube
(iv) Unexplained primary or secondary infertility
(v) Ovarian failure: using donor oocytes
(b) Process
(i) Ovarian hyperstimulation
(ii) Oocyte retrieval: usually transvaginal
(iii) Laparoscopy with tubal transfer of sperm and oocytes (usually four)
(c) Outcome
(i) Approximately 30% ongoing pregnancy rate
(ii) Approximately 4% ectopic pregnancy rate
c. Zygote intrafallopian transfer (ZIFT) and tubal embryo transfer (TET)
(1) Indications
(a) Severe male factor: allows fertilization to occur before laparoscopy
(b) Immunologic infertility
(c) Endometriosis
(d) Oocyte donation
(e) Unexplained infertility
(2) Process
(a) Ovarian hyperstimulation
(b) Oocyte retrieval
(c) Oocyte insemination fertilization
(d) Laparoscopic zygote embryo transfer (24 to 56 hours after retrieval)
(3) Outcome: a 30% to 35% ongoing pregnancy rate
d. Oocyte donation
(1) Indications
(a) Ovarian failure
(b) Genetic abnormalities
(c) Gonadal dysgenesis
(d) Poor oocyte quality
(2) Process
(a) Ovarian hyperstimulation of the donor
(b) Uterine preparation of the recipient
(c) Fertilization of the oocytes
(d) Transcervical embryo transfer (GIFT, ZIFT)
(3) Outcome: pregnancy rates approach 50%
7. Ovarian failure: surgical therapy with oocyte donation. (See previous section.)
8. Unexplained infertility: surgical therapy.
a. Assisted reproductive technologies

(1) IVF
(2) GIFT
(3) ZIFT/TET

6.2 Male Infertility

Philip J. Aliotta

Of patients presenting for fertility evaluation for their first pregnancy, 15% will fail to achieve pregnancy. Over 50% of all infertility cases can be ascribed to male factor involvement. Of these cases, the breakdown is as follows:

Male factor only	33%
Combined male and female factors	20%

The appropriate evaluation of the male partner is therefore very important.

EVALUATION

The evaluation of the male partner should include the following:

1. Historical review (Box 6-1).
   a. Childhood illnesses
   b. Existing medical disease review
   c. Prior surgeries
   d. Family history
   e. Sexual development
   f. Exposure to toxins
      (1) Alcohol
      (2) Heat
      (3) Radiation
      (4) Toxic fumes
      (5) Tobacco use
      (6) Drug and recreational drug use (marijuana, cocaine, hallucinogens, etc.)
2. Physical examination: A "fertility-focused" examination should seek to identify physical characteristics within organ systems that may contribute to or identify the male factor in a couple's infertility (Table 6-1).
3. Tests.
   a. Urinalysis and postejaculate urine: Rule out urinary tract infections, retrograde ejaculation, and medical renal diseases.
   b. *Chlamydia* and gonorrhea cultures (optional and where indicated).
   c. Endocrine evaluation: Knowledge of the hypothalamic–pituitary–gonadal (H–P–G) axis is important in the evaluation of the subfertile and infertile male. The H–P–G axis is a negative-feedback loop; the entire system is directed by pulsatile release from the hypothalamus of GnRH, which causes pituitary release of FSH and LH. The FSH acts on the Sertoli component of the testis with the release of inhibin, whereas the LH stimulates the Leydig cell component to release testosterone. The combination of high intratesticular levels of testosterone plus the effect of FSH on Sertoli cells is responsible for spermatogenesis. Both enter into

BOX 6-1 Factors in Male Infertility History

History of Infertility

Duration
Prior pregnancies
  Present partner
  Another partner
Previous treatments
Evaluation and treatment of wife

Sexual History

Potency
Lubricants
Timing of intercourse
Frequency of intercourse
Frequency of masturbation

Childhood and Development

Undescended testicles, orchiopexy
Herniorrhaphy
Y-V plasty of bladder
Testicular torsion
Testicular trauma
Onset of puberty

Medical History

Systemic illness (e.g., diabetes mellitus, multiple sclerosis)
Previous or current therapy

Surgical History

Orchiectomy (testis cancer, torsion)
Retroperitoneal surgery
Pelvic injury
Pelvic, inguinal or scrotal surgery
Herniorrhaphy
Y-V plasty, transurethral prostate resection

Infections

Viral, febrile
Mumps orchitis
Venereal
Tuberculosis, smallpox (rare)

Gonadotoxins

Chemicals (pesticides)
Drugs (chemotherapeutic, cimetidine, sulfasalazine, nitrofurantoin, alcohol, marijuana, androgenic steroids)

Box continued on following page

> **BOX 6-1 Factors in Male Infertility History** *(Continued)*
>
> Thermal exposure
> Radiation
> Smoking
>
> **Family History**
>
> Cystic fibrosis
> Androgen receptor deficiency
>
> **Review of Systems**
>
> Respiratory infections
> Anosmia
> Galactorrhea
> Impaired visual fields

From Sigman M, Lipshultz LI, Howards SS: The evaluation of the subfertile male. In Lipshultz LI, Howards SS, editors: *Infertility in the male*, ed 2, St. Louis, 1991, Mosby.

the systemic circulation and, through negative feedback, inhibit the release of GnRH. The endocrine evaluation allows for the categorization of male patients as follows[1]:

(1) Eugonadotropic
   (a) Normal FSH
   (b) Normal LH
   (c) Normal testosterone
(2) Hypogonadotropic (hypogonadotropic hypogonadism)
   (a) Low FSH
   (b) Low LH
   (c) Low testosterone
(3) Hypergonadotropic (hypergonadotropic hypogonadism)
   (a) Elevated LH → Leydig cell dysfunction → gonadal failure
   (b) Decreased testosterone → Leydig cell dysfunction → gonadal failure
   (c) Elevated FSH → spermatogenic dysfunction → gonadal failure
(4) Only in conditions associated with obstructive azoospermia or retrograde ejaculation are all hormonal levels within normal limits.

d. Semen analysis: Normal semen, as defined by the World Health Organization, is an admixture of spermatozoa suspended in secretions from the testes and epididymes, which are mixed at the time of ejaculation with secretions from the prostate, seminal vesicles, and bulbourethral glands. The final composition is a viscous fluid that comprises the ejaculate.[2]
   (1) Requirements are as follows:
      (a) 48 to 72 hours of abstinence.
      (b) Multiple analyses (minimum of three recommended) separated by 2-week to 4-week intervals.

Table 6-1 Focal Points of the Male Physical Examination

Examine	Look For	Suspect
1. Habitus	Eunuchoid proportions	Klinefelter's syndrome
2. Vital signs	Orthostatic hypotension	Autonomic insufficiency
3. Head, eyes, and nose	Diminished beard	Androgen deficiency
	Bitemporal hemianopsia	Pituitary tumor
	Retinopathy	Diabetes mellitus
	Anosmia	Kallmann's syndrome
4. Neck	Thyromegaly	Hypothyroidism or hyperthyroidism
5. Lungs	Wheezes, rhonchi, rales	Cystic fibrosis
		Young's syndrome
		Kartagener's syndrome
6. Breasts	Gynecomastia	Hyperprolactinemia
		Alcoholism
		Klinefelter's syndrome
		Reifenstein's syndrome
		Estrogen excess
7. Abdomen	Hepatomegaly	Alcoholism
	Inguinal hernia	Prior cryptorchidism
8. Genitalia		
a. Penis	Decreased length*	
Meatus	Ventral	Hypospadias
	Occluded	Urethral distortion
		Partial urethral obstruction
Foreskin	Phimosis	Local infection
		Dyspareunia

Table continued on following page

Table 6-1 Focal Points of the Male Physical Examination *(Continued)*

Examine	Look For	Suspect
Shaft	Lateral deviation*	Peyronie's disease
b. Testes		
Volume	Bilateral decrease	Primary or secondary hypogonadism
		Selective germinal cell aplasia
	Unilateral decrease	Prior cryptorchidism or torsion
	Bilateral increase	Congenital adrenal hyperplasia
Scrotum	Varicocele	Varicocele
Epididymus	Pain	Acute epididymitis
	Painless mass	Chronic epididymitis
Vas deferens	Asymmetry	Bilateral absence of vas deferens
9. Prostate	Boggy, tender, enlarged	Prostatitis

From Spark RF: *The infantile male: The clinician's guide to diagnosis and treatment*, New York, 1988, Plenum, p. 186.
*Not evident in flaccid penis. Apparent only during spontaneous or pharmacologically induced erection.

(c) A specimen: Generally obtained through masturbation and delivered to the laboratory within 2 hours in a wide-mouth container (usually silicone); should be kept as close to body temperature as is possible.
(d) Postejaculate urine: Tested to rule out retrograde ejaculation and possible retention of semen in the urethra secondary to obstruction.[3]
(e) Collecting jar: Cap or top must not have a rubber lining because this will kill whatever spermatozoa are present.
(f) Collection, avoid the following:
  (i) Ordinary condoms: interfere with sperm viability
  (ii) Coitus interruptus: high potential loss of first part of the ejaculate, a possibility of cellular and bacterial contamination, and acid vaginal pH affects sperm motility
(g) Safe handling: Semen may contain harmful agents (e.g., human immunodeficiency virus, hepatitis viruses, herpes simplex viruses, *Chlamydia*, gonorrhea) and must be handled with care.
(2) Box 6-2 shows the differential diagnosis based on sperm count.
(3) Macroscopic examination.
  (a) pH of semen
    (i) The pH of normal semen should be measured at a uniform time, usually within 1 hour of ejaculation, and should be in the range of 7.2 to 8.0.
    (ii) If the pH is less than 7.0 in a sample with azoospermia, dysgenesis of the vas deferens, seminal vesicles, or epididymis may be present.
  (b) Color
    (i) Opaque to opalescent is normal.
    (ii) Clear or translucent is oligospermia.
    (iii) Rust or red is hematospermia.
    (iv) Yellow, creamy, or milky is pyospermia.
    (v) In jaundice, the semen is bright yellow.
(4) Liquefaction: In humans, semen forms a gel-like clot after ejaculation, but within 15 to 20 minutes liquefaction of this clot has occurred. Coagulation of the human semen depends on the presence of a fibrinogen-like substance that is manufactured by the seminal vesicles and that is acted on by the enzyme vesiculase produced by the prostate. Breaking down of the clot and the associated fibrin takes place as a result of the activities of a series of proteolytic enzymes secreted by the prostate. These include proteases, pepsinogen, amylase, and even hyaluronidase. Concomitant release of transaminase enzymes can cause further peptide breakdown. Therefore, both clotting and liquefaction are induced by prostate secretions. Liquefaction of semen usually occurs within 10 to 20 minutes after ejaculation.[4]
  (a) Liquefaction is usually assessed visually. Grade 1: Semen that fails to liquefy forms a gel-like coagulum.

BOX 6-2 **Differential Diagnosis Based on Sperm Count in the Infertile Male**

1. Azoospermia—severe oligospermia
   a. Central
      (1) Hypogonadotropic hypogonadism
      (2) Hyperprolactinemia
      (3) Hemochromatosis
      (4) Panhypopituitarism
      (5) Hypothalamic and pituitary sarcoidosis
   b. Genetic
      (1) Klinefelter's syndrome and variants
      (2) Noonan's syndrome (XX male)
      (3) Ring Y chromosome mosaicism
   c. Testicular
      (1) Anorchia
      (2) Cryptorchidism
      (3) Primary hypogonadism secondary to orchitis
      (4) Other causes
         (a) Germ cell dysfunction
         (b) Androgen resistance syndromes
         (c) Germ cell aplasia
         (d) Radiotherapy
         (e) Sertoli cell–only syndrome
         (f) Chemotherapy
   d. Obstruction or aplasia of the ductal system
      (1) Congenital
         (a) Aplasia of vas deferens
         (b) Aplasia of the epididymis
      (2) Acquired
         (a) Preepididymal
         (b) Epididymal
         (c) Postepididymal
      (3) Vas deferens occlusion
         (a) Vasectomy
         (b) Young's syndrome
   e. Retrograde ejaculation
      (1) Autonomic insufficiency
      (2) Ganglionic blockers
2. Oligospermia
   a. Central
      (1) Hypogonadotropic hypogonadism
      (2) Hypothalamic and pituitary sarcoidosis
      (3) Hemochromatosis
      (4) Panhypopituitarism

> BOX 6-2 Differential Diagnosis Based on Sperm Count in the Infertile Male *(Continued)*
>
>   (5) Hyperprolactinemia
> b. Other causes
>   (1) Selective germ cell dysfunction
>   (2) Chemotherapy
>   (3) Androgen resistance syndromes
>   (4) Germ cell aplasia
>   (5) Radiotherapy
>   (6) Sertoli cell–only syndrome
> c. Varicocele
> d. Idiopathic
> 3. Normospermia
> a. Immunoinfertility
> b. Varicocele
> c. Unrecognized female factors
> d. "Normal but infertile"

From Spark RF: *The infantile male: The clinician's guide to diagnosis and treatment,* New York, 1988, Plenum, p. 195.

    Grade 2: Partially liquefied semen will contain many small gel-like clots. Grade 3: Fully liquefied semen has no gel-like clots and the semen is completely fluid.
    (b) Treatment of liquefaction defects includes the following:
        (i) Alpha-amylase
        (ii) Alpha-chymotrypsin
        (iii) Lysozyme
        (iv) Hyaluronidase
(5) Viscosity.
    (a) Viscosity is defined as the quality of semen that allows it to be poured drop by drop out of a container.
        (i) The viscosity of the seminal fluid can vary from sample to sample.
        (ii) Increased viscosity may be associated with infertility.[4]
    (b) Treatment of hyperviscous semen includes the following:
        (i) Passage through a wide-bore needle
        (ii) Mixing viscous semen with sperm-free seminal fluid from another patient
(6) Count.
    (a) There is a large variance in the normal sperm count.
    (b) Often cited are 20 million/mL to 200 million/mL.
    (c) The World Health Organization established a count of 20 million/mL as the line between "normal" and "abnormal or infertile."

(d) The sperm concentration takes no account of total number of sperm in the overall ejaculate, because volumes can and do vary.
(e) It is known, too, that in a single individual, counts per milliliter can vary from some number less than 20 million/mL or exceed 200 million/mL.
(f) For that reason, at least three analyses, done at least 1 week or more apart, with 2 days of abstinence are recommended.
(g) Sperm counts can vary with the type of counting chamber used (Table 6-2). With respect to accuracy and using 35 million beads per milliliter as a standard, the following chambers were tested for their accuracy:
  (i) Cell VU: mean count 35.1 ± 2.5
  (ii) Microcell: mean count 36.2 ± 9.3
  (iii) Neubauerhemacytometer: mean count 51.4 ± 12.8
  (iv) Makler: mean count 51.2 ± 7.4
(h) Nomenclature for semen variables
  (i) Normozoospermia: normal ejaculate
  (ii) Oligozoospermia: sperm concentration less than 20 million/mL
  (iii) Azoospermia: no spermatozoa in the ejaculate
  (iv) OligoAsthenoTeratozoospermia: disturbance of all three variables—count, motility, and morphology
  (v) Teratozoospermia: fewer than 30% spermatozoa with normal morphology
  (vi) Asthenozoospermia: fewer than 50% spermatozoa with forward progression of 3 or 4
  (vii) Aspermia: no ejaculate
  (viii) Polyzoospermia: sperm concentration in excess of 250 million/mL
  (ix) Necrospermia: dead sperm
(7) Motility.
(a) Sperm must be able to move in such a manner as to demonstrate forward progression. This type of movement is necessary for a sperm to enter and pass through the female genital tract and also for it to achieve fertilization.
(b) Sperm movement is evaluated both quantitatively and qualitatively.[5]
(c) Quantitation motility (viability) is defined as the average percentage of sperm moving in 10 random high-power microscopic fields.
(d) Qualitative assessment of sperm movement is based on the pattern displayed by the majority of motile spermatozoa.
  (i) 0 is none. No forward progression.
  (ii) 1 is poor. Sluggish forward progression.
  (iii) 2 is moderate. Definite forward progression.
  (iv) 3 is good. Good forward movement with progression.
  (v) 4 is excellent. Vigorous rapid forward progression.

Table 6-2 **Comparison of Chambers for Counting Sperm**

	Cell VU	Hemacytometer	Makler	Microcell
Cells counted	Body fluids/sperm	Body fluids/sperm	Sperm	Body fluids/sperm
Disposal	Disposable	Nondisposable	Nondisposable	Disposable
Chamber depth	20 μm	100 μm	10 μm	12 and 20 μm
Grid	100 squares each 0.1×0.1 mm	Ruled Neubauer	100 squares each 0.1×0.1 mm	None (micropereticle required)

From Seaman E, Bar-Chama N, Fisch H: Semen analysis in the clinical evaluation of infertility. In Carson CC III, Cooner WH, editors: *Mediguide to urology*, New York, 1994, Lawrence DellaCorte.

(e) If motility is under 50%, a viability stain is done using eosin Y with nigrosin as counterstain. Greater than 50% of sperm should be viable. Abnormalities in motility and quality of movement can be seen with the following[6]:
    (i) Infection
    (ii) Antisperm antibodies
    (iii) Partial ejaculatory duct obstruction
    (iv) Gonadotoxin exposure
    (v) Varicoceles
    (vi) Protein–carboxyl methylase deficiency (induced by radiation exposure or environmental toxin)
    (vii) Immotile cilia—Kartagener's syndrome
(8) Morphology.
    (a) According to the World Health Organization, a morphologically normal semen sample contains 50% normal forms, defined as sperm with oval heads and no neck or tail abnormalities (Figs. 6-1 and 6-2).
    (b) The advanced technology of in vitro fertilization has made it necessary to redefine sperm morphologic criteria that may correlate with fertilization outcomes.
        (i) According to "strict criteria" established by Kruger et al., a normal spermatozoon has an oval configuration with a smooth contour; an acrosome comprising 40% to 70% of the distal part of the head; no abnormalities of the neck, midpiece, or tail; and no cytoplasmic droplets of more than half of the sperm head.
        (ii) Borderline forms are abnormal.[5,7]
    (c) Kruger et al. grouped together the normal and borderline forms to obtain the "morphology index"; they proposed that more than 4% morphologically normal sperm and a morphology index greater than 30% predict a good fertilization outcome. Fertility rates per oocyte with a strict criteria score of under 4% was 7.6% compared to a fertility rate per oocyte of 64% with strict criteria score of greater than 4%.[5,7]
(9) Agglutination.
    (a) Simply put, motile spermatozoa stick to each other. These agglutinates can be as follows:
        (i) Head to head
        (ii) Tail to tail
        (iii) Midpiece to midpiece
        (iv) Mixed
    (b) The adherence of immotile sperm to each other or of motile sperm to mucus threads, cells other than spermatozoa, or debris is considered to be "nonspecific aggregation" rather than agglutination.
    (c) The presence of agglutination is suggestive of, but not sufficient evidence for, an immunologic cause of infertility.
    (d) Sperm tend to agglutinate spontaneously with fairly high frequency. This phenomenon is observed in sperm of both fertile and infertile men.

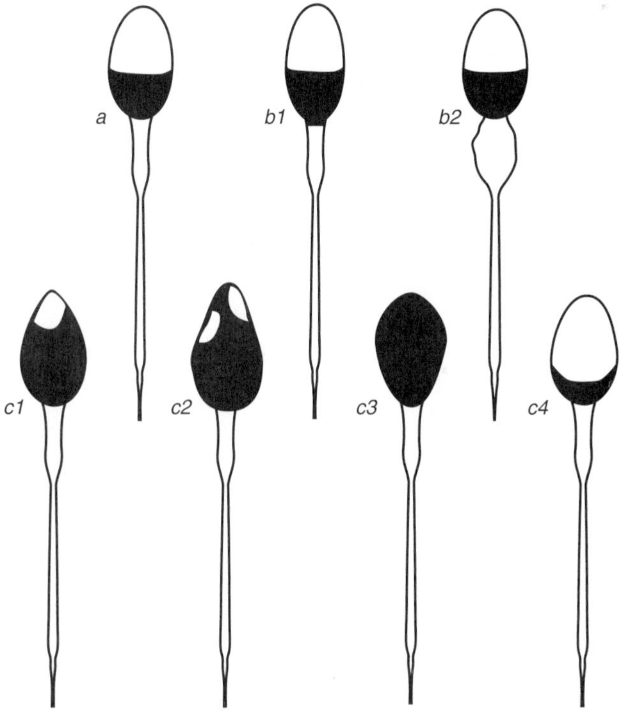

Figure 6-1 Diagrammatic representation of Diff-quick stained spermatozoa. *a*, Normal form. *b*, Slightly amorphous forms: *1*, head slightly elongated, loss of oval shape, *2*, thick neck but normal-shaped head. *c*, Severely amorphous forms: *1* and *2*, abnormally small acrosome; *3*, no acrosome; *4*, acrosome greater than 70% of head. (From Seaman E, Bar-Chama N, Fisch H: Semen analysis in the clinical evaluation of infertility. In Carson CC III, Cooner WH, editors: *Mediguide to urology*, New York, 1994, Lawrence DellaCorte Publications.)

- (e) Agglutination can occur with exposure of sperm to the following:
  - (i) Infection
  - (ii) Fungi
  - (iii) Antibodies
  - (iv) Steroids: testosterone → tail to tail agglutination; progesterone → head to head agglutination
- (f) The severity of agglutination can be approximated as follows:
  - (i) + = fewer than 33% of sperm agglutinated
  - (ii) ++ = 33% to 66% of sperm agglutinated
  - (iii) +++ = greater than 66% of sperm agglutinated

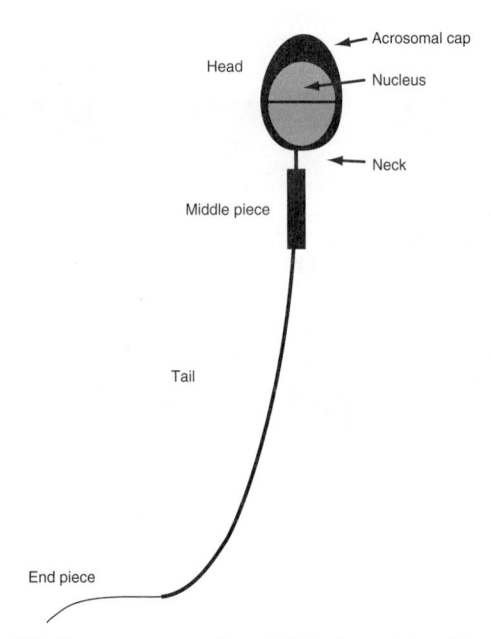

162   Practical Guide to the Care of the Gynecologic/Obstetric Patient

Figure 6-2 Basic components and morphologic characteristics of the normal spermatozoa. Note the following normal characteristics: oval-shaped head with regular outline; acrosomal cap covering greater than ⅓ of head surface; head length between 3 and 5 μm; head width between 2 and 3 μm; width must be between ½ and ⅔ of length; middle piece less than ⅓ width of head, 7 to 8 μm long; and tail is uncoiled and at least 45 μm in length. (From Gilbert BR, Cooper GW, Goldstein M: Semen analysis in the evaluation of male factor subfertility. In *AUA update 1992*, vol 11 no. 32, Houston, 1992, American Urological Association, pp. 250-255.)

- (g) Furthermore, clinicians should endeavor to describe the nature of the agglutination (i.e., head to head, etc.).
- (10) Antibody-agglutination testing (Box 6-3) should be done for the following[3]:
  - (a) Agglutination of spermatozoa
  - (b) Agglutination of motile dimers
  - (c) Idiopathic infertility
  - (d) Abnormal postcoital tests
  - (e) Historical factors that increase the risk of antibody formation:

Vasectomy	Testicular biopsy
Infection	Trauma
Obstruction	Torsion
Cryptorchidism	Cancer
Varicocele	Genetic predisposition

> BOX 6-3 Tests for Agglutination and Antisperm Antibody[2,4,6]
>
> 1. Gel agglutination test (Kibrick): detects IgG or IgM
> 2. Sperm microagglutination test (Franklin-Dukes): detects clumping of motile sperm (>10% is considered positive for sperm antibodies); IgG, IgM, IgA
> 3. Sperm immobilization test (Isojima/SIT): detects those antibodies that interact with the surface of sperm, are complement dependent, and cause sperm immobilization; IgM and IgG; IgA does not activate complement
> 4. Mixed agglutination reaction (MAR test): detects IgA and IgG
> 5. Immunobead test: detects IgG and IgA
> 6. Indirect immunofluorescence: detects IgG and IgA
> 7. Sperm–cervical mucus contact test (SCMC or Kremer): IgA and occasionally IgG within cervical mucus
> 8. Spermocytotoxicity tests: detect IgM and IgG
> 9. Enzyme-linked assay (ELISA)

(11) Cellular components of semen.
  (a) White blood cells (WBCs) and pyospermia
    (i) White blood cells are present in small numbers in normal semen. As a general guide, the normal ejaculate should not contain more than 5 to 10 WBCs per HPF.
    (ii) An abnormal number of WBCs in the semen is called pyospermia. The presence of WBCs lying together in aggregates is diagnostic of infection. Any sample demonstrating these findings must be cultured.
    (iii) Increased numbers of WBCs in the semen may also be the result of prostatic abnormalities.
    (iv) The four main sites for infection in the male genital tract are: epididymis, seminal vesicles, prostate, and urethra and periurethral glands. By doing split ejaculate analysis and culture, the site of infection can be localized using the physiology of the emission and ejaculation process[4]:
    Emission: derived from the accessory or periurethral glands.
    Ejaculation: The first part of the ejaculate derives from the testicular component, followed by secretions from the prostate; the last part derives from the seminal vesicles.
    (v) Another method for detecting infection in the prostate is prostatic massage for expressed prostatic

secretions (EPS). The sample can be examined under the microscope as well as sent for culture. A microscopic count of ± greater than or equal to 10 WBCs per HPF is indicative of prostatitis.[4]

(vi) Infection alters semen quality in the following ways: Ductal damage with resultant obstruction, interference with accessory gland secretion, and impaired motility of spermatozoa.

(vii) The most common organisms associated with pyospermia are as follows[4]:

Escherichia coli	*Mycobacterium tuberculosis*
Enterococci	*Chlamydia trachomatis*
Staphylococci	*Trichomonas vaginalis*
Neisseria gonorrheae	*Candida albicans*
Mycoplasmas	Viruses

(b) Epithelial cells
(c) Red blood cells
  (i) Hematospermia
  (ii) Can be a manifestation of infection and malignant disease or can be idiopathic
(d) Germ cells
  (i) Germ cells are generally considered normal in the semen.
  (ii) The exact number of these immature cells felt to be abnormal has yet to be defined.
(e) Lymphocytes
(f) Particulate matter
  (i) Spermine crystals
  (ii) Prostatic calculi

e. Tests of sperm function[3]: Of the many tests of sperm function available, none unequivocally identify functional spermatozoa. These tests are not performed as a matter of routine examination of the subfertile male. They are highly selective.
  (1) Sperm penetration assay (SPA): This test uses the golden hamster egg, which is unusual in that removal of its zona pellucida results in loss of all species specificity to egg penetration. It is used to yield information relative to sperm fertilization potential.
    (a) The SPA measures are as follows:
      (i) Capacitation
      (ii) The acrosome reaction
      (iii) Sperm oolemma fusion
      (iv) Sperm incorporation into the ooplasm
      (v) Decondensation of chromatin
    (b) The SPA *does not* test for the following:
      (i) Penetration of the zona pellucida
      (ii) Normal embryonic development
    (c) The *positive* SPA test cannot therefore do the following:
      (i) Guarantee fertilization of intact human eggs

(ii) Guarantee embryonic development of fertilized human eggs
- (d) The *negative* SPA test has not been found to correlate with poor fertilization in human IVF.
- (2) The acrosin assay: This test measures acrosin, which is thought to be responsible for penetration of the zona pellucida and for triggering the acrosome reaction.
- (3) The hemizona assay.
  - (a) This test measures the binding of sperm to the zona pellucida of human eggs.
  - (b) In the human hemizona assay, unfertilized oocytes obtained through donation are bisected and the number of sperm tightly bound to the outer surface is counted.
  - (c) The major advantages are as follows:
    - (i) Using the two halves of the hemizona allows for controlled comparisons of binding.
    - (ii) The limited number of human oocytes is amplified.
  - (d) The results of this test show good correlation with Kruger "strict" morphology criteria and IVF fertilization rates.
- (4) The hypoosmotic swelling test.
  - (a) This test measures the membrane integrity of sperm, important for metabolism but also for the successful union of male and female gametes.
  - (b) When viable sperm are exposed to hypoosmotic conditions, water enters the sperm, resulting in swelling. This places the tail fibers under tension, causing curling of the tails.
- (5) Cervical mucus penetration.
  - (a) This test quantitates the sperm–mucus interaction and yields information regarding the motility of the spermatozoa.
  - (b) The PCT is done at midcycle when the cervical mucus is less of a barrier to sperm. A good PCT done within 12 hours after coitus is defined as greater than 10 motile sperm per HPF.
  - (c) Female factors affecting the PCT are as follows:
    - (i) Inadequate estrogen priming
    - (ii) Deficient endocervical tissue
    - (iii) Previous surgery to the cervix
  - (d) Male factors affecting the PCT are as follows:
    - (i) Anatomical abnormality (i.e., hypospadias, resulting in inadequate delivery of sperm)
    - (ii) Oligozoospermia
    - (iii) Asthenozoospermia
    - (iv) Antibodies

REFERENCES

1. Gangi GR, Nagler HM: Clinical evaluation of the subfertile man, *Infertil Reprod Med Clin North Am* 3:299, 1992.
2. World Health Organization: *WHO laboratory manual for the examination of human semen and sperm-cervical mucus interaction*, Cambridge, England, 1992, Cambridge University Press.

3. Gilbert BR, Cooper GW, Goldstein M: Semen analysis in the evaluation of male factor subfertility. In AUA *update 1992*, vol 11 no. 32, Houston, 1992, American Urological Association, pp. 250-255.
4. Jequier A, Crich J: *Semen analysis: A practical guide*, St. Louis, 1986, Blackwell Mosby Book Company.
5. Seaman E, Bar-Chama N, Fisch H: Semen analysis in the clinical evaluation of infertility. In Carson CC III, Cooner WH, editors: *Mediguide to urology*, New York, 1994, Lawrence DellaCorte Publications.
6. Spark RF: *The infertile male: The clinician's guide to diagnosis and treatment*, New York, 1988, Plenum.
7. Kruger TF et al: Predictive value of abnormal sperm morphology in in vitro fertilization, *Fertil Steril* 49:112, 1988.

Amenorrhea

Ivan D'Souza

Amenorrhea is defined as the absence of menses for 6 consecutive months. Primary amenorrhea refers to a female who has never menstruated. Secondary amenorrhea is the cessation of menses after previous normal menses.

7.1 Classification

The classification of amenorrhea is given in Box 7-1.

1. Physiologic amenorrhea
   a. Physiologic amenorrhea can occur shortly after menarche, during pregnancy and lactation, and after menopause.
   b. All states except pregnancy are associated with a hypoestrogenic state with all the attendant clinical ramifications.
   c. Confirmation is with pregnancy test and pelvic examination.
2. Primary amenorrhea
   a. Absence of menses after age 16 indicates primary amenorrhea.
   b. Absence of pubertal development before age 14 may also indicate gonadal dysfunction.
   c. Gonadal abnormalities
      (1) Of patients with primary amenorrhea, 60% have gonadal abnormalities:
         (a) Failure of gonadal differentiation
         (b) Inappropriate gonadal function during fetal and neonatal life; usually results in abnormal external genitalia
      (2) Up to one third of primary amenorrhea patients may be genetic males.
      (3) If a Y chromosome is present in dysgenic gonads, the gonads need to be removed for prophylaxis against malignant degeneration. Karyotyping is therefore an important part of the workup.
      (4) Gonadal dysgenesis (Turner's syndrome).
         (a) 1:2700 of newborn phenotypic females
         (b) Karyotypes: 45X, 45X/46XX, 45X/46XY
         (c) Clinical features are as follows:
            (i) Short stature (< 150 cm)
            (ii) Webbed neck
            (iii) Shield chest
            (iv) High-arched palate

> BOX 7-1 The Classification of Amenorrhea

Physiologic

Pathologic

PRIMARY:

Gonadal abnormalities
  Gonadal dysgenesis (Turner's syndrome)
  Pure gonadal dysgenesis
  XY gonadal dysgenesis (Swyer's syndrome)
  Mixed gonadal dysgenesis
  Ovarian insensitivity syndrome (Savage syndrome)
  17-OH deficiency
Extragonadal abnormalities
  Congenital anatomic defect of genital tract
  Male pseudohermaphroditism
  Female pseudohermaphroditism
  Abnormal hypothalamic–pituitary function

SECONDARY WITH THE FOLLOWING:

Normal ovarian function
Increased gonadotrophins
Normal or decreased gonadotrophins
  Psychogenic
  Weight related
  Exercise induced
  Pseudocyesis
  Postpill
  Central nervous system lesions
  Endocrinopathies
  Drug induced
  Acute or chronic illness
  Estrogen-producing tumors
Androgen excess

(v) Neck hairline low
(vi) Cubitus vulgus
(vii) CVS and renal abnormalities
(viii) Gonads replaced by streaks of fibrous tissue in stroma without germ cells
(ix) May have transient ovarian function if mosaic with 46XX; therefore variable sexual maturation

(5) Pure gonadal dysgenesis (all sexually immature).
  (a) Height greater than 150 cm
  (b) Karyotyp 46XX or 46XY
  (c) Streak gonads

- (d) Increased incidence in siblings
- (e) Higher incidence of Y chromosome presence than in Turner's syndrome
- (6) XY gonadal dysgenesis (Swyer's syndrome).
  - (a) Phenotypic females; normal female external and internal genitalia
  - (b) Karyotype XY
  - (c) Streak gonads; high incidence of malignant degeneration
- (7) Mixed gonadal genesis (rare).
  - (a) Germ cell tumor or testis on one side and streak or no gonad on the other
  - (b) Abnormal external genitalia with pubertal virilization
  - (c) Y gonad: should be removed immediately
- (8) Ovarian insensitivity syndrome (Savage syndrome).
  - (a) Phenotypic females, normal external and internal genitalia, and normal appearing ovaries
  - (b) Functional ovarian failure resulting from possible receptor defect that makes them unresponsive to gonadotrophins
- (9) 17-OH deficiency: unable to synthesize androgens, estrogens, and some adrenal steroids
  - (a) Infantile external genitalia
  - (b) Hypertension, hypokalemic alkalosis
  - (c) Increased desoxycorticosterone, follicle stimulating hormone (FSH), luteinizing hormone (LH), and progesterone
  - (d) Ovarian function: cannot be restored

d. Extragonadal anomalies account for 40% of primary amenorrhea. There is normal ovarian functional capacity.
  - (1) Congenital anatomic defect of the genital tract
    - (a) Failure of normal Müllerian or urogenital sinus differentiation may lead to outlet obstruction or uterine agenesis.
    - (b) Phenotypic and genotypic females with normal external genitalia.
    - (c) Congenital absence of uterus and upper vagina is the most common defect (Mayer-Rokitansky-Kuster-Hauser syndrome). Incidence is 1:4000 female births. There is an association with renal abnormalities.
    - (d) Imperforate hymen or agenesis or stenosis of the proximal vagina, distal vagina, or cervix and transverse septa of the vagina are also contributing causes.
    - (e) Outlet obstruction results in retained menses with subsequent cyclic pain, hematocolpos, hematometra, and endometriosis.
    - (f) Physical examination and ultrasound will often make the diagnosis. Intravenous pyelogram (IVP) should be ordered.
    - (g) Surgical correction of the lower tract is often possible and should be done as soon as possible.
  - (2) Male pseudohermaphroditism
    - (a) Male pseudohermaphroditism results from inadequate androgenic influence on the development of external genitalia in a genetic male.

(b) Androgen insensitivity syndrome or testicular feminization (absence of testosterone receptors) is the most common cause. Clinical features include the following:
   (i) Normal external genitalia
   (ii) Blind vagina
   (iii) Absent uterus
   (iv) Scant pubic or axillary hair
   (v) Normal breasts with immature, pale areolae
   (vi) Often inguinal testis
(c) Testosterone levels are in the normal male range with normal gonadotrophins.
(d) Incomplete forms result from the presence of some functional androgen.
   (i) Chromosomal abnormalities are often found. The spectrum varies from almost normal males with minor abnormalities of the external genitalia to almost normal females with Turner's syndrome manifestations.
   (ii) Causes include chromosomal mosaicism (45X and a cell line with a Y chromosome).
   (iii) Enzymatic anomalies if steroid production with androgen overproduction, incomplete androgen insensitivity syndrome, hypospadias, multiple malformation syndromes, Müllerian derivative persistence, agonadia, and Leydig cell agenesis.
   (iv) Breast development must always raise the suspicion of an estrogen-producing tumor.

(3) Female pseudohermaphroditism
   (a) Female pseudohermaphroditism results from anomalous production of androgen in genetic females.
   (b) Congenital adrenal hyperplasia is the most common cause, usually secondary to 21-hydroxylase or 11-beta-hydroxylase deficiency. Incomplete forms may manifest as amenorrhea in virilized females. Adequate treatment results in normal menses.
   (c) Androgen-producing tumors of the adrenals and ovaries can also result in virilization of external genitalia and amenorrhea.

(4) Hypothalamic–pituitary dysfunction
   (a) Destruction or abnormal development of the hypothalamus or anterior pituitary would result in hypogonadotrophic hypogonadism.
   (b) Craniopharyngiomas are the most common destructive lesion in this area, but primary and metastatic lesions need to be ruled out if this diagnosis is being considered. These are uncommon causes of primary amenorrhea.
   (c) Kallmann's syndrome: isolated gonadotrophin deficiency with anosmia.

7.2 Clinical Assessment

1. History
   a. Intrauterine environment to rule out teratogen
   b. Chronologic pubertal development, including growth spurt, pubarche, and thelarche
   c. Dietary habits or preferences, body weight perception and changes, psychosocial stress
   d. Family history: pubertal delay, menstrual patterns
   e. Social skills, school achievement
2. Physical examination
   a. External genitalia maturity, virilization, pubic hair distribution
   b. Internal genitalia, inguinal hernial sites
   c. Pubertal features: degree of pubic hair and breast development, galactorrhea
   d. Skin: consistency, acne, hair distribution, bruising and pigmentation
   e. Growth: height and weight
   f. Thyroid
3. Diagnostic procedures (Fig. 7-1)
   a. Ultrasound may be used to assess internal genitalia when office examination is difficult. It will also rule out flow-tract abnormalities and assess adnexal status.
   b. Progesterone withdrawal: Provera 10 mg PO for 5 days (or 100 mg progesterone in oil); bleeding within 1 week indicates significant endogenous estrogen and normal outflow tract and a likely diagnosis of anovulation.
   c. Karyotyping (or buccal smear chromatin) should be ordered, and if necessary human Y antigen assay (occasionally leukocyte karyotyping does not detect all forms of mosaicism).
   d. FSH + LH (high levels = ovarian failure), thyroid-stimulating hormone (TSH), and prolactin are frequently also needed and can be used to assess pituitary status.
   e. Ambiguous genitalia.
      (1) With Y chromosome presence, a gonadal biopsy is needed (differential diagnosis male pseudohermaphrodite, mixed gonadal dysgenesis, or true hermaphrodite).
      (2) Without Y chromosome, consider virilizing tumors or 17-hydroxylase deficiency (late onset may require ACTH stimulation test).
   f. Elevated prolactin (> 50 ng/mL) warrants magnetic resonance imaging (MRI) or a computed tomography (CT) scan.
4. Treatment
   a. The cause should be treated if possible (i.e., dexamethasone for 17-OH deficiency).
   b. Phenotypic status should be attained with plastic surgery (i.e., clitoral recession for clitoromegaly and neovagina for blind nonfunctional vaginal pouches).
   c. Fertility should be achieved when possible and desired (i.e., parlodel for pituitary microadenomas, gonadotrophins for Kallmann's

7—Amenorrhea

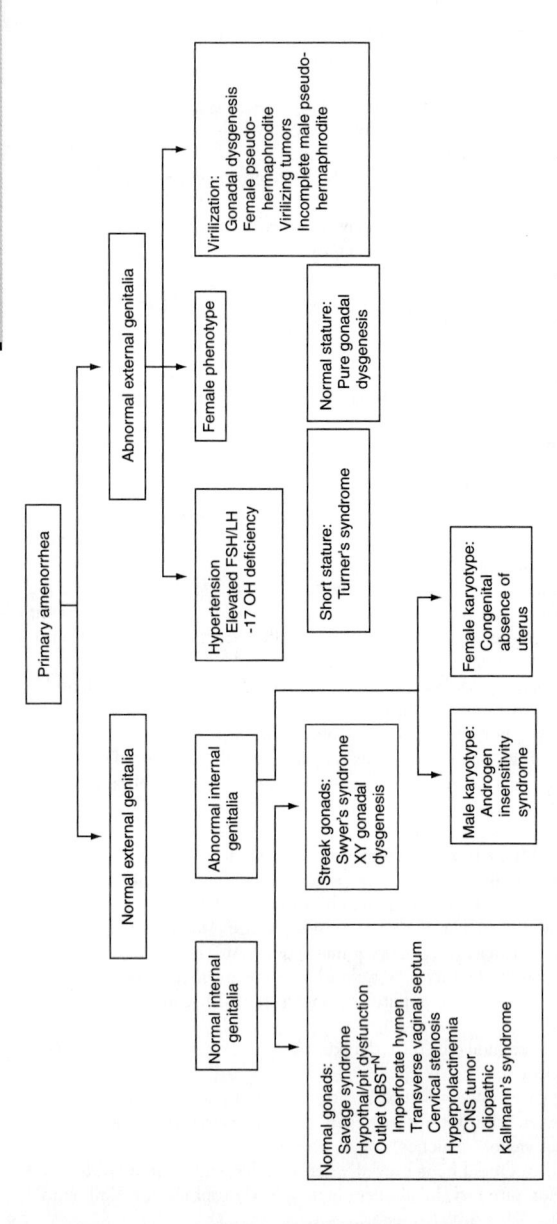

Figure 7-1 Steps in the assessment of primary amenorrhea. *CNS*, Central nervous system; *FSH*, follicle stimulating hormone; *LH*, luteinizing hormone; *OBST*, obstruction.

Primary amenorrhea

- **Normal external genitalia**
  - **Normal internal genitalia**
    - Normal gonads:
      - Savage syndrome
      - Hypothal/pit dysfunction
      - Outlet OBST
      - Imperforate hymen
      - Transverse vaginal septum
      - Cervical stenosis
      - Hyperprolactinemia
      - CNS tumor
      - Idiopathic
      - Kallmann's syndrome
  - **Abnormal internal genitalia**
    - Streak gonads: Swyer's syndrome XY gonadal dysgenesis
    - Male karyotype: Androgen insensitivity syndrome
    - Female karyotype: Congenital absence of uterus
- **Abnormal external genitalia**
  - Hypertension Elevated FSH/LH -17 OH deficiency
  - Short stature: Turner's syndrome
  - **Female phenotype**
    - Normal stature: Pure gonadal dysgenesis
  - Virilization:
    - Gonadal dysgenesis
    - Female pseudohermaphrodite
    - Virilizing tumors
    - Incomplete male pseudohermaphrodite

syndrome, in vitro fertilization for vaginal agenesis, donor eggs for gonadal dysgenesis, etc.).
   d. Excision of gonads in Y chromosome–positive individuals should be performed because of the increased risk of germ cell tumors. In testicular feminization, surgeons should wait until after puberty to allow normal long bone development. In others, surgery should occur before puberty to minimize risk of malignancy and virilization.
   e. Estrogen replacement therapy can be used for hypoestrogenic states.

7.3 Secondary Amenorrhea

Secondary amenorrhea is defined as the absence of menses for 6 months in a female who has had previous normal menstrual function.

CLASSIFICATION

The classification of secondary amenorrheas appears in Box 7-2.

1. Functional ovaries.
   a. Asherman's syndrome
      (1) Asherman's syndrome is the result of intrauterine synechiae, usually after curettage in association with endometritis (incomplete abortion or postpartum hemorrhage), but may occur with any operative procedure involving the uterine canal (myomectomy, septum resection, etc.).
      (2) Diagnosis is made by hysteroscopy or, less reliably, by hysterosalpingogram.
      (3) Asherman's syndrome is divided into grades (grade 1, mucosal adhesions, to grade 4, uterine cavity obliteration), which reflect on surgical correctability and subsequent pregnancy rate.
      (4) Degree of menstrual flow or Provera withdrawal bleeding depends on amount of functional endometrium.
      (5) Treatment consists of hysteroscopically directed lysis of adhesions with 90% probability of menstrual return and 35% to 50% pregnancy rate.
   b. Endometrial destruction
      (1) By radiation or by infectious organisms (tuberculosis and schistosomiasis).
      (2) Uterine cavity may be maintained but is replaced by nonfunctional epithelium.
2. Hypergonadotrophic amenorrhea.
   a. FSH and LH are increased and estrogen levels are low.
   b. Ten percent of secondary amenorrheas are caused by premature ovarian failure (menopause before age 40).
   c. It is associated with autoimmune disease, especially hypothyroidism.
   d. Antiovarian antibodies are present in 30% to 50%.
   e. Other causes include radiotherapy, chemotherapy (especially alkylating agents), chromosomal abnormalities, galactosemia, and postadnexal surgery.
   f. Reports of spontaneous remission and pregnancy are found in the literature, but the condition is usually irreversible.

> **BOX 7-2 The Classification of Secondary Amenorrheas**
>
> ### Functional Ovaries
>
> Asherman's syndrome
> Endometrial destruction
>   Infectious
>   Iatrogenic
>
> ### Hypergonadotrophic
>
> Premature ovarian failure
> Iatrogenic ovarian failure
>
> ### Eugonadotrophic
>
> Hypothalamic–pituitary dysfunction
>   Psychogenic
>   Nutritional
>   Eating disorders
>   Starvation
>   Exercise induced
>   Pseudocyesis
>   Central nervous system lesions
>   Nongonadal endocrinopathy
>   Pharmacologic
>   Acute and chronic disease
>   Idiopathic
> Central nervous system disease
> Feminizing ovarian tumors
>
> ### Androgen Excess
>
> Polycystic ovarian disease
> Masculinizing ovarian tumors

g. In vitro pregnancy with donor eggs or zygotes is an option for those requesting pregnancy.
3. Eugonadotrophic amenorrhea.
    a. The majority of patients with secondary amenorrhea have eugonadotrophic amenorrhea.
    b. Hypothalamic–pituitary dysfunction is the most common cause but is a diagnosis of exclusion.
    c. Mechanism is likely a slowing of the hypothalamic gonadotropin-releasing hormone (GnRH) pulse generator with increased CRF (corticotropin), growth hormone, and nocturnal melatonin.
    d. There is a blunted response to GnRH stimulation.
    e. Prognosis is usually good if the underlying cause is treatable.
        (1) Psychogenic amenorrhea.

(a) Increased CRF leads to decreased GnRH and therefore decreased LH.
(b) The cause may be acute or chronic stress.
(c) Treatment includes the following:
   (i) Stress management
   (ii) Antidepressants
   (iii) Psychopharmaceutical
   (iv) Estrogen replacement
   (v) If necessary, ovulation induction
(2) Weight loss–induced amenorrhea.
   (a) A minimum of 17% body fat is required for menarche.
   (b) Menstrual maintenance requires 22% body fat, but body fat is not the only determinant.
   (c) Anorexia nervosa is an extreme example and is associated with increased conversion of estradiol to catecholestrogens, which suppresses the hypothalamus.
   (d) Treatment includes the following:
      (i) Dietary counseling
      (ii) Behavior modification
      (iii) Estrogen replacement
      (iv) Ovulation induction (should be carried out only after careful consideration of underlying pathology)
(3) Exercise-induced amenorrhea.
   (a) A combination of stress, weight loss, loss of body fat, and dietary control causes this.
   (b) Individuals' responses of CRF axis exercise intensity are important variables.
   (c) No consistent relationship to endogenous opiates exists.
   (d) Bone loss has been documented in amenorrheic athletes.
   (e) Treatment includes the following:
      (i) Decreasing exercise
      (ii) Increasing body fat
      (iii) Estrogen replacement
      (iv) Pregnancy counseling (should be carried out before ovulation induction)
(4) Pseudocyesis.
   (a) All the symptoms and many of the signs of pregnancy are present.
   (b) Increased pulses of LH and prolactin with normal FSH are seen.
   (c) The LH/FSH ratio is high (> 2).
   (d) Treatment includes counseling and ovulation induction.
(5) Postpill amenorrhea.
   (a) Hypothalamic oversuppression syndrome.
   (b) Postpill amenorrhea occurs in less than 1% of women on the birth control pill (BCP).
   (c) There is no relationship to dose or duration of BCP use.
   (d) Spontaneous recovery may take years.
   (e) Treatment includes ovulation induction or sequential cyclic hormonal replacement.

- (6) Central nervous system (CNS) lesions.
    - (a) These are most often pituitary or parapituitary lesions.
    - (b) Amenorrhea with galactorrhea is a common presentation, but hyperprolactinemia can occur without galactorrhea.
    - (c) Hyperprolactinemia requires a search for a pituitary microadenoma, especially with amenorrhea.
    - (d) Pituitary gummas, nonfunctional pituitary tumors, postpartum ischemia (Sheehan's syndrome), and internal carotid aneurysms can cause pituitary insufficiency and present as amenorrhea.
    - (e) Destructive lesions of the hypothalamus usually have neurologic symptoms preceding the amenorrhea.
    - (f) Treatment requires an accurate diagnosis.
        - (i) Parlodel is the treatment of choice for prolactin-producing pituitary microadenomas.
        - (ii) Radiation or surgery is used for macroadenomas or other microadenomas.
        - (iii) Parlodel use has been shown to shrink the size of pituitary adenomas.
- (7) Amenorrhea with other endocrinopathies.
    - (a) Thyroid dysfunction (usually hyperthyroidism) often presents with amenorrhea.
    - (b) Juvenile diabetes mellitus and adrenocortical dysfunction may also cause amenorrhea.
- (8) Drug-induced amenorrhea.
    - (a) Dopamine antagonists (phenothiazines, metoclopramide, etc.) can cause amenorrhea by elevation of prolactin.
    - (b) Cytotoxic agents, especially alkylating agents, can cause ovarian follicular destruction that is often irreversible. Increased duration of therapy and patient age worsen prognosis.
    - (c) Depo-Provera has been associated with prolonged amenorrhea.
    - (d) Drug addiction has also been associated with amenorrhea.
- (9) Chronic and acute disease: Often caused by nutritional or stress factors, but a variety of metabolic pathways may also be involved. Correction of the underlying disease often results in return of menses.
- (10) Estrogen-producing tumors: These tumors are rare but should be considered if endometrial hyperplasia is noted.

4. Amenorrhea with androgenic excess: The source of androgen may be ovarian or adrenal.
    a. Polycystic ovarian disease
    - (1) This is the main cause of ovarian hyperandrogenic state.
    - (2) Results from altered feedback at hypothalamic level resulting in excessive suppression of FSH. Higher LH levels result in increased androgen production by theca cell layer in developing follicles.
    - (3) Oligomenorrhea, obesity, hirsutism, and infertility are often present.

- (4) Ovaries often have the characteristic smooth, thick, white capsule with multiple small developing follicles. This appearance can also be detected by ultrasound.
- (5) Increased LH/FSH ratio (> 2), increased androstenedione, and free testosterone are present.
- (6) Treatment involves the following:
  - (a) Cyclic progesterone (protection against endometrial hyperplasia)
  - (b) Birth control pills (endometrial protection, suppression of ovarian androgenic production, and increased sex hormone–binding globulin)
  - (c) Ovulation induction
- b. Late-onset congenital hyperplasia
  - (1) It presents with hirsutism and dysfunctional uterine bleeding.
  - (2) Increased frequency is seen in Eastern European Jews and Hispanics.
  - (3) Diagnosis is made by adrenocorticotropic hormone (ACTH) stimulation test.
  - (4) Treatment requires replacement therapy with prednisone or dexamethasone.
- c. Masculinizing ovarian tumors usually have high androgen levels.

DIAGNOSTIC WORKUP

1. Ovulation
   a. If present, indicates unresponsive endometrium.
   b. Suggested by the presence of cyclic events (e.g., mittelschmerz, premenstrual complaints).
   c. Diagnosed by basal body temperature charts, progesterone level, or endometrial biopsy.
2. Estrogenic status
   a. Hypoestrogenic states are associated with osteoporosis regardless of cause.
   b. Suggested by hot flushes and vaginal dryness.
   c. Lack of Provera withdrawal suggests hypoestrogenic state but 10% to 15% of hypoestrogenic females will have some bleeding.
   d. Estradiol is useful only when the estradiol level is high (estrogen tumor).
   e. Vaginal cytology is helpful.
3. Androgen excess
   a. Suggested by oily skin or hair, hirsutism, clitoromegaly, and defeminization
   b. Testosterone (50% ovarian, 50% adrenal), androstenedione (50% ovarian, 50% adrenal), dehydroepiandrosterone (DHEAS) (90% adrenal)
   c. 17-hydroxyprogesterone levels as necessary
4. Pituitary status
   a. Suggested by galactorrhea, visual field defects.
   b. FSH, LH, TSH, and prolactin: necessary for evaluation.

c. Most patients require blood for FSH, LH, TSH, and prolactin.
    (1) A progesterone withdrawal confirms outflow tract integrity and suggests normal endogenous estrogen.
    (2) Absence of bleeding to even sequential estrogen and progesterone necessitates a hysteroscopy or hysterosalpingogram.
d. Testosterone and DHEAS levels are useful when androgenic features are present.
e. GnRH stimulation test will be diagnostic for pituitary failure.
f. CT scans and MRI are necessary with hyperprolactinemia.
g. Counseling is imperative with eating or weight disorders.

TREATMENT MODALITIES

1. Cyclic progesterone (Provera 10 mg or Prometrium 400 mg, for a minimum of 10 days for a minimum of every 2 months) helps protect against the development of endometrial hyperplasia and endometrial carcinoma.
2. BCP.
    a. BCPs are useful when contraception is necessary but also protect against endometrial hyperplasia.
    b. BCPs improve hirsutism (reducing ovarian androgen production and increasing sex hormone–binding globulin that does reduce free androgen).
    c. This is a useful and convenient method of estrogen replacement therapy.
    d. Certain BCPs are not acceptable by athletic organizations because of androgenic activity.
3. Ovulation induction.
    a. Clomiphene citrate: There are increased incidence of symptomatic functional cysts, of multiple pregnancies, and a marginally increased risk of ovarian cancer.
    b. Pulsatile GnRH agonist therapy most closely mimics normal follicular development but is expensive and cumbersome.
    c. Gonadotrophin therapy is involved and expensive, with a higher risk of hyperstimulation, multiple pregnancy, and possibly ovarian carcinoma.
4. Hysteroscopic surgery often allows resumption of menses. Pregnancy rates depend on severity of the adhesions.
5. Prolactin antagonists are treatment of choice in pituitary microadenomas, idiopathic hyperprolactinemia, and pretherapy for macroadenomas (which usually require surgery or targeted radiation).
6. Estrogen therapy should be considered in all cases of hypoestrogenic states.
    a. Tamoxifen can be used in patients with breast cancer.
    b. Small doses of testosterone may improve quality of life and bone status.
7. Egg and zygote donation can be considered if pregnancy is desired in the presence of nonfunctional ovaries.

Abnormal Uterine Bleeding

George T. Danakas
Diane J. Sutter

Abnormal uterine bleeding (AUB) is defined as any bleeding that significantly deviates from the usual menstrual pattern. Normal menstruation varies among women in the amount and duration of blood flow and by the intervals between menstrual cycles. The average range of intervals between cycles is 21 and 35 days; the duration of normal menses is 3 to 7 days; blood lost during a normal cycle varies from 25 to 80 mL.

8.1 Etiology

1. Uterine bleeding can be divided into two major categories: organic and dysfunctional.
2. Dysfunctional uterine bleeding (DUB) is abnormal bleeding from the uterine endometrium that is unrelated to anatomic lesions of the uterus.
   a. In perimenopausal women, hypothalamic-pituitary dysfunction results in less predictable ovulation.
   b. Without adequate progesterone, the endometrium becomes unstable and fragile.
   c. Anovulatory bleeding can often be diagnosed by the patient's history of erratic bleeding that is painless and unpredictable in volume.
   d. If endometrial proliferation or hyperplasia without atypia is found on endometrial biopsy, progestin-based medical management is indicated with follow-up evaluation after 3 to 4 months.
3. Organic causes can be subdivided into systemic disease and reproductive tract disease.
   a. Endometrial polyps and uterine fibroids are very common causes of anatomic conditions causing AUB in the perimenopausal period.
   b. Endometrial atrophy is the most common cause of postmenopausal bleeding.
   c. All postmenopausal bleeding is considered abnormal and needs evaluation.

8.2 Definitions of Abnormal Bleeding

1. Amenorrhea: Absence or abnormal cessation of the menses
2. Hypermenorrhea: Menorrhagia, prolonged or profuse menses
3. Hypomenorrhea: A diminution of the flow or a shortening of the duration of menstruation
4. Menorrhagia: Excessively profuse or prolonged menstruation

5. Metrorrhea: Irregular, acyclic bleeding from the uterus, particularly between periods
6. Menometrorrhagia: Irregular or excessive bleeding during menstruation and between menstrual periods
7. Oligomenorrhea: Scanty menstruation; menses occurring at intervals greater than 35 days
8. Polymenorrhea: The occurrence of menstrual cycles of greater than usual frequency—usually at intervals less than 21 days

8.3 Diagnosis

1. History.
   a. Frequency, duration, and amount of bleeding
   b. Current pregnancy?
   c. Contraceptive history
   d. Systemic diseases (Box 8-1)
   e. List of medications
   f. Any recent surgical or gynecologic surgery

BOX 8-1 Systemic Diseases That Can Cause Abnormal Bleeding

I. Blood Dyscrasia

Thrombocytopenia purpura
von Willebrand's disease
Leukemia
Increased fibrinolysin (endometrium)

II. Hepatic Disease

Impaired synthesis of coagulation factors
Impaired metabolism of sex steroids (i.e., estrogen)
Impaired synthesis of sex hormone–binding globulin

III. Renal Disease

Impaired excretion of estrogens
Obesity

IV. Iatrogenic Causes

Anticoagulants, digitalis, oral contraceptives (breakthrough bleeding), aspirin, intrauterine device (IUD)

V. Endocrine

Hypothyroidism or hyperthyroidism
Diabetes mellitus

Adapted from Copeland LJ: *Textbook of gynecology*, Philadelphia, 1993, Saunders.

2. Physical examination.
   a. A complete physical examination, including a careful pelvic examination, should be performed. There are many anatomic causes of nonuterine bleeding (Box 8-2) and anatomic uterine abnormalities (Box 8-3).
   b. Examination should include the following:
      (1) Thyroid
      (2) Breasts

BOX 8-2 Anatomic Causes of Nonuterine Bleeding

Cervix

Neoplasia (polyps or carcinoma)
Cervicitis
Ectropion and eversion
Ulceration
Condylomatous lesions
Endometriosis

Vagina

Neoplasia (carcinoma, sarcoma)
Adenosis
Trauma
Foreign body
Atrophic vaginitis
Infection (vaginitis)
Condylomas

Vulva

Trauma
Infections or inflammations
Neoplasia
Condylomas
Dystrophy
Varices

Urinary Tract

Urethral caruncle
Urethral diverticulum
Hematuria

Gastrointestinal Tract

Hemorrhoids
Anal fissure
Colorectal lesions

Adapted from Copeland LJ: *Textbook of gynecology*, Philadelphia, 1993, Saunders.

> **BOX 8-3 Anatomic Uterine Abnormalities**
>
> 1. Endometrial hyperplasia
> 2. Endometrial or cervical carcinoma
> 3. Leiomyomas
> 4. Polyps: endometrial and endocervical
> 5. Infections: endometritis, cervicitis, vaginitis
> 6. Foreign bodies (e.g., IUD, tampon)
> 7. Pregnancy abnormalities
> 8. Estrogen-producing ovarian tumors
> 9. Medications: hormone replacement therapy, oral contraceptives (OCs)

    (3) Liver
    (4) Presence or absence of ecchymotic lesions on the skin
    (5) Obesity
    (6) Hirsutism
    (7) Inspection of vulva and vagina
    (8) Inspection and palpation of cervix and uterus
    (9) Determination of the size and shape of uterus
   (10) Palpation of adnexa for mass and to check for ovarian pathology

3. Diagnostic studies: Some of the following may be indicated depending on the history and findings on physical exam.
   a. Hemoglobin and hematocrit
   b. Serum iron level and serum ferritin level
   c. Chemistry profile including liver function tests
   d. Serum human chorionic gonadotropin (HCG)
   e. Thyroid profile
   f. Coagulation profile
   g. Luteal phase progesterone
   h. Prolactin, follicle-stimulating hormone (FSH), luteinizing hormone (LH)
   i. Serum androgens
   j. Stool for occult blood
   k. Urinalysis for hematuria
   l. Papanicolaou smear
   m. Pelvic ultrasound; include measurement of endometrial thickness
   n. Hysterogram or hysteroscopy
   o. Endometrial sampling

8.4 Management

In most patients, abnormal uterine bleeding is a recurrent problem and long-term management depends on correct diagnosis for treatment (see Box 8-3). Systemic and anatomic causes should be managed with their specific treatments.

MEDICAL THERAPY

1. Estrogen-progestin contraceptives
    a. Oral contraceptives containing low doses of estrogen (≤35 μg ethinyl estradiol)
        (1) First-line therapy for healthy, nonsmoking perimenopausal women with AUB
        (2) Variable effectiveness for women with fibroids
    b. Vaginal ring releasing etonogestrel and ethinyl estradiol
2. Continuous progestin-only contraceptives
    a. Depot injection of medroxyprogesterone acetate (Depo-Provera)
    b. Levonorgesterol intrauterine device (IUD) (Mirena)
3. Postmenopausal estrogen plus progestin therapy (EPT) (with sufficient progestin sufficient to inhibit ovulation)
    a. 17beta estradiol 1 mg plus 0.5 mg Norethindrone acetate (Activella)
    b. Ethinyl estradiol 5 μm plus 1 mg Norethindrone acetate (Femhrt)
4. Other therapies
    a. Cyclic oral progestogen alone
    b. Parenteral estrogen
    c. Danazol
    d. Gonadotropin-releasing hormone (GnRH) agonists such as leuprolide acetate (Lupron)

SURGICAL THERAPY

1. Dilation and curettage (D&C)
    a. This surgical procedure is now considered obsolete for the treatment of AUB because it can miss localized disease such as polyps.
    b. D&C does not completely remove intracavitary tissue.
2. Endometrial ablation
    a. Endometrial histologic evaluation should take place before endometrial ablation.
    b. Some approaches do not involve visualization of the endometrial cavity and may not effectively treat AUB caused by anatomic lesions such as submucous fibroids or polyps.
3. Hysterectomy
    a. Used to be the only definitive treatment for AUB.
    b. Postoperative complication rate is approximately 30%.

SUGGESTED READINGS

American College of Obstetricians and Gynecologists: Management of anovulatory bleeding. In *ACOG practice bulletin 2000*, no. 14, Washington, DC, 2000, ACOG.

North American Menopause Society: *Menopause practice: A clinician's guide*, Cleveland, OH, 2006, North American Menopause Society.

Speroff L, Fritz M: *Clinical gynecologic endocrinology and infertility*, ed 7, Baltimore, MD, 2005, Lippincott Williams & Wilkins.

Endometriosis

Ronald E. Batt
Germaine M. Louis

Endometriosis is an extraordinarily complex, enigmatic chronic disease, although some investigators believe that some endometriotic lesions may be physiologic. Clinicians and scientists are unable to predict in which patients the endometriosis will progress to moderate, severe, or extensive disease. While the etiology, pathophysiology, and natural history of endometriosis are being studied, therapeutic trials with a "no-treatment" control arm are essential to discern treatment efficacy.

9.1 Definition

Sampson defined endometriosis as "the presence of ectopic tissue which possesses the histologic structure and function of the uterine mucosa. It also includes the abnormal conditions which may result, not only from the invasion of organs and other structures by this tissue, but from its reaction to menstruation."[16] In light of new immunologic, biochemical, and physiologic findings, this pathologic definition of endometriosis is no longer adequate. A functional definition is needed to reflect prognostic and therapeutic issues.

9.2 Epidemiology

Traditionally, women with endometriosis were reported to be largely white, career-minded women of upper socioeconomic status who voluntarily delayed childbearing. This profile was based largely on convenient samples of women seeking treatment for infertility or pelvic pain associated with endometriosis. These early clinical studies did not fully adjust for biases arising from the selection of cases and other issues pertaining to medical care-seeking behaviors of affected women. More recent evidence suggests that endometriosis affects approximately 10% of women of reproductive age regardless of race, socioeconomic status, or childbearing intentions. Although limited in scope, findings from recent studies suggest that various factors may be associated with an increased or decreased risk of endometriosis, and these are summarized as follows.

PURPORTED RISK FACTORS

1. Reproductive age
   a. Mean age at diagnosis is 25 to 29 years.[2]

Practical Guide to the Care of the Gynecologic/Obstetric Patient 185

    b. Adolescents are more likely to have Müllerian duct anomalies or cervical or vaginal obstruction.[3]
    c. Postmenopausal women are more likely to be on estrogen replacement therapy.[4]
2. Socioeconomic status: suggestion of greater risk for upper socioeconomic status (difference possibly from health care–seeking behaviors)[5]
3. Family history: primarily first-degree relatives (mother, sister, first cousin), although no clear inheritance pattern[6]
4. Menstrual characteristics: shorter cycles (< 27 days), longer flow (> 7 days), and greater menstrual pain[7,8]
5. Somatotype
    a. Weight: peripheral predominance of body fat among affected women under 30 years of age (i.e., risk inversely related to waist-to-hip and waist-to-thigh ratios)[9]
    b. Height: greater risk for tall women (> 166 cm)[10]
6. Reproductive history: history of infertility and impaired fecundity (e.g., spontaneous abortion)[11]

FACTORS DECREASING RISK

1. Strenuous exercise: physical exercise, especially if begun early and practiced regularly[7,10]
2. Cigarette smoking: early and regular use. (Careful interpretation of these preliminary findings is warranted, especially in light of health hazards associated with smoking.)[7,10]

9.3 Theories of Histogenesis

1. General theories include the following:
    a. Coelomic metaplasia
    b. Transplantation of shed endometrium
    c. Direct extension, hematologic, and lymphatic spread
    d. Impaired immune system
2. Special theory of histogenesis to explain endometriosis in peritoneal pockets.
    a. Embryologic rudimentary duplication Müllerian ducts[12]

9.4 Clinical Manifestations[13]

ENDOMETRIOSIS-ASSOCIATED PAIN

1. Acquired dysmenorrhea: possibly as early as third menstrual cycle in adolescents
2. Three or more emergency visits for unexplained pelvic pain
3. Low central backache and lower abdominal pain
4. Midcycle pain: mittelschmerz
5. Deep dyspareunia resulting from endometriosis of uterosacral ligaments and rectovaginal pouch of Douglas
6. Deep dyspareunia, worse before menses
7. Pain with bowel movements before and during menses

ENDOMETRIOSIS-ASSOCIATED INFERTILITY

1. Primary infertility: never pregnant
   a. Affects roughly 41% of women with endometriosis
   b. Monthly fecundity reduced
2. Secondary infertility: previously pregnant
   a. Roughly 35% of women with endometriosis state difficulty conceiving and carrying pregnancy to term.
3. Outcome of first pregnancy before diagnosis of endometriosis
   a. Decreased live births
   b. Increased spontaneous abortions
   c. Increased elective abortions
   d. Infrequent ectopic pregnancies

ENDOMETRIOSIS-ASSOCIATED HEALTH PROBLEMS

1. Profuse, unremitting menorrhagia
   a. Risk of multiple blood transfusions
   b. Risk of pituitary ischemia
   c. Risk of multiorgan hormonal replacement
2. Intractable pelvic pain associated with frozen pelvis
3. Bowel pain or obstruction
4. Ureteral obstruction
   a. Risk of hydroureter and hydronephrosis
   b. Risk of hypertension
   c. Risk of autonephrectomy
   d. Risk of renal failure if obstruction is bilateral
5. Osteoporosis
   a. Risk increased by endometriosis
   b. Risk increased by gonadotropin-releasing hormone (GnRH) ovarian suppression
   c. Risk increased by early bilateral oophorectomy
   d. Risk increased by withholding estrogen replacement
6. Pneumothorax and hemothorax
7. Malignant transformation endometriosis posterior fornix
   a. Risk increased by unopposed estrogen replacement
   b. Risk removed by excising endometriosis

9.5 Physical Examination[13]

1. Inspection by examiner sitting at eye level of cervix
   a. Cervix displaced 1 cm or more lateral to midline
   b. Outflow obstruction favoring retrograde menstruation
      (1) Cervical stenosis
      (2) Imperforate hymen
      (3) Transverse vaginal septum
      (4) Uterine anomaly with blind uterine horn
   c. Tender, fixed angulation of rectum at sigmoidoscopy
2. Palpation: bimanual pelvic, rectovaginal, rectal examination
   a. Tenderness on stretching shortened cardinal ligament
   b. Tender rectovaginal pouch of Douglas

c. Tender uterosacral ligaments
d. Tender nodules in uterosacral ligaments
e. Fixed retroverted uterus

9.6 Tools for Assessment[13]

1. Existing medical records (e.g., office, operative, pathology)
2. History and physical examination
3. Female anatomic grid map to localize pain graphically
4. Color duplex Doppler ultrasound of ovarian cysts
5. *Chlamydia* and *Neisseria* antibody titers
6. Hysterosalpingogram and hysteroscopy (selective)
7. Diagnostic laparoscopy
   a. Systematic inspection of abdomen and pelvis and palpation of suspicious lesions
   b. Photo documentation
   c. Biopsy confirmation
8. American Fertility Society Revised Classification of Endometriosis for pelvic pain and infertility
9. Dictation of operative report immediately after each surgery
10. Intravenous pyelogram (IVP) for ureteral involvement, left-frozen-pelvis, frozen pelvis
11. Sigmoidoscopy for bowel involvement
12. Original staging: benchmark from which to measure the regression, stability, or progression of the disease (as in cancer)
13. Staging: essential to establish early the clinical course of the disease in each patient

9.7 Findings at Laparoscopy[13]

ORGANS AT RISK

1. Common organ involvement corresponds to those organs bathed in pelvic peritoneal fluid.
   a. Bladder
   b. Round ligaments
   c. Uterus
   d. Uterosacral ligaments
   e. Broad ligaments
   f. Ovaries
   g. Fallopian tubes
   h. Lateral pelvic peritoneum
   i. Rectovaginal pouch
   j. Rectum
   k. Sigmoid colon
   l. Cecum
   m. Appendix
   n. Distal ileum
2. Uncommon organ involvement
   a. Episiotomy
   b. Transverse colon

c. Sciatic nerve
   d. Trigone of bladder
   e. Lung
3. Rare organ involvement
   a. Pancreas
   b. Liver
   c. Brain
   d. Skin

ASYMMETRY

1. Anteroposterior asymmetry: Endometriosis is common in the vesicouterine pouch when the uterus is sharply anteverted, and in the rectovaginal pouch when the uterus is retroverted.
2. Lateral asymmetry: Endometriosis tends to be more severe on one side of the pelvis, with sparing or relative sparing of the other side.

INVASION

1. Endometriosis elicits a foreign body reaction, fibrosis, to encapsulate and contain the disease.
2. Deep nodules form in the rectovaginal pouch and uterosacral ligaments.
3. Endometriotic cysts form in the ovaries.

ACUTE AND CHRONIC ENDOMETRIOSIS

1. Acute endometriosis: exhibits red, angry, inflammatory host response to ruptured ovarian endometrioma, or aggressively active disease
2. Chronic endometriosis: exhibits firm, enveloping fibrosis in a quiescent pelvis

PERITONEAL POCKETS WITH ENDOMETRIOSIS

1. Located in broad ligaments and rectovaginal pouch of Douglas
2. Associated medial displacement of ureter(s) in some cases
3. Endometriosis presents as tan brim nodules and spider lesions

9.8 Host Responses to Endometriosis[13]

HYPERTROPHY AND RELAXATION

1. Uterine and ovarian hypertrophy, leiomyomas
2. Relaxation of round, uterosacral, utero-ovarian ligaments
3. Allow uterus and ovaries to adhere to rectovaginal pouch

SCLEROSIS OF SOLID ORGANS

1. Uterine sclerosis
2. Ovarian sclerosis: cartilaginous consistency

STENOSIS TO OCCLUSION OF HOLLOW ORGANS

1. Cervical stenosis
2. Cornual angle fallopian tube obstruction
3. Perifimbrial tubal stenosis
4. Fimbrial tubal phimosis
5. Ureteral stricture, obstruction
6. Bowel stricture, obstruction

INFLAMMATION

1. Retrograde menstruation
2. Ruptured endometriomas
3. Autoimmune changes

ADHESIONS

1. Endometriotic adhesions
2. Surgical adhesions
3. Adhesions from sexually transmitted diseases
4. Adhesions from malignancy

9.9 Disease Patterns[13]

1. Simple disease pattern: corresponds to stages I and II disease
   a. Normal pelvic architecture serves as a platform for subtle and conspicuous endometriotic lesions.
   b. In our referral center, 75% of cases are simple.
      (1) Subtle forms of endometriosis
         (a) Peritoneal pockets with endometriosis (Müllerianosis)
         (b) Nonpigmented peritoneal and ovarian endometriosis
         (c) Slightly enlarged "normal ovary" with deep endometrioma
         (d) Ovarian endometriosis hidden by surface adhesions
         (e) Early bowel endometriosis
      (2) Conspicuous form of endometriosis
         (a) Deeply pigmented peritoneal and ovarian lesions
         (b) Ovarian endometriomas
         (c) Constricting endometriotic lesions of ileum and colon
2. Complex disease patterns: corresponds to stages III and IV
   a. Distorted pelvic architecture: There are thresholds of increased complexity until irreversible damage occurs. The surgeon must understand the evolution and development of complex disease patterns to resolve them successfully by surgery.
   b. In our referral center, 25% of cases are complex.
      (1) Centrifugal pattern: obliterated rectovaginal pouch with rectum and ovaries attached to retroverted uterus
      (2) Left-frozen pelvis: sigmoid colonic adhesions obliterate the left adnexa, which is also densely adherent to left pelvic wall
      (3) Obliterated rectovaginal pouch of Douglas: rectum densely adherent to posterior uterus
      (4) Centripetal pattern: ovaries adherent laterally with or without an obliterated rectovaginal pouch of Douglas
      (5) Complete frozen pelvis

9.10 Complications of Treatment of Complex Disease Patterns

1. Despite meticulous dissection by skilled surgeons, the following complications may occur when operating and reoperating severe and extensive pelvic endometriosis:
   a. Premature menopause

b. Ovarian remnant syndrome
  c. Ligation or severance of a ureter(s)
  d. Ureterovaginal fistula
  e. Vesicovaginal fistula
  f. Rectovaginal fistula
  g. Coloperitoneal fistula with abscess
  h. Bowel obstruction
  i. Sciatic nerve injury
  j. Major arterial or venous injury
2. The risk of such complications may be minimized by the following:
  a. Meticulous preoperative preparation
  b. Mechanical and antibiotic bowel preparation
  c. An experienced operative team
  d. Good surgical exposure
  e. Meticulous operative technique using dissection of retroperitoneal spaces
  f. Ureteral catheters selectively

9.11 Options for Treatment

ENDOMETRIOSIS-ASSOCIATED PAIN[13-16]

The objective is to excise all visible endometriosis and treat with postoperative danocrine or GnRH for 3 months, then maintain the patient with combination oral contraceptive pills such as Orthonovum, 1/35-21 day, cyclically.

1. Stages I and II
  a. Danazol or GnRH in selected cases
  b. Laparoscopic surgery with postoperative danazol or GnRH
  c. Conservative surgery by laparotomy with preoperative danazol
2. Stage III: moderate disease
  a. Laparoscopic surgery with postoperative danazol or GnRH
  b. Conservative surgery by laparotomy with preoperative danazol
3. Stage IV: severe and extensive disease
  a. Conservative surgery by laparotomy with preoperative danazol
  b. Laparoscopic surgery with postoperative medical suppression

ENDOMETRIOSIS-ASSOCIATED INFERTILITY[13-16]

When surgery is indicated, the objective is to excise all visible endometriosis, and then allow the patient to conceive, using assisted reproductive technologies as indicated. Older patients and couples with prolonged infertility should be offered assisted reproductive therapies early.

1. Stages I and II
  a. Expectant treatment selectively
  b. Laparoscopic surgery with excision of endometriosis
  c. Menopausal gonadotropin or human chorionic gonadotropin (HCG) and intrauterine insemination
  d. Gamete intrafallopian transfer (GIFT), in vitro fertilization (IVF), and endotracheal tube (ET)

2. Stage III: moderate disease
   a. Laparoscopic surgery with excision of endometriosis
   b. Conservative surgery by laparotomy with preoperative danazol
   c. Menopausal gonadotropin or HCG and intrauterine insemination
   d. GIFT, IVF, and ET
3. Stage IV: severe and extensive disease
   a. Conservative surgery by laparotomy with preoperative danazol
   b. Laparoscopic surgery selectively
   c. GIFT, IVF, and ET

ENDOMETRIOSIS-ASSOCIATED HEALTH PROBLEMS[13-16]

The objective of treatment is to control symptoms promptly and, where surgery is indicated, to excise all visible endometriosis.

1. Stages I and II
   a. Laparoscopic surgery with postoperative danazol or GnRH
   b. Conservative surgery by laparotomy with preoperative danazol or GnRH
   c. Excision of all endometriosis, hysterectomy with or without bilateral salpingo-oophorectomy (SO)
2. Stage III: moderate disease
   a. Laparoscopic surgery with postoperative danazol or GnRH
   b. Conservative surgery with preoperative danazol or GnRH
   c. Excision of all endometriosis, hysterectomy with or without bilateral
   d. Salpingo-oophorectomy with preoperative danazol or GnRH
3. Stage IV: severe and extensive disease
   a. Conservative surgery with preoperative danazol or GnRH
   b. Excision of all endometriosis, hysterectomy, bilateral salpingo-oophorectomy with postoperative estrogen or estrogen and progesterone hormone replacement (postoperative danazol or GnRH selectively)

SYMPTOMATIC BOWEL ENDOMETRIOSIS[14]

In all cases, sigmoidoscopic examination for tender, fixed angulation of bowel is followed by double contrast barium enema. Selective colonoscopy. Mechanical and antibiotic bowel preparation in all cases. Estrogen hormone replacement therapy in patients without ovaries.

1. Conservative surgery for endometriosis and extraluminal, wedge, or segmental bowel resection
2. Excision of all pelvic endometriosis and hysterectomy with ovarian conservation and extraluminal, wedge, or segmental bowel resection
3. Excision of all pelvic endometriosis and hysterectomy, bilateral salpingo-oophorectomy, and extraluminal, wedge, or segmental bowel resection
4. Partial bowel obstruction
   a. Frozen section to rule out malignancy
   b. Wedge or segmental bowel resection
   c. Primary anastomosis if possible, colostomy if necessary
5. Complete bowel obstruction
   a. Frozen section to rule out malignancy

b. Colostomy to relieve bowel obstruction
c. Secondary bowel resection and closure of colostomy

SYMPTOMATIC URETERAL ENDOMETRIOSIS[13-16]

IVP, sonogram of kidneys, and renal function studies selectively.

1. Ureterolysis or ureterovesical implantation and excision of all pelvic endometriosis
2. Ureterolysis or ureterovesical implantation and excision of all pelvic endometriosis with hysterectomy and ovarian conservation
3. Ureterolysis or ureterovesical implantation and excision of all pelvic endometriosis with hysterectomy, bilateral salpingo-oophorectomy, and hormone replacement therapy
4. Nephrectomy selectively, and appropriate pelvic surgery, dialysis, and kidney transplant selectively

MALIGNANT ENDOMETRIOSIS

Malignant ovarian endometriosis and malignant endometriosis of the posterior vaginal fornix should be treated by a gynecologic oncologist or by appropriate surgery and chemotherapy in consultation with a gynecologic oncologist.

OSTEOPOROSIS

Women with endometriosis are prone to osteoporosis. The object of treatment is removal of all endometriosis followed by estrogen or combined estrogen and progesterone hormone replacement therapy. The importance of excising all endometriosis at surgery cannot be overemphasized, so that patients can receive the benefits of hormonal replacement therapy.

9.12 Physician–Patient Follow-Up from Diagnosis Until Postmenopause

1. Examine periodically.
2. Educate patient.
3. Maintain good physician records.
4. Ensure patient maintains good records also.
5. Minimize retrograde menstruation.
   a. Combination birth control pills cyclically or continuously
   b. Danazol selectively
   c. GnRH selectively
   d. Pregnancy when appropriate
   e. Lactation when desired
   f. Tubal ligation selectively
6. Repeat laparoscopic conservative surgery selectively.
7. Apply new research insights to patient care.

9.13 Overview of Management

1. Patient education to encourage active informed cooperation is a must.
2. The diagnosis should be made early and accurately.
3. The disease should be staged by the most up-to-date classification system.

4. Immediate and long-term treatment options should be discussed with patient.
5. Patient priorities should be respected: pain relief, fertility, health.
6. An appropriate treatment plan should be agreed on.
7. Copy of operative report and pathology reports should go to patient.
8. Endometriosis Association membership should be encouraged.

REFERENCES

1. Olive DL, Haney AF: Endometriosis. In Decherney AH, editor: *Reproductive failure*, New York, 1986, Churchill Livingstone, pp. 153-203.
2. McCann SE et al: Endometriosis and body fat distribution, *Obstet Gynecol* 83:545-549, 1983.
3. Houston DE et al: Evidence for the risk of pelvic endometriosis by age, race and socioeconomic status, *Epidemiol Rev* 6:167-191, 1984.
4. Djursing H, Petersen K, Weberg E: Symptomatic postmenopausal endometriosis, *Acta Obstet Gynecol Scand* 60:529-530, 1981.
5. Goldman MB, Cramer DW: The epidemiology of endometriosis. In Chadra DR, Buttram VC Jr, editors: *Current concepts in endometriosis*, New York, 1990, Alan R. Liss.
6. Hulka JF, Reich H: *Textbook of laparoscopy*, ed 2, Philadelphia, 1994, WB Saunders.
7. Cramer DW et al: The relation of endometriosis to menstrual characteristics, smoking and exercise, *JAMA* 255:1904-1908, 1986.
8. Darrow SL et al: Menstrual cycle characteristics and risk of endometriosis, *Epidemiology* 4:135-142, 1993.
9. Malinak LR, Wheeler JM: Endometriosis. In Aiman J, editor: *Infertility: diagnosis and management*, New York, 1984, Springer-Verlag, pp. 255-275.
10. Godlee F: Endomertrisis, *Clinical Evidence*, BMJ Publishing Group, 2006.
11. Darrow SL et al: Sexual activity, contraception, and reproductive factors in predicting endometriosis, *Am J Epidemiol* 140:500-509, 1994.
12. Batt RE et al: A case-series study of peritoneal pockets and endometriosis: Rudimentary duplications of the Müllerian system, *Adoles Pediatr Gynecol* 2:47-56, 1989.
13. Batt RE, Wheeler JM: Endometriosis: Advanced diagnostic laparoscopy. In Hunt RB, editor: *Atlas of female infertility surgery*, ed 2, St. Louis, 1992, Mosby–Year Book.
14. Batt RE, Udagawa SM, Wheeler JM: Endometriosis: microconservative surgery. In Hunt RB, editor: *Atlas of female infertility surgery*, ed 2, St. Louis, 1992, Mosby–Year Book, pp. 454-481.
15. Huffman JW: Endometriosis in young teenage girls, *Pediatr Ann* 10:44-49, 1981.
16. Sampson JA: The development of the implantation theory for the origin of peritoneal endometriosis, *Am J Obstet Gynecol* 40:549, 1940.

Gynecologic Infections

D. Michael Slate II
Lawrence J. Gugino

10.1 Gonorrhea

ETIOLOGY

Neisseria gonorrhoeae, a gram-negative diplococcus, is the causative agent for this disease.

1. Incidence
   a. Has been decreasing since 1975; fewer than 119 cases/100,000 in 2003.
   b. Most commonly reported communicable disease in United States; more than 330,000 reported cases in 2003, which represents approximately one half of new infections.
2. Prevalence
   a. Urban sexually transmitted disease (STD) clinics, 10% to 30% of cases.
   b. Female family planning clinics, 0.5% to 5% of cases.
   c. Female private doctor's office, 0% to 2% of cases.
   d. Of all female infections, 75% occur in age group 15 to 24 years.
3. Transmission
   a. By sexual contact
   b. Most efficiently by vaginal or anal intercourse
   c. Risk
      (1) Male to female: 80% to 90%
      (2) Female to male: 20% to 25%
4. Risk markers
   a. Homosexual male: 10 times greater incidence
   b. Unmarried
   c. Urban residence
   d. Lower socioeconomic status
   e. Illicit drug use
   f. Prostitution
   g. Previous gonorrhea
   h. No contraception or use of nonbarrier methods
   i. Nonwhite race
5. Incubation period
   a. Short
   b. Urethritis, 2 to 5 days
   c. Cervicitis, 5 to 10 days

SIGNS AND SYMPTOMS

1. Ten percent of males and 20% to 40% of females are asymptomatic.
2. Uncomplicated anogenital female: Endocervix, urethra, Skene's gland, Bartholin's gland, and anus sites may be infected.
3. Common symptoms.
   a. Urethral or vaginal discharge.
   b. Dysuria, abnormal bleeding.
   c. Mucopurulent endocervical exudates.
   d. Nongenital symptoms may result from direct or contiguous spread and bloodstream dissemination.
      (1) Pelvic inflammatory disease (PID) occurs in 15% to 20% of women with uncomplicated anogenital gonorrhea.
      (2) Anorectal infection: 30% to 40% of patients with positive endocervical gonorrhea culture (GC) will have positive anorectal cultures.
      (3) Perihepatitis (Fitz-Hugh–Curtis syndrome) may occur.
      (4) Conjunctivitis may occur as well.
      (5) Pharyngitis occurs in 10% to 20% of women with genital tract gonorrhea; it is most often asymptomatic.
   e. Disseminated gonorrhea occurs when an infection of the genital tract, pharynx, or rectum invades the bloodstream.
      (1) Prevalence: 0.1% to 0.3% of total gonorrhea
      (2) The disease's two stages are as follows:
         (a) Bacteremia
            (i) Chills
            (ii) Fever 38° to 39° C
            (iii) Skin lesions: erythematous macules 1 to 5 mm in diameter located on extremities secondary to gonococcal emboli
            (iv) Positive blood cultures in 50%
            (v) Endocarditis or meningitis may ensue
         (b) Septic arthritis
            (i) Purulent synovial effusion
            (ii) Knees, ankles, and wrists: erythema, edema, and pain
            (iii) Negative blood cultures

GONOCOCCAL INFECTION IN PREGNANCY

1. Perinatal implications.
   a. Postabortal endometritis and salpingitis
   b. Acute salpingitis in pregnancy
      (1) Very rare and difficult to diagnose
      (2) Occurs in first trimester
2. Perinatal complications.
   a. Increased incidence of premature rupture of membranes
   b. Preterm delivery
   c. Chorioamniotis
   d. Neonatal sepsis
   e. Postpartum sepsis
   f. Neonatal conjunctivitis in 30% to 40%

3. All pregnant patients should be screened for *N. gonorrhoeae* at initial prenatal visit. The test should be repeated early in the third trimester.

LABORATORY DIAGNOSIS

1. Gram-stain exudate
   a. Polymorphonuclear leukocytes (PMNs) intracellular gram-negative diplococci
   b. Diagnostic 90% male, 60% female
   c. Not useful for pharyngeal infection
2. Culture
   a. Isolation of organism in selective media (Thayer-Martin) is the gold standard.
   b. Culture detects 80% to 90% cervical, rectal, and pharyngeal infections.
   c. Culture all symptomatic sites: Recovery of *N. gonorrhoeae* is improved by two consecutive endocervical specimens or combination endocervical and anal specimens.
3. Other tests: antigen detection (gonozyme)
   a. Polymerase chain reaction (PCR)–based tests (Gen-probe)—becoming gold standard of testing
   b. Unable to measure antimicrobial susceptibility

TREATMENT OF UNCOMPLICATED ANOGENITAL GONORRHEA

1. Of gonococcal strains in the United States, 15% to 50% have a relative or absolute resistance to penicillin (PCN) or tetracycline (TCN).
2. 2002 Centers for Disease Control and Prevention (CDC) guidelines.
   a. Ceftriaxone, 125 mg intramuscular (IM), single dose
   b. Cefixime, 400 mg orally (PO), single dose
   c. Ciprofloxacin, 500 mg PO, single dose
   d. Ofloxacin, 400 mg PO, single dose
   e. Levofloxacin, 250 mg PO, single dose
   f. Treatment for coinfection with *Chlamydia trachomatis* add:
      (1) Azithromycin, 1 g PO, single dose, *or*
      (2) Doxycycline, 100 mg PO, bid × 7 days

TREATMENT OF DISSEMINATED GONORRHEA

1. 2002 CDC guildelines: Ceftriaxone, 1 g IM or intravenous (IV), q24h
2. Alternative initial regimens
   a. Cefotaxime, 1 g IV, q8h
   b. Ceftizoxime, 1 g IV, q8h
   c. Ofloxacin, 400 mg IV, q12h
   d. Levofloxacin, 250 mg IV, qd
3. β-Lactam allergic persons
   a. Spectinomycin, 2 g IM, q12h
   b. Continue all regimens for 24 to 48 hours after improvement, then switch to one of the following regimens to complete a full week of therapy:
      (1) Cefixime, 400 mg PO, bid
      (2) Ciprofloxacin, 500 mg PO, bid

(3) Ofloxacin, 400 mg PO, bid
(4) Levofloxacin, 500 mg PO, qd

10.2 Chlamydia

ETIOLOGY

Chlamydia is caused by *Chlamydia trachomatis*, an obligate intracellular parasite with 15 different serotypes.

1. The chlamydial organism has two forms.
   a. Elementary body (infectious): serotypes
      (1) L1, L2, L3: lymphogranuloma venereum
      (2) A, B, Ba, C: endemic blinding trachoma
      (3) D, E, F, G, H, I, J, K: oculogenital and STD strains
   b. Reticulate body (multiplies to form inclusions)
2. Epidemiology (Box 10-1).
   a. Emerging as most common STD
   b. Four million cases per year
   c. Prevalence three to four times more than GC
   d. Overall prevalence 3% to 5% (low risk), but greater than 20% of cases in STD clinics
   e. Transmission exclusively by sexual contact or perinatal contact
   f. Incubation period 6 to 14 days
3. Risk factors for acquiring *C. trachomatis*.
   a. Unmarried and sexually active
   b. Multiple sexual partners
   c. Use of oral contraceptives
   d. Use of intrauterine device (IUD)
   e. History of previous sexually transmitted disease
   f. Known exposure with partner having an STD
   g. Presence of concomitant STD especially *N. gonorrhoeae*
   h. Spotting after intercourse
   i. Intermenstrual spotting
   j. Vague complaints of lower abdominal pain

BOX 10-1 2002 CDC Screening Criteria for Chlamydia

Mucopurulent cervicitis
Sexually active fewer than 20 years
20 to 24 years age (one criterion)
Greater than 24 years age (both criteria)
  Inconsistent barrier contraception
  New partner or more than 1 partner in last 3 months

CDC, Centers for Disease Control and Prevention.

LOWER GENITAL TRACT INFECTION

1. May often be asymptomatic and progress to upper genital tract disease
2. Bartholinitis: 33% of chlamydial infections
3. Endocervicitis: most common
   a. Mucopurulent cervicitis
   b. Specific for most nonciliated columnar or cuboidal epithelia (i.e., conjunctiva, urethra, endocervix, endometrium, fallopian tube mucosa)
4. Diagnosis suggested by the following:
   a. Positive swab test: a Q-Tip inserted into the endocervix stains yellowish-green
   b. Greater than 10 PMNS/oil immersion field gram stain
   c. Friable cervix
5. Acute urethral syndrome
   a. Indicated by dysuria and urinary frequency.
   b. Develops from 25% of cases of *C. trachomatis*.
   c. Sterile pyuria is found on urinalysis, or pyuria is found but with fewer than 10^5 organisms/mL.
   d. Culture cervix and urethra for diagnosis.
   e. *C. trachomatis* will not be recovered from urine.

UPPER GENITAL TRACT INFECTION

1. Nonpuerperal endometritis
   a. Clinical signs of salpingitis are present.
   b. Patient has positive endometrial cultures or negative endocervical cultures.
   c. Infection is an intermediate step between endocervicitis and salpingitis.
2. PID
   a. The majority of serious acute illness and morbidity resulting from *Chlamydia* infections in women are caused by PID.
   b. Eight percent of females with *Chlamydia* have overt salpingitis.
   c. Chlamydia is found isolated or with other microorganisms in 5% to 50% of women with symptoms of PID.

DIAGNOSIS

1. Cell cultures are the gold standard as specificity approaches 100%. This is essential for medical–legal situations.
2. Nonculture tests can detect *Chlamydia* antigens with 97% to 99% specificity.
   a. Direct fluorescent antibody (Micro Trak)
   b. Enzyme immunoassay (Chlamydiazyme)
   c. Nucleic acid hydridization (deoxyribonucleic acid [DNA] probes)
   d. PCR
      (1) Gold standard of the future
      (2) Sensitivity greater than 95%, specificity near 100%
         (a) Male and female urine
         (b) Female endocervix

(c) Swabs: 90% to 100% sensitivity, specificity approaches 100%
(d) Urine: 95% sensitivity
3. Disadvantages of cell culture.
   a. Expensive
   b. Technically difficult
   c. Requires 3 to 7 days to obtain result
   d. Special transport media and storage temperatures required
4. Serology is rarely useful in clinical settings for genital tract infections.

CHLAMYDIA TREATMENT REGIMEN, 2002 CDC GUIDELINES

1. Recommended
   a. Doxycycline, 100 mg PO, bid × 7 days
   b. Azithromycin, 1 g PO, single dose
2. Alternative
   a. Ofloxacin, 300 mg PO, bid × 7 days
   b. Erythromycin base, 500 mg PO, qid × 7 days
   c. Erythromycin ethylsuccinate, 800 mg, qid × 7 days
   d. Levofloxacin, 500 mg PO, qd × 7 days
3. Pregnancy
   a. Erythromycin base, 500 mg PO, qid × 7 days
   b. Erythromycin ethylsuccinate, 800 mg PO, qid × 7 days
   c. Amoxicillin, 500 mg PO, tid 7 days
   d. Azithromycin, 1 g PO, single dose

FOLLOW-UP

1. Test of cure culture is not necessary unless symptoms persist or reinfection is suspected.
2. Test of cure culture is recommended for pregnancy.
3. Reculture more than 3 weeks after initial treatment.

10.3 Lymphogranuloma Venereum

ETIOLOGY

1. Lymphogranuloma venereum (LGV) is a sexually transmitted systemic disease.
2. *C. trachomatis* is the causative agent.
3. There are three serotypes: L1, L2, and L3.
4. LGV is rare in the United States (285 cases reported in 1993).
5. LGV is endemic in Africa, India, parts of Southeast Asia, South America, and the Caribbean.
6. Primary stage.
   a. Primary lesion is caused by multiplication of organism at site of infection.
   b. Papule, shallow ulcer.
   c. Herpetiform lesion at site of inoculation (most common).
   d. Incubation period is 3 to 21 days.

    e. Most common site of lesion in women is the posterior wall, fourchette, or vulva.
    f. Healing is spontaneous without scar.
 7. Second stage: Inguinal syndrome: Inguinal adenopathy is characteristic.
    a. Begins 1 to 4 weeks after primary lesion.
    b. Syndrome is the most frequent clinical sign of the disease.
    c. Inguinal adenopathy is unilateral in 70% of cases.
    d. Symptoms include painful, extensive adenitis (bubo), and suppuration may occur with numerous sinus tracts.
    e. "Groove sign" signals femoral and inguinal node involvement (20%); most often seen in men.
    f. Involvement of deep iliac and retroperitoneal lymph nodes in women may present as a pelvic mass.
 8. Third stage (anogenital syndrome).
    a. Subacute: proctocolitis
    b. Late: tissue destruction or scarring sinuses, abscesses, fistulas, strictures of perineum, elephantiasis

DIAGNOSIS

1. Positive Frei test
   a. Intradermal chlamydial antigen
   b. Nonspecific for all *Chlamydia*
   c. No longer available (historical significance only)
2. Complement fixation test
   a. Titer greater than 1:64 in active infection.
   b. Convalescent titers no difference.
3. Cell culture of *Chlamydia*: Aspiration of fluctuant node yields highest rates of recovery.

TREATMENT

1. Doxycycline, 100 mg PO, bid × 21 days (treatment of choice)
2. Erythromycin base, 500 mg PO, qid × 21 days
3. Surgical
   a. Aspirate fluctuant nodes
   b. Incise and drain abscesses

10.4 Syphilis

ETIOLOGY

1. Syphilis is a chronic sexually transmitted infection.
2. *Treponema pallidum* is the causative agent and is corkscrew shaped, microaerophilic, nonculturable, 10 to 14 μm length, 0.15 μm diameter, and very fragile.
3. Episodes of active clinical disease interrupted by periods of latency are characteristic of syphilis.
4. Transmission.
   a. Direct contact with infectious lesion is required for infection. Organism does not survive outside the body.
   b. Incubation period is 9 to 90 days (2 to 6 weeks average).

5. Primary stage characteristics.
   a. Painless, indurated chancre (genital, anal, oral)
   b. Firm, nontender, regional adenopathy
   c. Lasts 1 to 5 weeks
   d. Heals spontaneously if untreated
6. Secondary syphilis characteristics.
   a. Systemic infection: all major organ systems
   b. Headache, fever, malaise: may precede rash
   c. Generalized rash: macular (10%), papular (34%), pustular (6%), or maculopapular (51%); may be confused with other dermatoses
   d. Generalized lymphadenopathy (86%)
   e. Mucous patches (10%)
   f. Condylomata lata (10%)
   g. Persisting or unhealing chancre (15%)
   h. Alopecia; liver or kidney involvement
   i. Lasts 2 to 6 weeks; resolves spontaneously
   j. Recurrent secondary symptoms possible within 1 year for 25% of cases
7. Latent syphilis characteristics.
   a. Clinical manifestations will be absent.
   b. Positive serologic tests for syphilis are the mainstay of diagnosis.
      (1) Less than 1 year duration: early latent
      (2) More than 1 year duration: late latent
   c. Two thirds of patients with untreated syphilis remain in the latent phase for life.
8. Tertiary syphilis: If untreated, 33% of patients will progress to the tertiary stage.
   a. Late benign (gumma) (15%): Complete resolution is possible with treatment; bone, skin, cartilage, and internal organs are involved.
   b. Cardiovascular (10%): Ascending aorta is involved and results include the following:
      (1) Aortitis
      (2) Aortic insufficiency
      (3) Aneurysm
   c. Neurosyphilis (symptomatic) occurs in 8% of patients.
9. Congenital syphilis.
   a. Caused by transplacental transmission
      (1) Can occur at any time during gestation
      (2) Can occur at any stage of syphilis
         (a) Early active: 75% to 90% transmission
         (b) Late latent: 30% transmission
   b. Can result in the following:
      (1) Spontaneous abortion (second trimester)
      (2) Stillbirth
      (3) Infant with active or latent syphilis

DIAGNOSIS

There is no gold standard and no culture technique is available. Diagnosis must rely on the following:

1. Clinical manifestations
2. Identification of *T. pallidum* from lesions using darkfield microscopy

3. Serology
   a. Nontreponemal.
      (1) It measures immunoglobulin M (IgM) and immunoglobulin G (IgG) antibody directed against cardiolipin–lecithin–cholesterol antigen.
      (2) It is nonspecific for *T. pallidum*.
      (3) It is used to determine antibody titer and monitor therapy. Rising titer indicates an active infection that may be any one of the following:
         (a) New infection
         (b) Reinfection
         (c) Reactivation of the latent disease
      (4) Types of tests include the following:
         (a) Venereal Disease Research Laboratory (VDRL)
         (b) Rapid plasma reagin (RPR)
   b. Treponemal.
      (1) Measures IgM and IgG antibody against *T. pallidum*–specific antigens
      (2) Types are as follows:
         (a) Fluorescent treponemal antibody test (FTA-ABS)
         (b) *T. pallidum*–hemoglutinating antibody tests (MHA-TP, TPHA)
   c. Specific treponemal antibody tests may remain active after adequate therapy.

TREATMENT

1. Primary and secondary syphilis therapy. 2002 CDC guidelines
   a. Benzathine penicillin G, 2.4 million units IM, single dose
   b. Penicillin allergy
      (1) Doxycycline, 100 mg, bid × 2 weeks, *or*
      (2) Tetracycline, 500 mg orally, qid × 2 weeks
2. Latent and tertiary syphilis therapy. 2002 CDC guidelines
   a. Benzathine penicillin G, 2.4 million units IM, three doses at 1-week intervals
   b. Penicillin allergy
      (1) Doxycycline, 100 mg PO, bid × 4 weeks
      (2) Tetracycline, 500 mg PO, qid × 4 weeks
   c. Alternate drugs: should only be used after cerebrospinal fluid (CSF) examination to rule out neurosyphilis
3. Neurosyphilis therapy. 2002 CDC guidelines
   a. Aqueous crystalline penicillin G, 18 to 24 million units IV daily for 10 to 14 days
   b. Procaine penicillin G, 2.4 million units IM daily, plus Probenicid, 500 mg, qid for 10 to 14 days
   c. Penicillin allergy
      (1) Ceftriaxone, 2 g IM or IV, qd × 10 to 14 days
      (2) Desensitize and treat with penicillin
4. Syphilis therapy in pregnancy
   a. Penicillin is the drug of choice. Therapy should be appropriate for the woman's stage of syphilis.

b. Penicillin allergy in pregnancy.
   (1) There are no alternatives to penicillin.
   (2) The patient should be desensitized and treated with penicillin.
   (3) Tetracycline and doxycycline are contraindicated during pregnancy.
   (4) Erythromycin does not effectively cross the placenta and cannot be relied on to cure an infected infant.

10.5 Chancroid

ETIOLOGY

1. *Haemophilus ducreyi*, a pleomorphic gram-negative facultative anaerobic bacillus, is the causative agent.
2. The disease is common in tropical countries.
3. It is now common in the United States.
4. Disease is a cofactor for human immunodeficiency virus (HIV) transmission: 10% coinfection rate.
5. Approximately 10% of patients are coinfected with *T. pallidum* or herpes simplex virus (HSV).
6. Sexual contact is the only known method of transmission.

SIGNS AND SYMPTOMS

1. Incubation period is 2 to 10 days; with a median of 4 to 7 days.
2. "Soft chancre" is the primary clinical sign.
   a. Shallow, tender, nonindurated ulcer with purulent base
   b. Multiple ulcers in women: lesions on fourchette, labia, vestibule, and clitoris
3. Unilateral or bilateral inguinal adenopathy (bubo) present in 50% of cases.
   a. Unilateral, 70%
   b. Spontaneous rupture if untreated
4. In HIV patients ulcers are larger, persist longer, and have less extensive lymphadenopathy.

LABORATORY DIAGNOSIS

1. *H. ducreyi* should be isolated from lesion or node aspirate.
2. Gram stain is insensitive and nonspecific, revealing a pleomorphic gram negative "school of fish" pattern.
3. Cultures require special media, are 60% to 80% sensitive, and difficult to grow.
4. Rule out HSV, syphilis, and LGV.
5. Diagnostic criteria:
   a. Isolation of *H. ducreyi* is definitive.
   b. Otherwise, clinical diagnosis should include the following:
      (1) One or more painful genital ulcers
      (2) Negative darkfield examination, negative RPR
      (3) Negative HSV, negative LGV
   c. Painful ulcer along with tender inguinal adenopathy is suggestive of chancroid.

TREATMENT

1. Azithromycin, 1 g PO, single dose
2. Ceftriaxone, 250 mg IM, single dose
3. Erythromycin base, 500 mg, qid × 7 days
4. Ciprofloxacin, 500 mg PO, bid × 3 days

10.6 Donovanosis (Granuloma Inguinale)

ETIOLOGY

1. The infectious agent is *Calymmatobacterium granulomatis*, a gram-negative bacillus that reproduces within PMNs, plasma cells, and histiocytes, causing the infected cells to rupture 20 to 30 organisms.
2. Epidemiology
   a. Rare in the United States (<50 cases reported annually) and other developed countries
   b. Endemic in Australia, India, Caribbean, and Africa
3. Pathogenesis
   a. Indurated nodule is the primary lesion.
   b. Lesion erodes to granulomatous heaped ulcer, progresses slowly.
   c. Pathogenic features are as follows:
      (1) Large infected mononuclear cell containing many Donovan bodies
      (2) Intracytoplasmic location

SIGNS AND SYMPTOMS

1. Incubation period is 8 to 80 days.
2. Lesions bleed easily.
3. Lesions are sharply defined and painless.
4. Secondary infection may ensue.
5. Inguinal involvement causes pseudobuboes; true lymph node involvement is unusual.

DIAGNOSIS

1. Check for clinical manifestation
2. Obtain stained crushed prep from lesion. Wright stain: Donovan bodies; organisms in vacuoles within macrophages
3. Screen for other STDs
4. Exclude other causes of lesions
5. Differential diagnosis
   a. Carcinoma
   b. Secondary syphilis: condylomata lata
   c. Amebiasis: necrotic ulceration
   d. Concurrent infections

TREATMENT

1. Doxycycline, 100 mg PO, bid × 3 weeks
2. Trimethoprim-sulfamethoxazole, 800/160 mg PO, bid × 3 weeks
3. Ciprofloxacin, 750 mg PO, bid × 3 weeks

Practical Guide to the Care of the Gynecologic/Obstetric Patient 205

4. Erythromycin base, 500 mg PO, tid × 3 weeks
5. Azythromycin, 1 g PO, qwk × 3 weeks
6. Continue therapy until complete healing of all lesions

10.7 Genital Herpes Simplex Virus

HERPES SIMPLEX VIRUS INFECTION IN THE NONPREGNANT WOMAN

1. Biology and epidemiology.
   a. HSV is an exclusively sexually transmitted disease.
   b. It is a double-stranded DNA virus.
   c. Its two types are as follows:
      (1) HSV-1: Gingivostomatitis is the major clinical presentation but HSV-1 also causes 15% of primary genital herpes cases.
      (2) HSV-2: HSV-2 primarily affects the genital area.
   d. HSV is endemic in the United States with 500,000 new cases per year.
   e. Incidence is approximately 1% to 2% of the population.
   f. Genital HSV is prevalent: 50 million cases currently in the United States.
   g. About 50% to 80% of adults have antibodies to HSV-1 or HSV-2.
   h. The highest frequency of HSV occurs in the 15-year-old to 29-year-old age group.
   i. HSV is often associated with other STDs.
   j. HSV may present as a primary, latent, or recurrent disease.
2. Signs and symptoms: There are three distinct syndromes associated with HSV.
   a. First episode primary genital herpes refers to the initial genital HSV infection and includes the following:
      (1) No evidence of HSV-1 or HSV-2 antibodies
      (2) Severe local symptoms
      (3) Multiple painful lesions, vesicles, ulcers, inguinal adenopathy
      (4) Systemic symptoms such as fever, malaise, nausea, myalgia
      (5) First episode primary herpes is defined as three or more of the following:
         (a) At least two extragenital symptoms
         (b) Multiple bilateral genital lesions
         (c) Persistence of genital lesions more than 16 days
         (d) Distal HSV lesions on the fingers, buttocks, or oropharynx
   b. First episode nonprimary genital herpes is defined by the following:
      (1) Initial clinical episode
      (2) Antibodies to HSV-1 and HSV-2 present
      (3) Less severe clinical course
      (4) Symptoms similar to recurrent genital herpes
   c. Recurrent herpes simplex infection involves the following:
      (1) Milder and shorter duration
      (2) Caused by reactivation of latent virus, not reinfection
      (3) Usual unilateral distribution of recurrent lesions
      (4) Typical lesion outbreak (preceded by prodromal symptoms such as paresthesias, itching, or pain)

(5) Recurrent infection finished in 5 to 10 days
(6) Systemic manifestations absent with few lesions
3. Clinical diagnosis.
   a. Classical appearance of genital lesions is painful vesicles and ulcers in various stages of progression.
   b. History of prodrome and recurrences supports diagnosis.
4. Laboratory tests.
   a. Viral culture is the gold standard for diagnosis; most positive cultures are identifiable in 48 to 72 hours.
      (1) More likely positive in first episode than recurrence
      (2) Positive culture more likely in early vesicle lesions than later ulcerative crusted lesions.
   b. Tzanck smear is a cytologic test.
      (1) Presence of intranuclear inclusions and giant cells
      (2) Low sensitivity
   c. A negative Tzanck smear or negative culture does not exclude HSV.
   d. Indirect and direct immunoperoxidase stains are more sensitive than a Tzanck smear.
   e. The monoclonal antibody test with type-specific assays for HSV-specific glycoprotein G1 or G2 can also be used.
      (1) Positive predictive value: 93%
      (2) Negative predictive value: 92%
   f. Enzyme-linked immunosorbent assay (ELISA) is also a testing option.
5. Treatment.
   a. Acyclovir (Zovirax) was the first effective chemotherapeutic agent for genital herpes. The drug interferes selectively with viral thymidine kinase and ultimately inhibits viral DNA synthesis.
   b. 2002 CDC treatment guidelines:
      (1) First clinical episode of genital herpes
         (a) Acyclovir, 400 mg PO, tid × 7 to 10 days
         (b) Acyclovir, 200 mg PO, five times a day × 7 to 10 days
         (c) Famciclovir, 250 mg PO, tid × 7 to 10 days
         (d) Valacyclovir, 1 g PO, bid × 7 to 10 days
         (e) May extend therapy if incomplete healing
      (2) Recurrent episodes
         (a) Treatment instituted during prodrome or first 2 days of onset of lesions may provide limited benefit from therapy.
         (b) Recommended regimen is as follows:
            (i) Acyclovir, 200 mg PO, five times a day × 5 days
            (ii) Acyclovir, 400 mg PO, tid × 5 days
            (iii) Acyclovir, 800 mg PO, bid × 5 days
            (iv) Famciclovir, 125 mg PO, bid × 5 days
            (v) Valacyclovir, 500 mg PO, bid × 3 to 5 days
            (vi) Valacyclovir, 1 g PO, qd × 5 days
      (3) Daily suppressive therapy
         (a) This therapy indicated in patients with frequent (≥6) recurrences per year.

- (b) Therapy may reduce frequency of HSV recurrence 70% to 80%.
- (c) Should consider discontinuation of therapy to reevaluate frequency of recurrences after 1 year of suppressive therapy.
- (d) Recommended regimens:
  - (i) Acyclovir, 400 mg PO, bid
  - (ii) Famciclovir, 250 mg PO, bid
  - (iii) Valacylovir, 500 mg PO, qd
  - (iv) Valacyclovir, 1 g PO, qd
- (4) Severe disease
  - (a) Patients can be treated with intravenous therapy if indicated for complications of HSV such as encephalitis, pneumonitis, disseminated infection, or hepatitis.
  - (b) Recommended regimen is acyclovir, 5 to 10 mg/kg body weight IV, q8h × 5 to 7 days or until clinical resolution followed by an oral regimen for at least 10 days.
- (5) Other management
  - (a) Infected patients should abstain from sex during periods of active genital lesions.
  - (b) Use of condoms during all sexual exposures should be encouraged.
  - (c) Patients should be informed about the risks of neonatal infection.

HERPES SIMPLEX VIRUS IN PREGNANCY

1. Epidemiology
   a. HSV shedding occurs in 0.1% to 0.4% of deliveries.
   b. Frequency of neonatal infection is 0.01% to 0.04% of deliveries.
   c. Transmission rate of primary maternal infection to exposed neonate is estimated at 30% to 50%.
   d. Transmission rate with recurrent maternal infection is estimated less than 1%.
   e. The risk of asymptomatic lower genital tract HSV infection on day of delivery is 1.4% in women with a confirmed history of recurrent herpes.
   f. Nosocomial infection may also cause neonatal infection, most often HSV-1, at a rate of approximately 10%. Parents, family members, and health care workers may transmit the disease.
2. Neonatal infection
   a. Infection may result from HSV-1 or HSV-2.
   b. Neonatal complication is severe with third-trimester maternal infection.
   c. Seventy percent of neonates with severe HSV infection are delivered from asymptomatic mothers.
   d. The risk of neonatal herpes from an asymptomatic mother with a history of recurrent genital herpes infection is estimated at less than 1 in 1000.
3. Neonatal complications of perinatal HSV
   a. Active HSV infection leads to a 50% chance of complications in primary episode HSV infection.

b. Neonatal death may occur in 60% of cases.
  c. Fifty percent of surviving neonates have significant sequelae, including the following:
     (1) Microcephaly
     (2) Mental retardation
     (3) Seizures
     (4) Microophthalmia
     (5) Retinal dysplasia
     (6) Chorioretinitis
     (7) Meningitis
     (8) Encephalitis
  d. Onset of neonatal herpes is often insidious. Delay in diagnosis without lesions approximates 72 hours.
4. Management: The American College of Obstetricians and Gynecologists has endorsed the following recommendations for pregnant women with HSV infections or a history of HSV infections:
  a. Antepartum
     (1) Cultures should be done when a women has active HSV lesions during pregnancy to confirm the diagnosis. If there are no visible lesions at the onset of labor, vaginal delivery is acceptable.
     (2) Weekly surveillance cultures of pregnant women with a history of HSV infection, but no visible lesions, are not necessary and vaginal delivery is acceptable.
     (3) Amniocentesis in an attempt to rule out intrauterine infection is not recommended for mothers with HSV at any stage of gestation.
  b. Intrapartum
     (1) Cesarean section in women with active infection will significantly decrease but not eliminate the risk and incidence of neonatal HSV infection.
     (2) The American College of Obstetricians and Gynecologists recommends that term patients who have visible lesions and are in labor, or who have ruptured membranes, should undergo cesarean delivery.
     (3) Cultures for HSV obtained at delivery in women with a history of HSV may aid in identifying potentially exposed neonates.
  c. Medical therapy
     (1) The safety of systemic acyclovir therapy among pregnant women has not been established.
     (2) Acyclovir is indicated for life-threatening and disseminated HSV infection (e.g., encephalitis, pneumonitis, hepatitis).

10.8 Pelvic Inflammatory Disease

DEFINITION

Pelvic inflammatory disease (PID) is a spectrum of inflammatory disorders of the upper genital tract, including a combination of any of the following:
1. Endometritis, salpingitis, tuboovarian abscess, or pelvic peritonitis.

2. It results from an ascending lower genital tract infection.
3. It is not related to obstetric or surgical intervention.

EPIDEMIOLOGY

1. Incidence or prevalence.
   a. There are an estimated 600,000 to 1 million cases annually in the United States.
   b. Disease is diagnosed in 2% to 5% of women seen in STD clinics.
   c. PID is the most common cause of female infertility and ectopic pregnancy.
   d. Indirect and direct costs attributed to PID were estimated to be in excess of $4 billion in 1990.
2. Risk factors.
   a. Adolescent sexually active females under age 20 (1:8 risk)
   b. Nonwhite race
   c. Previous episode of gonococcal PID
   d. Multiple sexual partners (more than two partners within 30 days)
   e. Vaginal douching (associated with 2× increased risk of PID)
   f. Use of IUD (Users have a threefold to fivefold increased risk of developing acute PID.)
3. Risk reduction: Other contraceptives reduce risk of PID.
   a. Oral contraceptives
   b. Condoms
   c. Diaphragms with spermicide

MICROBIAL ETIOLOGY

1. *N. gonorrhoeae*
   a. This bacteria causes many cases of PID in populations with high incidence rates of gonorrhea (i.e., inner city).
   b. Acute PID is developed in 10% to 20% of women with endocervical gonorrhea.
2. *C. trachomatis*
   a. This organism is an important cause of PID.
   b. It is the predominant etiologic agent among patients of middle and upper socioeconomic status with PID in the United States.
   c. More than 50% of PID cases are caused by *N. gonorrhoeae*, *C. trachomatis*, or both.
3. Polymicrobial infection: Other microorganisms exist as causative agents for the disease, including facultative and anaerobic bacteria such as the following:
   a. *Escherichia coli*
   b. *Gardnerella vaginalis*
   c. *Bacteroides species*
   d. *Haemophilus influenza*
   e. *Mycoplasma hominis*
4. *Mycobacterium tuberculosis* is an important cause of chronic PID in developing countries.

SIGNS AND SYMPTOMS

1. Lower abdominal pain: usually bilateral, most common presenting symptom
2. Abnormal vaginal discharge
3. Abnormal uterine bleeding
4. Dysuria: 20% of patients
5. Dyspareunia: common
6. Nausea and vomiting: may suggest peritonitis
7. Fever
8. Right upper quadrant tenderness (perihepatitis): 5% of PID cases

LABORATORY FINDINGS

1. Leukocytosis
2. Elevated acute phase reactants: erythrocyte sedimentation rate (ESR), C-reactive protein
3. Gram stain of endocervical exudate: greater than 30 PMNs per high-power field (HPF) correlates with chlamydial or gonococcal infection
4. Endocervical cultures for *N. gonorrohoeae* and *C. trachomatis*
5. Fallopian tube aspirate or peritoneal exudate culture if laparoscopy performed

DIAGNOSIS

1. Differential diagnosis
   a. Ectopic pregnancy
   b. Appendicitis
   c. Urinary tract infection (cystitis or pyelonephritis)
   d. Renal calculus
   e. Adnexal torsion
   f. Proctocolitis
2. Additional diagnostic procedures
   a. Human chorionic gonadotropin (β-HCG): to rule out ectopic pregnancy
   b. Endometrial biopsy: abnormal histology in 90% of patients with laparoscopic evidence of salpingitis
   c. Endocervical ultrasonography
      (1) Detects tuboovarian abscesses
      (2) May detect early salpingitis if tubal dilation, intratubal fluid, and tubal wall thickening found
   d. Laparoscopy
      (1) Gold standard for diagnosis of acute salpingitis
      (2) Should be considered when the diagnosis of PID is unsure
3. Diagnostic considerations
   a. Clinical diagnosis of PID is difficult and imprecise.
   b. Clinical diagnosis of symptomatic PID has a positive predictive value of 65% to 90% when compared with laparoscopy as the standard.
   c. No single historical, physical, or laboratory finding is both sensitive and specific for the diagnosis of PID.

4. 2002 CDC diagnostic criteria for PID
   a. Empiric treatment of PID should be initiated based on the presence of all of the following minimum criteria:
      (1) Lower abdominal pain
      (2) Adnexal tenderness
      (3) Cervical motion tenderness
   b. The following additional routine criteria may be used to increase the specificity of the diagnosis of PID in women with severe clinical signs:
      (1) Oral temperature greater than 38.3° C
      (2) Abnormal cervical or vaginal discharge
      (3) White blood cells (WBCs) in vaginal secretion on saline microscopy
      (4) Elevated ESR
      (5) Elevated C-reactive protein
      (6) Laboratory documentation of cervical infection with *N. gonorrhoeae* or *C. trachomatis*
   c. Elaborate criteria for diagnosing PID are as follows:
      (1) Laparoscopic abnormalities consistent with PID
      (2) Histopathologic evidence of endometritis on endocervical biopsy
      (3) Tuboovarian abscess, fluid-filled tubes with or without free pelvic fluid on transvaginal sonography

MANAGEMENT

1. Most patients are treated as outpatients.
2. Few studies exist comparing outpatient versus inpatient management.
3. Criteria for hospitalization (2002 CDC) (Table 10-1) are as follows:
   a. The diagnosis is uncertain.
   b. Pelvic abscess is suspected.
   c. Patient is pregnant.
   d. Patient is an adolescent.
   e. Patient is HIV positive.
   f. Severe illness, nausea, or vomiting precludes outpatient management.
   g. Patient cannot tolerate outpatient regimens.
   h. Patient has failed to respond clinically to outpatient therapy.
   i. Clinical follow-up within 72 hours of initiating antibiotic treatment cannot be arranged.
4. Outpatient treatment
   a. Regimen A
      (1) Ofloxacin, 400 mg PO, bid × 14 days, *or*
      (2) Levofloxacin, 500 mg PO, qd × 14 days
      (3) The above may be combined with the following:
         (a) Metronidazole, 500 mg PO, bid × 14 days, *or*
         (b) Doxycycline, 100 mg PO, bid × 10 to 14 days
   b. Regimen B
      (1) Ceftriaxone, 250 mg IM, single dose, *or*
      (2) Cefoxitin, 2 g IM, single dose, and Pribenecid, 1 g PO, single dose, *or*

Table 10-1 **Regimens for Treatment of Pelvic Inflammatory Disease Recommended by the CDC 2002**

Inpatient Treatment	Comment
Regimen A Cefoxitin, 2 g IV, q6h, *or* Cefotetan, 2 g IV, q12h, *plus* Doxycycline, 100 mg IV or PO, q12h	Regimen should be continued for at least 24 hours after substantial clinical improvement, after which doxycycline, 100 mg PO, two times a day, should be continued for a total of 14 days.
Regimen B Clindamycin, 900 mg IV, q8h, *plus* Gentamycin, loading dose IV or IM (2 mg/kg of body weight), followed by a maintenance dose (1.5 mg/kg) q8h	Regimen should be continued for at least 24 hours after substantial clinical improvement, after which doxycycline, 100 mg PO, two times a day, or clindamycin, 450 mg PO, four times a day, to complete a total of 14 days of therapy.

CDC, Centers for Disease Control and Prevention; *IV,* intravenously; *PO,* orally.

(3) Third-generation cephalosporin (e.g., ceftizoxime or cefotaxime) plus doxycycline, 100 mg bid × 14 days, with or without metronidazole, 500 mg PO, bid × 14 days

FOLLOW-UP

1. Hospitalized patients receiving IV therapy should show significant clinical improvement characterized by defervescence, decreased abdominal tenderness, and decreased uterine, adnexal, and cervical motion tenderness within 3 to 5 days.
2. If no clinical improvement occurs, further diagnostic workup is necessary, including possible surgical intervention.
3. Clinical improvement for outpatient therapy should be observed within 72 hours.
4. Evaluation and treatment of male sex partners is essential.
5. Long-term sequelae of PID are as follows:
    a. Recurrent PID
    b. Chronic pelvic pain
    c. Ectopic pregnancy
    d. Infertility
6. The risk of tubal infertility related to episodes of PID is as follows:
    a. First episode: 8%
    b. Second episode: 20%
    c. Third episode: 40%

10.9 Bacterial Vaginosis (Table 10-2)

ETIOLOGY

1. Polymicrobial clinical syndrome
2. Disturbance of vaginal ecology
3. *Lactobacillus* replaced by anaerobes
4. Altered vaginal pH
5. Abnormal vaginal secretions
6. Most common vaginal disorder (35% to 45%)
7. Majority of cases: sexually active patients ages 15 to 44 years
8. Prevalence: general population (20% to 25%)
9. Normal vaginal ecosystem
   a. *Lactobacillus* predominant
   b. Usually fewer than 10^7 organisms/g
   c. Ratio of anaerobes to aerobes: 2:1 to 5:1
   d. *Gardnerella vaginalis*: 5% to 60%
   e. *Mobiluncus* spp.: 0% to 5%
   f. *Mycoplasma hominis*: 15% to 30% of sexually active women
10. Vaginal ecosystem in bacterial vaginosis
    a. Few hydrogen peroxide–producing lactobacilli
    b. 10^{11} organisms/g
    c. Ratio of anaerobes to aerobes: 100:1 to 1000:1
    d. *Gardnerella vaginalis*: 95%
    e. *Mobiluncus* spp.: 50% to 70%
    f. *Mycoplasma hominis*: 60% to 75%
11. Possible causes
    a. Intercourse
    b. Spermicides
    c. Hormones
    d. Douches
    e. IUDs
    f. Other infections

SIGNS AND SYMPTOMS

1. Vaginal discharge evident at introitus (main symptom)
2. Foul vaginal odor
3. Vulvovaginal irritation less severe than other forms of vaginitis

DIAGNOSIS

1. No single marker
2. Amsel's criteria
   a. pH greater than 4.5
   b. Clue cells present
   c. Milky discharge
   d. Positive "whiff" test (fishy odor before or after addition of 10% potassium hydroxide [KOH])
   e. No diagnostic value of demonstrating *Gardnerella vaginalis* on culture
3. Do not treat based solely on *Gardnerella vaginalis* culture (40% to 60% of women's natural vaginal flora)

Table 10-2 **Diagnostic Features of Vaginitis**

	Normal	Yeast Vulvovaginitis	Trichomonal Vaginitis	Bacterial Vaginosis
Symptoms	None	Vulvar pruritis, discharge	Purulent discharge, vulvar pruritis	Malodor, discharge
Discharge				
Amount	Variable to scant	Scant to moderate	Profuse	Scant to moderate
Color	Clear or white	White or yellow	Yellow	White
Consistency	Floccular, nonhomogeneous	Clumped or adherent plaques	Homogeneous, frothy	Homogeneous, smooth or coats vaginal mucosa
Inflammation (Vulva/Vagina)	None	Erythema vagina, introitus, vulva	Erythema vagina, vulva or petechiae, ectocervix	None
pH Vaginal Fluid	<4.5	<4.5	>5.0	>4.7
Amino Odor (KOH)	None	None	Present	Present
Microscopy	Normal epithelial cells, lactobacilli	Leukocytes, yeast pseudomycelia	Leukocytes, motile trichomonads	Clue cells, mixed flora, few lactobacilli

KOH, Potassium hydroxide.

BACTERIAL VAGINOSIS–ASSOCIATED DISEASES

1. Gynecologic
   a. Abnormal vaginal discharge
   b. Mucopurulent cervicitis
   c. Urinary tract infections
   d. Postoperative infections
   e. Cervical dysplasia
   f. Nonpuerperal endometritis
   g. PID
2. Obstetric
   a. Chorioamnionitis
   b. Premature labor
   c. Premature rupture of membranes
   d. Postpartum endometritis

TREATMENT

1. Metronidazole, 500 mg PO, bid × 7 days
2. Metronidazole, 2 g PO, single dose
3. Clindamycin cream 2%, 5 g intravaginal, qhs × 7 days
4. Metronidazole gel 0.75%, 5 g intravaginal, qd × 5 days
5. Clindamycin, 300 mg PO, bid × 7 days
6. Clindamycin ovules, 100 g intravaginal, qhs × 3 days
7. Bacterial vaginosis in pregnancy
   a. Metronidazole, 250 mg PO, tid × 7 days.
   b. Clindamycin, 300 mg PO, bid × 7 days.
   c. Treatment may reduce risk of adverse pregnancy outcomes.

10.10 Vulvovaginal Candidiasis (see Table 10-2)

ETIOLOGY

1. Vulvovaginal candidiasis (VVC) is the second most common cause of vaginitis in the United States.
2. *Candida* spp. can be isolated in 5% to 55% of asymptomatic women of childbearing age.
3. Hormonal dependence of infection: This is rare in premenarchal and in postmenopausal women.
4. There are three subpopulations of women with VVC.
   a. Those who never develop symptomatic VVC
   b. Those who suffer infrequent isolated episodes
   c. Those who have repeated, recurrent, often chronic infection (more than three episodes of symptomatic VVC annually)
      (1) Vulvovaginal candidiasis will be experienced by 75% of all women at least once.
      (2) Two or more episodes will be experienced by 40% to 50% of these women.
      (3) Fewer than 5% of women experience recurrent vulvovaginal candidiasis.
5. Microbiology.
   a. *Candida albicans* causes 85% to 90% of cases.

b. Other *Candida* spp. (*C. glabrata*, *C. tropicalis*) can also cause the disease.
c. Nonalbicans species of *Candida* are more resistant to conventional therapy.
d. Uniquely virulent strains of *Candida* have not been identified.
6. Dimorphism of *Candida*.
   a. Blastospores
      (1) Transmission or spread
      (2) Asymptomatic colonization
   b. Mycelia
      (1) Germination
      (2) Tissue invasive form
      (3) Symptomatic disease
7. *Candida* virulence factors.
   a. *C. albicans* adhere to vaginal epithelial cells in very high numbers.
   b. Germination enhances colonization and tissue invasion.
8. Pathogenesis.
   a. *C. albicans* may be a commensal or a pathogen in the vagina.
   b. Changes in the vaginal environment are necessary before disease is induced.
9. Predisposing factors.
   a. Pregnancy
   b. Oral contraceptives
   c. Diabetes mellitus
   d. Antibiotics
   e. Hygiene
   f. Immunosuppression
10. Source of infection.
    a. Intestinal reservoir: major source of vaginal colonization
    b. Sexual transmission: probable limited contribution; treatment of male partners rare
    c. Vaginal relapse: incomplete eradication of vaginal colonization after treatment
11. Natural vaginal defense mechanisms.
    a. Humoral immunity: IgM, IgG, IgA
    b. Phagocytic system: PMNs and monocytes absent from vaginal fluid
    c. Cell-mediated immunity: reduced T-lymphocyte reactivity to *Candida* antigen
    d. Vaginal flora: most important defense

SIGNS AND SYMPTOMS

1. Acute pruritus
2. Erythematous vulva and vagina
3. White vaginal discharge, white or yellow raised vaginal plaques
4. Dyspareunia
5. Dysuria
6. Minimal odor

DIAGNOSIS

1. Signs and symptoms with low specificity
2. Pruritus without discharge (38% positive predictive value [PPV])
3. Microscopic examination: saline, 10% KOH, wet preparation, confirmed by observing mycelia or pseudohyphae (2.3% false-positive and 6.2% false-negative results)
4. Vaginal pH
5. Cultures: only if KOH negative and patient symptomatic (to exclude yeast)
6. Do not treat solely on presence of *Candida* on culture (10% to 20% normal vaginal flora)

TREATMENT

1. Topical.
   a. Nystatin: 70% to 80% cure rate
   b. Imidazoles: 80% to 90% cure rate
2. Oral.
   a. Ketoconazole
   b. Fluconazole (FDA approved for treatment of VVC, 1994)
3. Uncomplicated: short course.
4. Severe: more than 1-week regimen.
5. Recommended regimens (2002 CDC guidelines): All azole preparations, both oral and vaginal, have the same efficacy of cure: 90%.
   a. Intravaginal preparation:
      (1) Butoconazole 2% cream, 5 g intravaginally, × 3 days*
      (2) Butoconazole 2% cream, 5 g (Butoconazole-1—sustained release) intravaginally, single dose
      (3) Clotrimazole 1% cream, 5 g intravaginally, × 7 to 14 days*
      (4) Clotrimazole, 100 mg vaginal tablet, × 7 days
      (5) Clotrimazole, 100 mg vaginal tablet, two tablets × 3 days
      (6) Clotrimazole, 500 mg vaginal tablet, one tablet, single application
      (7) Miconazole 2% cream, 5 g intravaginally, × 7 days*
      (8) Miconazole, 200 mg vaginal suppository, one suppository × 3 days*
      (9) Miconazole, 100 mg vaginal suppository, one suppository × 7 days*
      (10) Nistatin, 100,000-unit vaginal tablet × 14 days
      (11) Tiocinazole 6.5% ointment, 5 mg intravaginally, a single application*
      (12) Terconazole 0.4% cream, 5 g intravaginally, × 7 days
      (13) Terconazole 0.8% cream 5 g intravaginally, × 3 days
      (14) Terconazole, 80 mg suppository, one suppository × 3 days
   b. Oral preparation: Fluconazole, 150 mg, one single oral dose, the only FDA-approved oral agent for vulvovaginal candidiasis

---

*These preparations are available over the counter. Self-medication should be advised only for women who have been previously diagnosed with vulvovaginal candidiasis and have experienced a recurrence of the same symptoms.

c. Side effects
   (1) Vaginal preparations
      (a) Local burning or irritation
      (b) Usually free from systemic effects
   (2) Oral agents
      (a) Nausea
      (b) Abdominal pain
      (c) Headache
d. Alternative agents
   (1) Boric acid, 600 mg, qid × 2 weeks
   (2) 1% gentian violet, two times a week × 2 weeks
6. Treatment of recurrent vulvovaginal candidiasis (RVVC).
   a. Optimal treatment has not been established.
   b. All cases should be confirmed by culture before therapy.
   c. All cases should be evaluated for predisposing conditions (e.g., diabetes mellitus, immunosuppression).
   d. Clinical trials have involved continuing therapy between episodes.
      (1) Ketoconazole, 100 mg PO, qd for up to 6 months (monitor for hepatotoxicity)
      (2) Clotrimazole, intravaginally, weekly
      (3) Fluconazole, 100-150 mg PO, weekly
      (4) Itraconazole, 400 mg PO, monthly
      (5) Itraconazole, 100 mg PO, qd

10.11 Trichomoniasis

ETIOLOGY

1. *Trichomonas vaginalis* is the etiologic agent.
2. It is an anaerobic flagellated protozoan.
3. Humans are its only known hosts.
4. Epidemiology.
   a. Trichomoniasis is responsible for 25% of all cases of clinically evident vaginitis.
   b. Incidence or prevalence is as follows:
      (1) 5% family planning clinics
      (2) 25% gynecology clinics
      (3) 75% prostitutes
   c. The disease is transmitted sexually.
   d. It often coexists with other STDs.
   e. Pathogenesis is uncertain for the disease.
   f. The disease is associated with preterm labor and premature rupture of membranes.

SIGNS AND SYMPTOMS

1. Incubation period variable
2. Female: vagina, urethra, endocervix, or bladder infected
3. Male: most often asymptomatic, primary vector for transmission
4. Symptoms: profuse, malodorous vaginal discharge, postcoital bleeding

5. Signs: cervical "strawberry patches"; vaginal mucosal erythema; labial erythema

DIAGNOSIS

1. Clinical manifestations
2. Laboratory diagnosis
   a. pH ≥5
   b. Wet mount: motile trichomonads, PMNs; diagnostic 60% to 70%
   c. Culture for *T. vaginalis* in rare circumstances of treatment failures
3. Differential diagnosis
   a. Bacterial vaginosis
   b. Vulvovaginal candidiasis
   c. Mucopurulent cervicitis
   d. Chemical vaginitis

MANAGEMENT

1. Metronidazole, 2 g PO, single dose
2. Metronidazole, 500 mg, bid × 7 days
3. Metronidazole gel: not effective
4. Concurrent treatment of sex partner
5. Screen for other STDs
6. Alcohol with metronidazole: avoid (disulfuram-like reaction may ensue)

FOLLOW-UP

1. Not necessary if patient becomes asymptomatic.
2. If treatment fails, retreat with metronidazole, 500 mg, bid × 7 days.
3. If treatment fails repeatedly, do the following:
   a. Treat with metronidazole, 2 g PO, daily × 3 to 5 days.
   b. Consider culture for possible resistant strain of *T. vaginalis*.
   c. Evaluate the patient's sex partner.
4. Special considerations.
   a. Allergy: There is no effective alternative. Clotrimazole may inhibit growth of *T. vaginalis* but does not eradicate it.
   b. Pregnancy: Metronidazole is contraindicated in first trimester. Use cautiously in second and third for truly symptomatic cases.
   c. HIV positive: Treat with same regimen as patients who are HIV negative.

SUGGESTED READINGS

American College of Obstetricians and Gynecologists: Gonorrhea and chlamydial infections, ACOG Technical Bulletin 190, Washington, DC, 1994, ACOG.

American College of Obstetricians and Gynecologists: Gynecologic herpes simplex virus infections, ACOG Technical Bulletin 119, Washington, DC, 1988, ACOG.

American College of Obstetricians and Gynecologists: Perinatal herpes simplex virus infections, ACOG Technical Bulletin 122, Washington, DC, 1988, ACOG.

Andrews EB, et al: Acyclovir in pregnancy register: Six years experience, *Obstet Gynecol* 79:7-13, 1992.

Cates W: Epidemiology and control of sexually transmitted diseases: strategic evaluation, *Infect Dis Clin North Am* 1:1-23, 1987.

Centers for Disease Control: 2002 sexually transmitted diseases treatment guidelines, *MMWR* 51(RR-6), 2002.

Centers for Disease Control: Summary of notifiable diseases, United States 2003, MMWR 52(54), 2005.

Faro S: Lymphogranuloma venereum, chancroid, and granuloma inguinale, *Obstet Gynecol Clin North Am* 16:517, 1989.

Faro S: Review of vaginitis, *Infect Dis Obstet Gynecol* 1:158-161, 1993.

Gibbs RS, Amstey MS, Lezotte DC: Role of cesarean delivery in preventing neonatal herpes virus infection (editorial), *JAMA* 270:94-95, 1993.

Gibbs RS et al: Management of genital herpes infection in pregnancy, *Obstet Gynecol* 71:779-780, 1988.

Hager WD et al: Criteria for the diagnosis and grading of salpingitis, *Obstet Gynecol* 61:113-114, 1983.

Handsfield HH: Bacterial sexually transmitted diseases. In Handsfiels HH, editor: *Color atlas and synopsis of sexually transmitted diseases*, New York, 1992, McGraw-Hill, pp. 9-66.

Handsfield HH: Pelvic inflammatory disease. In Handsfield HH, editor: *Color atlas and synopsis of sexually transmitted diseases*, New York, 1992, McGraw-Hill.

Handsfield HH: Vaginal infections. In Handsfield HH, editor: *Color atlas and synopsis of sexually transmitted diseases*, New York, 1992, McGraw-Hill.

Holmes KK: Lower genital tract infections in women: cystitis, urethritis, vulvovaginitis, and cervicitis. In Holmes KK, Mardh PA, Sparling PF, editors: *Sexually transmitted diseases*, ed 2, New York, 1990, McGraw-Hill.

Klein EJ et al: Anorectal gonococcal infection, *Ann Intern Med* 86:340-346, 1977.

Martens MG: Herpes simplex in pregnancy. In Gilstrat L, Faro S, editors: *Infections in pregnancy*, New York, 1990, Alan R. Liss, pp. 143-150.

McCormack W: Current concepts: Pelvic inflammatory disease, *N Engl J Med* 330(4):115-118, 1994.

McGregor JA, French JI, Seo K: Premature rupture of membranes and bacterial vaginosis, *Am J Obstet Gynecol* 169:463-466, 1993.

Morales MJ: Gonococcal infections in pregnancy. In Mead PB, Hager DW, editors: *Infection protocols for obstetrics and gynecology*, 1992, Medical Economics Publishing, pp. 42-46.

Randolph GA, Washington AE, Prober CG: Cesarean delivery for women presenting with genital herpes lesions, *JAMA* 270:77-82, 1993.

Rein MF, Muller M: Trichomonas vaginalis and trichomoniasis. In Holmes KK, Mardh PA, Sparling PF, editors: *Sexually transmitted diseases*, ed 2, New York, 1990, McGraw-Hill.

Ronald AR, Albritten W: Chancroid and Haemophilus ducreyi. In Holmes KK, Mardh PA, Sparling PF, editors: *Sexually transmitted diseases*, ed 2, New York, 1990, McGraw-Hill, pp. 263-271.

Sobel JD: Candidial vulvovaginitis, *Clin Obstet Gynecol* 36(1):153-165, 1993.

Soper DE: Bacterial vaginosis and postoperative infections, *Am J Obstet Gynecol* 169:467-469, 1993.

Soper D: Diagnosis and laparoscopic grading of acute salpingitis, *Am J Obstet Gynecol* 164:1370-1376, 1991.

Stamm WE, Holmes KK: Chlamydial infections in the adult. In Holmes KK, Mardh PA, Sparling PF, editors: *Sexually transmitted diseases*, ed 2, New York, 1990, McGraw-Hill, pp. 181-193.

Sweet RL: Acute salpingitis: diagnosis and management, *J Reprod Med* 19:21-30, 1977.

Sweet RL, Gibbs RS: Herpes simplex virus infection. In Sweet RL, Gibbs RS, editors: *Infectious diseases of the female genital tract*, ed 2, Baltimore, 1990, Williams & Wilkins, pp. 144-157.

Sweet RL, Gibbs RS: Infectious vulvovaginitis. In Sweet RL, Gibbs RS, editors: *Infectious diseases of the female genital tract*, ed 2, Baltimore, 1990, Williams & Wilkins.

Sweet RL, Gibbs RS: Sexually transmitted diseases. In Sweet RL, Gibbs RS, editors: *Infectious diseases of the female genital tract*, ed 2, Baltimore, 1990, Williams & Wilkins, pp. 45-74, 109-143.

Thin RN: Early syphilis in the adult. In Holmes KK, Mardh PA, Sparling PF, editors: *Sexually transmitted diseases*, ed 2, New York, 1990, McGraw-Hill, pp. 221-230.

Thomason JL, Gelbart SM: *Bacterial vaginosis: current concepts*, Kalamazoo, Michigan, 1990, The Upjohn Company.

Thomason JL, Gelbart SM, Scaglione NJ: Bacterial vaginosis: current review with indications for asymptomatic therapy, *Am J Obstet Gynecol* 165:1210-1217, 1991.

Wager G: Lymphogranuloma venereum. In Mead PB, Hager DW, editors: *Infection protocols for obstetrics and gynecology*, 1992, Medical Economics Publishing, pp. 184-188.

Westrom L et al: Pelvic inflammatory disease and fertility: a cohort study of 1844 women with laparoscopically verified disease and 657 control women with normal laparoscopic results, *Sex Transm Dis* 19:185-192, 1992.

Westrum L, Mardh PA: Acute pelvic inflammatory disease. In Holmes KK, Mardh PA, Sparling PF, editors: *Sexually transmitted diseases*, ed 2, New York, 1990, McGraw-Hill.

HIV Infection in Women

D. Michael Slate II
Lawrence J. Gugino

11.1 Background

1. The rate of human immunodeficiency virus (HIV) infection continues to increase dramatically among women.
2. Current estimates are that 1 million individuals in the United States are infected with HIV.
3. The rate of new infection in women has been more rapid than in any other risk group.
4. Obstetrician-gynecologists provide reproductive care to HIV-positive women and those at risk for HIV infection.

11.2 Epidemiology

1. There were more than 11,000 cumulative acquired immune deficiency syndrome (AIDS) cases in women as of 2003.
2. Women represented 27% of all AIDS cases reported in 2003.
3. Approximately 7000 infants are born to mothers who are HIV positive in the United States each year.
4. African American and Hispanic women are disproportionately affected, accounting for greater than 55% of AIDS cases for women, although they collectively represent only 20% of the population of U.S. women.

11.3 Major Routes of Transmission of HIV-1

1. Blood and body fluids
2. Sexual contact
3. Perinatal transmission

PRIMARY TRANSMISSION CATEGORIES IN WOMEN

1. Injection drug use
2. Heterosexual contact
3. Transfusion recipient
4. Unknown

MODES OF TRANSMISSION

1. As of 2004, 34% women with AIDS acquired it by injection drug use.
2. As of 2004, 67% women with AIDS acquired it by heterosexual sex.

11.4 Pathophysiology

1. HIV is a retrovirus (RNA virus) converted to DNA copy by enzyme reverse transcriptase.
2. It preferentially infects cells with CD4+ receptor antigen, especially helper lymphocytes, but also cells of the placenta.
3. HIV infection results in progressive debilitation of the immune system.
4. Acute HIV infection may result in acute mononucleosis-like syndrome.
5. HIV antibodies may be detected in most individuals by 12 weeks after exposure (latent "window period").
6. The median time from HIV infection to development of AIDS is greater than 10 years.

11.5 HIV Testing and Counseling in Women

TESTS FOR HIV

1. Antibody (enzyme-linked immunosorbent assay, ELISA) HIV-1 and HIV-2
   a. Detects antibodies, not virus
   b. Screening test only
   c. Highly sensitive and specific test
   d. Needs confirmation by specific test: Western blot or indirect immunofluorescence assay (IFA)
   e. Negative result: infection unlikely
2. Antigen tests (p24)
3. Viral culture
4. Polymerase chain reaction (PCR)
5. Rapid tests (OraQuik—oral fluid and plasma specimen test for HIV-1 and 2 antibodies); sensitivity 99.3% and specificity 99.8%

"WINDOW PERIOD"

1. Three months after infection with HIV, 95% of individuals seroconvert.
2. Six months after infection with HIV, 99% of individuals seroconvert.
3. A negative HIV test done today is indicative of the absence of HIV infection 6 months previously.
4. Twelve months after infection with HIV, there is a 1:5000 false-negative rate.

WHY TEST FOR HIV INFECTION?

1. Allows early HIV medical intervention
2. Assists in diagnosis
3. Assists in pregnancy decisions
4. Reinforces high-risk behavior change
5. Relieves anxiety of not knowing personal HIV status

6. Decreases pediatric HIV infection
7. Prevents HIV transmission to others

WHO SHOULD BE TESTED FOR HIV?

1. Women with current or past injection drug use
2. The current or past sexual partner of an injection drug user, a bisexual, or a person known to be HIV positive
3. Women with a history of blood or blood product transfusions between 1978 and 1985
4. Women with a history of multiple sexual partners
5. Women with a history of sexually transmitted disease

A WIDESPREAD APPROACH TO HIV COUNSELING AND TESTING

1. A targeted approach to testing may fail to identify 50% to 70% of infected women.
2. Women may be unaware of their risk status.
3. Women may refuse testing to avoid the stigma of high-risk behaviors.
4. A universal approach to HIV counseling and testing is indicated for all women, regardless of the geographic prevalence of HIV.

11.6 Clinical Manifestations and Diagnosis

INITIAL CLINICAL MANIFESTATIONS

1. Symptoms are nonspecific in most women.
2. Constitutional symptoms such as night sweats, low-grade fevers, anorexia, and weight loss are common.
3. Recurrent, chronic, refractory vaginal candidiasis may be a sentinel indicator of HIV infection.

CENTERS FOR DISEASE CONTROL AND PREVENTION (CDC)–DEFINED AIDS DIAGNOSIS

The following is the CDC 1999 revised classification system for HIV infection case definition:

1. Positive HIV antibody test with conformation with Western blot *or*
2. Detection of nucleic acids (DNA or RNA) *or*
3. Detection of p24 antigen *or*
4. HIV isolation by culture

GYNECOLOGIC MANIFESTATIONS

1. Menstrual disorders
   a. Amenorrhea, oligomenorrhea, metrorrhagia are anecdotally reported as common.
   b. Irregular bleeding may cause difficulty in predicting early pregnancy.
   c. Increased risk of transmission of HIV from menstrual blood.
2. *Candida* vaginitis
   a. Most common gynecologic infection in HIV-positive women
   b. Often presents as chronic and refractory to treatment

c. May be a sentinel marker for HIV positivity
d. Occurs with highest frequency with CD4 counts less than 100
e. Treatment
   (1) Uncomplicated: topical antifungal agent for 7 days—advise abstinence during treatment due to decreased effectiveness of condoms and other barrier methods by oil-based antifungals
   (2) Recurrent or unresponsive candidiasis: oral imidazole agents
      (a) Ketoconazole, 400 mg, qd *or*
      (b) Fluconazole, 200 mg, qd for 14 days
   (3) Chronic recurrence: consider maintenance therapy
      (a) Ketoconazole, 100 mg, qd—contraindicated with several HIV drugs (e.g., Delavirdin, indinavir, etc.)
      (b) Ketoconazole, 100 to 200 mg, 5 days each month at menses
      (c) Fluconazole, 200 mg, qod
3. Herpes simplex
   a. Herpes simplex (HSV) type 2 is the most clinically significant.
   b. Outbreaks may be more severe and persistent.
   c. Recurrence may be frequent and more severe.
   d. Patients should be cultured for HSV and a serologic test for syphilis obtained before treatment.
   e. Acyclovir therapy for acute episodes may require higher doses (400 mg, five times per day).
   f. If recurrences are frequent, suppressive acyclovir therapy (400 mg bid) should be considered.
   g. If lesions do not resolve, the possibility of acyclovir-resistant HSV should be considered.
4. Syphilis and other genital ulcers
   a. Genital ulcers facilitate HIV transmission and acquisition secondary to interruption of epithelial barrier and presence of inflammatory cells in ulcer.
   b. Syphilis.
      (1) Serologic titers may be higher than expected for the stage of disease.
      (2) False-negative serologic tests or delayed seroreactive tests have been reported.
      (3) Both treponemal and nontreponemal serologic tests for syphilis are accurate for the majority of patients with syphilis and HIV coinfection.
      (4) Alternative tests such as lesion biopsy and darkfield examination may be helpful to confirm diagnosis if clinical suspicion suggests syphilis but serology is nonconfirmatory.
      (5) Neurosyphilis should be considered in the differential diagnosis of neurologic disease in the female who is HIV positive.
      (6) Women who are infected with HIV and have early syphilis may have increased neurologic complications and higher treatment failures.
      (7) Careful follow-up after treatment for all stages of syphilis is essential.

(8) Treatment of primary and secondary syphilis is the same as for individuals who are infected with HIV.
(9) Patients with latent syphilis and HIV infection should undergo cerebrospinal fluid (CSF) examination before treatment.
(10) Latent syphilis, HIV infection, and a normal CSF examination should be treated with benzathine penicillin G, three weekly doses of 2.4 million units each.

c. Chancroid.
(1) Patients coinfected with HIV should be closely monitored.
(2) Healing may be slower, and treatment failures occur.
(3) Longer courses of therapy may be required than standard CDC regimens.
(4) Azithromycin or ceftriaxone should be used only if follow-up is ensured.
(5) Some authorities recommend erythromycin base, 500 mg PO, four times daily for 7 days.

5. Pelvic inflammatory disease (PID)
   a. HIV seropositive rate is high in patients presenting with PID (6.7% to 13.6% in communities endemic for HIV).
   b. HIV infection does not predispose to PID.
   c. Clinical presentation may be altered in the following ways:
      (1) Lower abdominal tenderness scores
      (2) Lower admission white blood cells (WBC) (<10,000)
      (3) More likely to require surgical intervention
   d. Management should be based on the same diagnostic criteria and management protocols as for women who are HIV negative.
   e. Patients should receive inpatient treatment for PID when HIV positive.

6. Condylomata acuminata
   a. Human papillomavirus (HPV) is the causative agent.
   b. Exophytic anogenital warts are most often caused by types 6 or 11.
   c. Disease is sexually transmitted.
   d. Disease can cause anogenital condylomata (warts) and anogenital dysplasia.
   e. The clinical course of anogenital condylomata may be accelerated.
   f. There is a high frequency of recurrence or persistence of infection.
   g. Disease may be confused with condylomata lata of secondary syphilis.
   h. These lesions may resist conventional treatment. If so, biopsy is indicated before therapy.
   i. Management.
      (1) Goal of treatment is removal of exophytic warts and amelioration of signs and symptoms.
      (2) Current treatment modalities are 22% to 94% effective, with high recurrence rates with all modalities.
      (3) Regimens.
         (a) Cryotherapy with liquid nitrogen or cryoprobe.

(b) Trichloroacetic acid (TCA), 80% to 90%, should be applied only to warts. Repeat weekly if necessary. If warts persist after 6 weeks, reevaluate therapy.
(c) Podophyllin 10% to 25% in tincture of benzoin should be applied only to warts. Wash off in 1 to 4 hours. Systemic toxicity if absorbed. If warts persist after 6 weekly applications, reevaluate therapy. Podophyllin is contraindicated during pregnancy.
(d) Podofilox 0.5% solution, is used for self-treatment (genital warts) only. Apply to warts two times per day for 3 days followed by 4 days of no therapy. May be repeated for a total of four cycles. Podofilox is contraindicated during pregnancy.
(e) Surgical excision or CO_2 laser vaporization is useful in the management of extensive anogenital warts or for those patients who have not responded to other regimens.

7. Cervical neoplasia
   a. Women with impaired cellular immunity from other causes (e.g., renal transplant) have been shown to be more susceptible to HPV infection and cervical neoplasia.
   b. HPV infection is more common among women infected with HIV.
   c. HPV types 16, 18, 31, 33, and 35 are associated more often with cervical intraepithelial neoplasia.
   d. There is a 31% to 63% incidence of abnormal cervical cytology in women who are HIV positive.
   e. Cervical intraepithelial neoplasia (CIN) is increased in women infected with HIV by 8 to 49 times compared with women who are HIV negative.
   f. CIN may be more severe and extensive and may present with a higher grade (i.e., CIN II, CIN III, carcinoma in situ [CIS]) as compared with women who are HIV negative.
   g. The natural history of CIN may be more aggressive with decreased time to progression of high-grade CIN or malignancy.
   h. Management.
      (1) A Papanicolaou smear is an integral component of the initial comprehensive medical evaluation of a woman who is HIV positive.
      (2) If initial Papanicolaou smear results are within normal limits, repeat in approximately 6 months.
      (3) Repeat Papanicolaou smear annually when the initial two Papanicolaou smears are normal and reliability of follow-up is reasonably certain.
      (4) Papanicolaou smear should be repeated every 6 months when there is a history of the following:
         (a) HPV infection
         (b) Previous Papanicolaou smear showing squamous intraepithelial lesion (SIL) or other cellular abnormalities
         (c) Symptomatic HIV infection

(5) If inflammation is noted, the patient should be evaluated and treated, and a repeat Papanicolaou smear should be collected within 3 months.
(6) If Papanicolaou smear sampling is inadequate, repeat immediately.
(7) If any Papanicolaou smear shows SIL or atypical squamous cells of undetermined significance (ASCUS), refer for colposcopic examination of the lower genital tract.
(8) Treatment of CIN should be by standard modalities. Cryotherapy has been reported to have a higher failure rate.
(9) There is a high likelihood of recurrence of CIN (40%) after standard therapy.

11.7 HIV Infection in Pregnancy

1. Perinatal transmission accounts for the majority of pediatric AIDS cases (≈90% in 2004).
2. There are an estimated 7000 infants born to mothers infected with HIV yearly.
3. The estimated vertical transmission rate of HIV is 14% to 32% in developed countries.
4. Thus, 1000 to 2000 infants are born HIV infected each year.
5. Prevention of HIV infection of the fetus or infant is the most important current strategy.

VERTICAL TRANSMISSION OF HIV

1. Antepartum (transplacental): estimated at 30% to 50% of all cases
2. Intrapartum: exposure to maternal blood and cervical or vaginal secretions, estimated 50% to 70% of all cases
3. Postpartum: breast-feeding may increase risk of vertical transmission by 2% to 14%

FACTORS ASSOCIATED WITH AN INCREASED RISK OF MOTHER-TO-CHILD TRANSMISSION OF HIV

1. Advanced maternal HIV stage
2. Increased maternal viral load
3. Decreased CD4+ lymphocytes
4. Presence of immune complex dissociated (ICD) p24 antigen
5. Preterm labor
6. Premature rupture of membranes
7. Chorioamnionitis

HIV COUNSELING AND TESTING OF PREGNANT WOMEN

1. Recommend HIV testing to all prenatal patients.
2. Perform HIV risk assessment.
3. Women at high risk for HIV infection include those who have the following:
   a. Current or past history of injection drug use
   b. Sexual partners who are injection drug users
   c. Partners who are HIV positive

d. Bisexual partners
e. Current or past history of STDs
f. Multiple sexual partners
g. Past history of receiving blood products before 1985
4. Provide risk reduction counseling if HIV negative.

COUNSELING OF PREGNANT WOMEN WHO ARE HIV POSITIVE

1. Perinatal transmission rate of HIV is 14% to 32%, but can be decreased significantly with therapy.
2. Effect of HIV disease on pregnancy outcome: The same prevalence of intrauterine growth restriction (IUGR), prematurity, and early neonatal disease exists as for seronegative injection drug users.
3. Effect of pregnancy on the course of HIV disease: Studies have not demonstrated a significant influence on the course of HIV disease.
4. Information regarding measures to prevent perinatal transmission, including information on use of Zidovudine (ZDV) should be provided (see Obstetric Management).
5. No evidence exists that HIV is teratogenic.
6. Informed choice about continuing pregnancy should be respected by caregivers.
7. Referrals for pregnancy termination should be made when the option is chosen by the patient.
8. Referral for HIV follow-up and prenatal care should be provided when appropriate.

OBSTETRIC MANAGEMENT

1. Antepartum
   a. The standard approach to the care of women with HIV who are asymptomatic and symptomatic, including laboratory tests, skin tests, vaccinations, and treatments should not be altered because of pregnancy.
   b. Screen for other STDs, including gonorrhea, chlamydia, syphilis, and hepatitis B (present and past exposure).
   c. Pneumovax and hepatitis B vaccine are recommended.
   d. Rubella vaccine is contraindicated.
   e. Intradermal skin test for tuberculosis should be applied with two or more antigen controls (*Candida,* mumps, tetanus toxoid).
   f. Monitor CD4 counts once per trimester and more frequently if clinically indicated.
   g. At 10 to 12 weeks gestation, offer patients the option of ZDV to prevent perinatal transmission.
      (1) Dose.
         (a) Antepartum: ZDV 200 mg PO, three times daily *or* 300 mg, two times daily, until labor
         (b) Intrapartum: ZDV loading 2 mg/kg over 1 hour, then 1 mg/kg/hr maintenance until delivery
         (c) Postpartum: neonate older than 35 weeks gestation to receive oral ZDV syrup, 2 mg/kg, four times daily, for

6 weeks as per pediatrician *or* if younger than 35 weeks, start with 2 mg/kg two times daily
- (2) Maternal monitoring: complete blood count, liver function tests, and serum creatinine monthly.
- (3) Discontinue ZDV therapy if the following occur:
  - (a) Hemoglobin less than 8 mg/dL
  - (b) Platelet count less than 100,000/mm^3
  - (c) Absolute neutrophil count less than 750/mm^3
  - (d) Serum glutamic oxaloacetic transaminase (SGOT) or serum glutamic pyruvate transaminase (SGPT) greater than 5 times normal
  - (e) Serious cardiac, respiratory, neurologic, or gastrointestinal sequelae
- (4) Physicians should consider initiating ZDV for maternal indications when CD4 count is between 200 and 500 and patient is symptomatic or when CD4 count less than 200.
- (5) Lamivudine (3TC) and Nevirapine are second-line therapies.
- (6) If CD4 count less than 200/mm^3 or percentage CD4 less than 20%, begin *Pneumocystis carinii* pneumonia prophylaxis:
  - (a) Double-strength trimethoprim sulfamethoxazole qd or 3 days each week. This drug remains the first-line agent.
    - (i) Sulfonamides pose a theoretical risk of kernicterus to fetus.
    - (ii) Benefits of therapy outweigh its possible risks.
  - (b) Dapsone.
    - (i) Risk of hemolytic anemia in glucose-6-phosphodiesterase (G6PD)—deficient individuals
    - (ii) G6PD level measured before initiating therapy
  - (c) Aerosolized pentamidine, 300 mg, once per month.
- (7) Treatment of opportunistic infections.
  - (a) Recognize the possibility of opportunistic infections and obtain rapid consultation, diagnosis, and management.
  - (b) These infections generally occur with increasing immunosuppression and decreasing CD4 counts less than 200/mm^3.
  - (c) Aggressive therapy rarely needs to be altered because of pregnancy.
  - (d) Provider and patient must weigh the benefits and possible fetal risks of each therapy.
2. Intrapartum
   a. Mode of delivery should be for obstetric indication only.
   b. Fetal scalp sampling or electrode placement is to be avoided if possible.
   c. Prolonged rupture of membranes may increase the chance for vertical transmission of HIV.
   d. Universal blood and body fluid precautions should be practiced:
   - (1) Needles should not be resheathed.
   - (2) Water barrier gowns should be worn.
   - (3) Double gloving should be used in the operating room.
   - (4) Goggles should be used.
   - (5) Mouth-operated suction traps should not be used.

e. ZDV prophylaxis should be considered immediately if occupational exposure occurs.
3. Postpartum
   a. Continue universal blood and body fluid precautions.
   b. Counseling is against breast-feeding in the United States.
   c. Pediatric HIV follow-up should be arranged.
   d. Maternal HIV and gynecology referrals should be given.
4. Contraceptive counseling
   a. Contraceptive options should be discussed with all patients.
   b. Education about safer sexual practices should be provided.
   c. Barrier contraception (condoms and spermicide) should be recommended for vaginal, anal, and oral intercourse to reduce transmission of HIV.
   d. Hormonal contraception is not contraindicated in women who are HIV positive. Barrier techniques should accompany hormonal methods.
   e. Intrauterine devices (IUD) may be contraindicated in women with HIV infection. There is an increased susceptibility to PID, a greater risk of transmission because of increased blood flow, and the possibility of microabrasions on the head of the sexual partner's penis caused by the tail of the IUD.
   f. The option of surgical sterilization should be discussed with fully informed consent. It should neither be denied nor encouraged.

SUGGESTED READINGS

American College of Obstetricians and Gynecologists: Human immunodeficiency virus infections. In ACOG *Technical Bulletin 169*, Washington, DC, 1992, ACOG.

Carpenter CC et al: Human immunodeficiency virus infection in North American women: experience with 200 cases and a review of the literature, *Medicine* (Baltimore) 70:307-325, 1991.

Centers for Disease Control: MMWR 39(47), 1990.

Centers for Disease Control: Update: acquired immunodeficiency syndrome—United States, 1992, MMWR 42(28), 1993.

Centers for Disease Control: 2002 Sexually transmitted disease guidelines, MMWR 51(RR-6), 2002.

Centers for Disease Control: Update: barrier protection against HIV infection and other sexually transmitted diseases, MMWR 42(30), 1993.

Centers for Disease Control: Revised guidelines for HIV counseling, testing and referral, MMWR 50(RR19), 2001.

Centers for Disease Control: Revised recommendations for HIV screening of pregnant women, MMWR 50(RR19), 2001.

Centers for Disease Control: Revised surveillance case definition for HIV infection, MMWR 48(RR-13), 1999.

Centers for Disease Control: U.S. Public Health Service Task Force recommendation for the use of antiretroviral drugs in pregnant HIV-1 infected women for maternal health and intervention to reduce perinatal HIV-1 transmission in the U.S., 2005.

Center for Disease Control: Guidelines for use of antiretroviral agents in HIV-1 infected adults and adolescents, 2005.

Centers for Disease Control: Update: AIDS among women—United States, 1994, MMWR 44, 1995.

Centers for Disease Control: USPHS/IDSA guidelines for the prevention of opportunistic infection in persons infected with human immunodeficiency virus: a summary, *MMWR* 44(RR-8), 1995.

Chin S, Wortley P: Epidemiology of HIV/AIDS in women, In Minkoff H, Dehovitz JA, Duerr A, editors: *HIV infection in women,* New York, 1995, Raven Press.

Clinical management of the HIV infected adult, 2003.

Dehovitz JA: Natural history of HIV infection in women, In Minkoff H, Dehovitz JA, Duerr A, editors: *HIV infection in women,* New York, 1995, Raven Press.

European Collaborative Study: Risk factors for mother-to-child transmission of HIV-1, *Lancet* 339:1007, 1992.

Gwinn M et al: Prevalence of HIV infection in childbearing women in the United States, *JAMA* 265:1704-1708, 1991.

Hoegsberg B et al: Sexually transmitted diseases and human immunodeficiency virus among women with pelvic inflammatory disease, *Am J Obstet Gynecol* 163:1175-1179, 1990.

Hook III EW: HIV/sexually transmitted disease interactions in women, In Minkoff H, Dehovitz JA, Duerr A, editors: *HIV infection in women,* New York, 1995, Raven Press.

Maiman M et al: Human immunodeficiency virus infection and cervical neoplasia, *Gynecol Oncol* 38:377-382, 1990.

Maiman M et al: Colposcopic evaluation of human immunodeficiency virus-seropositive women, *Obstet Gynecol* 70:84-88, 1991.

Mandelblatt JS et al: Association between HIV infection and cervical neoplasia: implications for clinical care of women at risk for both conditions, *AIDS* 6:173-178, 1992.

Minkoff H: Exposing offspring to HIV infection, *Contemporary Ob/Gyn* 40(4):60-66, 1995.

New York State Department of Health, AIDS Institute, Medical Care Criteria Committee, Women's HIV Care Subcommittee, Health Care Services for Women with HIV Infection, July 1995.

Safrin S et al: Seroprevalence and epidemiologic correlates of human immunodeficiency virus infection in women with acute pelvic inflammatory disease, *Am J Obstet Gynecol* 163, 1993.

Safety and toxicity of individual antiretroviral agents in pregnancy, 2005.

Trends in HIV/AIDS diagnosis in 33 states 2001-2004, *MMWR* 54(RR45), 2005.

Villari P et al: Cesarean section to reduce perinatal transmission of human immunodeficiency virus: potential benefits and costs, *T Online J Curr Clin Rev Document* 74, 1993.

Worth LA: HIV infection in women, In Cohen PT, Sande MA, Volberding PA, editors: *The AIDS knowledge base,* ed 2, Boston, 1994, Little, Brown.

Evaluation of Lower Abdominal and Pelvic Pain

Avi Sklar • Farkad Balaya

Lower abdominal and pelvic pain are the most common symptoms encountered in gynecologic practice and are clinically challenging despite recent technologic advances in pregnancy testing, diagnostic imaging, and endoscopy. In fact, most women will experience some type of pelvic pain during the course of their lives. A detailed and thorough history, physical examination, selective use of diagnostic tests, and a well-considered differential diagnosis usually lead to an accurate diagnosis and appropriate therapy.

It is important to differentiate acute pain from chronic pelvic pain (CPP) that has been present for 6 months or more. CPP is further classified as episodic (e.g., dysmenorrhea) or continuous that waxes and wanes but is rarely or never completely absent. In each category, causes are further subdivided by gynecologic or nongynecologic origin. Some conditions (e.g., endometriosis) may be acute, episodic, or chronic. In the reproductive age, *pregnancy-related events must always be considered.*

12.1 Anatomy and Physiology

1. Stimuli that produce pain from lesions within the pelvic and lower abdomen arise from the following:
   a. Distension and subsequent high-amplitude contractions of a hollow viscus (e.g., bowel obstruction)
   b. Rapid stretching of an organ capsule (e.g., hematosalpinx)
   c. Chemical irritation of the parietal peritoneum (e.g., ruptured ovarian cyst)
   d. Tissue ischemia (e.g., degenerating fibroids)
   e. Neuritis secondary to inflammatory, neoplastic, or fibrotic processes in adjacent organs
2. Lesions involving the lower uterine segment, cervix, bladder trigone, or rectum tend to incite pain localized to the lower sacral area or the buttocks, with occasional radiation down the leg (sacral nerve roots 2 through 4).
3. Stimuli from the uterine fundus, adnexa, bladder dome, distal ileum, cecum, and appendix produce pain localized in the lower abdomen (hypogastric plexus).

4. Sensations from somatic structures (e.g., external genitalia and vagina) can be distinctly localized by the cerebral cortex, whereas those from visceral structures are poorly localized.
5. Pain originating in any organ is felt in a skin area supplied by the corresponding spinal nerve (dermatome) rather than in the specific organ site. This lack of correlation between perceived site and organ of origin contributes to the difficulties encountered in the diagnosis of pelvic pain.

12.2 Assessment

1. History
   a. Onset: Pain of sudden onset usually indicates an acute intraperitoneal event that exposes the pelvic peritoneum to blood, pus, bowel contents, ovarian cyst contents, or ischemic infarction. Events include hemorrhage, torsion, or rupture of an adnexal mass, bowel perforation, acute inflammation, ureteric calculi, and bowel obstruction. Pain of gradual onset suggests a more chronic process such as endometriosis or neoplasm.
   b. Character: Pain may be intermittent or constant, sharp or dull.
      (1) Intermittent pain of a colicky nature suggests obstruction of a hollow viscus such as bowel, ureter, uterus, or fallopian tube.
      (2) An intraperitoneal catastrophe is associated with acute sharp pain.
      (3) Dull pain is usually associated with inflammation.
      (4) Constant pain is more likely caused by intraperitoneal hemorrhage, ischemia of a pelvic or abdominal organ, or ovarian cyst rupture.
   c. Degree: Severe pain usually denotes peritoneal irritation, tissue infarction, and colic of the uterus, ureter, and intestine.
   d. Duration.
      (1) An acute incident (e.g., rupture, viscus perforation) causes the woman to present shortly after the onset.
      (2) Inflammatory conditions (e.g., pelvic inflammatory disease [PID], acute appendicitis) usually have a more indolent onset.
      (3) The duration of CPP is variable and often present for years.
   e. Relationship to menstrual cycle.
      (1) In the reproductive age group, any pain following a short period of amenorrhea must be assumed to be a complication of pregnancy until disproved.
      (2) Cyclic pelvic pain is often functional in nature, related to ovulation, premenstrual tension, or dysmenorrhea.
   f. Radiation: Pain radiation is often indicative of the degree of parietal peritoneal involvement.
   g. Associated symptoms.
      (1) Gastrointestinal symptoms
         (a) Anorexia
         (b) Nausea
         (c) Vomiting
         (d) Diarrhea

- (e) Tenesmus
- (f) Dyschezia
- (g) Bloody stools
- (2) Urinary symptoms
  - (a) Frequency
  - (b) Urgency
  - (c) Dysuria
  - (d) Hesitency
  - (e) Hematuria
  - (f) Flank pain
- (3) Shoulder tip pain: secondary to diaphragmatic irritation from blood or puss
- (4) Syncope: not uncommon with intraperitoneal bleeding, even in small amount
- (5) Modifiers of the pain, including relieving and aggravating factors (e.g., medications)
- (6) Fever and chills often indicate an infectious disorder (e.g., salpingitis, pyelonephritis, appendicitis)
- (7) Dyspareunia
- (8) Vaginal bleeding or spotting
- h. Past medical, surgical, menstrual, sexual, social, and contraceptive history must be noted.
- i. Review records from previous hospitalizations, surgeries, endoscopy, colonoscopy, and radiological investigations (especially for the patient with CPP).

2. Physical examination
  a. General appearance and vital signs.
  b. Heart and lung examination: Abdominal pain may be referred from pulmonary and cardiac disease, which must be ruled out.
  c. Abdominal examination.
    (1) Inspection for distension, contour, color changes (e.g., Cullen's sign), scars, area of greatest pain (patient should indicate where)
    (2) Auscultation for absent, hypoactive, or hyperactive bowel signs
    (3) Palpation for mass, tenderness, peritoneal signs (focal or diffuse), guarding, rebound tenderness, reflex rigidity, costovertebral angle tenderness (site of maximum pain should be evaluated last)
    (4) Percussion for ascites, shifting dullness
  d. Pelvic examination.
    (1) Inspection of external genitalia and cervix for evidence of trauma, infection, discharge, hemorrhage, or asymmetry
    (2) Palpation of the vaginal wall for tenderness and palpation of the cervix for cervical motion tenderness
    (3) Bimanual examination starting with the side of least tenderness and noting the size, shape, location, tenderness, mobility, and consistency of any mass and position and mobility of the uterus
    (4) Rectovaginal examination including stool for occult blood and assessment of the uterosacral ligaments and rectovaginal septum

(5) Presence of a pelvic or abdominal tumor: should not necessarily lead to the conclusion that the pain is secondary to the lesion (e.g., a patient with a multinodular fibroid uterus is subject to a variety of acute pelvic processes unrelated to the myomas)
(6) Absence of palpable pathology: does not rule out the presence of organic disease (e.g., endometriosis)

3. Investigations: If a firm diagnosis cannot be made, a differential diagnosis should facilitate selection of the appropriate investigations among the following list (Box 12-1):
   a. Complete blood count with differential.
      (1) An increased white blood cell count, especially with a left shift, may indicate systemic infection.
      (2) Decreased hemoglobin levels may indicate blood loss (internally or externally).
   b. Urinalysis: Presence of bacteria, white blood cells, or red blood cells suggests urinary involvement.
   c. Blood type and antibody screen.
      (1) Blood should be typed and screened for any surgical case.
      (2) Rhogam should be administered to unsensitized Rh-negative patients with miscarriages or ectopic pregnancies.
   d. Pregnancy test: Urine human chorionic gonadotropin (HCG) immunoassay is quick and sensitive to 50 mIU/mL. Serum (β-HCG) can be quantitated and followed serially.
   e. Cervical cultures for gonorrhea and chlamydia testing (enzyme immunoassays or antigen detection systems) are indicated when pelvic infection is suspected.
   f. Culdocentesis may be helpful in evaluating the peritoneal cavity for the following:
      (1) Blood (ectopic pregnancy, ruptured hemorrhagic ovarian cyst, ruptured spleen).
      (2) Free fluid (ruptured functional cyst).
      (3) Pus (PID, appendicitis).
      (4) Fixed mass in the cul-de-sac is a contraindication for this test.
   g. Erythrocyte sedimentation rate is nonspecific in an acute-phase C-reactive protein that indicates an inflammatory reaction when elevated.
   h. Ultrasound (U/S).
      (1) Transvaginal U/S avoids the thick abdominal wall and urine-filled bladder and generally has better resolution as the probe moves closer to the pelvic contents unobstructed by layers of fat and muscle.
      (2) A large pelvic-abdominal mass may be missed unless an abdominal U/S is performed.
      (3) U/S is helpful in the workup of early intrauterine pregnancy, ectopic pregnancy, adnexal mass, and in patients who cannot be examined otherwise because of pain, obesity, vaginal stenosis, or other conditions.
   i. Laparoscopy.
      (1) Laparoscoy is a valuable tool to diagnose and initiate therapy especially with ectopic pregnancy, salpingitis, appendicitis,

BOX 12-1 Differential Diagnosis of Pelvic and Lower Abdominal Pain

Acute

EARLY PREGNANCY COMPLICATIONS
Spontaneous abortion
Septic abortion
Ectopic pregnancy
Hemorrhagic corpus luteum of pregnancy
Gestational trophoblastic disease
Uterine incarceration

PELVIC INFECTIONS

PAIN OF ADNEXAL ORIGIN
Rupture
Hemorrhage
Torsion
Ovarian hyperstimulation syndrome

LEIOMYOMAS
Degeneration
Pedunculated myoma torsion
Aborting submucous myoma

INTESTINAL SOURCES OF PAIN
Appendicitis or hernia
Inflammatory bowel disease
Intestinal obstruction
Gastroeneritis diverticulitis
Meckel's diverticulitis colon fumors
Torsion of appendices epiploicae

URINARY SOURCES OF PAIN
Overdistended bladder
Acute cystitis
Ureteral calculi
Pelvic kidney
Urethral syndrome
Interstitial cystitis

VASCULAR SOURCES OF PAIN
Pelvic thrombophlebitis
Mesenteric occlusion

SYSTEMIC CAUSES OF PAIN
Sickle cell disease
Diabetes mellitus
Drug withdrawal
Acute intermittent porphyria
Connective tissue diseases

Box continued on following page

> **BOX 12-1 Differential Diagnosis of Pelvic and Lower Abdominal Pain** *(Continued)*
>
> Familial Mediterranean fever
> Henoch-Schönlein purpura
> Systemic lupus erythematous
> Hereditary angioneurotic edema
> Periarteritis nodosa
>
> **ENDOCRINE DISORDERS**
> Hyperthyroidism
> Addisonian crisis
> Hyperparathyroidism
>
> **INFECTIONS**
> Syphilis
> Tubercular peritonitis
> Herpes zoster virus
>
> ### Chronic
>
> Dysmenorrhea
> Endometriosis
> Adenomyosis
> Adhesions
> Mittelschmerz
> Ovarian remnant syndrome
> Pelvic congestion syndrome
> "Trigger point" abdominal wall pain
>
> **FUNCTIONAL BOWEL DISORDERS**
> Irritable bowel syndrome
> Chronic constipation
> Chronic pelvic pain syndrome

   adnexal accidents (ruptured cyst), endometriosis, and adhesions.
   (2) Contraindications include hypovolemic shock, bowel obstruction, and large pelvic-abdominal masses.
 j. Patients clearly in need of urgent laparotomy may proceed directly to the operating room for diagnosis and management.

12.3 Early Pregnancy Complications

Pregnancy-related complications should be highly suspected in any women of reproductive age with acute or subacute pelvic and lower abdominal pain.

1. Abortions are characterized by vaginal bleeding and suprapubic crampy lower abdominal pain of variable intensity.
   a. Spontaneous abortions
      (1) Threatened abortion is a frequent complication of pregnancy: presented with vaginal bleeding or spotting and a closed cervical os.
      (2) Inevitable abortion: painful uterine cramps/contractions, cervix is dilated, bleeding is increasing.
      (3) Incomplete abortion: partial passage of tissue through an open cervical os.
      (4) Complete abortion: complete passage of products of conception, usually resulting in resolution of symptoms (uterus is small and well contracted with an open cervix, scant vaginal bleeding, and only mild cramping).
   b. Induced abortions: Subsequent to an induced abortion, pelvic pain can occur secondary to the following:
      (1) Incomplete evacuation
      (2) Septic abortion
         (a) Septic abortion is associated with fever and sepsis secondary to infection of the uterine contents.
         (b) Treatment consists of obtaining appropriate cultures, broad-spectrum antibiotics, resuscitative measures, and evacuation of the uterine contents. Delay in evacuation may be fatal.
2. Ectopic pregnancy.

12.4 Ectopic Pregnancy

DEFINITION

An ectopic pregnancy (EP) is one in which a fertilized ovum implants outside the endometrial lining of the uterus; 97% are tubal, 78% ampullary, 12% isthmic, 2% to 3% interstitial, 1% ovarian, 1% to 2% abdominal, 0.5% cervical.

EPIDEMIOLOGY

1. The incidence of ectopic pregnancy increased lately, which correlated strongly with the increased incidence of PID.
   a. Plateauing at approximately 19 per 1000 pregnancies in the early 1990s until now
   b. Increasing number of EPs in the United States: 17,800 reported cases in 1970 and 108,000 in 1992
   c. Decreasing case fatality rate because of advances in diagnosis and therapy: 35.5 per 10,000 EP in 1970; 3.4 per 10,000 EP in 1987
2. Still, EP is the leading cause of pregnancy-related maternal death in the first trimester and accounts for approximately 10% of all pregnancy-related deaths, despite improved diagnostic methods leading to earlier detection and treatment.

ETIOLOGY

1. Anatomic obstruction to zygote passage

2. Abnormalities in tubal motility
3. Transperitoneal migration of the zygote

RISK FACTORS

1. Salpingitis (laparoscopic proven)
   a. One episode: 5.3%
   b. Multiple episodes: 19%
2. Previous EP: 10% to 20%
3. Previous tubal sterilization: 16%
4. Previous tuboplasty: 17% to 20%
5. Intrauterine device: 3% to 16%
6. Progestin-only pill: 2% to 3%
7. Assisted reproductive techniques: 5% to 17%

SIGNS AND SYMPTOMS

1. Presenting symptoms: over 50% of women are asymptomatic before tubal rupture and do not have an identifiable risk factor for ectopic pregnancy.
   a. Abdominal pain: 87% to 99%
   b. Abnormal bleeding: 48% to 64%
   c. Amenorrhea: 61% to 79%
   d. Pregnancy symptoms: 23%
   e. Syncope: 6% to 37%
   f. Shoulder pain: 5% to 22%
   g. Tissue passage: 6% to 7%
2. Presenting signs
   a. Abdominal tenderness: 97% to 99%
   b. Adnexal tenderness: 87% to 99%
   c. Peritoneal signs: 71% to 76%
   d. Adnexal mass: 33% to 53%
   e. Enlarged uterus: 6% to 30%
   f. Shock: 2% to 17%

DIFFERENTIAL DIAGNOSIS

1. Corpus luteum cyst
2. Rupture of torsion of ovarian cyst
3. Threatened or incomplete abortion
4. PID
5. Appendicitis
6. Gastroenteritis
7. Dysfunctional uterine bleeding
8. Degenerating uterine fibroids

DIAGNOSTIC MODALITIES (Fig. 12-1)

1. Pregnancy test.
   a. Monoclonal urine HCG (enzyme-linked immunosorbent assay [ELISA])
   b. Serum QHCG
      (1) Of normal intrauterine pregnancies, 85% have a mean doubling time for the hormone from 1.4 to 2.1 days.

    (2) Abnormal gestations shows less than 66% increase of QHCG within 2 days.
    (3) Of EP, 13% may have a normal doubling time.
  2. Progesterone.
     a. Decreased production in EP
     b. Single determination
     c. Progesterone less than 5 ng/mL: strongly predictive of abnormal pregnancy 99.8%
     d. Progesterone greater than 25 ng/mL: strongly predictive of normal intrauterine pregnancy 98% to 99%
  3. U/S: The sensitivity of detecting an EP can be increased by using both transvaginal ultrasound (TVS) and color-flow Doppler technology.
     a. Presence of an intrauterine pregnancy rules out EP (heterotopic pregnancy is rare in the nonreproductive-assisted pregnancy, approximately 1 per 30,000).
     b. Normal intrauterine gestation seen when QHCG greater than discriminatory-zone (DZ):
        (1) DZ for abdominal U/S: 6000 mIU/mL (international reference preparation [IRP])
        (2) DZ for transvaginal U/S: 6000 mIU/mL (IRP)
     c. U/S findings in EP include the following:
        (1) Empty uterus
        (2) Increased decidual response
        (3) Adnexal mass or ring
        (4) Free peritoneal fluid
        (5) Fetal sac or pole in the tube
        (6) Active fetal heart in adnexa
  4. Culdocentesis.
     a. It is clinically useful when other diagnostic modalities are not readily available.
     b. Positive tap means nonclotting blood with hematocrit (Hct) greater than 12%. Positive tap in up to 70% of EP, of which 65% are unruptured.
     c. Negative tap means clear or blood-tinged fluid.
     d. Nondiagnostic tap means clotted blood or no fluid.
  5. Dilation and curettage (D&C).
     a. D&C may be useful with low progesterone or abnormal serial QHCG levels.
     b. Products of conception on pathology rules out EP.
  6. Diagnostic laparoscopy.
     a. Can diagnose and treat EP in the hemodynamically stable patient.
     b. If performed too early, can miss the EP.

THERAPEUTIC OPTIONS

Before initiation of any protocol, Rh(D) immune globulin should be administered if the woman is Rh(D)-negative and the blood group of her male partner is Rh(D)-positive or unknown.

1. Expectant management is not recommended, as a higher chance of morbidity and mortality is a complication to this management.

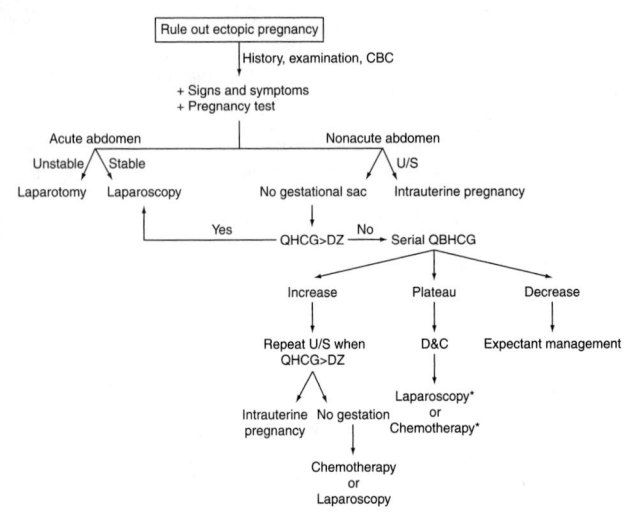

Figure 12-1 Steps in the diagnosis and treatment of lower abdominal or pelvic pain. *If clinically indicated. CBC, Complete blood count; D&C, dilation and curettage; DZ, discriminatory zone.

2. Medical management.
   a. Intramuscular (IM), intravenous (IV), or oral (per os; PO) methotrexate: Most common regimen is methotrexate 50 mg/m^2 body surface area.
   b. Selection criteria:
      (1) Compliant stable patient
      (2) No contraindication to methotrexate (hepatic or renal disease, thrombocytopenia, leukopenia, significant anemia)
      (3) Less than 3.5 cm mass
      (4) QHCG less than 10,000 mIU/mL (IRP)
      (5) No evidence of hemoperitoneum on transvaginal sonogram
   c. An 87% success rate with minimal side effects (stomatitis, elevated hepatic transaminases, leukopenia, dermatitis).
   d. Require second dose or surgical intervention if QHCG increases or plateaus after 7 days.
   e. Tubal mass may take up to 3 months to resolve.
3. Salpingiocentesis: direct injection of chemotherapy (e.g., methotrexate, 25 mg) into EP via laparoscopy, transvaginal U/S, or hysteroscopy.
4. Surgery (laparoscopy or laparotomy).
   a. Laparoscopy has the advantage of decreased recuperation time and shorter hospitalization.
   b. Alspingostomy or segmental resection depends on tubal location and size of EP.
      (1) In ampullary EP, the trophoblast has invaded the mucosa and propagated in the extraluminal, subserosal space.

(2) In contrast, isthmic pregnancies tend to propagate within and disrupt the lumen.
   c. Isthmic EP: Segmental resection is followed by delayed microsurgical anastomosis.
   d. Ampullary and fimbrial EP: Linear salpingostomy should be performed.
   e. Interstitial EP: Pregnancy should be resected with tubal preservation followed by delayed microsurgical anastomosis.
5. Salpingectomy.
   a. Recurrent EP in the same tube
   b. Patient not desiring future fertility
   c. Uncontrolled bleeding from the implantation site
   d. Severely damaged tube
   e. Large tubal pregnancy (i.e., greater than 5 cm)
6. Persistent EP.
   a. Persistent EP results from residual trophoblastic tissue or secondary implantation after surgery.
   b. Follow QHCG every week until less than 15 mIU/mL.
   c. Expect QHCG less than 20% preoperative level within 72 hours.
   d. If QHCG increases or plateaus, medical or surgical intervention is required.
   e. Occurs more often after salpingostomy performed at laparoscopy than at laparotomy, 8% versus 4%, respectively.

12.5 Hemorrhagic Corpus Luteum of Pregnancy

1. Rupture or hemorrhage of the corpus luteum occurs occasionally in the first trimester.
2. It is associated with acute onset of unilateral lower abdominal pain, with or without an adnexal mass.
3. When an intrauterine gestation is not seen on U/S, this condition may be confused with an EP.

12.6 Gestational Trophoblastic Disease

1. Molar pregnancy generally becomes symptomatic late in the first trimester or early in the second.
2. It often presents with abnormal bleeding and cramps, increased nausea and vomiting, suggesting a threatened abortion, and may be associated with uterine enlargement beyond that appropriate for dates, hyperthyroidism, preeclampsia before 20 weeks of gestation.
3. U/S is often diagnostic.
4. Bilateral ovarian enlargements caused by massive luteinization of both ovaries may be present and may become symptomatic if torsion occurs.

12.7 Pregnant Uterine Incarceration

1. This rare complication results from the continued growth of a retroflexed pregnant uterus trapped in the concavity of the sacrum between the twelfth and sixteenth week of pregnancy.
2. Symptoms and signs of threatened abortion occur.

3. They are generally relieved with repositioning of the uterus, which may require general anesthesia.
4. The condition is recognizable by the displacement of the cervix upward to a position directly behind the pubic symphysis, where it is found on pelvic examination to be firmly wedged.

12.8 Pelvic Infections

1. Pelvic infections include acute salpingitis and its complications of tuboovarian abscess, pyosalpingitis, and perhepatitis. Where an initial cervicitis can subsequently spread to cause an endometritis, salpingitis, and potentially peritonitis, intraabdominal suppuration may continue, producing a pelvic abscess. Most upper tract infections are presumed to be polymicrobial and should be treated with the same regard.
2. Classic presentation of acute PID includes a history of fairly acute lower abdominal pain, pyrexia, tachycardia, and sometimes gastrointestinal symptoms. The pain is usually poorly localized in the lower abdomen. There may be urinary frequency, dysuria, and often a vaginal discharge that may or may not be associated with vaginal bleeding.
3. On physical examination, the patient may appear flushed and distressed. The lower abdomen is very tender with guarding, but the epigastrium is usually soft. Pelvic examination is usually unsatisfactory because of the degree of bilateral adnexal tenderness and abdominal guarding. Cervical motion tenderness is present.
4. Early aggressive treatment may minimize the risks of sequels such as infertility, CPP, adhesions, and EP. Therefore, the clinician should have a lower threshold to hospitalize these patients for parenteral antibiotic therapy and interventional laparoscopic treatment, especially women of reproductive age.
5. It is important to note that many cases of salpingitis have attenuated or even an absence of symptoms and clinical findings.
6. It is often difficult to distinguish between PID and other causes of pelvic pain such as endometriosis, ovarian cyst rupture, and appendicitis. Frequently, these patients are treated with antibiotics without establishment of the correct diagnosis and mislabeled as having PID. (See full discussion of PID in Chapter 10.)

12.9 Pain of Adnexal Origin

The ovary is relatively insensitive to pain (e.g., an endometrioma may asymptomatically grow up to 15 cm in diameter because of the gradual nature of fluid accumulation). Pain in an adnexal mass is usually a result of rupture, intratumor hemorrhage, or torsion. Acute distension of the fallopian tube (e.g., EP, pyosalpynx) can cause intense colicky pain. An associated history of intercourse, intense physical activity, or abdominal trauma is commonly noted. U/S is often helpful in outlining an adnexal mass or fluid in the cul-de-sac because physical examination may be limited secondary to pain and abdominal guarding.

1. Ovarian cyst rupture
   a. Pain depends on the nature of the cyst's contents and the presence or absence of bleeding.
   b. Rupture or leakage of a benign cystic teratoma releases highly irritating material in the peritoneal cavity with potential development of the following:
      (1) Chemical peritonitis
      (2) Persistent spreading pelvic pain
      (3) Fever
      (4) Ileus
      (5) Abdominal distension
   c. Rupture of a follicular cyst is often painless or may cause only a temporary acute reaction that rapidly resolves.
   d. Corpus luteum cyst rupture is often associated with some degree of intraperitoneal bleeding and is frequently painful. This condition should be suspected in patients on anticoagulant therapy who have repeated bouts of abdominal pain during the luteal phase.
   e. The escape of old blood from endometriomas may produce repetitive acute attacks of pain.
      (1) Occurring with menses, they may be associated with fever up to 101° F (38.3°C) and may be mistaken for flare-ups of PID.
      (2) Because these attacks are self-limited, usually 7 to 10 days, mistakenly instituted antibiotic therapy appears to be repeatedly effective.
2. Internal hemorrhage
   a. Can cause sudden distension of a cystic or solid ovarian tumor producing a boring, throbbing pain of increasing severity.
   b. The mass usually has a tense consistency and is exquisitely tender.
   c. Delayed surgical intervention may result in infarction, tissue necrosis, and systemic toxicity.
3. Torsion of an ovarian or tubal mass
   a. Torsion may be intermittent, producing characteristic recurrent attacks of colicky pain, nausea, vomiting, and low-grade fever.
   b. It may also be persistent proceeding to thrombosis of the infundibulopelvic vessels beyond the twist site and tissue necrosis.
   c. Occasionally, torsion with necrosis of the tumor can be sufficiently walled off by the bowel and the omentum so that the process becomes low grade and chronic.

12.10 Ovarian Hyperstimulation Syndrome

1. Ovarian hyperstimulation syndrome (OHSS) is an iatrogenic cause of multiple follicular cysts in infertility patients as a consequence of ovulation induction, generally with gonadotropins and rarely with clomiphene.
2. The syndrome, which is self-limiting, is worsened and prolonged with conception because of the continued stimulation by HCG.
3. Signs and symptoms include the following:
   a. Abdominal pain
   b. Abdominal distension

c. Massive ovarian enlargement
d. Ascites
e. Pleural effusions
f. Dyspnea
g. Weight gain
h. Electrolyte imbalance
i. Hemoconcentration
j. Oliguria
k. Hypercoagulability

4. Patients usually respond to conservative management with particular attention to fluid status, correction of electrolyte imbalance, bed rest, and avoidance of any activity including coitus.
5. Mannitol may be used if renal failure is imminent and an ion-exchanged resin can reverse hyperkalemia.
6. Surgical intervention is rarely necessary except in cases of torsion or rupture.
7. The best treatment of OHSS is primary prevention: preventing the ovulation by withholding ovulation trigger medications (HCG, etc.).

12.11 Leiomyomas

1. Leiomyoma can be one or more tumors, with the size of millimeters to tens of centimeters. The size is usually described in menstrual weeks, as with the gravid uterus.
2. Leiomyoma is either asymptomatic in most cases or presents with vaginal bleeding, pelvic pressure, pain, or the complaint of infertility.
3. Uncomplicated uterine leiomyomas generally are asymptomatic. When acute pain is the presenting symptom, it is important to establish that no other coexisting pathology is involved. Complications of myoma that commonly cause acute pain include the following:
   a. Degeneration of the fibroid.
   b. Torsion of a pedunculated myoma leading to infarction produces acute colicky pain.
   c. Aborting submucous myoma comes with laborlike crampy pain and prolonged menstrual bleeding. Sometimes pain is accompanied by low-grade fever, increased white blood cell count, or peritoneal signs.
4. Treatment is:
   a. Surgical with the myoma sent for frozen section to rule out a mixed Millerian malignancy.
   b. Embolization of the uterine artery is used in some cases, with decrease of 50% per year of the fibroid size.
   c. Conservative if found accidentally or asymptomatic.

12.12 Intestinal Sources of Pain

1. Appendicitis.
   a. The pain of appendicitis usually starts as a vague, dull, lower epigastric or periumbilical discomfort.

b. After several hours, if the appendix is not retroperitoneal, the pain shifts to the right lower quadrant (RLQ), with the point of maximum tenderness at McBurney's point once the overlying parietal peritoneum becomes locally involved in the inflammatory process.
c. Associated symptoms include the following:
    (1) Anorexia
    (2) Nausea
    (3) Vomiting
d. Abdominal distension is unusual and bowel sounds are usually normal or slightly hypoactive.
e. Guarding, rebound tenderness, and Rovsing's sign (pain felt in the RLQ resulting from palpation in the left lower quadrant [LLQ]) are suggestive of the diagnosis.
f. The presence of adductor pain (that produced by passive internal rotation of the flexed thigh) or the psoas sign (an increase in pain from the passive extension of the right hip joint that stretches the iliopsoas muscle) may suggest both the anatomic location of the appendix and the progression of the inflammatory process.
g. It is often a difficult diagnosis because of the variable position of the appendix and the spectrum conditions with a similar form of presentation.
h. When the differential diagnosis cannot be effectively established, laparoscopy or exploratory laparotomy is indicated, because the risk of morbidity and mortality of appendiceal rupture is significant.

2. Inflammatory bowel disease.
    a. Ulcerative colitis involves the mucosa and submucosa of the gut and principally presents with lower abdominal cramping and diarrhea, often accompanied by rectal bleeding, tenesmus, and rectal urgency. The pain is usually LLQ and the initial course may be intermittent, with exacerbations or remissions lasting for up to a few months.
    b. Crohn's disease (ileitis) involves all tissue layers of the bowel.
        (1) The common symptoms include the following:
            (a) Diarrhea
            (b) Fever
            (c) RLQ pain
            (d) Sometimes associated with anorexia, nausea, vomiting, and perianal abscesses or fistulae
        (2) Although the disease is chronic, the initial symptoms are usually significant enough that the patient is evaluated for acute abdominal pain; often confused with appendicitis.

3. Intestinal obstruction.
    a. Pain is the primary complaint in all forms of small and large bowel obstruction arising from the following:
        (1) Adhesive bands
        (2) Tumors
        (3) Intussusception
        (4) Volvulus
        (5) Internal hernias

b. The pain of obstruction is intermittent, colicky, and usually accompanied by nausea, vomiting, progressive abdominal distension, and inability to pass flatus.
c. Bowel sounds are characteristically hyperactive and high pitched.
d. In distal small bowel or large bowel obstructions, the pain is less colicky and vomiting occurs late and often is feculent and foul smelling.
e. The diagnosis can be established by flat plate and upright films of the abdomen.

4. Gastroenteritis: This is a complex clinical syndrome characterized by colicky abdominal pain, diarrhea, and sometimes vomiting.
   a. Causal agents include enteric viral pathogens, *Salmonella*, and certain bacterial toxins.
   b. The pain is diffuse throughout the abdomen and may occur in various quadrants at different times.
   c. On physical examination, bowel sounds are found to be hyperactive, but not as high pitched as in bowel obstruction.
   d. The patient is often dehydrated.
   e. Stool studies for leukocytes, culture, ova, and parasites are indicated unless symptoms subside within 48 hours (staph infection).

5. Diverticulitis.
   a. Acquired diverticula are saclike profusions of the intestinal mucosa through the muscularis, which are covered only by the serosa.
   b. Most commonly located in the sigmoid, their frequency decreases as one ascends the intestinal tract.
   c. Diverticular disease's frequency increases with age, increasing from less than 5% at age 40, to 30% by age 60, to 65% by age 85.
   d. This is in contradiction to appendicitis and ileitis, which occur most frequently during the second and third decades of life.
   e. Diverticulitis results when diverticula become infected or perforate, which may lead to the formation of a pericolonic abscess.
   f. The principal symptom is LLQ abdominal pain, but if the sigmoid mesentery is elongated, the pain and tenderness may be in the RLQ. Right-sided diverticulitis occurs in only 1.5% of patients in Western countries but is more common in Asians (accounting for as many as 75% of cases of diverticulitis). Affected patients may present with RLQ pain.
   g. The patient may report prolonged periods of constipation, with intermittent episodes of lower abdominal pain sometimes relieved by defecation.
   h. On physical examination, the patient may appear clinically ill, with a fever of 101° to 102° F (38.3° to 38.9°C), and dehydrated.

6. Meckel's diverticulitis.
   a. Meckel's diverticulum is an embryologic remnant of the omphaloenteric duct.
   b. It is typically located on the antimesenteric border of the terminal ileum approximately 2 feet from the ileocecal valve.
   c. The diverticulum may be lined by astric mucosa or by exocrine pancreatic tissue and may produce painless gastrointestinal bleeding of obscure cause.

    d. If ulceration occurs, the diverticulum can become inflamed, producing lower abdominal pain with a midline or right of midline location.
    e. Seen infrequently, this condition is hard to differentiate from acute appendicitis, and the diagnosis of Meckel's diverticulitis is most often retrospective.
7. Colon tumors.
    a. Tumors of the colon (adenomatour polyps, villous tumors, adenocarcinomas, carcinoids, lymphomas, melanomas, and leiomyosarcomas) usually do not cause pain until they have progressed to the point of obstruction or invasion of the pelvic organs.
    b. The most frequent and early symptoms of bowel carcinomas are change in bowel habits and abdominal pain.
    c. There may also be tenesmus, melena, and weight loss.
    d. When a mass is present, it is often located at the pelvic brim and may be difficult to distinguish from the normal pelvic organs by palpation, but most rectal tumors can be palpated on rectal examination.
8. Torsion of appendices epiploicae.
    a. Rarely, the appendices epiploicae may twist and undergo necrosis. The resultant peritoneal irritation produces pain deep in the pelvis.
    b. This pain often has a rectal reference and is at times associated with tenesmus.
    c. The diagnosis is seldom made preoperatively.
9. Functional bowel disorder: see section on CPP later in this chapter.

12.13 Urinary Tract Sources of Pain

1. Overdistended bladder.
    a. Pain may simulate that produced by distension of a genital organ.
    b. On palpation, the tense bladder resembles a large ovarian cyst or pregnant uterus.
    c. This may occur in association with other conditions (e.g., acute urethritis, postoperative period).
2. Acute cystitis.
    a. Pain is suprapubic, related to micturition, and accompanied by a burning sensation at the external urethral meatus.
    b. Patients may initially present with lower abdominal pressure and soreness, urinary frequency, urgency, dysuria, and possibly hematuria.
    c. Urinalysis (U/A) reveals pyuria, and urine culture is subsequently positive.
    d. Symptoms usually respond to adequate hydration and antibiotics.
3. Ureteral calculi.
    a. Pain begins as an aching sensation that rapidly becomes severe, colicky, and radiates from the flank around the abdomen and down into the groin and labia majora, depending on the position of the stone in the upper urinary tract.
    b. Agitation and a constant search for a comfortable position with episodes of pain so severe as to interfere with respirations are common.

c. Unless obstruction is complete, hematuria is usually seen with or without pyuria.
d. Kidney, ureter, and bladder (KUB), IV pyelogram (IVP), or U/S will generally demonstrate the stone, particularly if it is radiopaque.
4. Pelvic kidney: A congenitally misplaced kidney located in the retroperitoneal area in front of the sacrum has an increased incidence of infectious complications because of stasis and retrograde reflux from the bladder.
5. Urethral syndrome.
   a. Symptoms of suprapubic pain, dysuria, urgency, frequency, dyspareunia, and absence of nocturia are prominent and the diagnosis is one of exclusion.
   b. A negative urine and urethral culture, sexually transmitted disease (STD), and vulvovaginitis evaluation should raise the suspicion of this syndrome.
   c. Urethrocystoscopic evaluation should be performed and urethral diverticulae, interstitial cystitis, and cancer of the bladder, urethra, vulva, cervix, or vagina should be ruled out.
   d. Treatment consists of a trial of antibiotics and, if without success, consideration for urethral dilation in the reproductive-aged women and vaginal estrogen for perimenopausal and postmenopausal women.
6. Interstitial cystitis (IC).
   a. IC is a chronic aseptic inflammation of the bladder of unknown etiology.
   b. Typical presentation is urinary frequency (day and nighttime), urgency, and pelvic or suprapubic pain often relieved by voiding.
   c. Dysuria is common.
   d. IC is often a diagnosis of exclusion and by cystoscopy with hydrodistension looking for Runner's ulcers and glomerulations.
   e. Workup: U/A is essential to determine the presence of pyuria or hematuria. Other considerations include urine culture, urethral culture, and cystoscopy.

12.14 Vascular Sources of Pain

1. Pelvic thrombophlebitis
   a. Pelvic thrombophlebitis may occur in the postoperative period or after obstetric complications of pelvic infection.
   b. Disease may be septic or primarily thrombotic, and pain may accompany severe disease.
   c. The presence of spiking temperatures, chills, tachycardia, an aching type of pelvic pain, and lack of response to antibiotics are suggestive of the diagnosis.
   d. The absence of a pelvic mass associated with pelvic wall tenderness tends to confirm the diagnosis, which may be imaged by venography or computed tomography (CT).
2. Small bowel mesenteric occlusion
   a. The pain produced by small bowel mesenteric occlusion (arterial, venous, or embolic) leading to bowel ischemia and necrosis is

initially colicky, periumbilical, and associated with hyperactive bowel sounds.
  b. If unrecognized, ischemia will progress to infarction with the development of an ileus, loss of bowel sounds, generalized peritonitis, sepsis, hemoconcentration, and shock.
  c. Patients often have a history of atrial fibrillation, extensive atherosclerosis, or poor tissue perfusion.
  d. Abdominal examination is notable for the presence of minimal tenderness, mild diffuse rebound, and the patient often appears sicker than the abdominal signs would suggest in the initial phase.
  e. Plain and erect abdominal films most often show evidence of an ileus and thickening of the bowel wall caused by mucosal edema or hemorrhage ("thumbprinting").
  f. Management requires immediate surgical intervention.

12.15 Systemic Causes of Abdominal Pain

Numerous medical conditions, including the following, may be associated with recurrent lower abdominal pain, but this is rarely an isolated or presenting symptom.

1. Sickle cell disease.
2. Diabetes mellitus with or without diabetic ketoacidosis.
3. Drug withdrawal.
4. Acute intermittent porphyria.
5. Connective tissue disease.
   a. Familial Mediterranean fever
   b. Henoch-Schönlein purpura
   c. Systemic lupus erythematosus
   d. Hereditary angioneurotic edema
   e. Periarteritis nodosa
6. Endocrine disorders: Untreated hyperthyroidism, Addisonian crisis, and hyperparathyroidism may be associated with vague and poorly localized lower abdominal pain.
7. Infections.
   a. Syphilis
   b. Tubercular peritonitis
   c. Herpes zoster virus
   d. Human immunodeficiency virus (HIV) infection
   e. Helminthic and other tropical infectious diseases

12.16 Dysmenorrhea

Primary dysmenorrhea is a recurrent, crampy lower abdominal pain that occurs during menstruation in the absence of pelvic pathology, and secondary dysmenorrhea when there is demonstrable organic pathology.

1. Primary dysmenorrhea: It is the most common gynecologic complaint among adolescent females.
   a. Primary dysmenorrhea is caused by prostaglandin-induced uterine contractions and ischemia.

b. Primary dysmenorrhea tends to occur with the onset of ovulatory cycles following menarche and usually improves with time; coincides with the onset of menstrual bleeding; and frequently is associated with other prostaglandin-mediated symptoms (e.g., nausea, vomiting, diarrhea, headache, and dizziness).
c. Pain is sharp, crampy, midline without a lower quadrant or adnexal component, but may have radiation to the lower back and upper thighs. Pelvic examination in a nonmenstruating patient is unremarkable.
d. Treatment is with nonsteroidal antiinflammatory drugs (NSAIDs) or oral contraceptives. Laparoscopy is indicated for failed medical management (rule out endometriosis).
2. Secondary dysmenorrhea: It is more common among women in the fourth and fifth decades of life. Begins in the 20s and progressively worsens, and may improve temporarily after childbirth.
a. Secondary dysmenorrhea is usually caused by endometriosis, adenomyosis, leiomyomas, and less commonly, chronic salpingitis, an intrauterine device, or congenital or acquired outflow tract obstruction, including cervical stenosis.
b. Pain is midline, may include one or both lower quadrants, and may begin long before menses and continue during or after it. Dyspareunia is common.
c. Bimanual pelvic-abdominal examination may demonstrate uterine or adnexal tenderness, fixed uterine retroflexion, uterosacral modularity, a pelvic mass, or an enlarged irregular uterus.
d. Treatment is aimed at evaluation and management of the underlying condition. U/S, laparoscopy, and hysteroscopy may be necessary to establish the diagnosis.

12.17 Endometriosis

Endometriosis is defined as the presence of endometrial glands and stroma outside the endometrial cavity and the uterine musculature.

1. There is a wide spectrum of presentation and clinical course, but the presentation is classically a gradual increase in the duration of dysmenorrhea, appearance of premenstrual pain, and cyclic dyspareunia that gradually becomes continuous but remains worst perimenstrually.
2. Symptoms may be acute (e.g., ruptured endometrioma with an acute abdomen), but they are typically of a gradually increasing and chronic nature.
3. Physical examination may reveal a tender, relatively immobile uterus and adnexa, adneal mass (endometrioma), fixed uterine retroflexion, or thickening and nodularity of the uterosacral ligament.
4. The severity of pain does not correlate with the amount of endometriosis.
5. Therapy is medical and surgical, depending on the severity of disease and the patient's reproductive plans. (Management is discussed in Chapter 9.)

Practical Guide to the Care of the Gynecologic/Obstetric Patient 253

12.18 Adenomyosis

1. Adenomyosis is a benign uterine disease characterized by the growth of endometrial glands and stroma in the uterine myometrium at a depth of at least 2.5 mm from the basalis endometrium layer.
2. The typical patient is multiparous in her later 30s or early 40s, with classic symptoms of progressive dysmenorrhea or menorrhagia.
3. During the premenstrual period, symptomatic patients describe pelvic heaviness, pressure, or an aching sensation.
4. With the onset of menses, the pain becomes more acute and crampy.
5. Pelvic examination is significant for a mildly enlarged, boggy, tender uterus, especially during menses.
6. It is important to note that adenomyosis is a common histologic finding in asymptomatic patients.
7. There is no long-term satisfactory medical treatment.
8. Success is variable with cyclic oral contraceptives and NSAIDs.
9. Gonadotropin-releasing hormone (GnRH) agonists may suppress adenomyosis growth, but any benefits last only as long as the drug is continued.
10. Conservative surgery for adenomyosis (ednomyometrial ablation, laparoscopic myometrial electrocoagulation, or excision of adenomyosis) is of limited use.
11. If a patient is perimenopausal with anticipated cessation of ovarian function, medical therapy with GnRH agonists may obviate the need for hysterectomy.
12. If appropriate for the woman's age, parity, and future reproductive plans, hysterectomy remains the definitive treatment.

12.19 Adhesions

1. The role of adhesions in abdominal and pelvic pain is controversial.
2. The pain may start within weeks of the physical insult responsible (e.g., pelvic infections, surgery).
3. In most instances, pain duration varies from moments to an hour or so, and may be related to physical activity.
4. Over time, pain originating with adhesions may spread, as intestinal, muscular, and chronic pain syndrome factors come into play.
5. The inability to diagnose adhesions accurately by U/S or other imaging techniques makes laparoscopy essential to the diagnosis and treatment.
6. Preoperative evaluation should include studies to exclude more acute causes of pain.
7. Bowel studies (endoscopy or barium enema) should be limited to those women exhibiting signs (e.g., hematachezia, mucus) as opposed to only symptoms of bowel disease.
8. Surgery (laparoscopy of laparotomy) is usually reserved for diagnostic purposes of pain with unknown etiology or attributed to adhesions causing pain with intestinal obstruction refractory to medical management.

12.20 Ovulatory Pain (Mittelschmerz)

1. Midcycle pelvic pain is usually a manifestation of peritoneal irritation caused by the release of blood or follicular fluid from the ovary at the time of ovulation.
2. Pain is generally unilateral, sharp, and dissipates within a few hours but may be intense and prolonged.
3. There may or may not be associated vaginal spotting.
4. When the pain is localized to the RLQ, the differential diagnosis of appendicitis can be challenging.
5. Less commonly, endometriosis or other organic conditions may be associated with isolated midcycle pain or midcycle exacerbation of continuous CPP.
6. Treatment is often expectant; otherwise NSAIDs, or ovarian suppression with oral contraceptives.

12.21 Ovarian Remnant Syndrome

1. Results from residual ovarian cortical tissue that is left in situ after a difficult oophorectomy (severe endometriosis or PID).
2. Often the patient has had multiple pelvic operations with the uterus and adnexa removed sequentially.
3. Patient usually complains of cyclic pelvic pain that may be accompanied by peritoneal signs and usually arises 2 to 5 years after surgery.
4. Pelvic examination may reveal a tender mass in the lateral region of the pelvis and U/S usually confirms a mass with sonographic characteristics of ovarian tissue.
5. Estradiol and follicle-stimulating hormone (FSH) assays reveal a premenopausal picture, although on occasion the remaining ovarian tissue may not be active enough to suppress FSH levels.
6. Medical treatment with danazol, progestins, or oral contraceptives has mixed results and GnRH agonist therapy is impractical for long-term therapy.
7. Surgical resection is usually the definitive therapy.

12.22 Pelvic Congestion Syndrome

1. Pelvic congestion syndrome is an ill-defined syndrome marked by the presence of continuous lower abdominal pain, premenstrual or menstrual accentuation of pain, postcoital aching, dyspareunia, low back pain, increased intensity while standing or jumping, and often associated with premenstrual syndrome.
2. Pelvic examination is usually unremarkable except uterine retroversion is common, and often there is tenderness in the posterior fornix.
3. Laparoscopy may show a normal pelvis or prominent, enlarged, broad ligament veins, the significance of which in the pathophysiology in the condition is uncertain.
4. Treatment is as with the CPP syndrome.

12.23 "Trigger Point" Abdominal Wall Pain

1. Trigger point pain is usually pinpoint, well localized, and of unknown etiology.
2. Diagnosis is confirmed if the patient's pain can be reproduced by pinching of the subcutaneous tissue directly beneath the point of maximal tenderness and by eliciting increased, rather than decreased, tenderness with palpation during voluntary guarding (rectus flexion).
3. Several treatment modalities have shown to be effective, including the following:
   a. Transcutaneous electric nerve stimulation (TENS)
   b. Acupuncture
   c. Massage
   d. Infiltration with a variety of agents (steroids and local anesthetics)
4. A common regimen is 5 to 10 cc of a long-acting topical anesthetic (e.g., bupivicaine, 0.25% to 0.5%) injected directly into the hyperpathic trigger point after it is first localized with the tip of a 25G ½-inch needle.
5. Injections are repeated on a biweekly to monthly basis initially, followed by longer intervals, until a long-term or permanent response is achieved.
6. The overall response rate is approximately 75% to 90%, with most patients requiring three to five injections.

12.24 Functional Bowel Disorders

1. Irritable bowel syndrome (IBS) and chronic constipation are symptomatic manifestations of altered bowel motility and are the most common medical diagnosis in women with CPP.
2. IBS is a common cause of lower abdominal pain that is usually intermittent, crampy, predominantly LLQ in location, but occasionally the pain is constant and often improved after defecation. IBS also accounts for a significant number of visits to primary care physicians, and is the second highest cause of work absenteeism after the common cold.
3. The pain may last for only a few minutes, but at least 50% of patients have pain for hours to days and 20% of patients may complain of pain for weeks or longer.
4. Associated symptoms include the following:
   a. Excessive flatulence
   b. Alternating diarrhea and constipation
   c. Passage of mucus
   d. Altered stool form
   e. Abdominal distension or bloating
5. Symptoms are usually worse during periods of stress, tension, anxiety, depression, and with the premenstrual and menstrual phases of the cycle.

6. The diagnosis is usually made by history and the exclusion of other disorders and therefore sigmoidoscopy and barium enema are often necessary.
7. IBS is a waxing and waning disorder and treatment consists of reassurance, dietary management (increase fiber intake, lactose-free diet, gluten-free diet, and exclusion of foods that increase flatulence [beans, onions, celery, carrots, raisins, bananas, apricots, prunes, brussels sprouts, wheat germ, pretzels, and bagels]), psychotherapy (stress reduction), and medical adjuncts, including anticholinergic agents.
8. Synthetic fiber supplements such as *polycarbophil* and *methylcellulose* are more soluble than natural fibers *(psyllium)* and could be used in the treatment.
9. To improve compliance, patients should be apprised of other advantages of a high-fiber diet, including reduced colon cancer and diverticular disease, and up to 15% mean reduction in serum cholesterol level.
10. Hypnosis, biofeedback, and psychotherapy help to reduce anxiety levels.
11. Care must be exercised to avoid exacerbation of symptoms or substitution of one problem (diarrhea) for another (constipation).
12. The chronic use of drugs should generally be minimized or avoided because of the lifelong nature of this disorder. Two medical adjuncts useful for treatment of unresponsive or severe IBS are dicyclomine and hyoscyamine.
13. Administration of these medications in the treatment of IBS should be on an as-needed basis.

12.25 Chronic Pelvic Pain

1. Facts
   a. Refers to noncyclic pain of at least 6 months duration, involves the region below the umbilicus, and causes functional disability or requires treatment.
   b. It accounts for about 10% of all ambulatory referrals to gynecologists and is one of the common indications for diagnostic and therapeutic surgery.
   c. Accounts for 20% of all hysterectomies performed for benign disease.
   d. Accounts for 40% of all laparoscopies performed annually in the United States.
   e. These patients are often distraught, angry, and demanding, and have a history of prolonged disability, loss of employment, sexual dysfunction, marital discord, divorce, and signs of depression (especially sleep disturbances).
   f. No significant difference was noted in regard to gravidity, parity, rates of elective abortion, race, or educational level.
2. Treatment
   a. Before treatment is initiated doctors should win patients' trust and confidence by listening to them, believing them, and assuring them that they will do all that they can to help.

b. Usually based on history and physical exam a list of differential diagnoses will be achieved with the help of laboratory and radiological tests. Even diagnostic surgery (laparoscopic or open) may be used trying to identify the specific cause.
c. If all previous steps were unable to confirm any diagnosis:
   (1) Heat therapy, especially for musculoskeletal pain.
   (2) Treat depression: It is common in women with CPP and warrants treatment. However, data regarding the efficacy of antidepressants in the treatment of pain in CPP are minimal.
   (3) Hysterectomy: often associated with long-term relief of CPP and is an option for women who have completed childbearing.
   (4) Nerve transection procedures: laparoscopic uterosacral nerve ablation (LUNA), presacral neurectomy (PSN).
   (5) Multidisciplinary approach should be considered (psychological contributors to pelvic pain and possible dependence on opiates are a major focus of most pain clinics).
      (a) Psychological counseling
      (b) Transcutaneous nerve stimulation device
      (c) Behavioral and relaxation feedback therapies
      (d) Implantable nerve stimulation device
      (e) Injection of affected sites with anesthetic medication

SUGGESTED READINGS

AGOG Technical Bulletin: Chronic pelvic pain, 2005.

Howard F: The role of laparoscopy in chronic pelvic pain: promise and pitfalls, *Obstet Gyn Surv* 46:357-386, 1993.

Peters AAW et al: A randomized clinical trial to compare two different approaches in women with chronic pelvic pain, *Obstet Gynecol* 77:740, 1991.

Rapkin AJ, Reading AE: Chronic pelvic pain: current problems in obstetrics, *Gynecol Fertil* 14:99-137, 1991.

Silen W: *Cope's early diagnosis of the acute abdomen*, Oxford University Press, 1991.

Stovall T, Ling F: clinical diagnosis and management, *Extrauterine pregnancy*, New York, McGraw-Hill, 1993.

Differential Diagnosis of Benign Gynecologic Conditions

13

Dennis M. Weppner

13.1 Abnormal Genital Tract Bleeding

PREMENARCHEAL
1. Trauma
2. Genital tract neoplasm
   a. Cervical
   b. Vaginal
   c. Uterine
3. Foreign body
4. Exogenous estrogen
5. Sporadic gonadotropin surge
6. Precocious puberty
7. Pseudopuberty
8. Neoplasm, hormone secreting
   a. Estrogen-granulosa cell tumor
   b. Human chorionic gonadotropin (HCG)–embryonal carcinoma
   c. Choriocarcinoma
9. Adrenal tumors
10. Craniopharyngioma
11. Albright's syndrome
12. von Recklinghausen's disease
13. Adrenal hyperplasia
14. Hypothyroidism
15. Idiopathic, gastrointestinal bleeding
16. Urinary tract bleeding

REPRODUCTIVE AGE
1. Menorrhagia
2. Hypermenorrhea
3. Metrorrhagia
4. Oligomenorrhea
5. Polymenorrhea
6. Hypomenorrhea

PREGNANCY

1. Intrauterine pregnancy with bleeding
   a. Placenta previa
   b. Vasa previa
   c. Abruptio placentae
   d. Spontaneous abortion
2. Ectopic pregnancy

NEOPLASIA

1. Genital tract
   a. Cervical
   b. Endometrial
   c. Gestational trophoblastic disease (GTD)
   d. Ovary: hormone producing
   e. Vaginal
   f. Vulvar
   g. Fallopian tube
2. Metastatic or contiguous involvement
3. Other
   a. Central nervous system (CNS)
   b. Adrenal
   c. Thyroid

POLYP

1. Cervical, endometrial
2. Leiomyoma: submucosal
3. Adenomyosis
4. Ectropion

INFECTION

Cervicitis: *Chlamydia trachomatis*

ENDOCRINE DYSFUNCTION

1. Hypothalamic or pituitary
2. Polycystic ovaries (PCO)
3. Adrenal
4. Hypothyroidism or hyperthyroidism

IATROGENIC

1. Intrauterine device (IUD)
2. Drug use
   a. Estrogens
   b. Progestins
   c. Androgens
3. Nonhormonal drugs
   a. Phenothiazines
   b. Tricyclic antidepressants
   c. Reserpine
   d. Alpha-methyldopa

BLOOD DYSCRASIAS
1. von Willebrand's
2. Thrombocytopenia
3. Disseminated intravascular coagulation (DIC)
4. Chronic anticoagulation
    a. Heparin
    b. Coumadin

DYSFUNCTIONAL UTERINE BLEEDING
1. Ovulatory
    a. Midcycle: inadequate proliferative estrogen
    b. Late cycle: inadequate progesterone production
2. Altered prostaglandin metabolism: increased PGI
3. Anovulatory
    a. Disturbance
        (1) Hypothalmic
        (2) Pituitary
        (3) Ovarian axis
    b. Emotional stress
    c. Anorexia
    d. Strenuous exercise
    e. Weight gain

POSTMENOPAUSAL BLEEDING
1. Neoplasm
    a. Endometrial hyperplasia
    b. Endometrial cancer
    c. Other tumors of uterus (see Section 13.12)
2. Other pelvic neoplasm
    a. Direct extension or metastatic
        (1) Vulva
        (2) Vagina
        (3) Cervix
        (4) Fallopian tube
        (5) Ovary
    b. Endometrial or cervical polyp
    c. Unopposed estrogen
        (1) Exogenous
        (2) Endogenous
            (a) Peripheral conversion
            (b) Tumor production
                (i) Granulosa cell tumor
                (ii) Thecoma
3. Trauma: vaginal
4. Infection
    a. Vaginitis
    b. Endometritis
    c. Vulvar dystrophy
    d. Vaginal atrophy

e. Idiopathic
  f. Urinary tract bleeding
     (1) Urinary tract infection (UTI)
     (2) Cystitis
     (3) Bladder tumor
  g. Gastrointestinal (GI) tract bleeding

13.2 Amenorrhea

PRIMARY AMENORRHEA (LIMITED OR NO SECONDARY SEXUAL DEVELOPMENT)

1. Gonadal defects
   a. Gonadal dysgenesis
      (1) Turner's syndrome
      (2) Turner's mosaic
      (3) Swyer's syndrome
   b. "Pure" gonadal dysgenesis
   c. Resistant ovary (Savage) syndrome
   d. Ovarian
      (1) Trauma
      (2) Postinfection
      (3) Radiation
   e. 17-Alpha-hydroxylase deficiency
   f. Androgen insensitivity syndrome
      (1) Testicular feminization
      (2) Alpha-reductase deficiency
2. Hypothalmic
   a. Pituitary dysfunction: pituitary dwarfs
      (1) Craniopharyngioma
      (2) Tuberculosis (TB)
      (3) Trauma
      (4) Sarcoidosis
   b. Systemic illness
   c. Anorexia nervosa
   d. Isolated gonadotropin deficiency: Kallmann's syndrome
   e. Hypothyroidism

PRIMARY OR SECONDARY AMENORRHEA (NORMAL SECONDARY SEXUAL DEVELOPMENT)

1. Hypothalamic
   a. Stress induced
      (1) Psychogenic
      (2) Nutritional
   b. Environmental stress
   c. Anorexia nervosa
   d. Weight loss
   e. Exercise related
   f. Bulimia

2. Tumors
    a. Craniopharyngioma
    b. Glioma
    c. Endodermal sinus tumor
3. Psychotropic drug therapy, pseudocyesis
4. Pituitary abnormalities
    a. Postpartum infarction: Sheehan's syndrome
    b. Simmond's syndrome
    c. Pituitary stalk section
    d. Tumor
        (1) Prolactinoma
        (2) Craniopharyngioma
        (3) Radiation
        (4) Surgery or trauma
5. Thyroid abnormalities
    a. Hypothyroidism
    b. Hyperthyroidism
6. Adrenal abnormalities
    a. Congenital adrenal hyperplasia
    b. 21-Hydroxylase deficiency
    c. 3β-01-Dehydrogenase deficiency
    d. 11β-Hydroxylase deficiency
    e. Cushing's syndrome
    f. Cushing's disease
    g. PCO
    h. Hyperthecosis
    i. Thecoma
    j. Adrenal tumor: hormone secreting
7. Ovarian abnormalities
    a. Ovarian failure
        (1) Constitutional
        (2) Chromosomally related
        (3) Postviral oophoritis
        (4) Postradiation
        (5) Postchemotherapy
    b. Polycystic ovary syndrome
    c. Premature ovarian failure
8. Neoplasm: hormone secreting
    a. Sertoli cell tumor
    b. Leydig cell tumor: androgen
    c. Granulosa cell tumor: estrogen
9. Endometrium and outflow tract: uterine synechiae (Asherman's syndrome)
10. Endometrial fibrosis
    a. TB
    b. Schistosomiasis
11. Endometrial atrophy
    a. Radiation
    b. Postmenopause
12. Congenital abnormality, uterus or outflow tract

    a. Imperforate hymen
    b. Transverse vaginal septum
    c. Atresia of vagina
    d. Absence of uterus and vagina
        (1) Complete agenesis
        (2) Müllerian aplasia
        (3) Rokitansky-Küster-Hauser syndrome

13.3 Ascites

1. Congestive heart failure
2. Portal vein obstruction
    a. Portal cirrhosis
    b. Hepatic amyloidosis
    c. Hilar lymphadenopathy, hepatic
3. Hepatic endothrombophlebitis
4. Budd-Chiari syndrome
5. Inferior vena cava thrombosis
6. Acute or chronic peritonitis
7. Neoplastic implant
8. Tuberculosis
9. Hydatid disease
10. Hypoproteinemia
    a. Nephrosis
    b. Anemia
11. Thoracic duct obstruction
    a. Injury thorax
    b. Abdomen
    c. Tuberculosis
    d. Filariasis
    e. Myxedema
    f. Primary amyloidosis
    g. Thiamine deficiency
    h. Wet beriberi
    i. Pancreatic ascites
    j. Pyogenic peritonitis
    k. Tuberculous peritonitis
    l. Neoplasm
        (1) Pelvic carcinomatosis
            (a) Ovarian
            (b) Peritoneal
    m. Ovarian hyperstimulation syndrome
12. Meigs' syndrome
13. Constrictive pericarditis, myxedema

13.4 Breast Inflammatory Lesion

1. Acute mastitis
    a. Infectious agent
        (1) *Staphylococcus aureus*

(2) Streptocci
(3) Foreign body
  b. Trauma
2. Chronic mastitis
3. Granuloma
  a. TB
  b. Actinomycosis
  c. Blastomycosis
  d. Cryptococcosis
4. Foreign body mastitis
  a. Suture
  b. Silicone mammoplasty
5. Plasma cell mastitis: duct ectasia
6. Fat necrosis
  a. Postbiopsy
  b. Trauma
  c. Injection
  d. Mammoplasty
7. Necrosis or infarction
  a. Anticoagulant therapy
  b. Pregnancy
  c. Lactation
  d. Atherosclerosis in elderly
8. Breast malignancy

13.5 Breast Mass

BENIGN

1. Stromal fibrosis
2. Adenosis
3. Intraductal hyperplasia
4. Atypical epithelial hyperplasia
5. Sclerosing adenosis
6. Lobular hyperplasia
7. Juvenile hypertrophy
8. Galactocele
9. Duct papilloma
10. Fibroadenoma
11. Cystosarcoma phyllodes
12. Tubular adenoma
13. Lactating adenoma
14. Granular cell myoblastoma
15. Hemangioma
16. Fibroma
17. Schwannoma
18. Lipoma

MALIGNANT

1. Ductal adenocarcinoma
  a. In situ

b. Infiltrating
2. Lobular adenocarcinoma
3. Variants of carcinoma
   a. Carcinoid
   b. Squamous cell
   c. Spindle cell
   d. Other
4. Sarcoma, carcinosarcoma

13.6 Endocrinopathies

HIRSUTISM

1. Regular menstruation
   a. Elevated alpha-reductase activity
   b. Genetic
      (1) Racial
      (2) Familial
   c. Physiologic
      (1) Premature pubarche
      (2) Precocious puberty
      (3) Puberty
      (4) Pregnancy
      (5) Menopause
   d. Idiopathic
   e. Local trauma
   f. Chronic skin irritation
   g. Drug related
      (1) Phenytoin
      (2) Diazoxide
      (3) Hexachlorobenzene
      (4) Adrenocorticotropic hormone
      (5) Corticosteroids
      (6) Progestogens
      (7) Anabolic agents
      (8) Androgen
   h. Hamartoma or nevi
      (1) Pigmented nevi with hair
      (2) Nevus pilosus
      (3) Pigmented hairy epidermal nevus
2. Irregular menstruation
   a. Adrenal origin
      (1) Congenital or adult-onset adrenal hyperplasia
      (2) Androgen-producing tumors
   b. Ovarian origin
      (1) PCO
      (2) Androgen-producing tumors
         (a) Arrhenoblastoma
         (b) Granulosa-theca cell tumor
         (c) Luteoma of pregnancy

(3) Hyperthecosis
(4) Chronic anovulation
   (a) Hypothalmic amenorrhea
   (b) Psychologic or emotional disorders
   (c) Hyperthyroidism
   (d) Hypothyroidism
  c. Pituitary origin
   (1) Cushing's syndrome
   (2) Acromegaly
   (3) Sheehan's syndrome
   (4) Simmond's syndrome
  d. Genetic
   (1) Male pseudohermaphroditism
   (2) Incomplete testicular feminization
   (3) Y-containing mosaics
   (4) Turner's syndrome

HYPERPROLACTINEMIA

1. Physiologic causes
   a. Sleep
   b. Nursing
   c. Breast stimulation
   d. Stress
   e. Vigorous exercise
   f. Coitus
   g. Pregnancy
2. Pharmacologic causes
   a. Phenothiazines
   b. Butyrophenones
   c. Thyrotrophin-releasing hormone (TRH)
   d. Opiates
   e. Endorphins
   f. Reserpine
   g. Metoclopramide
   h. α-Methyldopa
   i. Estrogens
3. Pathologic
   a. Hypothyroidism
   b. Idiopathic
   c. Pituitary adenoma
   d. Pituitary stalk section
   e. Chronic renal failure

PRECOCIOUS PUBERTY

1. True precocious puberty
   a. Constitutional: increased gonadotropins
   b. Idiopathic
   c. Cerebral lesion
      (1) Rickets
      (2) Skull fracture

                (3) Craniopharyngioma
                (4) Optic glioma
                (5) Astrocytoma
                (6) Suprasellar teratoma
                (7) Hypothalamic tumor
                (8) Pineal tumor
                (9) Hypothalamic trauma or surgery
            d. Postinflammatory reaction
                (1) Toxoplasmosis
                (2) Congenital syphilis
                (3) TB
                (4) Encephalitis
                (5) Meningitis
                (6) Hydrocephalus
            e. Hypothyroidism
            f. von Recklinghausen's disease
            g. McCune-Albright syndrome
            h. Polyostotic fibrous dysplasia
            i. Hypothalamic hamartoma
            j. Tuberous sclerosis
            k. Cushing's disease
    2. Precocious pseudopuberty: ectopic gonadotropin production
        a. Adrenal
            (1) Congenital adrenal hyperplasia
            (2) Steroid-producing adrenal tumor
        b. Ovarian
            (1) Dysgerminoma
            (2) Teratoma
            (3) Choriocarcinoma
        c. Exogenous
            (1) Ingestion of estrogen
            (2) Birth control pills (BCP)
            (3) Estrogen-containing tonics, lotions, creams
        d. Chorioepithelioma
        e. Hepatoblastoma

DELAYED PUBERTY

1. Hypergonadotropic hypogonadism: gonadal dysgenesis
    a. Turner's syndrome or Turner's mosaic
2. 17-Alpha-hydroxylase deficiency
3. Ovarian damage
    a. Torsion
    b. Inflammation
4. Hypogonadotropic hypogonadism
    a. Physiologic
    b. Weight loss
    c. Anorexia nervosa
    d. Hypothyroidism
    e. Congenital adrenal hyperplasma (CAH)
    f. Cushing's syndrome

g. Prolactinoma
h. Gonadotropin-releasing hormone (GnRH) deficiency
i. Hypopituitarism
j. Congenital CNS defects
k. Pituitary adenoma
l. Craniopharyngioma
m. Postsurgical hypopituitarism
5. Eugonadism
   a. Müllerian agenesis
   b. Vaginal septum
   c. Imperforate hymen
   d. Androgen insensitivity syndrome

13.7 Female Reproductive Tract Abnormalities

CONGENITAL STRUCTURAL DEFECTS

1. Vaginal septum
   a. Longitudinal
   b. Transverse
2. Imperforate hymen
3. Upper vaginal atresia
4. Rokitansky-Küster-Hauser syndrome
5. Pelvic kidney
6. Testicular feminization
7. Mesonephric duct remnants
   a. Appendix vesiculosa
   b. Epoophoron
   c. Paroophoron
   d. Gartner's duct cyst
8. Paramesonephric duct remnant: hydatid of Morgagni
9. Vaginal adenosis
10. Müllerian fusion defects
    a. Hypoplasia
    b. Agenesis
    c. Unicornuate
    d. Bicornuate
    e. Didelphus
    f. Arcuate
    g. Septate
    h. Diethylstilbesterol (DES) related

ACQUIRED STRUCTURAL DEFECT

1. Trauma perineal
2. Vaginal
3. Cervical
   a. Obstetric
      (1) Episiotomy: first-degree, second-degree, third-degree tear
      (2) Sulcus tear
   b. Coitus

       c. Sexual assault
       d. Fall
       e. Motor vehicle accident (MVA)
    4. Loss of pelvic support
       a. Hypoestrogenism
       b. Multiparity
       c. Congenital laxity of connective tissue
       d. Idiopathic
       e. Urethrocoele
       f. Cystocoele
       g. Rectocoele
       h. Enterocoele
       i. Uterine prolapse: first-degree, second-degree, third-degree
       j. Vaginal vault prolapse

GENITAL TRACT FISTULAE

1. Vesicocolic
2. Ureterocolic
3. Vesicouterine
4. Vesicocervical
5. Vesicovaginal
6. Ureterovaginal
7. Rectovaginal
8. Urethrovaginal
9. Vaginoperianal

13.8 Genital Discharge

1. Physiologic discharge
   a. Cervical mucus
   b. Vaginal transudation
   c. Bacteria
   d. Squamous epithelial cells
2. Individual variation
3. Pregnancy
4. Sexual response
5. Menstrual cycle variation
6. Infection (see Section 13.10)
7. Foreign body
   a. Tampon
   b. Cervical cap
   c. Other
8. Neoplasm (see Section 13.12)
9. Fistula
10. IUD
11. Cervical ectropion
12. Spermacide
13. Nongenital causes
    a. Urinary incontinence
    b. Urinary tract fistula

13.9 Infertility

MALE FACTOR

1. Abnormal semen
   a. History of testicular injury
   b. Surgery
   c. Mumps
   d. Heat
      (1) Sauna
      (2) Jockey shorts
   e. Allergy
   f. Radiation
   g. Industrial or environmental toxins
   h. Marijuana, cigarette smoking
   i. Cimetidine
   j. Spironolactone
   k. Furadantin
   l. Sulfasalazine
   m. Chemotherapy
   n. Ulcerative colitis: sulfasalazine
   o. Coital timing
   p. DES
   q. Immunologic
   r. Incompatible cervical mucus
   s. Abnormal sperm production
2. Anatomic
   a. Hypospadias
   b. Retrograde ejaculation
   c. Prostatectomy
   d. Obstruction or absence of vas deferens
   e. Congenitally absent fructose
   f. Hyalinization of seminiferous tubules
   g. Mumps orchitis
   h. Cryptorchidism
   i. Klinefelter's syndrome
   j. Infection
      (1) *Mycoplasma*
      (2) *Chlamydia*
   k. Varicocele
   l. Vasectomy
3. Endocrine
   a. Germ cell aplasia: increased follicle-stimulating hormone (FSH)
   b. Hypogonadotropic hypogonadism: decreased testosterone
   c. Hyperprolactinemia
   d. Hypothyroidism or hyperthyroidism
   e. Isolated gonadotropin deficiency

FEMALE FACTOR

1. Age
2. Delayed childbearing
3. Marriage postponement
4. Contraception
5. Abortion
6. Ovulatory disorders
   a. Intracranial tumor
   b. Stress
   c. Obesity
   d. Anorexia
   e. Systemic disease
   f. Physiologic
   g. Noncyclic production
      (1) FSH
      (2) Luteinizing hormone (LH)
      (3) Estrogen
   h. Abnormal ovarian or adnexal steroid production
   i. Luteal phase defect
7. Tubal peritoneal factors
   a. Tubal obstruction
      (1) Cornu
      (2) Isthmus
      (3) Fimbrial
      (4) Peritube or adhesions
   b. Pelvic adhesions
   c. Inflammatory bowel disease (IBD)
   d. Endometriosis
   e. Appendicitis
   f. Ovarian cyst rupture
      (1) Dermoid
      (2) Other
   g. Previous abdominal surgery
   h. Foreign body reaction
8. Cervical factors
   a. Cervical canal stenosis
   b. Abnormal or hostile mucus
   c. Endocervical polyp
   d. Endometriosis
   e. TB
   f. Surgical: cone or cautery
   g. Synechiae
   h. Preovulatory estrogen deficiency
   i. Endocervicitis
      (1) *Chlamydia*
      (2) Other
9. Uterine factors
   a. Polyp
   b. Myoma

c. Synechiae
   d. Asherman's anomaly
   e. Müllerian anomaly
      (1) Didelphys
      (2) Unicornuate
      (3) Septate
   f. Arcuate
   g. Bicornuate
   h. Hypoplasia or agenesis
   i. DES related
   j. Infection
      (1) *Mycoplasma*
      (2) *Toxoplasma gondii*
   k. Unexplained
   l. Idiopathic
   m. Immunologic
      (1) Sperm allergy
      (2) Antisperm antibody
   n. Hypothyroidism or hyperthyroidism
   o. Diabetes mellitus
   p. Collagen vascular disease (e.g., systemic lupus erythematosus)
   q. Disorders of ovulation
   r. Pituitary adenoma (see Section 13.6, Hyperprolactinemia)

13.10 Lower Reproductive Tract Infection

BACTERIAL

1. *Neisseria gonorrhoeae*
   a. Bartholin
   b. Skene
   c. Periurethral
2. *Chlamydia trachomatis*
   a. Cervicitis
   b. Lymphogranuloma venereum
3. *Treponema pallidum*: primary, secondary, tertiary, and congenital syphilis
4. *Gardnerella vaginalis*
   a. Bacteroides vivus
   b. Mobiluncus
5. *Hemophilus ducreyi*: chancroid
6. *Calymmatobacterium granulomatis*: granuloma inguinale
7. Donovanosis
8. *Corynebacterium minutissimum*: erythrasma
9. Lower genital tract abscess
   a. Bartholin gland or duct
   b. Skene's gland
   c. Follicular abscess
   d. Hydradenitis suppurativa
   e. Surgical or obstetric site infection

VIRAL

1. Human papillomavirus: high-risk or low-risk subtype
2. Herpes simplex virus (HSV): HSV-1, HSV-2
   a. Primary
   b. Recurrent
3. Mulloscum contagiosum
4. Human immunodeficiency virus (HIV)

FUNGAL

1. *Candida albicans*
2. *C. tropicalis*
3. *C. stellatoidea*
4. *C. krusei*
5. *C. (Torulopsis) glabrata*
6. *Trichophyton rubium:* tinea cruris
7. *Pityrosporum orbiculare:* pityriasis versicolor

PROTOZOAL

Trichomonas vaginalis

PARASITIC

1. *Sarcoptes scabiei:* scabies
2. *Phthirus pubis:* pediculosis pubis

13.11 Ovarian Failure

1. Menopause: climacteric
   a. Physiologic
      (1) Age
      (2) Heredity
      (3) Racial variation
      (4) Cigarette smoking
      (5) Nutritional status
2. Premature
   a. Genetic
   b. Turner's mosaic
   c. Iatrogenic
      (1) Surgical oophorectomy
      (2) Chemotherapy
      (3) Ionizing radiation
   d. Autoimmune endocrinopathy
   e. Idiopathic
3. Hypoestrogenemia
   a. Vasomoter instability
   b. Urogenital atrophy
   c. Psychosomatic complaints
   d. Osteoporosis
   e. Arteriosclerotic vascular disease
   f. Amenorrhea

13.12 Pelvic Mass—Gynecologic Causes

VAGINA

1. Benign tumor
   a. Imperforate hymen: hematocolpos
   b. Transverse septum
   c. Longitudinal septum
   d. Vaginal duplication
   e. Gartner's duct cyst
   f. Inclusion cyst
   g. Uterine prolapse
   h. Cystocoele
   i. Rectocoele
   j. Enterocele
   k. Prolapsed fallopian tube
   l. Polyp
   m. Leiomyoma
   n. Fibroma
   o. Rhabdomyoma
   p. Mixed tumor
   q. Granular cell tumor
   r. Endometriosis
2. Malignant tumor
   a. Squamous carcinoma
   b. Verrucous carcinoma
   c. Basal cell carcinoma
   d. Adenocarcinoma
   e. Sarcoma
   f. Leiomyosarcoma
   g. Embryonal rhabdomyosarcoma
   h. Mixed Müllerian tumor
   i. Endodermal sinus tumor
   j. Melanoma
   k. Metastatic tumor
   l. Clear cell adenocarcinoma

CERVIX

1. Benign
   a. Polyp
   b. Inclusion cyst
   c. Leiomyoma
   d. Hemangioma
   e. Adenofibroma
   f. Adenomyoma
   g. Fibroadenoma
   h. Papilloma
   i. Endometriosis
   j. Mesonephric remnant cyst

     k. Glioma
     l. Condyloma
     m. Cervical stenosis: hematometra
2. Malignant
    a. Squamous cell carcinoma
    b. Verrucous carcinoma
    c. Adenocarcinoma
        (1) Adenoma malignum
        (2) Adenoid cystic carcinoma
        (3) Mesonephric carcinoma
    d. Mixed epithelial
        (1) Adenosquamous carcinoma
        (2) Glassy cell carcinoma
        (3) Mucoepidermoid
        (4) Dual primary
    e. Neuroendocrine
        (1) Carcinoid
        (2) Small cell
    f. Metastatic tumors
    g. Rare tumors
        (1) Melanoma
        (2) Choriocarcinoma

UTERUS

1. Pregnancy
    a. Congenital Müllerian defects
        (1) Didelphys
        (2) Bicornuate
        (3) Rudimentary horn
        (4) Cervix atresia
2. Tumor
    a. Polyp
    b. Atypical polyploid adenoma
    c. Teratoma
    d. Brenner tumor
    e. Heterologous tumor
    f. Glioma
    g. Endometrial carcinoma
        (1) Papillary
        (2) Secretory
        (3) Ciliated cell
        (4) Adenocanthoma
        (5) Adenosquamous carcinoma
    h. Mucinous carcinoma
    i. Serous carcinoma
    j. Clear cell
    k. Squamous papillary serous
    l. Undifferentiated
    m. Mixed

n. Glassy cell
o. Metastatic
p. GTD
3. Sarcoma
    a. Homologous
        (1) Leiomyosarcoma
        (2) Stromal sarcoma
        (3) Angiosarcoma
    b. Heterologous
        (1) Rhabdomyosarcoma
        (2) Choridiosarcoma
        (3) Osteosarcoma
    c. Mixed
    d. Mixed Müllerian
    e. Malignant lymphoma
    f. Unclassified sarcoma leiomyoma variants
        (1) Myxoid
        (2) Vascular
        (3) Lipoid
        (4) With tubules
        (5) Intravenous
    g. Benign metastasizing leiomyoma
    h. Disseminated peritoneal leiomyomatosis
    i. Adeonmyosis
    j. Adenomyoma
    k. Adenomatoid mesothelioma
    l. Hemangioma
    m. Angiosarcoma
    n. Hemanogiopericytoma
    o. Pseudotumor

FALLOPIAN TUBE

1. Torsion
2. Pyosalpinx
3. Hydrosalpinx
4. Granulomatous salpingitis
5. Actinomycosis
6. Parasite salpingitis
    a. Enterbius vermicularis
    b. Schistosomiasis
    c. *Echinococcus granulosus*
7. Sarcoid
8. Crohn's disease
9. Foreign body
10. Ectopic pregnancy
11. Malignant
    a. Adenocarcinoma
        (1) Alveolar
        (2) Papillary
        (3) Medullary

b. Squamous
  c. Transitional cell
  d. Clear cell carcinoma
  e. Sarcoma
     (1) Carcinosarcoma
     (2) Mixed mesodermal
  f. Metastatic
  g. Lymphoma
  h. GTD

OVARY

1. Benign
   a. Supernumerary ovary
   b. Adrenal rest
   c. Splenic gonadal fusion
   d. Actinomycosis
   e. Granulomas
   f. Parasitic infection
   g. Inclusion cyst
   h. Follicular cyst
   i. Corpus luteum cyst
      (1) Ruptured or unruptured: hemorrhagic
   j. Lutein cyst of pregnancy
   k. Ovarian hyperstimulation
   l. Hyperreaction luteinalis
   m. PCO
   n. Hyperthecosis
   o. HAIR-AN (hyperandrogenism, insulin resistance, acanthosis nigricans) syndrome
   p. Fibromatosis
   q. Luteoma
   r. Torsion
   s. Endometrioma
   t. Retroperitoneal mucinous tumor
   u. Walthard rests
   v. Leiomyoma
   w. Mesothelioma
   x. Oophoritis
   y. Ovarian abscess
2. Serous tumor
   a. Benign and borderline
      (1) Cystadenoma
      (2) Papillary cystadenoma
      (3) Papilloma
      (4) Adenofibroma
      (5) Cystadenofibroma
   b. Malignant
      (1) Adenocarcinoma
      (2) Papillary adenocarcinoma
      (3) Papillary cystadenocarcinoma

(4) Papillary carcinoma
(5) Malignant adenofibroma
(6) Cystadenofibroma
3. Mucinous tumor
   a. Benign and borderline
      (1) Cystadenoma
      (2) Adenofibroma
      (3) Cystadenofibroma
   b. Malignant
      (1) Adenocarcinoma
      (2) Cystadenocarcinoma
      (3) Malignant adenofibroma and cystadenofibroma
4. Endometrial tumors
   a. Benign and borderline
      (1) Adenoma
      (2) Cystadenoma
      (3) Adenofibroma
      (4) Cystadenofibroma
   b. Malignant
      (1) Adenocarcinoma
      (2) Adenocanthoma
      (3) Malignant adenofibroma
      (4) Cystadenofibroma
      (5) Endometrial stomal sarcoma
      (6) Mixed Müllerian tumor
         (a) Homologous
         (b) Heterologous
5. Clear cell tumor
   a. Benign: Adenofibroma
   b. Borderline and malignant
      (1) Carcinoma
      (2) Adenocarcinoma
6. Brenner's tumor
   a. Benign
   b. Borderline
   c. Malignant
7. Mixed epithelial tumor
   a. Undifferentiated
   b. Unclassified
8. Granulosa stromal cell tumor: adult, juvenile
   a. Thecoma
      (1) Typical
      (2) Luteinized
   b. Fibroma, fibrosarcoma
      (1) Fibroma
      (2) Cellular fibroma
9. Sertoli stromal cell tumors: Sertoli cell, Leydig cell, mixed
   a. Gynadroblastoma
   b. Sex cord tumor with annular tubules
   c. Unclassified

    d. Hilus cell tumor
    e. Steroid cell tumor
    f. Carcinoid
    g. Zollinger-Ellison syndrome
    h. Small-cell carcinoma
10. Dysgerminoma
    a. Endodermal sinus tumor
    b. Embryonal carcinoma
    c. Polyembryoma
    d. Choriocarcinoma
    e. Teratoma
        (1) Immature
        (2) Mature-solid
        (3) Cystic-dermoid
        (4) Dermoid with malignant transformation
        (5) Struma ovarii
        (6) Carcinoid
        (7) Strumal carcinoid
        (8) Other
    f. Mixed forms
11. Fibroma
    a. Fibrosarcoma
    b. Leiomyoma
    c. Leiomyosarcoma
    d. Rhabdomyoma
    e. Rhabdomyosarcoma
    f. Hemangioma
    g. Lymphangioma
    h. Chordoma
    i. Osteoma
    j. Osteosarcoma
    k. Giant-cell tumor
    l. Neural tissue tumors
    m. Mesothelial tumors
    n. Lymphoma
    o. Burkitt's lymphoma
12. Metastatic tumors
    a. Uterus
    b. Vulva
    c. Vagina
    d. Fallopian tube
    e. Breast
    f. Intestinal
    g. Krukenberg
    h. Appendix
    i. Carcinoid
    j. Pancreas
    k. Gall bladder
    l. Liver
    m. Esophagus

n. Renal
o. Bladder
p. Ureter
q. Urethra
r. Adrenal gland
s. Melanoma
t. Lung
u. Mediastinum
13. Obstetric
    a. Pregnancy
    b. Multiple pregnancy
    c. Ectopic pregnancy
    d. Abdominal pregnancy
    e. Hydatiform mole
        (1) Complete
        (2) Partial
    f. Invasive mole
    g. Choriocarcinoma
    h. Placenta site trophoblastic tumor
    i. Placenta percreta
    j. Fetus papyraceus
    k. Retained placenta

13.13 Pelvic Mass—Nongynecologic Causes

1. GI tract
    a. Tuberculous granuloma
    b. Pericecal abscess
    c. Crohn's disease
    d. Carcinoma
    e. Constipation
    f. Obstipation
    g. Fecal impaction
    h. Polyp
    i. Bezoar
        (1) Tricho
        (2) Phyto
    j. Volvulus
    k. Intussusception
    l. Diverticular abscess
    m. Hemangioma
    n. Carcinoid
    o. Inguinal hernia
    p. Femoral hernia
2. Genitourinary (GU) tract
    a. Distended bladder
    b. Ectopic kidney
    c. Supernumerary kidney
    d. Horseshoe kidney
    e. Polycystic kidney

Practical Guide to the Care of the Gynecologic/Obstetric Patient 281

   f. Benign neoplasm
   g. Wilms' tumor
   h. Carcinosarcoma
   i. Pelvic carcinoma
3. Other
   a. Hematoma rectus abdominis
   b. Retained sponge or instrument after surgery
   c. Ectopic spleen
   d. Inguinal endometriosis
   e. Mistaken normal structure
   f. Pseudomyxoma peritonei
   g. Lymphoma
   h. Burkitt's lymphoma
   i. Aneurysm
   j. Retroperitoneal hematoma
      (1) Postoperative
      (2) Postlaparoscopy
   k. Procedentia
   l. Incisional or epigastric hernia
   m. Obturator or spigelian hernia
   n. Metastatic tumor

13.14 Pelvic Pain

ACUTE

1. Genital tract
   a. Pregnancy related
      (1) Abortion
         (a) Threatened
         (b) Inevitable
         (c) Complete
         (d) Induced
         (e) Septic
      (2) Ectopic pregnancy
         (a) Fallopian tube
         (b) Abdominal
         (c) Cervical
         (d) Ovarian
   b. Ovary
      (1) Ruptured cyst
      (2) Torsion of cyst
      (3) Hemorrhagic corpus luteum
         (a) Ruptured
         (b) Unruptured
      (4) Mittelschmerz
      (5) Ovarian hyperstimulation syndrome
         (a) Clomiphene
         (b) Human menopausal gonadotropin (HMG)
   c. Fallopian tube
      (1) Torsion

(2) Paratubal cyst
(3) Torsion of stump after sterilization
d. Uterus
(1) Fibroid degeneration
(2) Fibroid torsion
(3) Pyometria
(4) Retrograde menstruation
e. Acute pelvic inflammatory disease
(1) Endometriosis
(2) Salpingo-oophoritis
(3) Tuboovarian abscess
2. Nongenital tract
a. GI tract
(1) Appendicitis
(2) Meckel's diverticulitis
(3) Inflammatory bowel disease
(a) Crohn's disease
(b) Ulcerative colitis
(4) Mesenteric adenitis
(5) Bowel perforation
(6) Bowel obstruction
(7) Toxic megacolon
(8) Diverticulitis
b. Urinary tract
(1) Cystitis
(2) Pyelonephritis
(3) Renal calculus or colic
c. Other
(1) Abdominal wall hematoma: rectus
(2) Herpes zoster
(3) Acute intermittent porphyria
(4) Sickle cell crisis
(5) Idiopathic

CHRONIC

1. Cycle
a. Mittelschmerz
b. Primary dysmenorrhea
c. Secondary dysmenorrhea
(1) Endometriosis
(2) Endosalpingiosis
(3) Adhesive disease
(a) Chronic pelvic inflammatory disease (PID)
(b) Endometriosis
(c) Postsurgical
d. Uterine pathology
(1) Adenomyosis
(2) Leiomyoma
e. Congenital anomaly
(1) Hematometria

(2) Hematocolpos
    f. Imperforate hymen
    g. Transverse septum
    h. Noncommunicating uterine horn
    i. Acquired cervical stenosis
    j. Congenital cervical absence
    k. Other
        (1) Pedunculated myoma
        (2) Endometrial polyp
        (3) Intrauterine adhesions
        (4) Complete Asherman's
        (5) IUD use
        (6) Chronic PID
2. Acyclic
    a. Genital tract
        (1) Endometriosis
        (2) Pelvic adhesions
        (3) Pelvic congestion syndrome
        (4) Pelvic varicosities
        (5) Ovarian tumors
        (6) Leiomyoma
    b. Nongenital tract
        (1) Cystitis
        (2) Renal colic: renal calculi
        (3) Diverticulitis
        (4) Colitis
        (5) Spina bifida
        (6) Scoliosis
        (7) Osteoarthritis
        (8) Fibromyositis
        (9) Herniated intervertebral disc
3. No organic cause
    a. Sexual abuse
    b. Incest
    c. Spousal abuse
        (1) Physical
        (2) Mental
    d. Psychogenic etiologies
        (1) Borderline personality
        (2) Hypochondriasis
        (3) Depression
        (4) Hysteria
        (5) Munchausen syndrome

13.15 Premenstrual Syndrome

1. Normal physiology, psychologic factors, physiologic factors
    a. Estrogen excess
    b. Estrogen deficiency
    c. Progesterone deficiency

d. Vitamin deficiency
e. Disorder of renin–angiotensin–aldosterone
f. Disorder of melanocyte-stimulating hormone (MSH), β-endorphins
2. Abnormality of psychosocial adjustment

13.16 Sexual Dysfunction

DYSPAREUNIA

1. Introital
   a. Vaginismus
   b. Intact or rigid hymen
   c. Clitoral problems
   d. Vulvovaginitis
   e. Vaginal atrophy: hypoestrogen
   f. Vulvar dystrophy
   g. Bartholin or Skene gland infection
   h. Inadequate lubrication
   i. Operative scarring
2. Midvaginal
   a. Urethritis
   b. Trigonitis
   c. Cystitis
   d. Short vagina
   e. Operative scarring
   f. Inadequate lubrication
3. Deep
   a. Endometriosis
   b. Pelvic infection
   c. Uterine retroversion
   d. Ovarian pathology
   e. Gastrointestinal
   f. Orthopedic
   g. Abnormal penile size or shape

ORGASM DYSFUNCTION

1. Anorgasmia: inadequate stimulation or learning
2. Spinal cord lesion or injury
3. Multiple sclerosis
4. Alcoholic neuropathy
5. Amyotrophic lateral sclerosis
6. Spinal cord accident
7. Spinal cord trauma
8. Peripheral nerve damage
9. Radical pelvic surgery
10. Herniated lumbar disc
11. Hypothyroidism
12. Addison's disease
13. Cushing's disease
14. Acromegaly

15. Hypopituitarism
16. Pharmacologic agents

SEXUALITY DISORDERS

1. Primary or secondary sexual trauma
2. Incest
3. Abuse
4. Depression
5. Pharmacologic agents
    a. Anticholinergics
    b. Antiandrogens
    c. Alpha-blockers and beta-blockers
    d. Narcotics
    e. Sedatives
    f. Antidepressants
    g. Antihistamines
6. Malignancy
7. Hepatic renal disease
8. Chronic illness
9. Disfigurement
    a. Mastectomy
    b. Radical neck
    c. Burns
    d. Trauma
10. Multiple sclerosis
11. Cord injury
12. Diabetic nephropathy
13. Hypoadrenalism
14. Panhypopituitarism
15. Ovarian failure
16. Premenstrual syndrome

13.17 Upper Genital Tract Infection

1. PID
    a. Salpingitis
    b. Pyosalpinx
    c. Tuboovarian abscess
    d. Endomyometritis
    e. Parametritis
    f. Pelvic peritonitis
    g. Pelvic abscess
    h. Generalized peritonitis
    i. Fitz-Hugh–Curtis syndrome: perihepatitis
2. Ascending lower genital tract infection (see Section 13.10)
3. IUD: Dalkon shield
4. Postpartum endomyometritis
5. Postsurgical manipulation
    a. Hysteroscopy

b. Endometrial biopsy (EMB)
   c. Dilation and curettage (D&C)
   d. Hysterosalpingiogram (HSG)
6. Postsurgical procedure
7. Gynecologic procedure
   a. Hysterectomy
   b. Myomectomy
8. General surgical procedure
   a. Appendectomy
   b. Bowel resection
9. Adjacent ruptured viscus
   a. Appendicitis
   b. Diverticulitis
10. Hematogenous: pelvic tuberculosis
11. Chronic PID

13.18 Urinary Incontinence

INTERMITTENT

1. Genuine stress incontinence
2. Urethral sphincter incontinence
3. Detrusor instability
   a. Inflammatory
   b. Neurologic
   c. Idiopathic
4. Diabetes
5. Surgery
6. Drugs
7. Spinal cord lesion
8. Spina bifida
9. Multiple sclerosis
10. Overflow incontinence
11. Detrusor or sphincter dyssynergia
12. Psychogenic
13. Mixed

GENUINE STRESS INCONTINENCE (GSI)

1. Trauma
   a. Childbirth
   b. Pelvic surgery
   c. Injury
2. Pelvic relaxation
   a. Congenital
   b. Childbirth
   c. Other
3. Drugs: alpha-blockers (e.g., Minipress)
4. Menopause: hypoestrogenism

DETRUSOR INSTABILITY

1. Inflammatory

    a. Chronic UTI
    b. Interstitial cystitis
    c. Bladder stone
    d. Neoplasm
    e. Suture
2. Neurologic
    a. Cerebrovascular accident (CVA)
    b. Multiple sclerosis
    c. Spinal cord tumor
    d. Cerebral degeneration
3. Miscellaneous
    a. Urethral diverticulum
    b. Psychogenic
        (1) Depression
        (2) Anxiety
        (3) Emotional conflict regarding process of urination
    c. Neglect
    d. Inability to ambulate

CONTINUOUS

1. Fistula
    a. Congenital: ectopic ureter
    b. Acquired: pelvic surgery
        (1) Hysterectomy
        (2) Radical hysterectomy
        (3) Pelvic irradiation
        (4) Crohn's disease

13.19 Vulvar Lesions

RED LESION

Infection

1. Fungal infection
    a. *Candida*
    b. Tinea cruris
    c. Intertrigo
    d. Pityriasis versicolor
2. *Sarcoptes scabiei*
3. Erythrasma: *Corynebacterium minutissimum*
4. Granuloma inguinale: *Calymmatobacterium granulomatis*
5. Folliculitis: *Staphylococcus aureus*
6. Hidradenitis suppurativa
7. Behçet's syndrome

Inflammation

1. Reactive vulvitis
2. Chemical irritation
    a. Detergent
    b. Dyes

c. Perfume
   d. Spermacide
   e. Lubricants
   f. Hygiene sprays
   g. Podophyllun
   h. Topical 5-FU
   i. Saliva
   j. Gentian violet
   k. Semen
3. Mechanical trauma: scratching
4. Vestibular adenitis
5. Essential vulvodynia
6. Psoriasis
7. Seborrheic dermatitis

Neoplasm

1. Vulvar intraepithelial neoplasia (VIN)
   a. Mild dysplasia
   b. Moderate dysplasia
   c. Severe dysplasia
   d. Carcinoma in situ
2. Vulvar dystrophy
3. Bowen's disease
4. Invasive cancer
   a. Squamous cell carcinoma
   b. Malignant melanoma
   c. Sarcoma
   d. Basal cell carcinoma
   e. Adenocarcinoma
   f. Paget's disease
   g. Undifferentiated

WHITE LESION

1. Vulvar dystrophy
   a. Lichen sclerosis
   b. Vulvar dystrophy
   c. Vulvar hyperplasia
   d. Mixed dystrophy
2. VIN
3. Vitiligo
4. Partial albinism
5. Intertrigo
6. Radiation treatment

DARK LESION

1. Lentigo
2. Nevi (mole)
3. Neoplasm (see Neoplasm, Vulvar in this section)
4. Reactive hyperpigmentation
5. Seborrheic keratosis
6. Pubic lice

ULCERATIVE LESION

Infection
1. Herpes simplex
2. Vaccinia
3. Treponema pallidum
4. Granuloma inguinale
5. Pyoderma
6. Tuberculosis

Noninfection
1. Behçet's disease
2. Crohn's disease
3. Pemphigus
4. Pemphigoid
5. Hidradenitis suppurativa (see Neoplasm, Vulvar in this section)

Neoplasm
1. Basal cell carcinoma
2. Squamous cell carcinoma
3. Vulvar tumor less than 1 cm
    a. Condyloma acuminata
    b. Mulluscum contagiosum
    c. Epidermal inclusion
    d. Vestibular cyst
    e. Mesenephric duct
    f. VIN
    g. Hemangioma
    h. Hidradenoma
    i. Neurofibroma
    j. Syringoma
    k. Accessory breast tissue
    l. Acrocordon
    m. Endometriosis
    n. Fox-Fordyce disease
    o. Pilonidal sinus
4. Vulvar tumor greater than 1 cm
    a. Bartholin cyst or abscess
    b. Lymphogranuloma venereum
    c. Fibroma
    d. Lipoma
    e. Verrucous carcinoma
    f. Squamous cell carcinoma
    g. Hernia
    h. Edema
    i. Hematoma
    j. Acrocordon
    k. Epidermal cysts
    l. Neurofibromatosis
    m. Accessory breast tissue

Gynecologic Oncology

14

Alexander B. Olawaiye

14.1 Cervical Cancer

Worldwide, cervical cancer is the second most common cancer in women. In the United States, it is the third most common gynecologic malignancy behind ovarian and uterine cancers. In 2005, about 10,370 cases of invasive cervical cancer will be diagnosed in the United States and 3,710 women will die from this disease. Squamous cell cancer accounts for 80% of cervical cancers, the remaining are made up of adenocarcinomas (15%) and adenosquamous cancer (5%).

ETIOLOGY

The most important risk factor for cervical cancer is infection by the human papillomavirus (HPV), specifically, the "high-risk" types of HPV. These include HPV 16, HPV 18, HPV 31, HPV 33, and HPV 45, as well as some others. About half of all cervical cancers are caused by HPV 16 and HPV 18. These HPV types are passed from one person to another during skin-to-skin sexual contact, including oral and anal sex.

Certain sexual behaviors increase a woman's risk of developing cervical cancer; these include sex at an early age, having many sexual partners, and having sex with uncircumcised males.

Other risk factors for cervical cancer are smoking, human immunodeficiency virus (HIV) infection, chlamydia infection, oral contraceptive pills, in utero diethylstilbesterol (DES) exposure, diets low in fruits and vegetables, multiple pregnancies, low socioeconomic status, and family history.

CLINICAL PRESENTATION

Early cervical cancer is usually asymptomatic, underscoring the importance of cervical screening. The most common symptom is abnormal vaginal bleeding. This presents in a variety of ways, including disorganized vaginal bleeding, postcoital bleeding, or postmenopausal bleeding. Malodorous vaginal discharge is also common. In advance cases, low backache, pelvic pain, hematuria, or hematochezia may be reported at presentation. Clinical findings may range from a normal appearing cervix to one that is almost entirely replaced by tumor.

DIAGNOSIS AND STAGING

1. Diagnosis is confirmed by biopsy in women with grossly visible lesions. Symptomatic women without visible lesions and women with abnormal Papanicolaou smear require colposcopy, colposcopic-directed biopsy, and endocervical curettage (ECC).
2. In microinvasive disease, diagnostic conization is necessary to assess the depth of invasion. This could be done by cold knife, loop electrosurgical excision procedure, or laser.
3. The current International Federation of Gynecology and Obstetrics (FIGO) staging system (Table 14-1) is based on clinical assessment, including findings from pelvic examination under anesthesia, colposcopy, sigmoidoscopy, lesion biopsy, ECC, hysteroscopy, cystoscopy, proctoscopy, intravenous pyelography (IVP), barium enema, and x-rays of the lungs and skeleton. Information gained from higher order imaging (computed tomography [CT], magnetic resonance imaging [MRI], and positron emission tomography [PET]) or from surgery can be used in management decisions but *will not change the stage*.

TREATMENT

1. Treatment depends on the stage at diagnosis.
   a. Ia$_1$: Simple hysterectomy without nodal dissection or conization in selected cases.
   b. Ia$_2$: Radical hysterectomy and pelvic lymphadenectomy.
   c. Ib to IIa: Two choices: (i) primary surgical approach with radical hysterectomy and pelvic lymphadenectomy or (ii) primary radiation therapy with external-beam radiation and either high-dose-rate or low-dose-rate brachytherapy.
      (1) Pelvic lymphadenectomy and radical trachylectomy (provided all lymph nodes are negative) is now available to young women with early stage (stage Ib$_1$ or less) who wish to preserve their fertility. A permanent cervical circlage is inserted at the time of surgery. Initial reports of outcome are very encouraging.
   d. IIb to IV: Platinum-based chemoradiation.

PROGNOSIS

Five-year survival decreases as the FIGO stage at diagnosis increases: stage Ia, 97%; stage Ib, 70% to 85%; stage II, 60% to 70%; stage III, 30% to 45%; stage IV, 12% to 18%.

14.2 Uterine Cancer

The lifetime risk of developing endometrial cancer is 1 in 38 in the United States. Cancer of the endometrium is the most common gynecologic malignancy and accounts for 6% of all cancers in women. Estimated new cases and deaths from endometrial cancer in the United States in 2005 were 40,8880 and 7310, respectively. There are various histological types, distributed as follows: endometrioid (75% to 80%), mixed (10%), uterine papillary serous (<10%), clear cell (4%), mucinous (1%), squamous cell (<1%), and undifferentiated.

Table 14-1 FIGO Staging of Cervical Cancer

Stage 0 Carcinoma in situ, cervical intraepithelial neoplasia grade III.
Stage I The carcinoma is strictly confined to the cervix (extension to the corpus would be disregarded).
   Ia Invasive carcinoma that can be diagnosed only by microscopy
      Ia_1 Measured stromal invasion of not more than 3 mm in depth and extension of not more than 7 mm
      Ia_2 Measured stromal invasion of more than 3 mm and not more than 5 mm with an extension of not more than 7 mm
   Ib Clinically visible lesions limited to the cervix uteri or preclinical cancers greater than stage Ia
      Ib_1 Clinically visible lesions not more than 4 cm
      Ib_2 Clinically visible lesions more than 4 cm
Stage II Cervical carcinoma invades beyond the uterus, but not to the pelvic wall or to the lower third of the vagina.
   IIa No obvious parametrial involvement
   IIb Obvious parametrial involvement
Stage III The carcinoma has extended to the pelvic wall. The tumor involves the lower third of the vagina. All cases with hydronephrosis or nonfunctioning kidney are included, unless they are known to be due to other causes.
   IIIa Tumor involves lower third of the vagina, with no extension to the pelvic wall
   IIIb Extension to the pelvic wall or hydronephrosis or nonfunctioning kidney
Stage IV The carcinoma has extended beyond the true pelvis, or has involved (biopsy proved) the mucosa of the bladder or rectum.
   IVa Spread of the growth to adjacent organs (bladder or rectum or both)
   IVb Spread to distant organs

Data from FIGO Committee on Gynecologic Oncology: *Int J Gynecol Obstet* 70:207-312, 2000.
FIGO, International Federation of Gynecology and Obstetrics.

ETIOLOGY

1. The use of unopposed estrogen is clearly associated with the development of endometrial cancer. Additional risk factors have been identified and often appear to be related to estrogenic effects. Among these factors are obesity, a high-fat diet, reproductive factors like nulliparity, early menarche and late menopause, polycystic ovarian syndrome, and tamoxifen use.
2. Lynch II syndrome describes the association between hereditary nonpolyposis colorectal cancer (HNPCC) and endometrial cancer.

Among women who are HNPCC mutation carriers, the estimated cumulative incidence of endometrial cancer ranges from 20% to 60%.
3. The incidence of endometrial cancer is higher in Caucasian women than in African American women. However, endometrial cancer tends to be of higher grade and stage at diagnosis in the African American population and survival is comparatively lower.

PREVENTION

Unlike cervical cancer, there is currently no effective screening method that is applicable to the general population. However, in some cases the etiologic evidence has suggested strategies that may be pursued to reduce endometrial cancer risk in target populations.

Factors that have been associated with a decreased incidence of endometrial cancer include parity, lactation, use of combined oral contraceptives, a diet low in fat and high in plant foods, and physical activity.

CLINICAL PRESENTATION

The classic symptom of endometrial carcinoma is abnormal uterine bleeding; the possibility of endometrial cancer needs to be excluded in any woman with postmenopausal bleeding unrelated to hormone therapy. Overall, 5% to 20% of such women will have endometrial cancer; the probability of cancer increases with years beyond menopause. Premenopausal and perimenopausal women with menometrorrhagia also should be evaluated, particularly if they have other risks described above. The presence of endometrial cells (normal or abnormal) on the cervical cytology of asymptomatic women increases the risk of endometrial disease including carcinoma. Although this finding justifies further evaluation, Papanicolaou smear is not an effective screening method for endometrial cancer.

DIAGNOSIS

In women with postmenopausal bleeding, transvaginal ultrasound (TVS) to measure endometrial thickness is a very helpful initial evaluation approach. Endometrial thickness in excess of 5 mm should be followed with endometrial biopsy. TVS is not as helpful in postmenopausal women taking hormone replacement therapy or women who are still menstruating. Abnormal uterine bleeding in these settings should be evaluated with endometrial biopsy.

Office endometrial biopsy using Pipelle sampling is an effective diagnostic technique that is simple to perform, does not require anesthesia, and is generally well tolerated by the patient. Hysteroscopy with dilation and curettage remains the gold standard for the diagnosis of endometrial cancer and should be performed when office biopsy is impossible or a diagnostic conclusion can not be made from office biopsy findings.

STAGING

Endometrial carcinoma is surgically staged according to the joint FIGO (Table 14-2).

> **Table 14-2 FIGO Staging of Uterine Cancer**
>
> **Stage I   Tumor confined to the corpus uteri.**
> - IA Tumor limited to endometrium
> - IB Tumor invades up to or less than one half of myometrium
> - IC Tumor invades to more than one half of myometrium
>
> **Stage II Tumor invades cervix but doesn't extend beyond uterus.**
> - IIA Endocervical glandular involvement only
> - IIB Cervical stroma involvement
>
> **Stage III Local and/or regional spread.**
> - IIIA Tumor invades serosa and/or adnexa (direct extension or metastasis)
> - IIIB Vaginal involvement (direct extension or metastasis)
> - IIIC Metastasis to pelvic and/or paraaortic lymph nodes
>
> **Stage IV Involvement of bowel and/or bladder mucosa or distant metastasis.**
> - IVA Tumor invades bowel and/or bladder mucosa
> - IVB Distant metastasis

Data from FIGO Committee on Gynecologic Oncology: *Int J Gynecol Obstet* 70:207-312, 2000.
FIGO, International Federation of Gynecology and Obstetrics.

TREATMENT

1. There are ongoing debates about different aspects of uterine cancer treatment. A comprehensive discussion of such controversies is beyond the scope of this chapter.
2. Patients are generally divided into low-risk, intermediate-risk, and high-risk categories for disease recurrence, and treatment is based on the individual woman's risk category.
3. Low-risk patients have stage IB or less with grade I or grade II histology, stage IA with grade III histology. Also, the following additional criteria should be met:
   a. Disease confined to the uterine fundus.
   b. No involvement of the lymphovascular space.
   c. No evidence of lymph node metastases.
   d. These women are treated with total abdominal hysterectomy (TAH) and bilateral salpingo-oophorectomy (BSO) with the addition of vaginal brachytherapy if grade III histology.
4. Intermediate-risk patients have grade I or grade II tumor extending beyond one half of the myometrium (stage IC), or with invasion of the cervix or isthmus (stage II). Also, the following additional criteria should be met:
   a. No involvement of the lymphovascular space.
   b. No evidence of metastases.

c. The treatment for this group is complete surgical staging: extrafascial TAH and BSO, pelvic/paraaortic lymphadenectomy followed by adjuvant radiotherapy.
5. High-risk women have the following characteristics:
   a. Grade III cancer with any degree of myometrial invasion.
   b. Adnexal or pelvic metastases.
   c. Grade II disease with invasion beyond one half of the myometrium and isthmic or cervical involvement.
   d. Involvement of the lymphovascular space: The treatment for the high-risk group includes complete surgical staging (as described for the intermediate group) whenever possible. This is then followed by pelvic brachytherapy for organ-confined disease or whole pelvic radiotherapy if there is paraaortic lymph node involvement. Adjuvant chemotherapy is also a reasonable option, although the best chemotherapy regimen has not been defined.

PROGNOSIS

The overall 5-year survival is 86% and 60% for Caucasian and African American women, respectively. The prognosis is dependent primarily on stage of disease at diagnosis but if disease is confined to the uterus, prognosis is based on grade, histological cell type, and depth of invasion. The degree of lymphovascular space invasion and the patient's race and age are important independent prognostic factors.

14.3 Vaginal Cancer

BRIEF DESCRIPTION AND EPIDEMIOLOGY

The incidence of vaginal cancer in the United States is approximately 1 in 136,000. In 2005, 1069 women were expected to develop vaginal cancer and 378 deaths were expected to result from this rare form of genital cancer. Overall, it constitutes 1% to 2% of gynecologic malignancies and it is made up of two main histological subtypes: squamous cell carcinoma (85%) and adenocarcinoma (15%). Clear cell adenocarcinoma of the vagina is a very rare variant most often associated with in utero DES exposure.

ETIOLOGY

1. Vaginal cancer is rare, therefore less information is available about its etiology. In general, vaginal cancer is associated with the same risk factors as in cervical neoplasia: multiple lifetime sexual partners, early age at first intercourse, and current smoking.
2. Up to a third of the women diagnosed with vaginal cancer have been previously treated for other low genital malignancy, especially cervical. In addition, two thirds of biopsies from vaginal cancer test positive for high-risk HPV (16 and 18).
3. DES exposure in utero has been strongly associated with the development of vaginal adenosis and vaginal cancer.

PREVENTION

Vaginal intraepithelial neoplasia (VAIN) is a preinvasive lesion capable of progressing to vaginal cancer in 10% to 30% of cases. Screening for VAIN in at-risk women is a good strategy in the prevention of vaginal cancer. Women diagnosed with neoplasia elsewhere in the lower genital tract and those who have undergone hysterectomy for cervical intraepithelial neoplasia (CIN) are at risk for VAIN even years after the primary diagnosis and treatment. Another group of women at risk are those exposed in utero to DES. These high-risk groups of women need close surveillance with Papanicolaou smear and thorough colposcopic inspection.

Anti-HPV vaccination, once it becomes available, may potentially protect women against vaginal cancer.

CLINICAL PRESENTATION

The main presenting symptoms of vaginal cancer are abnormal vaginal bleeding, including postcoital and postmenopausal bleeding, watery vaginal discharge, vaginal pain, and vaginal lump. Physical examination may detect a mass, plaque, or ulcer in the vagina.

Vaginal cancer may be asymptomatic; sometimes it is discovered incidentally during evaluation for abnormal Papanicolaou smears.

DIAGNOSIS

Vaginal cancer is diagnosed by histology from biopsies. It is beneficial to use colposcopic guidance during biopsy of less obvious lesions. All suspected areas should be biopsied.

STAGING

The FIGO staging of vaginal cancer is clinical and it is based on findings from physical and pelvic examination, cystoscopy, proctoscopy, and chest and skeletal radiography (Table 14-3).

TREATMENT

Treatment is primarily based on disease stage but is influenced by tumor location in early stage disease.

Table 14-3 FIGO Staging of Vaginal Cancer

Stage	Description
Stage 0	Vaginal carcinoma in situ.
Stage I	Disease confined to vaginal mucosa.
Stage II	Submucosa infiltration by disease, does not extend to pelvic side wall.
	IIA Subvaginal infiltration, does not involve the parametrium
	IIB Parametrial involvement
Stage III	Pelvic side wall involvement by disease.
Stage IV	Involvement of bladder or rectal mucosa or extension outside the true pelvis or distant metastasis.
	IVA Bladder or rectal mucosa infiltration or extension outside the true pelvis
	IVB Distant metastasis

Data from FIGO Committee on Gynecologic Oncology: *Int J Gynecol Obstet* 70:207-312, 2000.
FIGO, International Federation of Gynecology and Obstetrics.

1. **Stage 0:** Standard treatment options include the following: wide local excision, partial or total vaginectomy with skin graft, topical 5% 5-fluorouracil, and intracavitary radiotherapy. All these treatments have equivalent cure rates.
2. **Stages I and II:** Standard treatments can either be (i) surgical—excision of lesion, which may sometimes require an exenteration with pelvic and/or inguinal lymphadenectomy in selected cases or (ii) radiation therapy—combination of brachytherapy and external-beam radiation.
3. **Stages III and IVA:** Combined interstitial, intracavitary, and external-beam radiation therapy. Rarely, surgery may be combined with radiotherapy.
4. **Stage IVB:** Palliative radiotherapy with or without chemotherapy.

PROGNOSIS

Prognosis is determined by stage of disease at diagnosis. The overall 5-year survival rate (all stages combined) is 61%. Stage-specific 5-year survival rates are 95% for stage 0, 67% for stage I, 39% for stage II, 33% for stage III, and 19% for stage IV.

14.4 Vulvar Cancer

BRIEF DESCRIPTION AND EPIDEMIOLOGY

Vulvar cancer is the fourth most common gynecologic malignancy, accounting for 5% of all cancers of the female genital tract. In 2005, 3870 new cases and 870 vulvar cancer deaths were anticipated in the United States. Vulvar cancer is primarily a disease of elderly women but has been observed in premenopausal women as well. It is most commonly squamous cell carcinoma in type. Although comparatively rare, other histological types do occur; these include melanoma, adenocarcinoma, extramammary Paget's disease, verrucous carcinoma, and basal cell carcinoma.

ETIOLOGY

1. Risk factors for vulvar cancer include cigarette smoking, vulvar dystrophy, vulvar intraepithelial neoplasia, HPV infection, immunodeficiency syndromes, a prior history of cervical cancer, and northern European ancestry.
2. Recent studies suggest that vulvar cancer can develop in at least two ways. In about 30% to 50% of cases, high-risk HPV infection appears to play a role. Women affected by HPV-associated vulvar cancer tend to have multiple areas of vulvar intraepithelial neoplasia (VIN) elsewhere on their vulvas, are usually smokers, and tend to be younger (age 35 to 55) than typical vulvar cancer patients.
3. The second process by which vulvar cancer develops does not involve HPV infection. This variant of vulvar cancer is usually diagnosed in older women (age 55 to 85) who rarely have VIN but often have lichen sclerosis.

PREVENTION

Avoidance of smoking, close monitoring and treatment of vulvar dystrophies, and VIN are good strategies for prevention. High vigilance is particularly important in high-risk women; these include women with immunodeficiency syndromes, smokers, women with prior history of cervical cancer, and women with established diagnosis of vulvar dystrophy.

CLINICAL PRESENTATION

1. The most common symptoms are a red, pink, or white bump or bumps with a wartlike or raw surface. An area of the vulva may appear white and feel rough.
2. About half of the women with vulvar cancer complain of persistent itching and a growth. Some also complain of pain, burning, painful urination, bleeding, and discharge not associated with the normal menstrual period. An ulcer that persists for more than a month is another sign.
3. The labia majora is the most common site of involvement and accounts for about 50% of cases. The labia minora accounts for 15% to 20% of cases. The clitoris and Bartholin's glands are less frequently involved.

DIAGNOSIS

Biopsies for histology should be taken from the central part of visible lesions and surrounding skin. Sometimes, no obvious lesions are seen during clinical inspection. If there is clinical suspicion, colposcopic examination of the vulvar with 5% acetic acid should be performed and acetowhite areas biopsied.

STAGING

The FIGO staging of vulvar cancer is surgical, based on thorough histological evaluation of biopsy and/or excision specimen as well as lymph nodes (Table 14-4).

TREATMENT

Treatment is based on the stage of disease at diagnosis. Standard therapy is discussed here; however, treatment is usually individualized for each patient in order to maximize efficacy and reduce morbidity.

1. Stage 0
   a. Wide local excision or laser beam therapy or a combination of both; *or*
   b. Skinning vulvectomy with or without grafting; *or*
   c. 5% fluorouracil cream.
2. Stages I and II
   a. Wide or radical local excision for microinvasive disease.
   b. Modified radical vulvectomy with unilateral or bilateral inguinofemoral lymphadenectomy for all others.
   c. If patient is unsuitable for surgery, radical radiation therapy may result in longtime survival.
3. Stage III and IV
   a. Radical vulvectomy/iguinofemoral lymphadenectomy. In selected patients a pelvic exenteration may be appropriate.
   b. Radical vulvectomy/inguinofemoral lymphadenectomy followed by radiation therapy. Sometimes, radiation therapy is administered first, followed by surgery.

Table 14-4 **FIGO Surgical Staging for Vulvar Cancer**

Stage 0 **Vulvar carcinoma in situ.**
Stage I **Tumor confined to the vulva or perineum, $\leq$2 cm in greatest dimension and negative nodes.**
  IA Tumor confined to the vulva or perineum, $\leq$2 cm in greatest dimension, negative nodes, and stromal invasion $\leq$1 mm
  IB Tumor confined to the vulva or perineum, $\leq$2 cm in greatest dimension, negative nodes, and stromal invasion >1 mm
Stage II **Tumor confined to the vulva or perineum, >2 cm in greatest dimension and negative nodes.**
Stage III **Tumor of any size with adjacent spread to the lower urethra or anus and/or unilateral inguinal lymph node involvement.**
Stage IV **Tumor spread to upper urethra, bladder or rectal mucosa, pelvic bone, both inguinal lymph node regions, and distant spread.**
  IVA Tumor invades any of the following: upper urethra, bladder or rectal mucosa, pelvic bone or bilateral inguinal lymph node metastasis
  IVB Any distant spread including pelvic lymph nodes

Data from FIGO Committee on Gynecologic Oncology: *Int J Gynecol Obstet* 70:207-312, 2000.
FIGO, International Federation of Gynecology and Obstetrics.

c. Patients unsuitable for surgery can be treated with radical radiation therapy, which may result in longtime survival.

PROGNOSIS

Survival is most dependent on the pathologic status of the inguinal nodes. In patients with operable disease without nodal involvement, the overall survival rate is 90%; however, in patients with nodal involvement, the overall 5-year survival rate is approximately 50% to 60%. The stage-specific 5-year survival, according to FIGO, is as follows:

1. 77% for stage I
2. 55% for stage II
3. 31% for stage III
4. 0% for stage IV

14.5 Ovarian Cancer

BRIEF DESCRIPTION AND EPIDEMIOLOGY

Overall, the age-adjusted incidence rate of ovarian cancer is 16 per 100,000 women. A woman's risk of getting ovarian cancer during her lifetime is 1.7%. The risk of developing and dying from ovarian cancer is higher for Caucasian women than for African American women. Several histological types of malignancies arise from the ovary. Epithelial carcinoma accounts for 90% of all cases and it is one of the most common gynecologic malignancies. Also, ovarian cancer is the fifth most frequent cause of cancer death in women. In 2005 alone, 22,220 new cases and 16,210 deaths were expected in the United States from ovarian cancer.

HISTOLOGICAL CLASSIFICATION

Ovarian cancer can be divided into three broad categories in accordance with their anatomic site of origin in the ovary, these are: epithelial (ovarian surface), sex cord (cells that surround the oocyte), and germ cell (oocyte) tumors. Each of these categories has further subdivisions but the rest of this discussion shall focus on the epithelial tumors, which constitute the overwhelming majority. Table 14-5 shows the subclassification of malignant ovarian tumors.

ETIOLOGY

1. The exact etiology of ovarian cancer is unknown. Hereditary cancers account for less than 10% of ovarian cancers. In this small fraction, germ line mutations in BRCA1 and BRCA2 genes, Lynch II syndrome,

Table 14-5 Ovarian Cancer Histological Classification

Epithelial Tumors

Classification	Cell Type	Organ/Structure Where Normally Found
Serous	Endosalpingeal	Fallopian tube
Mucinous	Endocervical	Uterine cervix
Endometrioid	Endometrial	Uterus
Clear cell	Renal	Kidney
Brenner	Transitional	Bladder
Mixed	Combination	Combination of two or more of above
Undifferentiated	N/A	N/A
Borderline	Any of the above	Any of the above without stromal invasion

Sex Cord Tumors

Granulosa cell tumor
Thecoma
Fibroma
Sertoli-Leydig

Germ Cell Tumors

Dysgerminoma (equivalent to seminoma in men)
Yolk sac (endodermal sinus tumors)
Embryona carcinoma
Nongestational choriocarcinoma
Immature teratoma

All shown is the cell type, with an indication of where these cell types are normally found for epithelial tumors.

and suppressor gene p53 mutation are some of the genetic pathways implicated as causes.
2. A few theoretical causes that have been suggested include incessant ovulation associated with surface epithelial trauma and repair which can lead to mutagenesis, excessive gonadotrophin levels with consequent high estrogen levels, and stromal hyperactivity.
3. Risk factors for ovarian cancer include family history, early menarche, late menopause, infertility, endometriosis, and postmenopausal estrogen replacement. Other risk factors include cigarette smoking, exposure to talc, and diet high in animal fat.

PREVENTION

1. Evidence from epidemiologic data indicates that the following are protective against ovarian cancer: combined oral contraceptive pills, breast feeding, tubal ligation, and to a lesser extent, hysterectomy. Evidence in support of exercise, weight reduction, fruit and vegetable consumption, use of antioxidants as protective factors are inconclusive.
2. In women at high risk for ovarian cancer, currently utilized preventive strategies include regular pelvic ultrasound, CA 125, and other tumor markers. Those who test positive for genetic mutations may consider risk-reducing surgery following appropriate counseling.
3. There is no effective routine screening for ovarian cancer in the general population. The U.S. Preventive Services Task Force, the American College of Obstetricians and Gynecologists, and the American College of Physicians all recommend against routine screening for ovarian cancer in asymptomatic women.

CLINICAL PRESENTATION

Ovarian cancer typically presents in the seventh decade of life. Generally, early stage ovarian cancer is asymptomatic. Up to 75% of women with ovarian cancer present in stages III and IV, by which time they have overt symptoms that include abdominal distention, nausea, anorexia, or early satiety due to the presence of ascites and omental or bowel metastases. Occasionally, they may be dyspneic due to a pleural effusion. Unfortunately, women with early stage ovarian cancer are usually asymptomatic, although vague symptoms are common. Examination may detect an irregular pelvic mass, ascites, and sometimes an upper abdominal mass indicative of omental cake.

DIAGNOSIS

It is impossible to confirm or refute the diagnosis of ovarian cancer with a noninvasive test. However, a combination of the presenting history, physical examination findings, serum tumor markers, and imaging tests would give a reasonable suspicion of malignancy in most cases. The glycoprotein CA 125, associated with epithelial ovarian cancer, is elevated in more than 80% of patients with stage II or higher disease. Unfortunately, the sensitivity of CA 125 in stage I disease is less than 50%. Other promising tumor markers from cDNA microarray technology are under investigation, these include osteopontin, YLK-40, and CA 15-3. Some tumor markers are helpful in nonepithelial tumors, e.g., lactate

Table 14-6 FIGO Surgical Staging of Ovarian Cancer

Stage I **Ovarian cancer is limited to the ovaries.**
- IA Tumor limited to one ovary; capsule intact, no tumor on ovarian surface. No malignant cells in ascites or peritoneal washings.
- IB Tumor limited to both ovaries; capsules intact, no tumor on ovarian surface. No malignant cells in ascites or peritoneal washings.
- IC Tumor limited to one or both ovaries with any of the following: capsule ruptured, tumor on ovarian surface, malignant cells in ascites or peritoneal washings.

Stage II **Tumor involving one or both ovaries with pelvic extension and/or implants.**
- IIA Extension and/or implants on the uterus and/or fallopian tubes. No malignant cells in ascites or peritoneal washings.
- IIB Extension to and/or implants on other pelvic tissues. No malignant cells in ascites or peritoneal washings.
- IIC Pelvic extension and/or implants (stage IIA or stage IIB) with malignant cells in ascites or peritoneal washings.

Stage III **Tumor involving one or both ovaries with microscopically confirmed peritoneal implants outside the pelvis. Superficial liver metastasis equals stage III. Tumor is limited to the true pelvis but with histologically verified malignant extension to small bowel or omentum.**
- IIIA Microscopic peritoneal metastasis beyond pelvis (no macroscopic tumor).
- IIIB Macroscopic peritoneal metastasis beyond pelvis ≤2 cm in greatest dimension.
- IIIC Peritoneal metastasis beyond pelvis >2 cm in greatest dimension and/or regional lymph node metastasis.

Stage IV **Tumor involving one or both ovaries with distant metastasis. If pleural effusion is present, positive cytologic test results must exist to designate a case to stage IV. Parenchymal liver metastasis equals stage IV.**

Data from FIGO Committee on Gynecologic Oncology: *Int J Gynecol Obstet* 70:207-312, 2000.
FIGO, International Federation of Gynecology and Obstetrics.

---

dehydrogenase (LDH) in dysgerminomas, alpha-fetoprotein (AFP) in immature teratomas, inhibin in granulosa cell tumors, and human chorionic gonadotropin (HCG) in nongestational trophoblastic tumors.

Ultrasonography, CT, and MRI are all helpful in the diagnostic evaluation of women with ovarian cancer. Ultrasonography has become a frontline investigation of any pelvic mass and it is usually combined with Doppler study of the blood flow pattern in and around the mass. Features suggestive of malignancy include the presence of a solid component, internal septation, irregularity, and suspicious blood flow pattern. In addition ultrasound may detect ascitis. CT and MRI are not required for the diagnosis of ovarian cancer but because they indicate the extent of metastatic spread may be helpful in planning management. Ultimately, the diagnosis is confirmed at surgery.

STAGING
The FIGO and the American Joint Committee on Cancer (AJCC) have designated staging for ovarian cancer (Table 14-6).

TREATMENT
1. The standard treatment for ovarian cancer is laparotomy with full staging; this includes peritoneal washing for cytology, systematic inspection of all pelvic and intraabdominal organs, palpation of retroperitoneal structures, TAH, and BSO. In addition, pelvic and paraaortic lymph nodes are dissected, smears of the diaphragmatic undersurface are taken, and an omentectomy is performed. The goal is to achieve optimal cytoreduction, which means no residual tumor or residual tumor is no more than 1 to 2 cm in diameter after surgery.
2. Patients are then given 4 to 6 cycles of platinum-based adjuvant chemotherapy (a combination of paclitaxel with either carboplatin or cisplatin).
3. In young patients with stage IA, grade I disease who desire fertility, a unilateral salpingo-oophorectomy (USO) combined with washings, systematic inspection, peritoneal and lymph node biopsies is an acceptable option. Adjuvant chemotherapy is not required in this setting.

PROGNOSIS
Favorable factors associated with good outcome in epithelial ovarian cancer include younger age, good performance status, cell type other than mucinous and clear cell, lower stage, well-differentiated tumor, smaller disease volume prior to any surgical debulking, absence of ascites, and smaller residual tumor following primary cytoreductive surgery.

The overall 5-year survival rates for epithelial ovarian cancer by stage are 77% for stage I, 70% for stage II, 40% for stage III, and 13% for stage IV.

Hirsutism

Arundathi G. Prasad

15.1 Definitions

1. Hirsutism is androgen-dependent excessive growth of sexual hair.
2. Virilization is hirsutism accompanied by the following:
   a. Temporal hairline recession
   b. Deepening of the voice
   c. Loss of female body contour, atrophy of the breasts
   d. Enlargement of the clitoris
   e. Development of male muscular pattern and body habitus in extreme cases
3. Hypertrichosis is characterized by excessive growth of nonsexual hair (hair on the forehead, lower leg, or forearm).

15.2 Physiology of Hair Growth

1. Definitions
   a. Vellus hairs: fine, short, nonpigmented hairs
   b. Terminal hairs: long, coarse, pigmented, and responsive to hormones in certain parts of the body
2. Hair growth cycle
   a. Anagen: growing phase
   b. Catagen: rapid involution phase
   c. Telogen: resting phase
3. Hair growth is influenced by the following:
   a. Genetics: Certain ethnic groups have more hair follicles per surface area of skin.
   b. Androgens initiate growth and increase rate of matrix cell mitosis; estrogens have the opposite effect.
   c. Ratio of growth phase to resting phase: Length of hair is determined by duration of the growth phase (anagen); shorter hair is produced by a short anagen, long telogen.
   d. Degree of asynchrony: marked synchrony.
      (1) All hair undergoes telogen at the same time, which leads to shedding, as seen in pregnancy.
      (2) Anagen at the same time produces increased hair growth.
   e. Once the pattern of hair growth is established, it persists despite withdrawal of androgens.

15.3 Androgen Production

1. Testosterone
   a. Normal female produces 0.2 to 0.3 mg per day.
   b. Peripheral conversion: 40% from androstenedione.
   c. Adrenal gland: 25%.
   d. Ovary: 25%.
   e. Bound to sex hormone–binding globulin (SHBG): 65% (strongly bound).
   f. Bound to albumin: 33% (weakly bound).
   g. Unbound: 1%, which is the free active portion that acts on the target cells.
   h. Testosterone is converted in the skin to dihydrotesterone (DHT), which stimulates the hair follicles. DHT is metabolized to androstenediol glucuronide.
2. Dehydroepiandrosterone sulfate (DHEAS): produced exclusively by the adrenal gland
3. Androstenedione: produced in both the adrenal glands and ovaries

15.4 Etiology of Hirsutism

The etiology of hirsutism can be divided into the following four categories.

ALTERED ANDROGEN METABOLISM

1. It is the idiopathic or familial form of hirsutism.
2. Caused by an increase in 5-alpha-reductase activity in the skin, which leads to an increased conversion of testosterone to DHT.
3. Diagnosed by measuring 3-androstanediol glucuronide, a metabolite of DHT, which correlates well with 5-alpha-reductase activity.

DECREASE IN ANDROGEN BINDING

1. SHBG
   a. Produced in the liver
   b. Decreased by androgen; therefore, men have decreased binding capacity and increased level of free testosterone
   c. Increased by estrogen and thyroid hormone
      (1) Therefore, binding capacity is increased in women, pregnancy, hyperthyroidism, and when taking estrogen-containing medications
      (2) Pathologic states with decreased binding capacity are as follows:
         (a) Hypothyroidism
         (b) Anorexia
         (c) Dermatomyositis
         (d) Porphyria

EXOGENOUS ANDROGEN INGESTION

1. Danazol: gonadotropin-releasing hormone (GnRH) agonist used to treat endometriosis
2. Anabolic steroids
3. Minoxidil: antihypertensive

4. Androgen-containing creams: used for vulvar dystrophies
5. Dilantin
6. Streptomycin
7. Penicillamine
8. Diazoxide
9. Cyclosporine

INCREASED ANDROGEN PRODUCTION

Increased androgen production arises from one of two sources: adrenal gland or ovary.

1. Adrenal gland
   a. Cushing's syndrome
      (1) Common reason for referral, but rare cause
      (2) Associated with cortisol hypersecretion
      (3) Related to malignant pituitary adrenocorticotropic hormone (ACTH)-producing tumor (Cushing's disease) or ectopic ACTH-producing tumor
      (4) Clinical signs and symptoms
         (a) Truncal obesity
         (b) Purple striae over abdomen
         (c) Buffalo hump
         (d) Hypertension
         (e) Easy bruisability
      (5) Diagnosis
         (a) Unlikely if clinical signs and symptoms are lacking
         (b) 24-hour urinary-free cortisol excretion; normal level: 20 to 90 µg
         (c) Single-dose overnight dexamethasone suppression test
            (i) There is a very low incidence of false results.
            (ii) Give 1 mg dexamethasone at 11 PM and measure 8 AM serum cortisol, which should be less than 5 µg/dL.
   b. Congenital adrenal hyperplasia (CAH)
      (1) Most commonly caused by 21-hydroxylase deficiency
      (2) May also result from 11-hydroxylase deficiency
      (3) Diagnosis
         (a) Increased DHEAS
            (i) Greater than 325 µg/dL considered elevated
            (ii) Greater than 700 µg/dL suspicious for tumor
         (b) Increased 17-hydroxyprogesterone
            (i) Greater than 200 µg/dL considered elevated
            (ii) Between 200 and 800 µg/dL suspicious for adult-onset CAH (perform ACTH stimulation test)
            (iii) Greater than 800 µg/dL virtually diagnostic for adult-onset CAH
   c. Androgen-producing tumors: rare, but should be suspected if testosterone level greater than 200 µg/dL
      (1) Adenomas
         (a) Usually benign
         (b) More common in reproductive age

(c) Characterized by acute onset of hirsutism
(d) Produce testosterone or DHEAS
(2) Carcinomas
  (a) Usually malignant
  (b) More likely to develop in postmenopausal women
  (c) Progressive onset of hirsutism
  (d) Rarely produce DHEAS, lack sulfotransferase enzyme activity to convert dehydroepiandrosterone (DHEA) to DHEAS
2. Ovary
  a. Polycystic ovarian syndrome or hyperandrogenic chronic anovulation.
    (1) Most common cause of excess androgen production.
    (2) Characterized by menstrual irregularity, hirsutism, obesity, and acne.
    (3) Increased risk for developing endometrial cancer at an early age.
    (4) Definition: endocrinologic disorder beginning soon after menarche consisting of inappropriate luteinizing hormone (LH) and follicle-stimulating hormone (FSH) secretion associated with increased GnRH pulse amplitude, which leads to chronically elevated LH and anovulation. Both adrenal and ovarian androgen hypersecretion are commonly present.
    (5) Diagnosis.
      (a) Increased levels of the following:
        (i) Testosterone
        (ii) DHEAS
        (iii) LH
        (iv) LH:FSH ratio greater than 2
        (v) Increased insulin resistance (Fasting insulin levels are elevated in 70% of the cases and diabetes mellitus is seen in approximately 13%.)
      (b) Decreased SHBG
    (6) HAIR-AN syndrome—subgroup of polyceptic ovaries (PCO) characterized by the following:
      (a) Hyperandrogenism
      (b) Insulin resistance
      (c) Acanthosis nigricans: velvety pigmented lesion found in the nape of the neck and intertriginous areas
  b. Ovarian neoplasms: Nearly every type of primary or metastatic tumor can have stromal cells that secrete excess amounts of androgens.
    (1) Krukenberg tumor: tumor metastatic to the ovary consisting of signet ring cells that usually originate from the gastrointestinal tract—stomach, colon
    (2) Brenner tumor: epithelial neoplasm that consists of cells resembling urothelium mixed with ovarian stroma
    (3) Germ cell tumors
      (a) Sertoli-Leydig cell tumors
        (i) Rare; less than 1%
        (ii) Most common in age group of 20-40 years
        (iii) Palpable ovarian mass in 85%

(b) Hilus cell tumor
  (i) Usually postmenopausal
  (ii) Not always palpable
  (iii) Diagnosis: testosterone level greater than two times normal with normal DHEAS
(4) Lipoid cell tumors: increase in testosterone, DHEAS, or both
(5) Granulosa-theca cell tumors: can occasionally produce increased testosterone in addition to increased estradiol

15.5 Evaluation

1. Complete history and physical.
2. Document extent of hirsutism (i.e., Ferriman-Galloway score), age of onset, and rapidity of onset.
3. Perform laboratory studies (purpose is to rule out neoplasm).
   a. Testosterone level: greater than 200 µg/dL indicates tumor
   b. DHEAS: adrenal is the only source; greater than 700 µg/dL indicates tumor
   c. 17-Hydroxyprogesterone: marker of late-onset congenital adrenal hyperplasia
   d. Prolactin: to rule out pituitary tumor
4. Perform additional laboratory studies: Other metabolic problems are very common in hirsute women and they have increased risk factors for heart disease.
5. Radiology.
   a. Ultrasound
   b. Computed tomography (CT)
   c. Selective adrenal or ovarian vein catheterization

15.6 Treatment

Once androgen-producing tumors, Cushing's syndrome, and CAH have been ruled out, medical treatment is generally successful in limiting new hair growth but does not affect existing hair.

1. Oral contraceptive pills.
   a. First-line therapy
   b. Very effective in the majority of cases
   c. Suppress ovarian function and decrease ovarian estrogen secretion
   d. Takes at least 6 months to get results
   e. Mechanism of action
      (1) Estrogen component decreases LH, which decreases testosterone production and, in turn, decreases free testosterone.
      (2) Estrogen component also increases SHBG, which increases testosterone binding capacity and thus decreases free testosterone.
      (3) Progestin component decreases plasma ACTH, which decreases adrenal androgen secretion.
2. Spironolactone.
   a. Inhibits 5-alpha-reductase
   b. Competes at the androgen receptor level in the hair follicle

    c. Dose-dependent: 100 to 200 mg PO daily
    d. Side effects: initial diuresis, mastodynia, and irregular menses (when used without oral contraceptive pills [OCPs]); hyperkalemia or hyponatremia is uncommon
    e. May combine peripheral action of spironolactone with OCPs for a more dramatic result (Yasmin)
    f. Acne: effectively treated with 2% to 5% spironolactone topical cream
3. Dexamethasone.
    a. Treatment of choice for patients with CAH (i.e., deficiency in 21-hydroxylase, 11-β-hydroxylase, or 3-β-hydroxysteroid dehydrogenase-isomerase)
    b. Mechanism: ACTH suppression decreases testosterone derived from adrenal steroid precursors
    c. Androgen more sensitive than cortisol
    d. May be effective in inducing ovulation when added to clomiphene citrate (Clomid)
4. Cimetidine, an H2-receptor antagonist, has weak antiandrogenic properties. It inhibits androgen receptor activity. Recent studies have shown little or no benefit in treatment of hirsutism.
5. GnRH agonist (Synarel, Lupron depot).
    a. May be required in addition to OCPs in severe cases
    b. Mechanism: down regulation of GnRH receptors leads to LH/FSH suppression and thus ovarian androgen decrease
6. Finasteride: inhibits 5-alpha reductase, the enzyme that converts testosterone to active DHT in the skin. It provides modest reduction in hirsutism over 6 months, but less effective than spironolactone. It is ineffective for androgen alopecia in women.
7. Flutamide: inhibits androgen receptor uptake and also suppresses serum androgen. Used with an oral contraceptive it appears to be more effective than spironolactone in improving hirsutism. Flutamide causes decreased renal cortisol clearance in CAH, causing lower hydrocortisone dosage requirements. Glucocorticoid replacement doses should therefore be reduced when flutamide is added for treatment of hirsutism. Hepatotoxicity has been reported but rare.
8. Cyproterone acetate: potent antiandrogen with progestational activity that is prescribed along with an oral contraceptive. It is not available in the United States. It is available as a progestin element in an oral contraceptive pill in Europe. (Dose: Diane-35: Ethinyl estradiol 35 μm with cyproterone acetate 2 mg)
9. Local treatments by shaving or depilatories, waxing, electrolysis, or bleaching should be encouraged. Laser therapy is an effective treatment for facial hirsutism, particularly for women with dark hair and light skin. Complications include skin hypopigmentation (rare) and hyperpigmentation, which occurs in 20% but usually resolves.
10. Antiandrogen treatments must be given only to nonpregnant women. Women must be counseled to take contraceptives when indicated and avoid pregnancy, because use during pregnancy causes malformations and pseudohermaphrodism in male infants.

Premenstrual Syndrome

George T. Danakas
Ibrahim Joulak

16.1 Definition

Premenstrual syndrome (PMS) is a cyclic recurrence during the luteal phase of the menstrual cycle of somatic, affective, and behavioral disturbances that are of sufficient severity to affect interpersonal relationships adversely or interfere with normal activities.

Premenstrual dysphoric disorder (PMDD) is the most severe form of PMS with prominence of anger, irritability, and internal tension.

16.2 Epidemiology

1. PMS is thought to be extremely prevalent, intermittently affecting approximately 75% of all women.
2. Approximately 50% have mild symptoms.
3. Approximately 2% to 10% of women with PMS are severely affected (PMDD).
4. Most women who seek treatment for PMS are in their 30s or 40s.
5. The natural history of PMS has yet to be clearly elucidated.

16.3 Diagnostic Criteria[1,2]

1. Cyclic, recurrent physical, emotional, and behavioral symptoms are present in the luteal phase of the menstrual cycle and remit shortly after the onset of menstruation.
2. The luteal phase symptoms are present in the majority of menstrual cycles.
3. The luteal phase symptoms do not represent simply a worsening of a chronic physical or emotional disorder.
4. Luteal phase symptoms are severe enough to cause physical or emotional distress or deterioration in psychosocial functioning.
5. The recurrent, cyclic nature of the disorder can be confirmed by prospective daily monitoring by the woman and her significant other for at least two menstrual cycles.

16.4 Etiology

The available evidence suggests that PMS results from the interaction of cyclic changes in ovarian steroids with central neurotransmitters, mostly serotonin, beta-endorphin, and gamma-aminobutyric acid (GABA).

16.5 Symptoms

1. The symptoms of PMS are diverse and potentially disabling.
2. There are more than 150 psychologic, physical, and behavioral symptoms associated with PMS.
3. Treatment is most frequently sought because of emotional symptoms.
4. The most common emotional symptoms are as follows:
   a. Depression
   b. Irritability
   c. Anxiety
   d. Mood swings
5. The most common physical (somatic) complaints are the following:
   a. Headache
   b. Bloating
   c. Cramps
6. The most common behavioral symptom is food cravings.

16.6 Diagnosis[1,2]

1. PMS is a diagnosis of exclusion (Box 16-1).
2. Symptoms should be restricted to the luteal phase.
3. Symptoms should be affecting the quality of life.
4. Other medical or psychologic disorders must be ruled out.
5. No laboratory test is available that can specifically confirm the diagnosis of PMS.
6. Premenstrual dysphoric disorder (PMDD) is a diagnostic category for PMS included in the Diagnostic and Statistical Manual of Mental Disorders[1] (DSM-IV TR) (Box 16-2).
7. Confirming PMS by symptom charting for 2 months (Fig. 16-1) is important to the diagnostic process.

16.7 Management[1,3,4]

1. The key to the management of PMS is early and correct diagnosis using prospective methods of documentation.
2. Initial management consists of education, support, and stress reduction.
3. Interventions should include psychosocial, nutritional, and pharmacologic approaches, with consideration for surgical intervention in severe cases.
   a. Psychosocial: Individualization of the treatment plan will maximize therapeutic response.
      (1) Education
      (2) Stress management
      (3) Environmental changes
      (4) Adequate rest and sleep
      (5) Regular exercise
      (6) Light therapy

> **BOX 16-1 Diagnostic Criteria for Premenstrual Syndrome**
>
> 1. Premenstrual syndrome can be diagnosed if the patient reports at least one of the following affective and somatic symptoms during the 5 days before menses in each of the three prior menstrual cycles:
>   a. Affective symptoms
>   (1) Depression
>   (2) Angry outbursts
>   (3) Irritability
>   (4) Anxiety
>   (5) Confusion
>   (6) Social withdrawal
>   b. Somatic symptoms
>   (1) Breast tenderness
>   (2) Abdominal bloating
>   (3) Headache
>   (4) Swelling of extremities
> 2. These symptoms are relieved within 4 days of onset of menses without recurrence until at least cycle day 13.
> 3. The symptoms are present in the absence of any pharmacologic therapy, hormone ingestion, or drug or alcohol use.
> 4. The symptoms occur reproducibly during two cycles of prospective recording.
> 5. The patient suffers from identifiable dysfunction in social or economic performance.

From American College of Obstetricians and Gynecologists: Clinical management guidelines for obstetricians-gynecologists: premenstrual syndrome. In ACOG *Practice Bulletin*, no. 15, Washington, DC, 2000, ACOG.

   b. Nutritional.
     (1) The American College of Obstetricians and Gynecologists recommends a complex carbohydrate diet and nutritional supplements including magnesium, vitamin E, and calcium.
     (2) Well-balanced meals should be eaten regularly.
     (3) Food should contain adequate amounts of protein, fiber, and complex carbohydrates and be low in fat.
     (4) Carbohydrate-rich foods and beverages may improve mood symptoms and food cravings because they increase the level of tryptophan, the precursor of serotonin.
     (5) Caffeine-containing beverages should be avoided because the stimulant effects of caffeine may worsen tension, irritability, and insomnia.
     (6) Alcohol and illicit drugs should be avoided because their use may worsen emotional lability.
     (7) Calcium supplementation (1.2 g/day) reduces the physical and emotional symptoms of PMS.

BOX 16-2 Criteria for Premenstrual Dysphoric Disorder

1. In most menstrual cycles during the past year, five (or more) of the following symptoms for most of the time during the last week of the luteal phase, began to remit within a few days after the onset of the follicular phase, and were absent in the week postmenses, with at least one of the symptoms being either a, b, c, or d:
   a. Markedly depressed mood, feelings of hopelessness, or self-deprecating thoughts
   b. Marked anxiety, tension, feelings of being "keyed up" or "on edge"
   c. Marked affective lability (e.g., feeling suddenly sad or tearful or increased sensitivity to rejection)
   d. Persistent and marked anger or irritability or increased interpersonal conflicts
   e. Decreased interest in usual activities (e.g., work, school, friends, hobbies)
   f. Subjective sense of difficulty in concentrating
   g. Lethargy, easy fatigability, or marked lack of energy
   h. Marked change in appetite, overeating, or specific food cravings
   i. Hypersomnia or insomnia
   j. Subjective sense of being overwhelmed or out of control
   k. Other physical symptoms, such as breast tenderness or swelling, headaches, joint or muscle pain, a sensation of "bloating," weight gain

   NOTE: In menstruating females, the luteal phase corresponds to the period between ovulation and the onset of menses, and the follicular phase begins with menses. In nonmenstruating females (e.g., those who have had a hysterectomy), the timing of luteal and follicular phases may require measurement of circulating reproductive hormones.

2. The disturbance markedly interferes with work or school or with usual social activities and relationships with others (e.g., avoidance of social activities, decreased productivity and efficiency at work or school).
3. The disturbance is not merely an exacerbation of the symptoms of another disorder, such as major depressive disorder, panic disorder, dysthymic disorder, or a personality disorder (although it may be superimposed on any of these disorders).
4. Criteria 1, 2, and 3 must be confirmed by prospective daily ratings during at least two consecutive symptomatic cycles. (The diagnosis may be made provisionally prior to this confirmation.)

From American Psychiatric Association: *Diagnostic and statistical manual of mental disorders*, ed 4, Text Revision (DSM-IV-TR), Washington, DC, 2000, APA.

Name:																																					
Day of cycle:		1	2	3	4	5	6	7	8	9	10	11	12	13	14	15	16	17	18	19	20	21	22	23	24	25	26	27	28	29	30	31	32	33	34	35	36
Date																																					
Menses																																					
Irritability																																					
Anxiety																																					
Nervous tension																																					
Mood swings																																					
Anger/Rage																																					
Violent behavior																																					
Depression																																					
Crying easily																																					
Despondency																																					
Overemotionality																																					
Fatigue																																					
Skin problems																																					
Swelling (legs, hands)																																					
Breast tenderness																																					
Abdominal bloating																																					
Headaches																																					
Migraine headaches																																					
Abdominal cramps																																					
General aches/pains																																					
Hot flushes																																					
Nausea																																					
Gastrointestinal																																					
Food cravings																																					
Insomnia																																					
Increased naps																																					

Figure 16-1 Example of a daily symptom calendar. The patient records her symptoms on a 1 to 3 severity scale for mild, moderate, and severe, respectively. Boxes are left blank if symptom severity is zero. (From Smith S: Diagnosis of premenstrual syndrome. In Smith S, Schiff I, editors: *Modern management of premenstrual syndrome*, New York, 1993, WW Norton.)

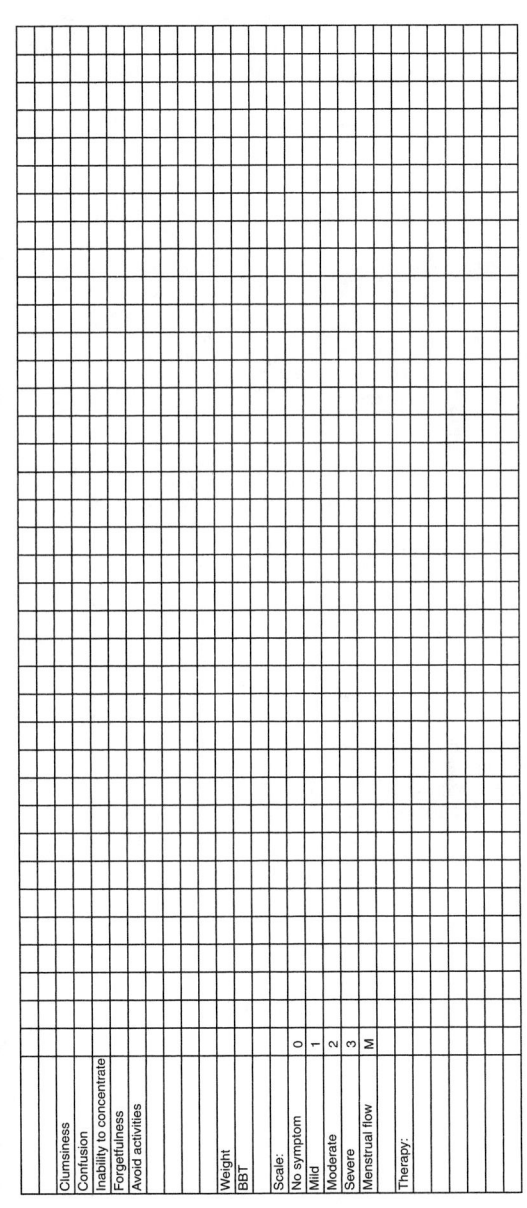

Practical Guide to the Care of the Gynecologic/Obstetric Patient 315

Figure 16-1, cont'd *BBT*, Basal body temperature.

Table 16-1 Alternative Treatments for Premenstrual Symptoms

Therapy/Supplement	Typical Dose	Efficacy	Level of Evidence*
Aerobic exercise		Yes	B
Bright light therapy		Likely yes	B
Guided imagery		Possible	C
Homeopathy		Possible	B
Massage		Possible	B
Relaxation response		Possible	B
Dietary manipulation		Unlikely	C
Caffeine avoidance		Possible	B
Calcium	1200-1600 mg/d	Yes	A
Magnesium	400-800 mg/day	Likely yes	B
Vitamin B$_6$	50-100 mg/day	Likely yes	B
Black cohosh	40 mg twice daily	Possible	C
Chasteberry	4-20 mg/day	Likely yes	B
Evening primrose oil	2-3 g/day	Unlikely	B
Ginkgo	80 mg twice daily	Likely yes	B
Kava[†]	100-300 mg/day	Possible	C
St. John's wort	300 mg 3 times/day	Possible	B

Modified from Girman A, Lee R, Klinger B: *Am J Obstet Gynecol* 188:S56-S65, 2003.
Level A: large high-quality, randomized, double-blind, placebo-controlled trials, meta-analysis; *Level B:* lesser quality randomized trials, retrospective studies, systematic reviews; *Level C:* expert opinion, case series, uncontrolled studies, consensus statements.
[†] Kava use not recommended at present—reports of liver failure being investigated.

---

(8) Magnesium (200 to 400 mg/day) reduces water retention and the negative affect associated with PMS.

(9) Vitamin E (400 IU/day) helps breast tenderness because it is recommended to treat mastalgia.

(10) Pyridoxine (vitamin B$_6$) has been shown to improve depression, fatigue, and irritability. Neurotoxicity (paresthesia, hyperesthesia, muscle weakness, numbness, bone pain), however, has been observed at 100-mg doses.

c. Pharmacologic.
  (1) Intervention needs to be individualized and targeted to the symptoms.
  (2) Pharmacotherapy should be initiated only after a diagnosis is made (based on medical evaluation and confirmed by prospective daily symptom ratings) and after psychosocial and nutritional strategies have been attempted[3,4] (Table 16-1).
  (3) Pharmacologic treatments include the following:
    (a) Although hormonal treatments have long been advocated, it is clear that progesterone (oral or intravaginal) is not effective.
      (i) Oral contraceptives are widely used but few data support their effectiveness. They should be considered

Table 16-2 Prescription Medications Used for Premenstrual Symptoms

Medication	Typical Dose	Efficacy	FDA Approved
GnRH agonists	Variable by product	Likely yes	No
Nonsteroidals	Variable by product	Likely yes	Dysmenorrhea only
Oral contraceptives	Variable by product	No	No
Progesterone	Variable by product	No	No
Spironolactone (Aldactone)	25-50 mg/day	Likely yes	No
Alprazolam (Xanax, −XR)	0.5-1 mg twice daily	Likely yes	No
Bupropion (Wellbutrin, −SR, −XL; Zyban)	Variable	Unlikely	No
Citalopram (Celexa)	10-20 mg/day	Yes	No
Clomipramine (Anafranil)	Variable	Yes	No
Escitalopram (Lexapro)	10 mg/day	Likely yes	No
Fluoxetine (Prozac, Sarafem)	10-20 mg/day	Yes	PMDD only*
Fluvoxamine (Luvox)	50 mg/day	Yes	No
Paroxetine (Paxil, −CR)	10-40 mg/day	Yes	No
Sertraline (Zoloft)	25-50 mg/day	Yes	PMDD only*
Venlafaxine (Effexor, −XR)	Variable	Yes	No

*Not approved for PMS, though commonly used off-label for PMS.
FDA, Food and Drug Administration; *GnRH*, gonadotropin-releasing hormone; *PMDD*, premenstrual dysphoric disorder.

if symptoms are primarily physical, not mood symptoms.
- (ii) The Food and Drug Administration (FDA)–approved treatments for PMDD include only fluoxetine and sertraline. The literature indicates that antidepressants that do not contain serotonin, namely bupropion and older tricyclic agents (except clomipramine) are not likely to help PMS.
- (iii) One serotonin norepinephrine reuptake inhibitor (SNRI): venlafaxine (Tables 16-2 and 16-3).
- (iv) Danazol (100 to 200 mg/day): 19-nortestosterone derivative with progesterone-like effects. Inhibits

Table 16-3 Recommended Treatment Strategies for Premenstrual Dysphoric Disorder*

Medication	Starting Dose (mg)	Therapeutic Dose (mg)	Common Side Effects
First-line: Selective Serotonin Reuptake Inhibitors (SSRIs)			
Fluoxetine	10-20	20	Sexual dysfunction (anorgasmia and decreased libido), sleep alterations (insomnia, sedation, or hypersomnia), and gastrointestinal distress (nausea and diarrhea)
Sertraline	25-50	50-150	Same as fluoxetine
Paroxetine	10-20	20-30	Same as fluoxetine
Citalopram	10-20	20-30	Same as fluoxetine
Second-line			
Clomipramine	25	50-75	Dry mouth, fatigue, vertigo, sweating, headache, nausea
Alprazolam	0.50-0.75	1.22-2.25	Drowsiness, sedation
Third-line			
Leuprolide	3.75	3.75	Hot flashes, night sweats, headache, nausea

*For SSRIs and clomipramine, the starting and therapeutic doses are administered once daily and are the same with luteal-phase and continuous administration. For luteal-phase administration, the medication should be initiated at time of ovulation (usually approximately 2 weeks before the expected onset of menses) and discontinued on the first day of menses. The therapeutic doses given for SSRIs are those that were reported in the randomized clinical trials. However, clinical experience has shown that a subgroup of patients with premenstrual dysphoric disorder may require slightly higher doses (up to 60 mg of fluoxetine; up to 150 mg or sertraline; up to 40 mg of paroxetine; and up to 40 mg of citalopram). If a patient is taking another SSRI and tolerating it well but has a partial response at the doses listed, it would be appropriate to increase the dose of the specific SSRI before switching to another agent. Alprazolam is administered three times a day; treatment should begin at 0.25 mg three times a day. Clinical trials of leuprolide used the depot form; leuprolide should be administered intramuscularly each month.

pituitary gonadotropin secretion and ovulation leading to symptomatic relief.

(v) Gonadotropin-releasing hormone (GnRH) agonists: Majority of studies show improvement of symptoms but the hypoestrogenic side effects and cost discourage its use. Also, the treatment should be limited to 6 months because of the risk of osteoporosis and cardiovascular disease.

(vi) Spironolactone (25 to 50 mg/day): Can be used for mild PMS. Effective in alleviating breast tenderness

and bloating. Side effects include antiestrogenic effects and hyperkalemia.
- (b) Prostaglandin-related treatments.
  - (i) Effective in alleviating various physical symptoms of PMS. Any nonsteroidal antiinflammatory drug (NSAID) should be effective.
  - (ii) Mefenamic acid (250 mg tid with meals).
  - (iii) Naproxen sodium (275 to 550 mg bid).
- (c) Nonprescription preparations (see Table 16-1).
  - (i) Chasteberry (4 to 20 mg/day), ginkgo (80 mg bid), St. John wort (300 mg tid)
  - (ii) Evening primrose oil (2 to 3 g/day)

d. Surgical.
  (1) Severe intractable PMS responds well to hysterectomy with bilateral ovariectomy.
  (2) Before surgery, a trial of GnRH therapy or danazol is recommended.
  (3) Estrogen replacement therapy is recommended postoperatively to reduce the risk of osteoporosis, heart disease, and genitourinary atrophy.

REFERENCES

1. American College of Obstetricians and Gynecologists: Clinical management guidelines for obstetricians-gynecologists: premenstrual syndrome. In *ACOG Practice Bulletin 2000*, no. 15, Washington, DC, 2000, ACOG.
2. American Psychiatric Association: Premenstrual dysphoric disorder. *In Diagnostic and statistical manual of mental disorders*, ed 4, Text Revision (DSM-IV-TR), Washington, DC, 2000, APA, pp. 771-774.
3. Dell DL: Premenstrual syndrome, premenstrual dysphoric disorder, and premenstrual exacerbation of another disorder, *Clin Obstet & Gynecol* 47(3):568-575, 2004.
4. Grady Weliky, Tana A: Premenstrual dysphoric disorder, *N Engl J Med* 348(4):33-438, 2003.

SUGGESTED READING

Goldstein S, Halbreich U: Psychotropic medications as treatment of dysphoric premenstrual syndrome, In Smith S, Schiff I, editors: *Modern management of premenstrual syndrome*, New York, 1993, WW Norton.

Menopause

Diane J. Sutter

17.1 Menopause

DEFINITIONS
1. Menopause: no menstrual periods for 1 year after age 40; permanent cessation of menses resulting from the loss of ovarian follicular activity.
2. Climacteric or perimenopause: reproductive stage of life marked by waxing and waning estrogen levels followed by decreasing ovarian function.
3. Premature ovarian failure: amenorrhea due to ovarian insufficiency before age 40; can be transient or permanent.

EPIDEMIOLOGY
1. Average age of menopause in the United States is 51.
2. Wide age range for spontaneous menopause: 40 to 58.
3. Age at which menopause occurs is genetically determined.
4. Smokers experience menopause an average of 1.5 years earlier than nonsmokers.
5. More than one third of a woman's life will be spent after menopause.

PATHOPHYSIOLOGY
1. Degenerating theca cells fail to react to endogenous gonadotropins.
2. Less estrogen is produced.
3. There is decreased negative feedback on the hypothalamic–pituitary axis.
4. There is increased follicle-stimulating hormone (FSH) and luteinizing hormone (LH) production.
5. Stromal cells continue to produce androgens as a result of increased LH stimulation.

MENOPAUSAL SYMPTOMS
1. Hot flashes (flushes)
   a. Definition: A hot flash is a sudden, transient sensation ranging from warmth to intense heat that spreads over the body, particularly over the chest, face, and head, typically accompanied by flushing and perspiration and often followed by a chill.
   b. Menopause as the cause for hot flashes can be documented by elevated FSH level.

c. Hot flashes are thought to be hypothalamic in origin but the precise cause is not known.
d. Seventy-five percent of women experience hot flashes; one third will require treatment of their symptoms.
e. Women typically experience hot flashes for 6 months to 2 years but they may last 10 or more years.
f. Hot flashes frequently occur at night and produce insomnia or disrupted sleep.
g. Hot flashes tend to be more frequent and severe after surgically induced menopause.
h. Clinician should determine the level of impact for the woman and how she is coping with them.
   (1) Estrogen is the most effective treatment (see Section 17.4 for treatment options).
   (2) Nonestrogenic prescription therapies:
       (a) Medroxyprogesterone (150 mg intramuscular [IM], each month)
       (b) Antidepressants: venlafaxine, paroxetine, or fluoxetine
       (c) Gabapentin, an anticonvulsant drug
       (d) Clonidine, alpha-adrenergic receptor agonist
   (3) Nonpharmacologic treatments may be helpful for mild symptoms and include the following:
       (a) Change in the ambient temperature (may ameliorate hot flashes and reduce night sweats)
       (b) Vitamin E
       (c) Paced respirations
       (d) Acupuncture
       (e) Exercise
       (f) Caffeine, alcohol, and spicy foods avoidance if they trigger hot flashes
2. Atrophic vaginitis
   a. Etiology: decreased maturation of the vaginal mucosal epithelium from estrogen deficiency, vagina shortens and narrows, vaginal walls become thinner and less elastic, are pale in color, and lose rugations.
   b. Symptoms are as follows:
      (1) Burning
      (2) Itching
      (3) Bleeding
      (4) Dyspareunia
      (5) Vaginal discharge
   c. Differential diagnosis: Physician should rule out other causes for vulvovaginitis such as the following:
      (1) Malignant and nonmalignant tumors (rare)
      (2) Infection
      (3) Trauma
      (4) Foreign body
   d. Treatment: Estrogen therapies delivered by vaginal creams, rings, or tablets are effective if only a local vaginal effect is desired.

(1) Once an initial therapeutic effect is reached, therapy should be reduced to maintain the desired response.
(2) Water-based lubricants such as KY jelly or Replens may be useful for temporary relief of vaginal dryness with intercourse.

3. Incontinence
   a. Definition: the demonstrable involuntary loss of urine that is a social or hygienic problem
   b. Etiology
      (1) The bladder and urethra are embryologically derived from estrogen-dependent tissues.
      (2) Hypoestrogenism leads to atrophy of these tissues, producing dysuria, urinary frequency and urgency, incontinence, and increased frequency of urinary tract infections.
      (3) Evaluation and treatment: Topical estrogen with or without systemic estrogen is helpful in alleviating the irritation and urgency symptoms.

4. Mood changes
   a. Etiology: Most women pass through the menopause transition without significant emotional or psychiatric problems.
   b. Women with a history of premenstrual syndrome, premenstrual dysphoric disorder, or psychiatric illness may experience an exacerbation of symptoms during the perimenopause.
   c. Differential diagnosis of mood disturbance during the perimenopause includes:
      (1) Untreated vasomotor symptoms
      (2) Recurrence of major depression or new episode of major depression
      (3) Hypothyroidism
      (4) Medications for an acute or chronic illness
      (5) Stressful life events
      (6) Adjustments to age-related social changes

5. Sleep disturbance
   a. Definition: difficulties falling asleep and disrupted sleep, usually because of hot flashes (Lack of sleep can cause fatigue and lead to irritability, impaired memory, and disrupted concentration; sleep is less efficient and there is longer time to the onset of rapid eye movement sleep.)
   b. Etiology
      (1) Hypothalamic alterations may cause vasomotor instability and sleep disruption.
      (2) Estrogen affects serotonin and norepinephrine, the neurotransmitters involved in sleep.

6. Sexual changes
   a. Sexual desire decreases in both sexes with age.
   b. Sexual function changes occur in women because of the loss of ovarian hormone production.
      (1) Decreased estrogen may lead to urogenital atrophy, vaginal dryness, and dyspareunia.
      (2) Testosterone, responsible for libido, declines to half the premenopausal level.

c. The impact of the loss of ovarian hormones is variable among women because of the multifactorial nature of sexual activity:
    (1) Medical illness in self or partner
    (2) Perception of sexuality and aging
    (3) Stressors: family, work, personal life
    (4) Incontinence
    (5) Sleep disturbance

17.2 Osteoporosis

DEFINITION

Osteoporosis is a systemic skeletal disease characterized by low bone mass and microarchitechural deterioration of bone tissue with a consequent increase in bone fragility and fracture.

EPIDEMIOLOGY

1. Osteoporosis-related fractures will occur in more than 40% of women over the age of 50.
2. In the United States, 1.2 million fractures a year result from osteoporosis.
3. Risk factors include the following:
    a. Northern European heritage
    b. Petite body frame
    c. Smoking
    d. Sedentary lifestyle
    e. Family history
    f. Low calcium intake
    g. Early menopause or oophorectomy
    h. History of long-term steroid use
    i. Hyperparathyroidism
4. Hip fractures represent one of the most devastating consequences of osteoporosis.
    a. In the United States, 250,000 hip fractures occur every year.
    b. Subsequent to the fracture, 50% of cases will not be able to ambulate independently; 25% will be confined to long-term care facilities, and 20% will die within 6 months.

PATHOPHYSIOLOGY

1. Estrogen promotes bone formation by the following mechanisms:
    a. Stimulating osteoblastic activity
    b. Enhancing calcium absorption from the gut
    c. Increasing blood levels of the active vitamin D metabolite, 1,25-dihydroxyvitamin D_3
2. Loss of ovarian function is associated with increased rate of bone loss, especially in the first 3 to 4 years of menopause, by increasing bone resorption.
3. Early loss is primarily trabecular bone, leading to vertebral crush fractures, followed by long-term loss of both cortical and trabecular bone, leading to other fractures such as those of the wrist and hip.

DIAGNOSIS

1. The World Health Organization defines osteopenia, or low bone density, as a bone mineral density between 1 and 2.5 standard deviations below the young adult mean. Osteoporosis is defined as bone mineral density 2.5 standard deviations below the young adult mean. Other authorities define osteoporosis as a bone mineral density more than 2.0 standard deviations below the young adult mean.
2. At the spine and hip, a 1 standard deviation decrease in bone mass is associated with approximately a twofold increase in fracture.
3. Dual x-ray absorptiometry (DXA) is now preferred by most authorities to determine bone density with minimal radiation exposure and high accuracy.
4. Computed tomography (CT) has been adapted for bone density measurement but radiation dosage, cost, and accessibility issues have limited its use.
5. X-ray film may pick up fractures occurring with no-impact or low-impact trauma.
6. Ultrasound bone mass measurement is a new technique that offers the advantage of avoiding ionizing radiation.
7. Measurement of current height and comparison to maximal adult height can help establish the diagnosis of osteoporosis. More than 1 inch of height loss, with or without the development of kyphoscoliosis (dowager's hump) is consistent with the diagnosis of osteoporosis.

DIFFERENTIAL DIAGNOSIS

1. Osteomalacia: This is a defect in collagen matrix mineralization caused by an abnormality in vitamin D metabolism. This may occur with renal failure, steatorrhea, vitamin D–resistant rickets, or severe hypophosphatemia (usually because of excess ingestion of phosphate-binding antacids).
2. Multiple myeloma: Plasma cells produce osteoclast-activating factor or transforming growth factor, which induce bone resorption.
3. Hyperparathyroidism and hyperthyroidism: Excess hormone induces bone resorption.
4. Carcinoma: Squamous cell, renal, bladder, and ovarian carcinomas may secrete humoral factors that induce bone resorption.
5. Hypercortisolism: Glucocorticoid excess causes osteoporosis by inhibiting intestinal calcium absorption, leading to a compensatory bone resorption.
6. Idiopathic postmenopausal osteoporosis is the most common form.
7. Evaluation of osteoporosis should include the following:
   a. Serum calcium
   b. Phosphorus
   c. Alkaline phosphatase
   d. Complete blood count
   e. Protein electrophoresis
   f. Thyroid function tests
   g. Parathyroid hormone
   h. Serum cortisol level
   i. 24-hour urinary calcium excretion

TREATMENT

1. With all osteoporosis agents, concomitant intake of adequate calcium and vitamin D is necessary for optimal response.
   a. Calcium supplementation reduces loss, deficiency causes bone loss.
      (1) 1500 mg elemental calcium orally (PO) per day is necessary to maintain zero calcium balance in postmenopausal women (1000 mg PO per day when taking hormone replacement therapy [HRT]).
      (2) Epidemiologic studies suggest that a lifetime of adequate calcium intake reduces fracture risk.
   b. Vitamin D_3.
      (1) In elderly women, vitamin D_3 deficiency may contribute to bone loss.
      (2) Treatment with vitamin D (800 IU, qd) and calcium has been shown to decrease hip fractures.
2. Antiresorptive agents.
   a. These agents inhibit osteoclastic bone resorption, preserve or increase bone density, and preserve skeletal structure. They do not rebuild damaged microarchitecture. All of these agents have been shown to reduce fracture risk.
      (1) Estrogens as recommended in Section 17.4. Several estrogen therapy (ET) and estrogen plus progestin therapy (EPT) preparations are approved for the prevention of bone loss after menopause but none are approved for treatment of women known to have osteoporosis.
      (2) Biphosphonates (Actonel, Boniva, Fosamax) reduce bone resorption by inhibiting differentiation of osteoclasts and speeding osteoclast cell death.
      (3) Selective estrogen receptor modulators (SERMs). The goal of SERM therapy is to provide the bone benefits of estrogen without an adverse effect on the breast or endometrium. Raloxifene reduces bone resorption by inhibiting osteoclasts.
      (4) Calcitonin nasal spray (Miacalcin, Fortical).
         (a) Inhibits osteoclasts and reduces bone resorption.
         (b) It is reserved as an alternative for women who cannot or choose not to use another treatment option because it is less potent than the other agents.
3. Anabolic agents: These stimulate bone formation and result in the accumulation of new bone tissue. Teriparatide (Forteo) is a recombinant parathyroid preparation given by daily subcutaneous injection.

17.3 Cardiovascular Disease

EPIDEMIOLOGY

1. Heart disease is the leading cause of death in postmenopausal women and causes more mortality than the next seven causes of death combined including breast cancer.
2. Cardiovascular disease (CVD) is an inclusive term that includes hypertension, coronary artery disease (CAD), stroke, valvular heart disease, and congestive heart failure.

3. CVD develops in women on average 10 years later in life compared with men, and this lag has been attributed to the protective effects of estrogen before menopause. Prior to the release of the Heart and Estrogen/Progestin Replacement Study (HERS) and the Women's Health Initiative (WHI) in 2002, 42% of women between 50 and 72 years were taking hormone therapy.
   a. HERS was the first published secondary prevention trial in 2763 women with known coronary heart disease (CHD) who were followed up for the primary outcome of the cardiovascular events of nonfatal myocardial infarction (MI) or CHD death. At a mean of 4.1 years, there was no significant difference in the hormone therapy (HT) arm versus the placebo arm and HT was associated with an increased risk for MI in the first year.
   b. The WHI is the largest (>16,000 women) randomized, placebo-controlled clinical trial to investigate whether HT conferred a primary cardioprotective effect. The study was stopped early because of a small increase in breast cancer among patients who were taking both conjugated equine estrogens (CEE) and medroxyprogesterone acetate (MPA) with no cardiovascular benefit.
   c. Selective reporting from the popular media and some scientific sources overemphasized the risks versus benefits of HT therapy and did not correctly report that, at least in the case of CHD, the overall risk of CHD did not achieve statistical significance.
   d. The risk for CHD is primarily in older women, many years from menopause, who have already developed atherosclerotic disease. The current position on HT and CVD according to the North American Menopause Society (NAMS):
      (1) HT is not effective for the treatment of CHD.
      (2) Younger, newly menopausal women may have some benefit but this concept awaits further clinical research.
      (3) HRT should not be initiated for the secondary prevention of CVD. The decision to continue or stop HRT in women with CVD who have been undergoing long-term HRT should be based on established noncoronary benefits and risks and patient preference.
      (4) If a woman develops an acute CVD event or is immobilized while undergoing HRT, it is prudent to consider discontinuance of the HRT or to consider venous thromboembolism (VTE) prophylaxis while she is hospitalized to minimize risk of VTE associated with immobilization. Reinstitution of HRT should be based on established noncoronary benefits and risks, as well as patient preference.

PATHOPHYSIOLOGY

1. Heart disease risk factors for women
   a. Advancing age
   b. African American race
   c. More than two alcoholic drinks per day
   d. Hypertension

e. Hypercholesterolemia: high-density lipoprotein (HDL) (>50 mg/dL) is a negative risk factor for CAD
f. Family history: CVD in a male younger than 55, in a female younger than 65
g. Weight more than 20% over ideal
    (1) There is a 60% lower risk of MI in women who maintain their ideal body weight.
    (2) Weight loss decreases blood pressure and low-density lipoprotein (LDL) cholesterol.
h. Diabetes
    (1) Diabetes is an independent risk factor for CVD.
    (2) Gestational diabetes predicts a 30% risk for developing overt diabetes later on in life.
i. Cigarette smoking
    (1) Smoking is the leading preventable cause of CVD.
    (2) After smoking cessation, the risk of CAD begins to decline and may reach the level of risk among nonsmokers within 3 to 5 years.
j. Early menopause (especially before age 35)
k. Physical inactivity: current recommendation is for 30 minutes of aerobic exercise every day
l. Stress

17.4 Hormone Replacement Therapy

INDICATIONS AND CONTRAINDICATIONS

1. Use of ET and EPT should be limited to the shortest duration consistent with the treatment goals, benefits, and risks for the individual woman, taking into account symptoms and domains (e.g., sexuality, sleep) that may impact on quality of life.
2. Treatment of moderate to severe menopausal symptoms (hot flashes, night sweats) is the primary indication for systemic ET and EPT.
3. All systemic and local estrogen products are Food and Drug Administration (FDA) approved for treating moderate to severe symptoms of vulvar and vaginal atrophy. When estrogen is considered solely for this indication, local ET is recommended.
4. The primary menopause-related indication for progestagen use is endometrial protection from unopposed estrogen.
    a. For all women with an intact uterus who are using ET, they must also be prescribed an adequate progestagen.
    b. Women without a uterus should not be prescribed a progestagen.
5. There is definitive evidence that EPT reduces the risk for postmenopausal osteoporotic fracture. Because of the potential risks associated with HT, alternative prevention and treatment options for osteoporosis should be considered.
6. Contraindications for ET/EPT:
    a. Undiagnosed abnormal genital bleeding
    b. Liver dysfunction or disease
    c. Active or history of deep vein thrombosis, pulmonary embolism

d. Known or suspected breast cancer except in appropriately selected patients
   e. Active or recent (within the past year) arterial thromboembolic disease (e.g., stroke, MI)
7. The relationship between breast cancer and HRT is still a controversial and widely debated topic. Although some studies indicate that there may be an increased risk of breast cancer associated with the prolonged use of estrogen and or progestagens, they are not randomized controlled studies.

METHODS OF HORMONE REPLACEMENT THERAPY

1. Oral estrogen preparations
   a. Conjugated equine estrogen (CEE) (Premarin)
      (1) The oldest estrogen on the market and the most widely studied
      (2) No generic equivalent
   b. Synthetic conjugated estrogens (Cenestin, Enjuvia)
   c. Esterified estrogens (Menest, Neo-Estrone)
   d. Estropipate (Ogen, Ortho-Est, generics)
   e. Ethinyl estradiol (Femhrt)
2. Transdermal estradiol (Vivelle Dot, Climara, generics)
   a. Transdermal estrogen products can be dosed lower because they are not subjected to the first pass mechanism of the liver.
   b. Unlike oral preparations, which are associated with fluctuating serum levels, transdermal administration is associated with relatively stable serum levels.
3. Progestagens
   a. Reduces the risk of endometrial hyperplasia and cancer associated with unopposed ET to a level found in women who never used ET.
   b. Progestagens may be given cyclically, 10 to 12 days of the month, to allow the patient to a have a withdrawal bleed, or they may be given continuously so that the patient does not have a bleeding episode.
   c. Progesterone is the steroid hormone produced by the ovary. Oral micronized progesterone (Prometrium) is an exogenous compound identical to endogenous progesterone. Before micronization, the rapid inactivation and poor bioavailability of orally administered progesterone led to the development of the progestins in the 1950s.
   d. Oral preparations.
      (1) Medroxyprogesterone acetate (Provera, MPA)
      (2) Norethindrone
      (3) Norethidrone acetate
      (4) Micronized progesterone
   e. Intrauterine system: levonorgesterol intrauterine device (Mirena).
   f. Vaginal: progesterone gel.

SUGGESTED READINGS

North American Menopause Society. *Menopause practice: a clinician's guide*, Cleveland, OH, 2006, North American Menopause Society.

Speroff L, Fritz M: *Clinical gynecologic endocrinology and infertility*, ed 7, Baltimore, MD, 2005, Lippincott Williams & Wilkins.

Labor, Delivery, and Obstetrics Pain Management

18

Farkad Balaya

18.1 Normal Labor and Delivery

Parturition is the process of giving birth. This process incorporates two major events: labor and delivery. Labor is defined as the progressive cervical dilation in response to repetitive uterine contractions. Delivery is the expulsion of the fetus as a result of uterine contractions and cervical dilation.

The initiation and maintenance of labor is complex. Prostaglandins, cytokines, and sex-steroid hormones appear to play pivotal roles in this process.

The gestational age is used to classify the type of delivery. Premature labor occurs before 37 weeks gestation. A delivery before 24 weeks of gestation is referred to as an abortion. Term labor is defined as labor occurring after 37 weeks gestation.

ESSENTIAL FACTORS

Before labor, several factors need to be considered to ensure good progress and to minimize risks to the fetus and mother. An abnormality of any one of these factors is often a contraindication to labor and results in dystocia.

1. Pelvic architecture: The classic work of Caldwell and Moloy in the 1930s provided the framework for the evaluation of the female bony pelvis. The four basic types of bony pelvis are characterized in Figure 18-1. Although most pelvises are mixed, these four types provide us with a basic configuration. The clinical evaluation of the bony pelvis has replaced x-ray pelvimetry over the years. The focus of the evaluation of the pelvis is on the true rather than the false pelvis. The true pelvis includes the pelvic inlet, the midpelvis, and the outlet. Figure 18-2 illustrates the pelvic landmarks.
   a. Pelvic inlet: The pelvic inlet is evaluated by measuring the diagonal conjugate diameter. The diagonal conjugate diameter is the distance between the lower edge of the symphysis and the sacral promontory. Subtracting 1.5 to 2 cm from the diagonal conjugate provides an estimate of the true conjugate diameter. The true conjugate should measure 11 cm or more. The critical distance is known as the obstetric conjugate diameter. This represents the

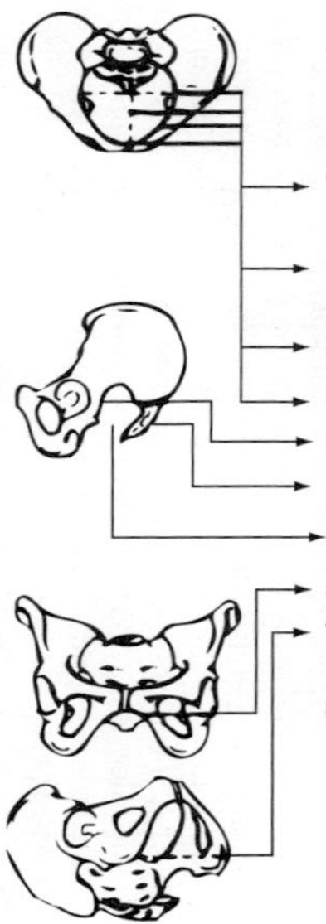

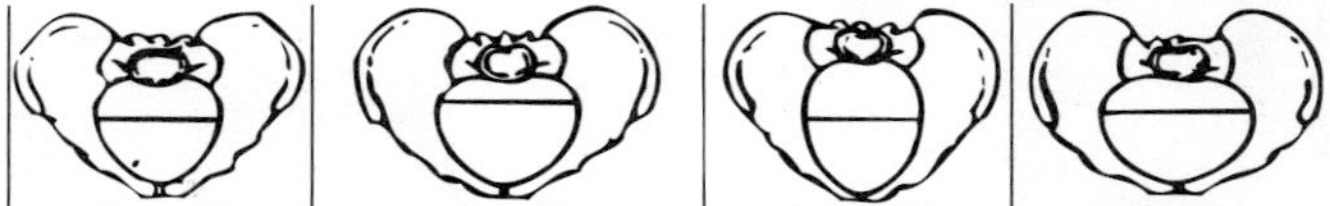

330　Practical Guide to the Care of the Gynecologic/Obstetric Patient

	Gynecoid	Android	Anthropoid	Platypelloid
Widest transverse diameter of inlet	12 cm	12 cm	<12 cm	12 cm
Anteroposterior diameter of inlet	11 cm	11 cm	>12 cm	10 cm
Side walls	Straight	Convergent	Narrow	Wide
Forepelvis	Wide	Narrow	Divergent	Straight
Sacrosciatic notch	Medium	Narrow	Backward	Forward
Inclination of sacrum	Medium	Forward (lower 1/3)	Wide	Narrow
Ischial spines	Not prominent	Prominent	Not prominent	Not prominent
Suprapubic arch	Wide	Narrow	Medium	Wide
Transverse diameter of outlet	10 cm	<10 cm	10 cm	10 cm
Bone structure	Medium	Heavy	Medium	Medium

Figure 18-1 Architecture and dimensions of the four basic pelvic types. (From Niswander KR: *Manual of obstetrics: diagnosis and therapy*, ed 3, Boston, 1987, Little, Brown.)

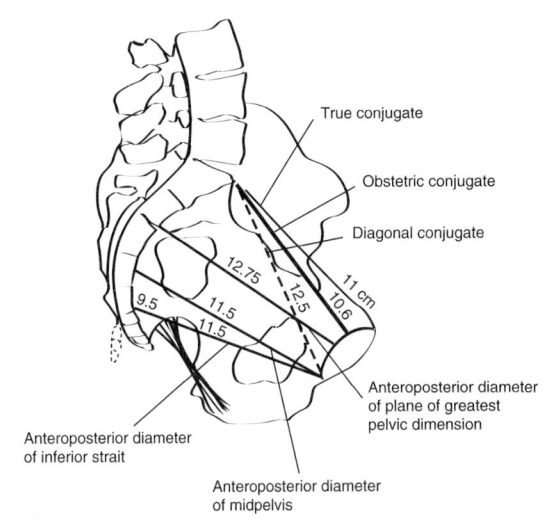

Figure 18-2 Obstetrical measurements of the bony pelvis. (From Niswander KR: *Manual of obstetrics: diagnosis and therapy*, ed 3, Boston, 1987, Little, Brown.)

shortest distance of the inlet and is measured just below the upper edge of the symphysis to the sacral promontory. A diagonal conjugate diameter greater than 12.5 cm has been shown to be a reliable estimate of the pelvic inlet.

b. Midpelvis: The midpelvis is the plane with the narrowest dimensions. The transverse diameter is measured between the ischial spines. The normal length is approximately 10 cm. Clinically, the evaluation has centered on the side walls. The side walls are determined by sweeping the digits laterally from the inlet to the intertuberous diameter during the pelvic examination. The side walls are normally straight. A converging side may limit descent of the fetal presenting part. Midpelvis contraction is also recognized if the distance between the spines is less than 9.5 cm. The sacral curvature should also be examined. A flat or prominent sacrum may result in either failure of the fetus to descend or inability to complete the rotation necessary.

c. Pelvic outlet: The pelvic outlet is evaluated by the angle of the pubic symphysis and the intertuberous diameter. The intertuberous diameter is the most critical and is normally 8 cm or greater. The angle of the symphysis should be equal to or greater than 90 degrees. It should be noted that contractions of both the midpelvis and the outlet are usually concomitant.

2. Fetal presentation: Fetal presentation refers to the part that lies over the pelvic inlet. At term, more than 95% of infants present as vertex. Breech presentation may occur in 3% to 5% of pregnancies at term.

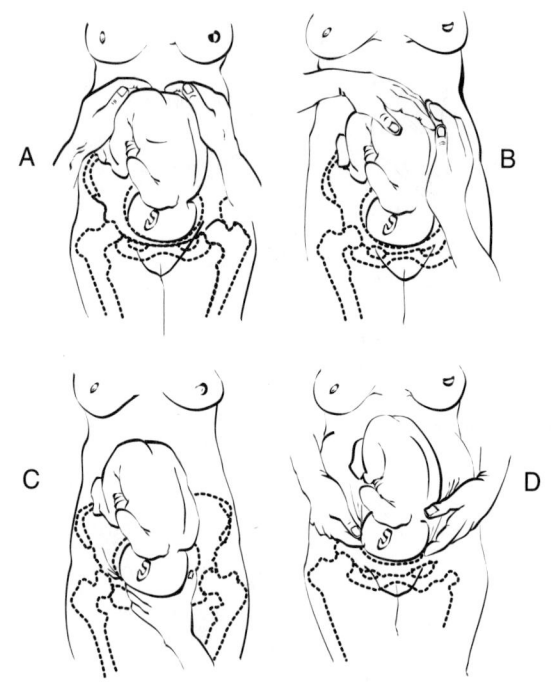

Figure 18-3 A-D, The four Leopold maneuvers. (From Niswander KR: *Manual of obstetrics: diagnosis and therapy*, ed 3, Boston, 1987, Little, Brown.)

Fetal position is defined as the relationship of the lowest presenting part to one of the four quadrants of the bony pelvis. In most cases, the fetal occiput is the lowest part and the position is described as occiput anterior or posterior. The left or right designation is given if the occiput is rotated to the right or left of the pelvis. Dystocia may occur if any malposition or malpresentation occurs. Leopold maneuvers and a pelvic examination in early labor are crucial to identify any malpresentations (Fig. 18-3). Leopold maneuvers assist in determining whether the presentation is vertex or breech. The pelvic examination confirms an abnormal presentation and identifies a face, brow, or compound presentation.

3. Fetal weight: Fetal macrosomia is defined as a birth weight greater than 4000 g (or 4500 g per the American College of Obstetricians and Gynecologists). The most common complications encountered are shoulder dystocia and postpartum hemorrhage; other complication are operative delivery, genital tract lacerations, and uterine rupture. Clinical and sonographic techniques have been used to identify macrosomic infants. Clinical assessment has been shown to be very

inaccurate. Sonography suffers from low sensitivity and high false-positive rates. Shoulder dystocia has been found to occur in more than 8% of infants weighing more than 4500 g. Also, the risk of fetal injury increases fourfold in infants over 4000 g. Nevertheless, attempts should be made to estimate fetal weight using both techniques. Women carrying a fetus weighing over 4500 g should be given the option of a cesarean delivery.

INITIAL EVALUATION

The initial evaluation should determine whether the woman is in labor and identify any conditions that will impact the labor and delivery process. A complete history and physical examination is required. Laboratory tests are also indicated before admission.

1. **History**
   a. Proper evaluation of the laboring patient should begin with a complete history. The gravidity and the gestational age should be determined. The gestational age may be determined from the last menstrual period and confirmed by any sonograms obtained during the pregnancy.
   b. The onset of contractions and their frequency and duration should be determined next. This assists in determining true labor from false labor. False labor, or Braxton-Hicks contractions, is usually mild, is irregular, and generally does not result in any cervical change.
   c. Any history of leakage of fluid or bleeding should be sought. Spontaneous rupture of membranes may be very obvious, with copious amounts of watery discharge from the vagina, or it may be very subtle. A woman may complain of only a small amount of moisture on her underpants. A history of bleeding or spotting may simply be a result of a "bloody show," or it may be something more ominous such as a placenta previa.
   d. Information should also be obtained regarding the antepartum course. Any problems, such as infections, hospitalizations, and medications used, may become relevant during the labor process. A history of abnormal glucose tolerance test and any treatment should be noted.
   e. History from any past pregnancies and general medical history need to be obtained. The past pregnancy outcomes need to be elicited to assess any risks to this labor. Attention should be paid to any history of preeclampsia, placental abruptio, and postpartum hemorrhage. Any general medical problems that may impact the labor should be identified. Women with pulmonary, cardiac, hematologic, or autoimmunologic disorders may need very careful observation and prophylactic therapy during labor.

2. **Physical examination**
   a. The physical examination during labor is usually brief, but it should be as thorough as possible.
   b. The abdominal examination should focus on the fundal height, the fetal presentation, and assessment of the fetal heart rate. The fundal height can be measured with a tape measure. Fundal height

measurement in centimeters is from the pubic symphysis to the top of the uterine fundus. This method is a good approximation of gestational age between 16 and 38 weeks.
   c. The fetal presentation can be assessed from Leopold maneuvers. The four maneuvers are shown in Figure 18-3. The first maneuver attempts to determine the fetal pole in the uterine fundus. The second step determines on which side of the maternal abdomen lies the fetal small parts or the fetal back. The third step is performed to determine the presenting part in the pelvis and whether engagement has occurred. The fourth maneuver confirms the presentation.
   d. The fetal heart rate can be determined by Doppler. The baseline heart rate and any decelerations or accelerations in relation to contractions should be noted. The pattern and frequency of contractions should also be determined to assist in the determination of an adequate labor pattern or an abnormal one.
3. **Pelvic examination**
   a. The pelvic examination begins by inspecting the perineum, vagina, and cervix. Close inspection is required to identify any herpetic lesions or other vaginal or cervical lesions. The diagnosis of ruptured membranes is often made by noting pooling of amniotic fluid in the posterior fornix; confirmation may be made by nitrazine test and ferning. Amniotic fluid air dried on a slide develops a "ferning" pattern under the microscope. The basic pH of amniotic fluid turns yellow nitrazine paper deep blue. A cotton swab is used to obtain the sample from the lateral and upper wall of the vaginal fornix. False-positive tests can be obtained from cervical mucus, blood, and urine. Any green discoloration to the amniotic fluid suggesting meconium should be noted.
   b. Digital examination of the cervix and vagina is carried out to determine the dilation and effacement. The dilation refers to the opening of the cervical os. The effacement describes the thinning of the cervix. This process has usually been described very subjectively in terms of percentage. The normal length of the cervix is usually approximately 3 to 4 cm long. When the cervix shortens to 1.5 to 2 cm long, it is usually described as 50% effaced. To add some consistency to the description, the length in centimeters is being used more frequently. The description in terms of percentage has been plagued with high interobserver variability, which often creates discrepancies during examination.
   c. The digital examination also assists in identifying the presenting part. The station should be noted. This refers to the relationship between the presenting part and the ischial spines. The level of the ischial spines is referred to as zero station. Each centimeter above the spines is termed minus and below the spines is termed plus. Therefore, a presenting part 2 cm below the spines is referred to as 2 station.
   d. Every attempt to evaluate the position of the presenting part should also be made. The landmark in a vertex presentation is the occiput, which is identified by the junction of the lamboidal and sagittal

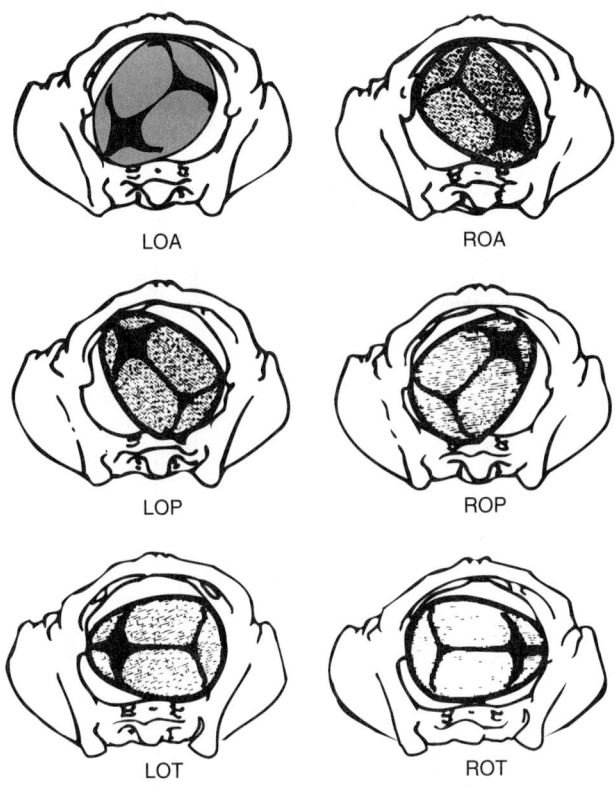

Figure 18-4 Fetal positions in the bony pelvis. *LOA,* Left occiput anterior; *LOP,* left occiput posterior; *LOT,* left occiput transverse; *ROA,* right occiput anterior; *ROP,* right occiput posterior; *ROT,* right occiput transverse. (From Pernoll ML, Benson RC: *Current obstetrics and gynecologic diagnosis and treatment,* ed 6, Norwalk, CT, 1987, Appleton & Lange.)

sutures. The term used for the position is the relationship between the occiput and the pelvis (Fig. 18-4).

LABOR

Labor has traditionally been divided into three stages. The first stage is recognized from the onset of labor until complete cervical dilation. The second stage is defined from complete dilation until the delivery of the infant. The interval from delivery of the infant until the delivery of the placenta is known as the third stage. Some have attempted to add a fourth stage, defined as the first hour following the delivery of the placenta, which carries an increased risk of hemorrhage (Fig. 18-5).

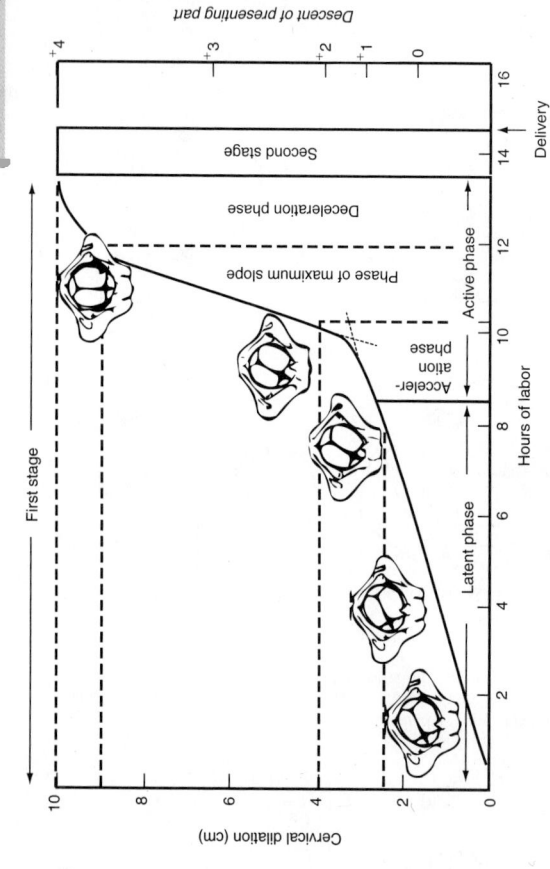

Figure 18-5 Normal labor curve and the fetal position. (From Niswander KR: *Manual of obstetrics: diagnosis and therapy*, ed 3, Boston, 1987, Little, Brown.)

1. Mechanism of labor.
   a. During labor, the fetus undergoes certain movements to maneuver through the pelvis. These movements are known as the seven cardinal movements of labor. They consist of engagement, flexion, descent, internal rotation, extension, external rotation, and expulsion. These movements apply to both vertex and breech presentations. These movements allow the fetus to pass through the pelvis with the least resistance.
   b. Engagement occurs early in labor or before labor. The presenting part reaches the level of the ischial spines. The most common position is occiput anterior. As engagement occurs, the head often rotates transversely. However, the position is usually dictated by the size of the pelvic inlet.
   c. Flexion allows the smallest diameter of the head to pass through the pelvis. Once again, this is dependent on the shape of the pelvis. A platypelloid pelvis may cause some deflexion in some cases and result in a brow or face presentation.
   d. Fetal descent progresses constantly. It is dependent on the uterine contractions and the size of the fetus. The position of the presenting part also plays a role.
   e. As descent takes place, the presenting part undergoes internal rotation. The fetal head rotates from a transverse position to an anterior or posterior position so as to maneuver through the ischial spines. The rotation is complete by the time the head reaches the perineum.
   f. At the level of the perineum, a combination of uterine contractions and maternal expulsive efforts assist in extension. The extension of the fetal head also allows it to maneuver under the pubic symphysis.
   g. The external rotation occurs after the head is delivered. The rotation restores the fetal head to the initial position it occupied when it became engaged.
   h. The complete expulsion of the infant occurs with the delivery of the shoulders and the rest of the body.
2. First stage.
   a. The first stage of labor is composed of two phases. The latent phase is the period of gradual cervical effacement and dilation. This period begins with the onset of labor and ends when cervical dilation is approximately 4 to 5 cm. The active phase begins at the conclusion of the latent phase and ends with complete cervical dilation. This period is recognized by rapid cervical dilation. Nulliparous women should dilate at least 1.2 cm/hour and multiparous women at least 1.5 cm/hour during the active phase. The average duration of the entire first stage in nulliparous women is 8 hours; in multiparous women it averages 5 hours (see Fig. 18-5).
   b. Analgesia is offered to a woman once labor has started and her level of pain has risen. The goal should be to allow her to participate as fully as possible in the labor process without compromising the fetus. Most women have been encouraged to take prenatal classes emphasizing the Lamaze method or another psychoprophylaxis method to alleviate stress and anxiety during labor.

c. Other methods, such as narcotics and regional anesthetics, are available. Some of the most common narcotics used, such as butorphanol or meperidine, are parenterally administered and have little effect on the progress of labor in the active phase. They generally are best avoided in the latent phase because of their effect of prolonging it. The most common regional block used is an epidural anesthesia. Similar to narcotic analgesics, epidurals are best used in the active phase of labor. Prolongation of the second stage and an increase in operative deliveries have been reported with the use of epidural anesthetics.

3. Second stage.
   a. The second stage is defined as the period between complete cervical dilation and delivery of the infant. Maternal expulsive efforts are usually spontaneous during this stage if no regional anesthetic is used. These expulsive efforts and the uterine contractions drive the presenting part to the pelvic floor. Delivery is anticipated as the perineum begins to distend.
   b. Delivery is generally performed with a woman in a lithotomy position, although in some European countries a left lateral position (Sims) is preferred for delivery. The goal is to control the delivery of the infant to avoid excessive force or a rapid release of pressure on the fetal head. A modified Ritgen maneuver is often used for control. A gloved hand covered with a towel is used to apply pressure on the fetal chin upward, and the other hand is used to control the extension of the fetal head superiorly.
   c. An episiotomy is performed to avoid any lacerations of the perineum and to provide an adequate space to minimize any soft tissue dystocia.
   d. As the head is delivered, external rotation follows. The rotation is often assisted and gentle traction is exerted downward to aid the progress of the anterior shoulder under the symphysis. It is imperative to avoid excessive traction on the head and neck to avoid a brachial plexus injury. The head is then lifted upward to deliver the posterior shoulder.
   e. After the shoulders, the rest of the infant is delivered by gentle traction.

4. Third stage.
   a. The period between the delivery of the infant and the delivery of the placenta is termed the third stage of labor. The placenta separates within 5 minutes following the delivery of the infant. This process is often assisted by administering oxytocin to the intravenous (IV) fluid. The separation of the placenta is believed to occur by the rapid reduction of the uterine size resulting in "buckling" of the placental surface area and forming a retroplacental bleed. This bleed eventually propagates and shears off the remaining surface of the placenta.
   b. Spontaneous separation of the placenta can be determined by certain signs. Three commonly noted signs are a change in the shape of the uterus, a flow of blood, and a relative lengthening of the

umbilical cord. A fourth sign often noted is a release of the tension on the umbilical vessels when gently compressed.
  c. Caution should be applied when traction is applied to the umbilical cord to deliver the placenta. Brandt-Andrews maneuver is a technique used to minimize any risk of a uterine inversion. With one hand placed on the abdomen, the uterus is gently massaged near the fundus; the other hand applies gentle traction to the umbilical cord once separation has started. As the placenta is delivered, the abdominal hand is lowered to the suprapubic area to identify any signs of a uterine inversion. A Credé maneuver has been described that uses the abdominal hand to massage the uterus and uses the fundus as a piston to drive the placenta out of the uterine cavity. This maneuver carries great risk for uterine hemorrhage and inversion. There is no role for this maneuver in modern obstetrics.
  d. Manual removal of the placenta may be indicated if the placenta has not separated after 20 minutes or if there is excessive vaginal bleeding. After adequate anesthesia is given, one hand is introduced into the uterine cavity and the other hand is placed on the uterine fundus. The intrauterine hand cleaves off the placenta from the uterine wall in a circumferential pattern. The uterus is then aggressively massaged to minimize any excessive bleeding.
  e. The placenta should always be examined to determine whether the entire placenta has been delivered. Missing cotyledons may suggest retention in the uterine cavity. The inspection should also note any placental pathology. Three vessels of the umbilical cord should be confirmed. Any evidence of succenturiate lobes or of circumvallate or marginal insertion of the umbilical cord should be documented.
5. Fourth stage: This stage has been recognized as the first hour following the delivery of the placenta. It appears to be a critical period for postpartum hemorrhage. The use of oxytocin and uterine massage will minimize any significant bleeding. The perineal region needs to be frequently noted for any signs of excessive bleeding.

EPISIOTOMY/LACERATIONS

Episiotomy is a surgical incision of the perineum performed during a delivery to provide sufficient area for the delivery of the infant and minimize or avoid lacerations of the perineum and rectum.

1. Types.
   a. Lacerations of the perineum have been classified as first, second, third, and fourth degree.
      (1) **A first-degree laceration** involves a tear of the vaginal mucosa but spares any underlying muscle and tissue.
      (2) **A second-degree laceration** is when the tear extends through the muscle and fascia.
      (3) **A third-degree laceration** is when the tear involves the rectal sphincter.
      (4) **A fourth-degree laceration** encompasses the entire thickness of the perineal body and into the rectal mucosa.
   b. Episiotomies are classified as either midline or mediolateral.

(1) Midline episiotomies are incisions directed downward from the middle of the fourchet, including the vaginal mucosa and the underlying fascia and muscle.
(2) A mediolateral episiotomy begins at the same point but is directed laterally to avoid the rectum.
   (a) Mediolateral episiotomies have the advantage of rarely extending, and damage to the rectal mucosa is avoided.
   (b) The disadvantage is an increase in blood loss and greater postpartum pain.

OXYTOCICS

The three commonly used oxytocics in modern obstetrics are oxytocin, methylergonovine maleate, and prostaglandin F2-alpha. They are used primarily in the third stage of labor to reduce blood loss and stimulate uterine contractions.

1. **Oxytocin**
   a. Oxytocin is an octapeptide commonly used to stimulate uterine contractions. It is often used for induction and augmentation of labor. Intravenously, its half-life is approximately 3 to 5 minutes.
   b. Administration is usually carried out using controlled infusion pumps, and the dose is diluted to avoid any side effects.
   c. The most common side effects are significant hypotension if given as a large IV bolus, or antidiuresis if given as a continuous infusion of greater than 20 mU/min.
2. **Methylergonovine**
   a. Methylergonovine is a synthetic alkaloid created from lysergic acid. It is a very potent uterotonic substance. Its use is primarily confined to the third stage of labor.
   b. Caution should be used because of its ability to cause vasoconstriction, resulting in hypertension.
   c. Its administration is confined to intramuscular (IM) dosing. IV administration is contraindicated.
3. **Prostaglandin F2**
   a. A 15-methyl derivative of prostaglandin F2 has been noted to be a potent oxytocic agent. Its use is limited for the control of postpartum hemorrhage.
   b. It is administered IM or directly into the myometrium.
   c. Some side effects reported have involved hypertension, diarrhea, vomiting, and fever.

18.2 Abnormal Labor

Abnormalities of labor are generally described as dystocia. Since 1980, the incidence of cesarean births has increased significantly in the United States. One of the major indications for cesarean births has been dystocia. The exact incidence has been difficult to ascertain because the definition has been vague and generalized. Frequently, generic terms such as cephalopelvic disproportion or failure to progress have been used to describe various dystocias. Every effort should be made to characterize the dystocia encountered precisely so that the correct diagnosis is made.

Dystocias can be classified into three categories. The categories are a result of problems with uterine contractions, the size of the maternal pelvis, or the size of the fetus. These have been referred to as abnormalities of the power, the passenger, and the passage.

1. **Power.**
    a. Normal uterine contractions during labor complete their purpose by developing a rhythmic pattern beginning in the fundus near a cornual end. The average resting tone is approximately 10 to 15 mm Hg. During the active phase of labor, contractions reach 40 to 60 mm Hg. One of the most common quantitative measurements developed to assess uterine contractions has been the Montevideo unit. The Montevideo unit is calculated by multiplying the average intensity of contractions by the number of contractions in a 10-minute window. Adequate contractions are recognized as more than 180 Montevideo units. Intrauterine pressure catheters are pivotal in evaluating the adequacy of uterine contractions.
    b. Abnormalities of the power are usually classified into protraction disorders, arrest disorders, or a prolonged latent phase. Understanding the definition of each assists in the proper diagnosis.
        (1) Prolonged latent phase
            (a) A prolonged latent phase is defined as a latent phase exceeding 20 hours in nulliparous women and 14 hours in multiparous women. The most common etiology is heavy sedation or early analgesia. False labor can be another common etiology.
            (b) Treatment is usually accomplished by sedating the patient with meperidine, butorphanol, or morphine. Oxytocin augmentation can be used to organize the frequency of the contraction pattern.
        (2) Protraction disorders
            (a) Protraction disorders can be a protraction either of cervical dilation or of fetal descent. In nulliparous patients, cervical dilation in the active phase should be at least 1.2 cm/hour (1.5 cm/hour in multiparous women). Fetal descent should also be 1 cm/hour for multiparous women and 2 cm/hour in multigravidas.
            (b) Common causes of protraction disorders are fetopelvic discrepancy from either size or fetal presentation abnormalities. Factors such as macrosomia, occiput transverse, brow presentation, or narrow inlet should be investigated. Heavy sedation or anesthesia may play a role in multigravidas.
            (c) Attempts should be made to determine the cause of the protraction. Macrosomic infants or fetal malpresentation may require a cesarean section. An intrauterine catheter should be inserted and the contractions quantified. Augmentation is attempted with oxytocin for hypotonic dysfunction.

(3) Arrest disorders
    (a) The most common arrest disorder recognized is an arrest of dilation. This is defined as failure to dilate in the active phase for 2 hours or more. It is found in approximately 5% of nulliparous labor. An arrest of descent is defined as failure to descend for 1 hour or more.
    (b) The most common causes of arrest disorders are fetopelvic discrepancy. Many are as a result of positional abnormalities such as occiput transverse or occiput posterior. Uterine dystocia also accounts for a large percentage of arrest disorders. Fetal macrosomia or pelvic contractions account for many of the abnormalities encountered with arrest of descent.
    (c) Intrauterine catheters should be placed in these cases to identify any evidence of uterine inertia. Oxytocin augmentation may be required. Careful pelvic examination may be required to assess the fetal position and sonography may be indicated to evaluate the estimated fetal weight.

2. **Passenger:** Dystocia from the fetus is usually caused by a large infant, malposition of the presenting part, or a malpresentation. Treatment for many of these disorders is often an operative delivery by a cesarean section or forceps.
   a. Macrosomia
      (1) Fetal macrosomia occurs in approximately 5% of infants and is defined as a fetal weight in excess of 4000 g. A fetal weight over 4500 g has been used by others for the definition. Several risk factors for macrosomia have been encountered. Women with previous macrosomic infants, diabetic women, obese women, women with postdate pregnancies, and those with a prolonged second stage are at increased risk. Unfortunately, clinical estimates of fetal weight have been poor. Sonographic evaluation has not provided sufficient sensitivity.
      (2) Macrosomic infants have a fivefold increased risk of perinatal mortality. Shoulder dystocia occurs in approximately 8% to 10% of infants weighing over 4500 g. A thorough review of the maneuvers performed in the event of a shoulder dystocia should be performed when a labor abnormality occurs.
   b. Malpresentation: Approximately 5% of all labors at term are complicated by malpresentations. These are abnormalities related to the fetal position, or presentation. Malpresentations are the most common cause of fetal dystocia.
      (1) Breech
         (a) A breech is an abnormal fetal lie in which the head of the infant lies in the uterine fundus. Breeches are described as frank, complete, or footling, based on the position of the fetal hips and knees (Fig. 18-6). A frank breech is a fetus that is lying with flexed hips and extended knees. If both the knees and the hips are flexed, it is referred to as a complete breech. When one or both hips are extended,

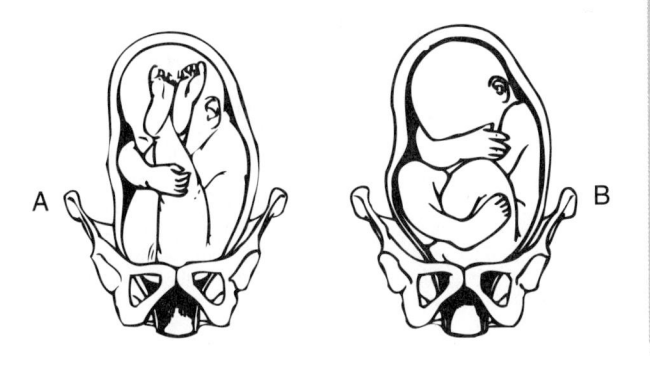

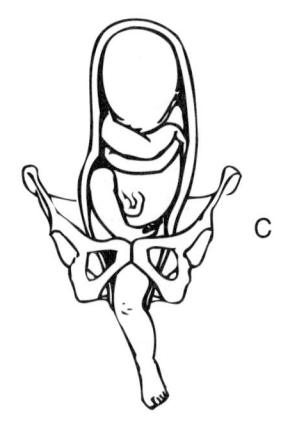

Practical Guide to the Care of the Gynecologic/Obstetric Patient 343

Figure 18-6 Breech presentations: **A,** Frank. **B,** Complete. **C,** Footling. (From Pernoll ML, Benson RC: *Current obstetrics and gynecologic diagnosis and treatment*, ed 6, Norwalk, CT, 1987, Appleton & Lange.)

a footling breech is identified. The infants may be designated as single or double footling breeches.
(b) The incidence of breech infants is dependent on the gestational age. Pregnancies less than 28 weeks have an incidence of approximately 25%. This decreases to 7% to 9% by 32 weeks. At term, the incidence of all breeches is 3% to 4%.
(c) Breech presentations have been associated with fetal and uterine anomalies. A careful sonographic evaluation is warranted in persistent breech infants to rule out any anomalies. The perinatal mortality rate of breech presentations

varies from 9% to 25%. However, controversy exists because many breeches have anomalies and are premature. The corrected estimates of perinatal mortality at term may not be different from those of infants presenting as vertex.
- (d) The mode of delivery remains controversial. A cesarean section should be considered for any breech between 800 and 1500 g. The optimal mode of delivery between 1500 and 2500 g has not clearly been established. A trial of labor may be considered with a breech presentation between 2500 and 3800 g. Box 18-1 demonstrates prerequisites needed for the management of a trial of labor.

(2) Occiput posterior
- (a) An occiput posterior occurs when the vertex fails to rotate once it has reached the pelvic floor. Dystocia occurs because of partial deflexion of the fetal head. It is often a result of a contracted pelvis, an anthropoid pelvis, or poor uterine contractions.
- (b) The diagnosis can be made on pelvic examination as the anterior fontanel is palpated on the anterior aspect of the pelvis. Confirmation may be made by palpating the orientation of the fetal ear.
- (c) Management may involve oxytocin augmentation if the contractions are inadequate. A vaginal delivery of a posterior occiput may be considered if fetal descent progresses. In skilled hands and with no evidence of fetal macrosomia, midforceps rotation and extraction may be considered. A cesarean section may be necessary if the vertex fails to descend and a rotation is not possible.

(3) Occiput transverse
- (a) The occiput transverse is considered to be a transient position. As labor progresses, the occiput rotates to either an anterior or a posterior position. The etiology may be a platypelloid pelvis or inadequate contractions. A deep transverse arrest occurs when the vertex has failed to negotiate the inlet.

BOX 18-1 Prerequisites for a Vaginal Delivery of a Breech

Estimated fetal weight between 2500 and 3800 g
  Frank breech
  Adequate x-ray pelvimetry
  Flexed head
  Continuous fetal monitoring
  Normal progress of labor
Experienced clinician

(b) The diagnosis is made on the pelvic examination. The axis of the sagittal suture is used for orientation.
(c) A cesarean section is indicated in infants with deep transverse arrest. In other cases of a transverse arrest, evaluation of the contractions may be warranted and, if adequate, patience may be necessary.

(4) Brow presentation
 (a) Brow presentations are also recognized as transient positions. They occur in approximately 0.06% of deliveries. Pelvic contractures, prematurity, and grand multiparity are associated with this position.
 (b) The diagnosis is made on pelvic or speculum examination.
 (c) Management is usually expectant. Spontaneous rotation occurs in most of the cases. Inadequate uterine contractions may be encountered in cases with a contracted pelvis.

(5) Face presentation
 (a) Face presentations are noted in approximately 0.2% of deliveries. In this position, the fetal head is deflexed from its longitudinal axis. The most common causes are fetal anomalies, prematurity, grand multiparity, and a contracted pelvis.
 (b) The diagnosis is often made on pelvic examination. The palpation of the fetal mouth, orbit, or malar prominence can often shock an examiner. The diagnosis of either a breech or umbilical cord can sometimes be made.
 (c) Management depends on the location of the mentum. Mentum posterior presentations are unable to extend any further and require a cesarean section. Infants with mentum anterior may be able to negotiate the pelvis; however, the presenting submentobregmatic diameter may be too large and dystocia may occur. No attempts should be made to flex the fetal head or manually rotate a mentum posterior.

(6) Shoulder dystocia
 (a) A shoulder dystocia is defined as when the anterior shoulder of the infant fails to maneuver the pubic symphysis after the head is delivered. The incidence is approximately 0.15%. The incidence rises to approximately 2% in infants over 4000 g.
 (b) The most common cause of a shoulder dystocia is maternal obesity, diabetes, fetal macrosomia, and a previous history of a shoulder dystocia.
 (c) Management should always be reviewed before any delivery, and the clinician should remain calm and proceed in a systematic fashion. Once the diagnosis is made, attention should be placed on the perineum, and a large episiotomy is made to ensure adequate space. An assistant and an anesthesiologist should be notified immediately. Suprapubic pressure is applied downward along with gentle traction downward on the fetal head. Fundal pressure should be

avoided because this can wedge the shoulder under the symphysis and also the risk of a uterine rupture is increased.
- (d) A McRoberts maneuver is next attempted if suprapubic pressure fails. The woman's legs are flexed extensively toward her abdomen and chest. This may rotate the symphysis cephalad and straighten the sacrum, allowing the anterior shoulder to be freed.
- (e) A Wood's screw maneuver may be tried after the McRoberts maneuver. In this procedure, the clinician places two fingers on the anterior aspect of the posterior shoulder and rotates the shoulder anteriorly and in an oblique position. This allows the posterior shoulder to be delivered and the anterior shoulder, which is now in the posterior space of the pelvis, is delivered.
- (f) Delivery of the posterior arm may also be performed by inserting a hand into the hollow of the sacrum and sweeping the posterior arm across the chest and out of the vagina. This often leads to clavicular or humeral fractures.
- (g) Birth asphyxia, clavicular or humeral fractures, and Erb's palsy may occur in up to 50% of cases of shoulder dystocia.

3. **Passage.**
   a. Dystocia from the passage should be considered in every woman with protraction or arrest disorders in labor. X-ray pelvimetry was used extensively to examine for any evidence of pelvic contractures. However, clinical pelvimetry has replaced x-ray pelvimetry in modern obstetrics. There is still some limited use for x-ray pelvimetry, particularly in cases of breech presentations.
   b. The contractions of the pelvis are defined by the location of the abnormality. They are described as either inlet, midpelvis, or outlet contractions.
      (1) Inlet dystocia
         (a) An inlet contraction is often suspected if the diagonal conjugate diameter is less than 12.5 cm. Other clinical indications may be a floating vertex failure of descent or deep transverse arrest.
         (b) Considerable molding is evident in these infants because of the prolonged use of oxytocin and the failure of fetal descent.
         (c) A caput succedaneum can often be misleading and the clinician may determine that descent is occurring.
         (d) Treatment is often a cesarean section.
      (2) Midpelvic–outlet dystocia
         (a) Contractions of the midpelvis and the outlet are very commonly indistinguishable. The diagnosis is often made on pelvic examination because the sidewalls are convergent, the ischial spines are prominent, and the pubic arch is 90 degrees or less.
         (b) The diagnosis is often confirmed by a prolonged second stage, a persistent occiput posterior, or a deep transverse arrest. A caput is often found on the fetus.

(c) As a result of the contracted pelvis, rotation and extension are often difficult. Careful applications of forceps may be attempted if the vertex has managed to descend to the pelvis floor. A cesarean section is often indicated in those infants who have failed to descend appropriately.
4. **Operative delivery:** An operative delivery is defined as any delivery requiring an active maneuver. The three most common methods are with forceps, by vacuum, or by a cesarean section.
   a. Forceps
      (1) The obstetric forceps is composed of two matched instruments. Each instrument consists of a blade, a shank, a lock, and a handle. The cephalic curve is the area of the blade that is applied to the infant's head. The area of the blade placed on the mother's pelvis is known as the pelvic curve. There is a left and a right blade on all forceps, which correspond to the left and right side of the mother's pelvis when placed.
      (2) There are a variety of classic and modern or special forceps available.
   b. Cesarean section
      (1) Cesarean section is a surgical incision through the abdominal wall and the uterus, performed to deliver a fetus. Its use has increased significantly over the past several years, and numerous attempts are underway to reduce the cesarean births in the United States. Most hospitals report a 10% to 35% cesarean birth rate.
      (2) Cesareans are classified as either classical or low cervical.
         (a) Classical cesarean section refers to a delivery of an infant through a vertical incision on the corpus of the uterus. It is associated with increased blood loss and an increased risk of uterine rupture in a subsequent pregnancy.
         (b) Low cervical cesarean sections apply to transverse incisions (Kerr incision) performed in the lower, noncontractile portion of the uterus.
      (3) Major risks during cesarean sections are infection, anesthetic complications, and hemorrhage. The mortality rate for cesarean section is approximately 5.8 per 100,000 live births.

18.3 Analgesia and Anesthetics in Obstetrics

CHARACTERISTICS OF LABOR PAIN
1. Severe, exceeded only by the following:
   a. Causalgia
   b. Traumatic amputation
   c. Terminal cancer pain
2. Labor pain is physiologic.
3. Variable in onset and severity. Not all parturients experience pain; however, 35% to 77% of parturients characterize their pain as severe or intolerable. Factors associated with increased severity are as follows:
   a. Nulliparity

b. Occiput posterior position
   c. History of severe dysmenorrhea
   d. Young maternal age
   e. Increased maternal and/or fetal weight
   f. Absence of supportive companion
   g. Unrealistic expectations
   h. Maternal fear and anxiety
4. Predictive: Early onset and increased severity may indicate dysfunctional labor and malpresentation of the fetus, resulting in a higher likelihood of operative or instrumented delivery.
5. Retrospectively devalued: Postpartum recall will minimize the intensity of the pain experienced.
6. Labor pain is treatable.

HARMFUL PHYSIOLOGIC EFFECTS OF LABOR PAIN

The pain is generally well tolerated by most parturients; however, for parturients with compromised cardiopulmonary function, the provision of adequate laboring analgesia can be life saving.

1. Cardiovascular
   a. Increased heart rate
   b. Increased stroke volume
   c. Increased systemic vascular resistance
   d. Increased cardiac output
   e. Increased myocardial workload and oxygen (O_2) requirements
2. Pulmonary (hyperventilation or hypoventilation syndrome)
   a. Maternal hyperventilation during contractions
      (1) Hypocarbia
      (2) Alkalemia
      (3) Deleterious leftward shift of the oxyhemoglobin dissociation curve
   b. Maternal hypoventilation between contractions
      (1) Maternal hypoxemia
      (2) Less O_2 available to the uteroplacental circulation
3. Metabolic
   a. Increased systemic O_2 consumption
   b. Decreased O_2 available to the uteroplacental circulation
4. Increased levels of circulating catecholamines
   a. Uterine artery vasoconstriction
   b. Decreased uteroplacental blood flow
5. Decreased uterine activity and delayed progress of labor
6. Increased maternal anxiety and fear

ANALGESIC OR ANESTHETIC INTERVENTIONS
(Table 18-1)

1. Psychoprophylactic or nonpharmacologic techniques
2. Systemic intravenous agents
   a. Intermittent bolus dosing
   b. Patient-controlled (demand) dosing
3. Inhalation analgesia

Table 18-1 A Comparison of Analgesic Techniques

Psychoprophylactic Nonpharmacologic Techniques	Systemic Intravenous Analgesia	Neuraxial Anesthesia (Epidural or Spinal)
May require specialized equipment, supportive partner, or attendance at prenatal classes	Technically easy to administer	Requires specialized equipment and personnel
Progressively ineffective, poor late first-stage efficacy, poor second-stage efficacy	Incomplete analgesia, improves tolerability of labor, poor second-stage efficacy	Superior laboring analgesia; offers excellent first-stage and second-stage analgesia
Maternal safety unquestioned	Maternal side effects	Procedural risks incurred
Avoids systemic medications, fetal or neonatal effects	Fetal or neonatal effects of systemically administered agents possible	Systemic absorption minimal; fetal or neonatal effects are rare
Has no effect on harmful physiologic effects of labor pain	Blunts the harmful physiologic changes of labor pain	Largely ablates the harmful physiologic changes of labor pain
Operative anesthesia absent	Operative anesthesia absent	Operative anesthesia capability readily inherent in continuous techniques

4. Neuraxial anesthesia
    a. Continuous techniques
        (1) Continuous lumbar epidural
        (2) Continuous subarachnoid catheter
        (3) Continuous caudal epidural
    b. Single-injection techniques
        (1) "Saddle" block
        (2) "Modified saddle" block
        (3) Spinal anesthesia
        (4) Intrathecal opioids
    c. Combined spinal and epidural
5. Paracervical block
6. Lumbar sympathetic block
7. Bilateral pudendal nerve blocks with or without local infiltration

PSYCHOPROPHYLACTIC OR NONPHARMACOLOGIC TECHNIQUES

1. Techniques are as follows:
   a. Lamaze and other childbirth preparatory classes
   b. Emotional support
   c. Massage or touch therapy
   d. Hydrotherapy
   e. Biofeedback and self-hypnosis
   f. Acupuncture
   g. Transcutaneous electrical nerve stimulation (TENS)
2. Purported advantages are hotly debated.
   a. Purported advantages not consistently demonstrated
      (1) Decreased use of systemic analgesics
      (2) Decreased use of regional anesthesia
      (3) Shorter labor
      (4) Decreased incidence of instrumented vaginal delivery
      (5) Decreased incidence of operative delivery
      (6) Decreased incidence of fetal distress
   b. Advantages
      (1) Increased maternal control or cooperation
      (2) Reduced maternal anxiety
      (3) Reduced perception of pain
3. Risks and disadvantages are as follows:
   a. Attendance at prenatal classes may be required.
   b. Presence of supportive partner may be required.
   c. Instructor bias may lead women to believe they have "failed" if they require additional analgesic techniques.
4. No psychoprophylactic or nonpharmacologic technique consistently provides the quality of relief provided by neuraxial analgesia.

SYSTEMIC INTRAVENOUS ANALGESICS

1. Opioids.
   a. Opioids are equally effective at equianalgesic doses; choice is largely a matter of provider preference.
   b. Adverse maternal effects occur with equal frequency or severity at equianalgesic doses.
   c. Morphine's longer duration of action and the heightened sensitivity of the neonate to its respiratory depressant effect limit its use in labor.
   d. Fentanyl's short duration of action and accumulative effect (loss of short duration of action with repeated dosing) limits its use in labor.
2. Opioid agonist or antagonists.
   a. Possess respiratory depressant "ceiling effect" (i.e., beyond a certain "ceiling" dose, increased effect no longer occurs)
   b. Possess analgesic ceiling effect
   c. Increased incidence of dysphoria relative to the opioids
3. Ketamine.
   a. Amnesia and short duration of action limit use for first-stage analgesia.

- b. Intense analgesia useful for the following:
    - (1) Painful vaginal delivery
    - (2) Instrumented vaginal delivery in the absence of regional anesthesia
    - (3) Adjunctive therapy when regional anesthesia is inadequate
- c. Neonatal depression, abnormal muscle tone, and low Apgar score occur at maternal doses greater than 1.5 to 2 mg/kg.
4. Ketorolac: The efficacy and safety of ketorolac for laboring analgesia is unproven.
5. Dosing (Table 18-2).
6. Intravenous analgesia, patient-controlled (demand) dosing (PCA).
    - a. To date none of the purported benefits (with the exception of higher patient satisfaction) have been consistently demonstrated in the obstetric population.
    - b. Purported benefits and advantages are as follows:
        - (1) Superior analgesia compared with intermittent dosing
        - (2) Decreased total drug requirements, resulting in decreased placental transfer and fetal or neonatal accumulation
        - (3) Decreased incidence of untoward side effects, particularly respiratory depression and nausea or vomiting
        - (4) Higher patient satisfaction
    - c. Risks and disadvantages are those of the agent chosen.

SYSTEMIC INTRAVENOUS ADJUVANTS

1. Commonly used adjuvant agents include the following:
    - a. Antihistamines (diphenhydramine, hydroxyzine)
    - b. Barbiturates (pentobarbital, secobarbital)
    - c. Benzodiazepines (diazepam, lorazepam, midazolam)
    - d. Narcotic antagonists (naloxone)
    - e. Phenothiazine derivatives (promethazine, propriomazine)
2. Indications
    - a. Treatment of untoward effects of systemic analgesics
        - (1) Opioid overdose (naloxone)
        - (2) Opioid-induced pruritus (diphenhydramine, naloxone, opioid agonist or antagonists)
        - (3) Nausea or vomiting (promethazine, propriomazine)
        - (4) Local anesthetic induced central nervous system (CNS) excitability (diazepam, lorazepam)
    - b. Sedation anxiolysis (pentobarbital, secobarbital, diazepam, lorazepam, midazolam)
    - c. Amnesia, generally an undesired effect (diazepam, lorazepam, midazolam)
    - d. Analgesic adjuvant (hydroxyzine)
3. Dosing (Table 18-3)

INHALATION ANALGESIA

1. Definition: Inhalational analgesia is the administration of subanesthetic doses of inhalational agents to provide analgesia.

Table 18-2 Systemic Analgesics

Drug	Dose	Onset	Duration
Fentenyl	IV: 25-50 µg	2-3 min	30-60 min
	IM: 50-100 µg	7-10 min	1-2 hr
Meperidine	IV: 25-50 mg	5-10 min	2-3 hr
	IM: 50-100 mg	40-50 min	3-4 hr
Morphine	IV: 2-5 mg	5-10 min	3-4 hr
	IM: 5-10 mg	20-40 min	4-6 hr
Butorphanol	IV: 1-2 mg	5-10 min	3-4 hr
	IM: 1-2 mg	5-10 min	3-4 hr
Nalbuphine	IV: 10-20 mg	2-3 min	3-4 hr
	IM: 10-20 mg	10-15 min	4-6 hr
Pentazocine	IV: 10-20 mg	2-3 min	2-3 hr
	IM: 20-40 mg	10-20 min	3-4 hr
Ketamine	IV: 10-20 mg	30-60 sec	2-5 min

IM, Intramuscular; *IV*, intravenous; *PO*, by mouth.

2. This is largely impractical for first-stage analgesia because of the following:
    a. Episodic crescendo—decrescendo pattern of labor pain
    b. Need for specialized vaporizers
    c. Environmental pollution by agent

Table 18-3 Adjuvant Agents

Drug	Dose
Dephenhydramine, antihistamine	IV: 12.5-25 ng
	IM: 25-50 mg
Hydroxyzine, antihistamine	IM: 25-50 mg
Pentobarbital, barbiturate	PO: 100-200 mg
	IM: 100-200 mg
Secobarbital, barbiturate	PO: 100 mg
	IM: 100 mg
Diazepam, benzodiazepine	IV: 2.5-5 mg
	IM: 5-10 mg
Lorazepam, benzodiazepine	IV: 1-2 mg
	IM: 2-5 mg
Midazolam, benzodiazepine	IV: 1-5 mg
	IM: 1-5 mg
Naloxone, opioid antagonist	IV bolus: 40-400 µg (in 40 µg increments)
	IV infusion: 5-10 µg/kg/min
	IM: 400 µg
Promethazine, phenothiazine	IV: 12.5-25 mg
	IM: 25-50 mg
Propriomazine, phenothiazine	IV: 10-20 mg
	IM: 20-40 mg

IM, Intramuscular; *IV*, intravenous; *PO*, by mouth.

    d. Undesirable maternal amnesia
    e. Potential for maternal overdose
3. Indications
    a. Painful vaginal delivery.
    b. Instrumented vaginal delivery in the absence of regional anesthesia.
    c. Adjunctive therapy when regional anesthesia is inadequate.
    d. Many prefer low doses of ketamine (0.10 to 0.25 mg/kg) titrated to lessen the risks of inhalational analgesia.
    e. Major risk of this technique is accidental maternal overdose with loss of protective airway reflexes and increased risk for maternal aspiration.

NEURAXIAL ANESTHESIA

Anatomy (Internal to External)

1. Spinal cord, terminating at L1 level (continues as the cauda equina)
2. Pia mater
3. Subarachnoid space containing the cerebrospinal fluid (CSF) and transversed by the spinal nerves as they exit or enter the spinal cord
4. Arachnoid membrane
5. Dura mater, a tough fibrous sheath tethered at the S2 level
6. Epidural space, transversed by the spinal nerves, and bounded by the following:
    a. Vertebral bodies and intervertebral discs anteriorly
    b. Vertebral pedicles laterally
    c. Vertebral laminae and spinous processes posteriorly
    d. Ligamentum flavum, connecting the anterior aspects of laminae and spinous processes, thus forming the posterior border of the epidural space in the interspinous space

Mechanism of Action

1. Epidural versus spinal (Table 18-4)
2. Epidural
    a. Local anesthetic diffuses through the dural sheath to exert its influence on the nerve roots as they exit the central neuraxis.
    b. Opioids diffuse through the dural membrane to enter the CSF and exert antinociceptive actions via interaction with spinal cord and higher CNS opioid receptors.
3. Subarachnoid
    a. Local anesthetic is directly injected into CSF to exert influence on spinal cord neural transmission.
    b. Opioids are directly injected into the CSF to exert antinociceptive actions via interaction with spinal cord and higher central nervous system opioid receptors.

Absolute Contraindications

1. Patient refusal
2. Localized infection at skin puncture site

Table 18-4 A Comparison of Neuraxial Techniques

Characteristic	Subarachnoid Administration (Single Injection)	Epidural Administration (Continuous)
Ease of administration	Technically easy	Technically more difficult than subarachnoid
Efficacy	Failure rate under 1%	Operative failure rate 2% to 4%
Onset	Rapid	Slower onset
Segmental level	Dependent on characteristics of technique	Segmental level titratable
Motor block	Dense	Dependent on local anesthetic concentration
Dose required	Less than epidural	Greater dosing requirement
Systemic absorption	Negligible to nonexistent	Does occur, but maternal, fetal, and neonatal effects are rare
Use a laboring analgesic	Dense motor block limits use as laboring analgesic	Superior laboring analgesic
Operative anesthetic	Operative anesthesia available with initial or repeat injection	Operative anesthetic capability present throughout labor

3. Septicemia
4. Coagulopathy
5. Increased intracranial pressure

Continuous Techniques

1. Continuous lumbar epidural (CLE)
    a. Analgesia
        (1) First stage: excellent
        (2) Second stage: variable; may require a "sitting" dose or a segmental level to T6 or greater to provide adequate sacral coverage or perineal anesthesia
        (3) Operative: capability present throughout duration of catheterization
    b. Technically easier to place than caudal epidural
    c. Motor block: can be minimized by using dilute local anesthetic
    d. Disadvantages: none, relative to other continuous techniques; surpassed only by combined spinal and epidural technique in its usefulness
    e. Dosing

(1) Local anesthetic only (intermittent dosing or continuous infusion)
    (a) Advantage is relatively long history of safety and efficacy.
    (b) Disadvantages are as follows:
        (i) Motor block usually presents at effective doses: decreases maternal satisfaction and may increase the likelihood of operative or instrumented delivery
        (ii) Increased incidences of hypotension
        (iii) Increased risk for local anesthetic toxicity
(2) Continuous infusion of local anesthetic and opioid combination
    (a) Advantages are as follows:
        (i) Decreased concentration (i.e., 0.0625% bupivicaine) of local anesthetic
        (ii) Minimal motor block
        (iii) May provide superior analgesia compared to infusion of local anesthetic only
        (iv) May provide superior second-stage analgesia without increasing the incidence of malrotation or instrumented vaginal delivery
    (b) Disadvantages include the following:
        (i) Maternal respiratory depression (less than with systemic administration)
        (ii) Increased incidence of opioid-induced pruritus
        (iii) Neonatal respiratory depression (less than with systemic administration, but more than with spinal administration)
(3) Continuous infusion of opioid only
    (a) Advantages: avoids local anesthetic effects entirely
    (b) Disadvantages are as follows:
        (i) Required analgesic doses can cause maternal and fetal or neonatal effects comparable to systemic opioids (epidural only; subarachnoid administration results in negligible maternal systemic uptake)
        (ii) Poor second-stage analgesia
        (iii) Not an operative anesthetic
    (c) Usually reserved for parturients with coexisting disease who would not tolerate even the minimal afterload reduction caused by a dilute local solution

2. Caudal epidural anesthesia
   a. Analgesia
      (1) First stage: excellent; requires significantly more infusate
      (2) Second stage: excellent; more effective sacral coverage than lumbar technique
      (3) Operative: capability present throughout duration of catheterization
   b. Advantages: particularly useful for parturients in whom lumbar techniques are technically difficult (e.g., parturients who have had prior back surgery)

c. Disadvantages
      (1) Technically more difficult or painful to place than lumbar epidural
      (2) Motor block: generally greater than lumbar, particularly pelvic floor
      (3) Potential for direct fetal injury with the needle
   d. Dosing: as for lumbar epidural
3. Continuous subarachnoid catheter
   a. Possesses characteristics of epidural or spinal depending on the dosing or infusion agent chosen.
   b. Can be dosed as "spinal" for operative anesthesia.
   c. Risks-and-benefits profile dependent on dosing agent.
   d. Systemic absorption of agents negligible.
   e. Major disadvantages are as follows:
      (1) Potential for unexpected high block
      (2) Potential avenue for infection directly into CNS
   f. Rarely used, but ideally suited for the following:
      (1) Continuous intrathecal opioids in parturients with coexisting disease who would tolerate neither the pain of labor nor regional blockade from local anesthetic (e.g., parturients with stenotic valvular disorders)
      (2) Neuraxial anesthesia when epidural placement is technically difficult or impossible (e.g., status post [s/p] back surgery, morbidly obese parturients)

Single-Injection Techniques

1. Subarachnoid block (SAB, "spinal," "saddle block")
   a. True saddle block (dense motor and sensory block S1-S5)
      (1) Second-stage analgesia.
      (2) Perineal anesthesia.
      (3) Patient must be sitting for placement.
      (4) First-stage analgesia is not provided.
      (5) Dense motor block may increase incidence of malrotation or instrumented vaginal delivery.
   b. Modified saddle block (dense motor and sensory block to T10 level)
      (1) First and second stages of analgesia.
      (2) Perineal anesthesia.
      (3) Dense motor block (to T10 level) limits use of this technique.
   c. Spinal (dense motor and sensory block to T4 level): indicated for operative anesthesia
2. Intrathecal opioids
   a. Opioids provide analgesia for the latent and early active phases of the first stage of labor.
   b. Opioids avoid local anesthetic (local anesthetic during early labor may increase the incidence of operative and instrumented delivery).
   c. Analgesia for the late first stage and second stage of labor are of doubtful effectiveness (intrathecal opioids appear ineffective past 6 to 8 cm of cervical dilation).
   d. Opioids do not provide surgical anesthesia.

e. With the advent of the combined spinal and epidural technique, the use of intrathecal opioids as sole laboring analgesic is rarely, if ever, indicated.
f. Maternal systemic absorption and fetal or neonatal effects are negligible.

Combined Spinal and Epidural

1. Combined spinal and epidural (CSE) possesses all the capabilities and benefits of the intrathecal single-injection techniques and continuous lumbar epidural techniques.
2. CSE is ideally suited for parturients who hurt early in labor. The combination of intrathecal narcotics for latent and early active laboring analgesia and epidural catheter placement for later laboring analgesia avoids local anesthetic or systemic analgesics in early labor and offers these patients their single best opportunity at an uncomplicated vaginal delivery while maintaining all the benefits of an epidural catheter.

GENERAL ANESTHESIA

1. Indications
   a. Dire fetal distress in the absence of preexisting epidural anesthesia
   b. Acute maternal hypovolemia
   c. Any patient for whom regional anesthesia is contraindicated or refused
   d. Inadequate regional anesthesia
   e. Need for uterine relaxation (e.g., difficult breech delivery, retained placenta), failing to respond to IV nitroglycerin
2. Advantages
   a. Rapid induction: allows surgery to begin immediately
   b. Optimal control of airway
   c. Decreased incidence of hypotension in the hypovolemic patient
3. Complications
   a. Maternal death or hypoxic brain injury caused by airway complications.
   b. Maternal aspiration.
   c. Maternal awareness: rare.
   d. Untoward effects of systemically administered agents.
      (1) Medication errors
      (2) Extension of physiologic effect
      (3) Allergic reactions
   e. Fetal or neonatal demise: Rare; perioperative fetal or neonatal demise is generally a result of the underlying condition necessitating operative delivery.
   f. Neonatal depression.
      (1) Preexisting uteroplacental insufficiencies
      (2) Prolonged uterine incision to delivery time
      (3) Systemically administered analgesics during labor
      (4) Rarely caused by placental transfer of general anesthetics unless skin incision to delivery time is prolonged

ANESTHESIA FOR OPERATIVE DELIVERY

1. General anesthesia
   a. Offers most rapid establishment of operating conditions
   b. Rarely contraindicated
2. Epidural anesthesia: establishment of dense motor and sensory block to T4 level
   a. Establishment of dense motor and sensory block to T4 segmental level using local anesthetic with or without opioids added.
   b. Extension with an in situ epidural catheter requires 5 to 10 minutes for operating conditions.
   c. De novo institution can require considerably longer than extension of preexisting epidural blockade.
   d. It is contraindicated in the following:
      (1) Acute maternal hypovolemia
      (2) Uterine rupture
      (3) Cord prolapse with fetal distress
      (4) Agonal fetal distress
3. Spinal anesthesia
   a. Establishment of dense motor and sensory block to T4 segmental level using local anesthetic with or without opioids added.
   b. Technically easy, rapid onset: Operating conditions can generally be established in 5 to 10 minutes.
   c. Technical ease and quicker onset allow de novo institution much more rapidly than epidural blockade.
   d. Contraindications are those of extension of preexisting epidural blockade.
4. Local infiltration
   a. Extremely rare
   b. Use 0.5% lidocaine
   c. Infiltrate
      (1) Intracutaneous (10 mL)
      (2) Subcutaneous (10 to 20 mL)
      (3) Intrarectus (40 to 50 mL)
      (4) Parietal peritoneum (5 to 10 mL)
      (5) Visceral peritoneum (10 mL)
      (6) Paracervical (5 to 10 mL, bilaterally)
   d. Disadvantages
      (1) Maternal distress
      (2) Potential for local anesthetic toxicity
      (3) Prolonged skin incision to delivery time
5. Anesthetic options
   a. Stat
      (1) Indications
         (a) Maternal hemorrhage
         (b) Ruptured uterus
         (c) Cord prolapse with fetal bradycardia
         (d) Agonal fetal distress, prolonged bradycardia, late decelerations without recovery of variability

- (2) Anesthesia (in order of preference)
    - (a) General anesthesia
    - (b) Local infiltration (only in instances where general anesthesia is unavailable)
- b. Urgent
    - (1) Indications
        - (a) Dystocia
        - (b) Failed forceps
        - (c) Active genital herpes with rupture of membranes
        - (d) Previous classical cesarean section and active labor
        - (e) Cord prolapse without fetal distress
        - (f) Variable decelerations with prompt recovery
        - (g) Abnormal fetal presentation with ruptured membranes (in active labor)
    - (2) Anesthesia (in order of preference)
        - (a) Extension of preexisting epidural blockade
        - (b) Spinal (Note: Provider should not persist if initial attempts at locating the subarachnoid space are unsuccessful.)
        - (c) General anesthesia
- c. Emergent
    - (1) Indications
        - (a) Chronic uteroplacental insufficiency
        - (b) Abnormal fetal presentation with ruptured membranes (not in active labor)
        - (c) Deteriorating maternal illness
    - (2) Anesthesia (in order of preference)
        - (a) Spinal or epidural
        - (b) General anesthesia
- d. Elective: anesthesia (in order of preference)
    - (1) Spinal or epidural
    - (2) General anesthesia

ANESTHESIA FOR NONOBSTETRIC SURGERY DURING PREGNANCY

1. General principles
    a. The surgical disease and maternal perioperative complications pose the greatest risk to the fetus.
    b. Physiologic changes of pregnancy increase maternal risk for anesthetic complications, most notably airway complications.
    c. Surgery and anesthesia do not increase the risk of congenital abnormalities. No anesthetic is a proven teratogen (use of nitrous oxide is controversial because it has been shown to be teratogenic is some animals when given in excessive, nonclinical doses).
    d. No anesthetic or anesthetic technique has shown a difference relative to maternal and fetal or neonatal outcome.
    e. Surgical disease or operative treatment located in or near the uterus will have an associated increased incidence of preterm labor or spontaneous abortion.
2. Anesthetic goals

a. Avoidance of hypoxemia, hypercarbia, hypocarbia, hypertension, hypotension, and other extremes of physiologic changes associated with surgery
b. Prevention of preterm labor

ANESTHETIC CONSIDERATIONS

1. For labor and vaginal delivery, small doses of narcotics will provide moderate pain relief.
2. Lumbar epidural block can provide excellent pain relief both for labor and delivery.
3. A separate intravenous line should be used for the rapid infusion of solutions not containing dextrose if necessary to treat hypotension without producing hyperglycemia.
4. The following criteria should be considered in the use of anesthesia for cesarean delivery in diabetic parturients:
    a. Acute hydration by nondextrose solution before induction of anesthesia. A separate intravenous line should be used for this purpose.
    b. Prompt treatment of hypotension with intravenous ephedrine (increments of 5 mg).
    c. Amide local anesthetics with long fetal or neonatal half-life (e.g., mepivacaine) should be avoided in these cases.
    d. Well-conducted general anesthesia can be used if necessary with good neonatal outcome.

SUGGESTED READINGS

Acker DB, Sachs BP, Friedman EA: Risk factors for shoulder dystocia, *Obstet Gynecol* 66:762-765, 1985.

American College of Obstetricians and Gynecologists: Operative vaginal delivery. In *ACOG Technical Bulletin 1991*, no. XX, Washington, DC, 1991, ACOG, p. 152.

American College of Obstetricians and Gynecologists: Fetal macrosomia. In *ACOG Technical Bulletin 1991*, no. XX, Washington, DC, 1991, ACOG, p. 159.

Bigrigg A, Chissell S, Read MD: Use of intra myometrial 15-methyl prostaglandin F2-alpha to control atonic postpartum haemorrhage following vaginal delivery and failure of conventional therapy, *Br J Obstet Gynaecol* 98:734-736, 1991.

Brandt ML: Mechanism and management of the third stage of labor, *Am J Obstet Gynecol* 25:662-663, 1933.

Caldwell WE, Moloy HC: Anatomical variations in the female pelvis and their effect in labor with a suggested classification, *Am J Obstet Gynecol* 26:479-483, 1933.

Caldwell WE, Moloy HC, D'Espo DA: Further studies on the pelvic architecture, *Am J Obstet Gynecol* 28:482-486, 1934.

Chestnut DJ: *Obstetric anesthesia: principles and practice*, St. Louis, 1994, Mosby.

Cunningham FG, et al: *Williams obstetrics*, ed 19, Norwalk, CT, 1993, Appleton & Lange.

Friedman EA: *Labor: clinical evaluation and management*, ed 2, New York, 1978, Appleton-Century-Crofts.

Gabbe SG, Niebyl JR, Simpson JL: *Obstetrics: normal and problem pregnancies*, ed 2, New York, 1991, Churchill Livingstone.

Harris AP, Michitsch RU: Anesthesia and analgesia for labor, *Curr Opin Obstet Gynecol* 4:813-817, 1992.

Keirse MJ: Therapeutic uses of prostaglandins, *Baillieres Clin Obstet Gynaecol* 6:787-808, 1992.

Okazaki T: Initiation of human parturition. XII. Biosynthesis and metabolism of prostaglandins in human fetal membranes and uterine decidua, *Am J Obstet Gynecol* 39:373-376, 1981.

Ott WJ: The diagnosis of altered fetal growth, *Obstet Gynecol Clin* 15:237-263, 1988.

Santos AC, Pedersen H: Current controversies in obstetric anesthesia, *Anesthesia Analgesia* 78:753-760, 1994.

Shnider SM: *Anesthesia for obstetrics*, ed 3, Baltimore, 1993, Williams & Wilkins.

Stoelting RK: *Pharmacology and physiology in anesthetic practice*, ed 2, Philadelphia, 1991, JB Lippincott.

Wittels B: Does epidural anesthesia affect the course of labor and delivery? *Sem Perinatol* 15:358-367, 1991.

Langer O, Berkus MD, Huff RW, Samueloff A: Should the fetus weighing >4,000 grams be delivered by cesarean section? *Am J Obstet Gynecol* 165:831, 1991.

High-Risk Obstetrics

19.1 Diabetes in Pregnancy

Bruce D. Rodgers

CLASSIFICATION OF DIABETES MELLITUS

1. Type I
   a. Accounts for 10% of all cases of diabetes
   b. Inadequate pancreatic insulin secretion
   c. Autoimmune destruction of pancreatic beta cells
   d. Body habitus thin
   e. Usually diagnosed under 30 years of age
   f. Patients usually symptomatic
   g. Strong predisposition to ketosis and ketoacidosis
   h. Some familial predisposition (common human leukocyte antigen [HLA] haplotypes)
   i. Therapeutic principles
      (1) Diet
      (2) Insulin
2. Type II
   a. Accounts for 90% of all cases of diabetes
   b. Heterogenous causes (one or more of the following):
      (1) Subnormal beta-cell function
      (2) Insulin resistance in muscle and adipose tissue
      (3) Increased hepatic production of glucose
   c. Body habitus usually obese
   d. Usually presents greater than 30 years of age
   e. Patients often asymptomatic and undiagnosed
   f. Little predisposition to ketosis
   g. Strong familial predisposition
   h. Often accompanied by hypertension and hyperlipidemia
   i. Therapeutic principles (one or combination of the following):
      (1) Diet
      (2) Weight loss
      (3) Oral hypoglycemic drugs
      (4) Insulin
3. Other type of diabetes
   a. Associated with other conditions or syndromes

b. Rare cause of diabetes
4. Impaired glucose tolerance and impaired fasting glucose
   a. Higher than normal plasma glucose levels
   b. Glucose levels not diagnostic of diabetes
5. Gestational diabetes
   a. Onset or discovery of glucose intolerance during pregnancy
   b. May include preconceptionally undiagnosed overt diabetes

CLASSIFICATION OF DIABETES DURING PREGNANCY

1. White classification of diabetes in pregnancy (Table 19-1)
   a. Basis of classification
      (1) Age of onset
      (2) Duration of diabetes
      (3) Presence of vascular disease
   b. Largely of historical interest
   c. Still used as a descriptive tool in clinical practice
2. A more clinically relevant classification scheme is as follows:
   a. Type I pregestational diabetes
   b. Type II pregestational diabetes
   c. Pregestational diabetes with vascular disease
      (1) Nephropathy
      (2) Retinopathy; background, proliferative
      (3) Arteriosclerotic heart disease
      (4) Renal transplant
      (5) Hypertension
   d. Gestational diabetes
      (1) Diet controlled
      (2) Medication required
         (a) Insulin
         (b) Glyburide
         (c) Metformin (pending results of clinical studies)

GESTATIONAL DIABETES

1. Risk assessment for gestational diabetes (American Diabetes Association) (Box 19-1)
   a. Performed in first trimester
   b. Universal screening
      (1) All patients screened at 24 to 28 weeks
      (2) High risk: screen as soon as possible; if negative, screen again at 24 to 28 weeks
   c. Selective screening based on risk assessment
      (1) Low risk: no screening required
      (2) Average risk: screen at 24 to 28 weeks
      (3) High risk: screen as soon as possible; if negative, screen again at 24 to 28 weeks
   d. Selective versus universal screening for detecting gestational diabetes

Table 19-1	**White Classification of Diabetes in Pregnancy**
Class	Description
A1	Gestational diabetes, diet controlled
A2	Gestational diabetes, requiring insulin
B	Age of onset ≤20 yr, or duration <10 yr
C	Age of onset 10-19 yr, or duration >10-19 yr
D	Age of onset <10 yr or duration ≥20 yr
F	Nephropathy
R	Proliferative retinopathy
H	Arteriosclerotic heart disease
T	Postrenal transplantation

   (1) Selective screening detects 97% of patients detected by universal screening.
   (2) Selective screening excludes only 10% of population from screening.
   (3) Universal screening may be more practical.
   (4) Universal screening prevents inadvertent exclusion of indicated screening.
   (5) Either screening method is acceptable.
2. Two-step screening (most patients)
   a. 50-gram glucola given randomly (no fasting required)
   b. Blood glucose drawn in 1 hour: threshold 130 or 140 mg/dL
      (1) Threshold: plasma glucose greater than or equal to 130 mg/dL
         (a) 90% sensitivity
         (b) 23% screen positive rate
      (2) Threshold: plasma glucose greater than or equal to 140 mg/dL
         (a) 80% sensitivity
         (b) 14% screen positive rate
   c. Positive screen: 3-hour oral glucose tolerance test
3. One-step screening
   a. Option for patients at high risk for gestational diabetes
   b. Go directly to 3-hour oral glucose tolerance test
4. Diagnosis
   a. Based on 3-hour oral glucose tolerance test (OGTT) (Table 19-2)
   b. National Diabetes Data Group (NDDG) criteria
      (1) Criterion modified from original O'Sullivan criteria
      (2) Modification based on plasma glucose measurements
   c. Carpenter and Coustan criteria (modified)
      (1) Also adjusts for inaccuracy of older laboratory technique for measuring glucose
      (2) Cutoffs lower then NDDG criteria
      (3) More sensitive for diagnosis of gestational diabetes
   d. Positive test: two or more values greater than or equal to cutoff values
   e. Borderline test: one value greater than or equal to cutoff value
      (1) Retest in several weeks, *or*
      (2) Treat as gestational diabetes

BOX 19-1 American Diabetes Association Recommended Screening Algorithm for Gestational Diabetes

Risk Assessment at First Prenatal Visit

1. **Low risk for gestational diabetes**
   a. Age <25 years
   b. Normal prepregnancy weight (BMI ≤25)
   c. Member of ethnic group with low prevalence of type 2 diabetes
   d. No history of carbohydrate intolerance
   e. No history of polycystic ovarian disease
   f. No known diabetes in first-degree relatives
   g. No history of prior adverse pregnancy outcome likely related to diabetes or gestational diabetes
2. *Average risk for gestational diabetes (one or more of the following)*
   a. Age >25
   b. Prepregnancy BMI >25
   c. Member of ethnic group with high prevalence of type 2 diabetes
      (1) African American
      (2) Hispanic
      (3) Southeast Asian
      (4) Native Islander
      (5) Native American
   d. First-degree relative with diabetes, especially type 2 diabetes
   e. Polycystic ovarian disease
   f. Prior adverse pregnancy outcome likely related to diabetes or gestational diabetes
3. **High risk for gestational diabetes** (one or more of the following)
   a. Morbid obesity
   b. Prior history of carbohydrate intolerance or gestational diabetes
   c. Strong family history of diabetes
   d. Glycosuria

Screening Assignment

1. Low-risk patients do not require screening.
2. Average-risk patients should be screened between 24 and 28 weeks.
3. High-risk patients should be screened as soon as possible. If the initial screen is negative, they should again be screened between 24 and 28 weeks.

Screening Methodology

1. **Two-step screen**: 50-g 1-hour glucola test followed by formal OGTT if positive.
2. **One-step screen**: go directly to OGTT.
3. **Patients with fasting glucose greater than or equal to 126 OR random glucose greater than or equal to 200** fulfill the diagnostic criteria for diabetes. This precludes the need for any form of additional glucose challenge screening.

Data from Gestational Diabetes: American Diabetes Association's fourth international workshop-conference of gestational diabetes mellitus. In *Diabetes Care* 2003, Suppl. 1(26), S103-S105.
OGTT, oral glucose tolerance test.

Table 19-2 **Three-Hour Glucose Tolerance Test Criteria (plasma glucose values; mg/dL)**

Time	NDDG Criteria	Modified Criteria
Fasting	≥105	≥95
1 hour	≥190	≥180
2 hour	≥165	≥155
3 hour	≥145	≥140

NDDG, National Diabetes Data Group.

5. Goals of treatment
    a. Attenuation and prevention of fetal hyperinsulinemia
    b. Prevention of macrosomia
    c. Prevention of fetal or neonatal birth trauma
    d. Reduction of need for cesarean section
    e. Prevention of neonatal complications
        (1) Hypoglycemia
        (2) Jaundice
        (3) Polycythemia
        (4) Respiratory distress syndrome
    f. Prevention of long-term complications
        (1) Childhood obesity
        (2) Type II diabetes in offspring
6. Risk
    a. Most common
        (1) Macrosomia
        (2) Shoulder dystocia
        (3) Neonatal hypoglycemia
    b. Less common
        (1) Intrapartum hypoxia or acidosis
        (2) Intrauterine fetal death
    c. High-risk gestational diabetes (Box 19-2)
        (1) Ten percent to 20% of gestational diabetes are high risk.
        (2) High-risk gestational diabetes may include patients with undiagnosed pregestational diabetes.
        (3) Risk may be similar to pregestational diabetes in some cases.
7. Treatment
    a. Maternal glycemic control
        (1) Diet
        (2) Selective insulin therapy
        (3) Selective glyburide therapy
    b. Fetal surveillance
        (1) Optional in low-risk gestational diabetes
        (2) Mandatory in high-risk gestational diabetes
    c. Elective delivery in select high-risk gestational diabetes
    d. Selective delivery by primary cesarean section
    e. Expert management of shoulder dystocia

> **BOX 19-2 High-Risk Gestational Diabetes**
>
> Maternal age >35 years
> Hypertension
> Previous intrauterine fetal death
> Noncompliance
> Poor glucose control
> Macrosomia
> Diabetic fetopathy
> Hydramnios
> Therapeutic insulin therapy
> Insulin dose >100 U/day

PREGESTATIONAL DIABETES

1. Differs from gestational diabetes
   a. Complexity of medical management
   b. Maternal risk
      (1) Hypoglycemia
      (2) Diabetic ketoacidosis
      (3) Infection
      (4) Poor wound healing
   c. Diversity and level of perinatal risk
   d. Risk of congenital anomalies
2. May require team approach
   a. Maternal-fetal medicine specialist
   b. Diabetic teaching nurse
   c. Medical endocrinologist
   d. Nephrologist
   e. Ophthalmologist
3. Goals of management
   a. Preconception counseling and diabetes management
   b. Establishment of the extent of maternal disease
   c. Establishment of pregnancy viability and gestational age
   d. Detection of congenital anomalies
   e. Prevention and treatment of preterm labor
   f. Prevention and treatment of fetal growth aberrancy
   g. Establishment of euglycemia
   h. Prevention of intrauterine fetal death (IUFD)
   i. Prevention of intrapartum asphyxia
   j. Prevention of fetal and maternal birth trauma
   k. Prevention and treatment of neonatal complications

PRECONCEPTION COUNSELING AND DIABETES MANAGEMENT

1. Establishment of extent of maternal disease and submission for treatment

- a. Presence of microvascular and macrovascular disease
  - (1) Nephropathy
  - (2) Retinopathy
  - (3) Coronary artery disease
- b. Neuropathy
- c. Gastroenteropathy
- d. Hypertension
2. Contraceptive counseling
3. Establish periconception glucose control
   - a. May reduce fetal anomaly risk
   - b. May reduce first-trimester pregnancy loss
   - c. Pregnancy standards of glucose control
     - (1) Insulin therapy
     - (2) American Diabetes Association (ADA) diet
     - (3) Risk of first-trimester hypoglycemia

ESTABLISHMENT OF THE EXTENT OF MATERNAL DISEASE

1. Formal eye ground examination
   - a. No retinopathy; examination repeated if clinically indicated
   - b. Background retinopathy; examination repeated each trimester
   - c. Proliferative retinopathy:
     - (1) Referral for treatment
     - (2) Frequent examinations
     - (3) May progress during pregnancy
2. Macular edema; referral for treatment
3. Spot urine for microalbumin/creatinine ratio
   - a. Normal: less than 29
   - b. Microalbuminuria: 30 to 299
   - c. Proteinuria: greater than or equal to 300
4. 24-hour urine collection
   - a. Creatinine clearance
   - b. Total protein excretion
     - (1) Greater than 300 mg: suspect nephropathy
     - (2) Greater than 500 mg: nephropathy present
5. Electrocardiogram
6. Hypoglycemia unawareness
   - a. Unawareness poses a significant risk for hypoglycemia and insulin coma.
   - b. Hypoglycemia is common in long-standing type I insulin-dependent diabetes mellitus (IDDM).
   - c. Patient should not live alone.
   - d. Family members should be trained to do the following:
     - (1) Recognize symptoms of hypoglycemia
     - (2) Treat hypoglycemia
     - (3) Administer glucagon
   - e. Avoid excessively rigid glucose control.
7. Hypertension
   - a. Medications

(1) Angiotensin-converting enzyme (ACE) inhibitors should be discontinued.
(2) Angiotensin receptor blockers (ARBs) should be discontinued.
(3) Beta-blockers should be avoided.
(4) Alpha-methyldopa, nifedipine, labetalol may be used.
(5) Diltiazem (calcium channel blocker):
   (a) May ameliorate proteinuria in diabetic nephropathy
   (b) May be used in pregnancy
 b. Consider preeclampsia prophylaxis; aspirin, 81 mg/day
 c. Long-standing or severe hypertension
   (1) Electrocardiogram (ECG)
   (2) Echocardiogram
8. Symptoms of coronary insufficiency
 a. Exertional chest pain or dyspnea
 b. Referred pain
 c. Arrhythmia
 d. Heart failure
 e. Treatment
   (1) ECG
   (2) Echocardiogram
   (3) Referral to cardiologist
9. Gastroenteropathy
 a. Intermittent constipation and diarrhea
 b. Emesis
 c. Early satiety
 d. Problems include the following:
   (1) Dehydration and ketoacidosis
   (2) Erratic blood sugar control
   (3) Hypoglycemia
   (4) Poor maternal weight gain

ESTABLISHMENT OF PREGNANCY VIABILITY AND GESTATIONAL AGE

1. Viability and gestational age
 a. Accurate dating imperative
   (1) Increased risk of later perinatal complications
   (2) Timing of delivery at term
 b. Increased risk of first-trimester pregnancy loss
   (1) Higher in pregestational diabetes
   (2) Early diagnosis important for diabetes management
   (3) Correlates with periconceptional hyperglycemia
2. Pregnancy dating
 a. Serum human chorionic gonadotropin (HCG)
 b. Vaginal probe ultrasound: 6 to 12 weeks
   (1) Date pregnancy accurately within ± 5 days.
   (2) Establish intrauterine pregnancy.
   (3) Rule out missed abortion.
   (4) Rule out multiple gestation.
   (5) Diagnose gross fetal anomalies.

DETECTION OF CONGENITAL ANOMALIES

1. Overall risk is twofold to threefold over general population.
2. All major organ systems may be involved.
3. Risk related to poor first-trimester glucose control.
4. Detection:
    a. First-trimester glycosylated hemoglobin
        (1) Elevated: increased risk of anomalies
        (2) Normal: risk approaches general population
    b. First trimester vaginal ultrasound
        (1) Ultrasound is performed at 10 to 12 weeks.
        (2) Detection of major anomalies is possible.
        (3) Sensitivity and specificity are not well defined.
    c. Maternal serum alpha-fetoprotein (AFP)
        (1) Performed at 14 to 16 weeks.
        (2) Level is lower in diabetic women.
        (3) Level is lower in obese women.
    d. Transabdominal ultrasound
        (1) Perform at 15 to 20 weeks
        (2) Fetal anomaly screen
        (3) Four-chambered cardiac view
    e. Fetal echocardiography
        (1) Echocardiography is performed at 22 to 24 weeks.
        (2) Fetal anomaly screen repeated.

PREVENTION AND TREATMENT OF PRETERM LABOR

1. Risk increased in diabetic pregnancy
    a. Hydramnios increases risk.
    b. Poor glucose control increases risk.
    c. Vascular disease increases risk.
2. Frequent prenatal visits
3. Patient education and counseling
4. Screening and treatment for bacteriuria
5. Treatment
    a. Avoid betasympathomimetic tocolytics
        (1) Cause hyperglycemia
        (2) May precipitate diabetic ketoacidosis
    b. Tocolytic agents
        (1) Nifedipine; first choice
        (2) Indomethacin; second choice; do not use after 32 weeks gestation
    c. Betamethasone or dexamethasone
        (1) Can be used for fetal lung maturation.
        (2) It may cause hyperglycemia.
        (3) It may precipitate diabetic ketoacidosis.
        (4) Careful monitoring of blood glucose is required.
        (5) Insulin drip may be necessary during acute phase of treatment.

FETAL GROWTH ABERRANCY

1. Macrosomia
   a. Neonatal weight greater than 90th percentile for gestational age
   b. Characterized by central obesity
   c. Associated with the following:
      (1) Poor maternal glucose control
      (2) Elevated third-trimester glycosylated hemoglobin
      (3) Excessive maternal weight gain
      (4) Maternal obesity
      (5) Diabetic classes A through C
      (6) Hydramnios
      (7) Previous macrosomic infant
   d. Increases risk of the following:
      (1) Neonatal metabolic complications
      (2) Neonatal physiologic complications
      (3) Intrauterine fetal death
      (4) Intrapartum hypoxia and acidosis
      (5) Fetal birth trauma and shoulder dystocia
      (6) Cephalopelvic disproportion and cesarean section
      (7) Maternal genital trauma
      (8) Uterine atony and postpartum hemorrhage
2. Intrauterine growth retardation (IUGR)
   a. Associated with the following:
      (1) Diabetic classes D, R, F, T, H
      (2) Hypertension
      (3) Vascular disease
      (4) Oligohydramnios
      (5) Preeclampsia
      (6) Chronic maternal hypoglycemia (mean daily glucose <95 mg/dL)
   b. Increased risk of the following:
      (1) Intrapartum and neonatal hypoxia or acidosis
      (2) Intrauterine fetal death
      (3) Long-term developmental impairment
      (4) Meconium aspiration syndrome

ESTABLISHMENT OF GLUCOSE CONTROL (TABLE 19-3)

1. Establishment defines most perinatal risk.
   a. Fetal anomalies
   b. First-trimester pregnancy loss
   c. Preterm labor
   d. Intrauterine fetal death
   e. Intrapartum hypoxia
   f. Macrosomia
   g. Neonatal metabolic and physiologic complications (e.g., hypoglycemia)
2. Perinatal outcome correlates better with postprandial glucose levels.

Table 19-3 Standards of Glucose Control in Diabetic Pregnancy

Time	Ideal Glucose Range (mg/dL)
Fasting	70 to 90-95
Premeal	70-95
1 hour postprandial	110-140
2 hour postprandial	80-120
2 AM to 6 AM	60-120

  a. 1-hour postprandial blood sugars correlate best with macrosomia risk
  b. 1-hour postprandials may be better then 2-hour postprandials
3. Self-monitoring of blood glucose
  a. Glucometer should be used.
  b. Daily blood sugars should be measured.
  c. Diary of blood sugars should be kept.
  d. Glucometers that report plasma glucose or plasma equivalents should be used.
  e. Standards are more stringent than in nonpregnant state.
4. Complications of glucose control
  a. Diabetic ketoacidosis: associations are as follows:
    (1) Patient noncompliance
    (2) Use of betasympathomimetic drugs
    (3) Use of betamethasone or dexamethasone
    (4) Emesis with dehydration
    (5) Maternal infection
    (6) Can occur more readily and at lower glucose levels in pregnancy
  b. Hypoglycemia
    (1) Hypoglycemia is more frequent in first trimester.
    (2) It is more frequent in type I IDDM.
    (3) It is associated with overzealous insulin administration.
    (4) Hypoglycemia is associated with maternal dietary noncompliance.
    (5) Insulin coma may result in face of hypoglycemia unawareness.
    (6) Chronic hypoglycemia may lead to IUGR (mean daily plasma glucose <95 mg/dL).

PREVENTION OF INTRAUTERINE FETAL DEATH

1. Risk is increased in complicated diabetes mellitus
  a. Poor third-trimester glucose control
  b. Maternal age greater than 35 years or teenage pregnancy
  c. Insulin requirement greater than 100 U/day
  d. Fetal macrosomia or diabetic fetopathy
  e. Maternal vascular disease
  f. Maternal hypertension
  g. Preeclampsia

h. Previous IUFD
   i. IUGR
   j. Hydramnios or oligohydramnios
   k. Patient noncompliance
   l. Fetal anomalies
2. Fetal surveillance
   a. Uncomplicated diabetes; to begin at 30 to 32 weeks
   b. Complicated diabetes; to begin at 28 to 30 weeks
   c. Ultrasound
      (1) Every 2 to 4 weeks after 20 weeks
      (2) Assessment of fetal growth and amniotic fluid volume
   d. Doppler ultrasound
      (1) Generally not predictive of fetal health in diabetic pregnancy
      (2) May be useful in presence of hypertension or vascular disease
      (3) Should be interpreted with caution
      (4) Should be interpreted in conjunction with other surveillance methods
3. Timed delivery
   a. No risk factors for IUFD, good glycemic control, compliant:
      (1) Vigilant expectancy until 40 weeks
      (2) Induction at 40 weeks if labor has not occurred
   b. Risk factors for IUFD, poor glycemic control, noncompliant:
      (1) Assess fetal lung maturity by amniocentesis.
      (2) Amniocentesis is generally performed between 37 and 38 weeks.
      (3) Induction at confirmation of fetal lung maturity.

PREVENTION OF INTRAPARTUM ASPHYXIA

1. Continuous fetal monitoring
2. Amniotomy
   a. Internal monitor placement
   b. Detection of meconium
3. Amnioinfusion
   a. Recurrent severe variable decelerations
   b. Presence of thick meconium
4. Skilled pediatric personnel in attendance at delivery

PREVENTION OF BIRTH TRAUMA

1. Primary cesarean section may be considered for either of the following:
   a. Estimated fetal weight is greater than 4000 g; head circumference to abdominal circumference ratio is less than 10th percentile.
   b. Estimated fetal weight is greater than 4200 g.
2. Attention to dysfunctional labors associated with cephalopelvic disproportion
   a. Protraction of descent or dilation
   b. Arrest of descent or dilation
   c. Failure of descent

3. Attention to pelvic findings associated with cephalopelvic disproportion
   a. Excessive fetal cranial molding
   b. Fetal caput
   c. Fetal cranium overriding maternal symphysis
4. Use of intrauterine pressure catheters for management of dysfunctional labor
5. Avoidance of unnecessary operative delivery with vacuum or forceps
   a. Especially in face of dysfunctional labor
   b. Especially if fetal macrosomia suspected
6. Anticipation and expert management of shoulder dystocia
   a. Selective use of formal delivery room setting
      (1) Large baby suspected clinically or by ultrasound
      (2) Risk factors for macrosomia present
   b. Rehearsed protocol for clinical management
   c. Anesthesia on standby
   d. Skilled pediatric personnel in attendance at delivery

PREVENTION AND TREATMENT OF NEONATAL COMPLICATIONS

1. Variables associated with complications
   a. Poor glycemic control
   b. IUGR
   c. Macrosomia
   d. Premature delivery
   e. Preeclampsia
   f. Maternal noncompliance
   g. Congenital anomalies
   h. Hyperglycemia during labor
   i. Complicated diabetes mellitus
2. Categories of complications
   a. Anatomic
      (1) Occult fetal anomalies
      (2) Birth trauma
   b. Metabolic
      (1) Hypoglycemia: most common and most immediate problem
      (2) Hypocalcemia
      (3) Hypomagnesemia
      (4) Polycythemia and hyperviscosity syndrome
      (5) Hyperbilirubinemia
   c. Physiologic
      (1) Respiratory distress
      (2) Renal vein thrombosis
      (3) Cardiomyopathy
      (4) Asphyxia
3. Prevention
   a. Glycemic control during pregnancy and labor
   b. Ultrasound detection of growth aberrancy
   c. Ultrasound detection of congenital anomalies
   d. Selective delivery at tertiary centers

(1) Complicated diabetes
(2) Poor glycemic control or noncompliance
(3) Premature gestational age
(4) Suspected IUGR or oligohydramnios
(5) Preeclampsia
(6) Suspected fetal anomalies
(7) Suspected extreme macrosomia (>4500 g)
(8) Premature labor
e. Confirmation of fetal pulmonary maturity before onset of labor
    (1) Less than 39 weeks gestation
    (2) Uncertain dating

GENERAL MANAGEMENT PRINCIPLES

1. Applicable to both gestational and pregestational diabetes
   a. Standards of glycemic control
   b. Perinatal risk assessment
   c. Fetal surveillance strategies
   d. Timing of delivery
   e. Intrapartum surveillance
2. Diet
   a. ADA diet
   b. Must minimize hyperglycemia
   c. Must meet nutritional needs of pregnancy (Box 19-3)
   d. Calories determined by maternal weight at time of diagnosis
      (1) 10% of calories at breakfast
      (2) 30% of calories at lunch
      (3) 30% of calories at dinner
      (4) 30% of calories as snacks
   e. Prevent excessive maternal weight gain (see Box 19-3)
3. Maternal glucose monitoring
   a. Blood glucose should be measured as least 4 times per day in gestational diabetes.
      (1) Fasting
      (2) 1 or 2 hours after each meal
   b. Blood glucose should be measured 4 to 8 times per day in pregestational diabetes.
      (1) Fasting
      (2) 1 or 2 hours after each meal
      (3) Before meals (AC)
   c. Standards of glycemic control.
      (1) Fasting glucose greater than 70 and less than 90 to 95 mg/dL
      (2) 1 hour postprandial less than 140 mg/dL
      (3) 2 hour postprandial less than 120
      (4) Before meal (AC) glucose 70 to 95 mg/dL
   d. Poor control: Mean daily plasma glucose greater than 120 mg/dL.
   e. Good control: Mean daily plasma glucose less than 100 mg/dL.
   f. Glycosylated hemoglobin determinations.

> ### BOX 19-3 Diet Composition—Pregnancy (Jovanovic-Peterson)
>
> **Suggested Diabetic Diet**
>
> | | |
> |---|---|
> | Carbohydrate | 35% to 40% of total calories |
> | Fat | 40% of total calories |
> | Protein | 20% of total calories |
>
> **Daily Caloric Intake**
>
> | | |
> |---|---|
> | 40 cal/kg of present pregnancy weight | Body mass index <22 |
> | 30 cal/kg of present pregnancy weight | Body mass index 22 to 27 |
> | 24 cal/kg of present pregnancy weight | Body mass index 27 to 29 |
> | 12 to 15 cal/kg of present pregnancy weight | Body mass index ≥30 |
>
> | Meal | Distribution of Calories (% of total calories) | Distribution of Carbohydrate (% of total carbohydrate) |
> |---|---|---|
> | Breakfast | 10 | 10 |
> | Lunch | 30 | 30 |
> | Dinner | 30 | 30 |
> | Snack | 30 | 30 |
>
> **Weight Gain During Pregnancy (Institute of Medicine, 1990)**
>
> | Status | Prepregnancy BMI | Pregnancy Weight Gain |
> |---|---|---|
> | Underweight | <18.5 | 28 to 40 lbs |
> | Normal | 18.5 to 24.9 | 25 to 35 lbs |
> | Overweight | 25 to 29.9 | 15 to 25 lbs |
> | Obese | >30 | 15 lbs |
> | Morbid | | No weight gain required |

Data from Jovanovic L: *Drugs* 64(13):1401-1417, 2004.
BMI, Body mass index (kg/m^2).

(1) Indicator of chronic glycemic control over prior 4 to 6 weeks
(2) Limited use in gestational diabetes
(3) Insensitive indicator of subtle but perinatally significant maternal hyperglycemia usually seen in gestational diabetes
(4) Measure every 6 to 12 weeks in pregestational diabetes
(5) Not a substitute for frequent maternal glucose measurement
4. Insulin therapy; pregestational diabetes
   a. Split dose insulin used

(1) Intermediate acting (neutral protamine hagedorn [NPH] preferred)
(2) Long-acting insulin (insulin glargine—not yet approved for pregnancy)
(3) Short-acting insulin (regular insulin)
(4) Rapid-acting insulin
  (a) Insulin lispro
  (b) Insulin aspart
(5) Rapid-acting insulins
  (a) May be taken before, with, or just after a meal
  (b) Peak sooner
(6) More rapid onset
(7) Superior for controlling 1-hour postprandial blood sugars
b. Human insulin used
c. First trimester: Dose = approximately 0.5 U/kg/day
d. Second trimester: Dose = approximately 0.8 U/kg/day
e. Third trimester: Dose = approximately 1 to 2 U/kg/day
5. Insulin therapy; gestational diabetes
 a. Therapeutic insulin treatment: NPH and rapid-acting insulin preferred
  (1) Failure to achieve glycemic control by diet in gestational diabetes
  (2) Human insulin used
  (3) Begin with 0.7 U/kg total insulin
   (a) $2/3$ total insulin in the morning: $2/3$ of this as NPH, $1/3$ as rapid-acting insulin
   (b) $1/3$ total insulin in the evening: $1/3$ of this as NPH, $1/3$ as rapid-acting insulin
  (4) Further dose adjustments according to initial dose response
6. Oral hypoglycemic agents and gestational diabetes
 a. Glyburide
  (1) Second-generation sulfonylurea
  (2) Stimulates pancreatic beta-cell insulin production
  (3) Does not cross placenta
  (4) Does not cause fetal anomalies, macrosomia, or neonatal hypoglycemia
  (5) Equally efficacious to insulin
 b. Glyburide dosing
  (1) 2.5 mg qd with breakfast
  (2) Increase to 2.5 mg bid
  (3) Incremental increase to maximum of 10 mg bid (20 mg/day)
 c. Metformin
  (1) Biguanide
  (2) Reduces hepatic production of glucose
  (3) Increases insulin sensitivity of tissues
  (4) Improves fertility in polycystic ovarian syndrome
  (5) Reduces miscarriage rate in polycystic ovarian syndrome
  (6) May prevent gestational diabetes in polycystic ovarian syndrome

(7) Does not cause fetal anomalies, macrosomia, or neonatal hypoglycemia
  d. Metformin use
    (1) Use in gestational diabetes presently awaiting clinical trials
    (2) Highly selective use in type 2 diabetes mellitus with extreme insulin resistance
7. Ultrasound surveillance
  a. First-trimester vaginal sonography
    (1) Principally for pregestational diabetes
    (2) Detect early pregnancy loss
    (3) Accurate pregnancy dating
    (4) Detection of gross fetal anomalies
  b. Second-trimester sonography
    (1) Pregnancy dating
    (2) Detect fetal anomalies in pregestational diabetes (15 to 18 weeks)
  c. Third-trimester sonography
    (1) Applicable for both pregestational and gestational diabetes
    (2) Detection of diabetic fetopathy
    (3) Detection of fetal macrosomia and cardiomyopathy
  d. Fetal echocardiography: pregestational diabetes
    (1) Four-chambered view (15 to 18 weeks)
    (2) Formal study (22 to 24 weeks)
    (3) Detection of diabetic cardiomyopathy (third trimester)
8. Ultrasound predictors of growth aberrancy
  a. Macrosomia
    (1) Third-trimester fetal abdominal circumference growth greater than 1.5 cm/week
    (2) Head circumference to abdominal circumference ratio less than 10th percentile
    (3) Femur length to abdominal circumference ratio less than 20%
    (4) Estimated fetal weight greater than 4200 g at term
    (5) Hydramnios
    (6) 28-week fetal abdominal circumference greater than 75th percentile
  b. IUGR: pregestational diabetes
    (1) Poor interval fetal abdominal circumference growth
    (2) Head circumference to abdominal circumference ratio greater than 90th percentile
    (3) Femur length to abdominal circumference ratio greater than 24%
    (4) Transcerebellar diameter to abdominal circumference ratio greater than 15%
    (5) Elevated umbilical artery Doppler systolic/diastolic (S/D) or pulsatility index
    (6) Decreased middle cerebral artery Doppler S/D or pulsatility index
    (7) Elevated uterine artery Doppler S/D ratio
    (8) Oligohydramnios

9. Congenital anomalies
   a. Anomalies are increased twofold to threefold in pregestational diabetes.
   b. This applies to all fetal organ systems.
   c. Most anomalies present by the seventh gestational week.
   d. There is no increased risk in gestational diabetes except if fasting glucose greater than or equal to 120 mg/dL.
   e. Risk correlates with first-trimester hyperglycemia.
      (1) Documented hyperglycemia by self-glucose monitoring
      (2) Elevated first-trimester glycosylated hemoglobin
   f. Independent risk is possibly related to vascular disease.
   g. Congenital abnormalities are the leading cause of perinatal mortality.
   h. Incidence has remained constant in diabetic pregnancies.
   i. Risk is not related to first-trimester hypoglycemia.
   j. No risk from first-trimester oral hypoglycemic drugs.
   k. Detection.
      (1) First-trimester sonography: limited to gross anomalies
      (2) Second-trimester sonography
      (3) Fetal echocardiography
      (4) Second-trimester maternal alpha-fetoprotein screening
   l. Prevention.
      (1) Preconception counseling and glycemic control
      (2) Planned pregnancy
      (3) Cannot be effectively prevented postconception
10. Diabetic fetopathy: refers to ultrasound-detected fetal somatic disproportion, reflecting accelerated growth of insulin-sensitive tissues (liver, adipose tissue, skeletal muscle) in response to fetal hyperinsulinemia
    a. Implies presence of fetal hyperinsulinemia
       (1) May suggest poor maternal glucose control
       (2) Increased risk of macrosomia
       (3) Increased risk of intrauterine fetal death
       (4) Increased risk of intrapartum hypoxia
       (5) Increased risk of neonatal morbidity
    b. Sonogram findings (one or more of the following):
       (1) Low head circumference to abdominal circumference (HC/AC)
       (2) Low femur to abdominal circumference (F/AC)
       (3) Accelerated third-trimester abdominal circumference growth (≥ 2 cm/wk)
       (4) Abdominal circumference greater than or equal to 90th percentile for gestational age
       (5) Estimated fetal weight greater than or equal to 90th percentile for gestational age
11. Hydramnios
    a. Frequent complication of pregestational and gestational diabetes
    b. Exact mechanism not well understood
    c. Sonographic findings

(1) Amniotic fluid index greater than or equal to 24 cm any time during gestation
(2) Amniotic fluid index greater than 2 standard deviations (SD) from mean for gestational age
d. Correlates somewhat with poor maternal glycemic control
e. Correlates somewhat with fetal macrosomia
f. May indicate the presence of a fetal anomaly
g. Increases risk of the following:
(1) Preterm labor, preterm rupture of membranes
(2) Maternal preeclampsia
(3) Intrauterine fetal death
(4) Fetal macrosomia
(5) Fetal malpresentation
(6) Cord prolapse
(7) Placenta separation
(8) Uterine atony
12. Surveillance of fetal well-being
a. Timing and intensity depends on risk of fetal death
(1) 32 to 34 weeks: all pregestational diabetics and high-risk gestational diabetics (see Box 19-2)
(2) Less than 32 weeks: selected pregestational diabetics
(3) 35 weeks: low-risk gestational diabetics
b. Fetal risk is increased by the following:
(1) Pregestational diabetes in general
(2) High-risk gestational diabetes
(3) Diabetic fetopathy or fetal macrosomia
(4) IUGR
(5) Hydramnios or oligohydramnios
(6) Poor maternal glucose control (especially third trimester)
(7) Poor prior pregnancy history
(8) Prior intrauterine fetal death
(9) Maternal hypertension
(10) Maternal vascular disease
(11) Abnormal umbilical artery Doppler indices
(12) Patient noncompliance
(13) Advanced maternal age (>35 years)
(14) Large doses of maternal insulin (>100 U/day)
(15) Maternal smoking
(16) Maternal substance abuse
c. Surveillance strategies
(1) Daily maternal fetal movement counts
(2) Formal fetal surveillance
d. Surveillance techniques
(1) No method has been definitively demonstrated superior
(2) One of three modalities can be used for pregestational and high-risk gestational diabetics:
(a) Weekly contraction stress testing (CST)
(b) Twice weekly biophysical profile assessment (BPP)
(c) Twice weekly nonstress testing (NST) with adjunctive BPP
e. Low-risk gestational diabetics: weekly NST

13. Umbilical artery Doppler ultrasound
    a. Poor predictor of perinatal outcome in diabetic pregnancy
    b. Some efficacy in diabetics with hypertension or vascular disease
        (1) Initial assessment at 28 weeks
        (2) Repeat at intervals depending on 28-week findings
14. Fetal lung maturity
    a. Lung maturity may be delayed in diabetic fetuses.
    b. Risk of delay is correlated to maternal glucose control.
    c. Amniotic fluid lung maturity should be confirmed before elective delivery under 39 weeks.
15. Timing of delivery
    a. Pregestational and high-risk gestational diabetes
        (1) Assessment of fetal lung maturity beginning at 37 to 38 weeks
        (2) Delivery at fetal lung maturity
    b. Gestational diabetes
        (1) Spontaneous labor should be allowed.
        (2) If undelivered at 40 to 41 weeks, labor should be induced.
    c. Low-risk pregestational diabetes
        (1) Allowing spontaneous labor should be considered.
        (2) Delivery should be considered in presence of fetal lung maturity and high cervical Bishop score.
        (3) If undelivered at 40 weeks, labor should be induced.
16. Mode of delivery
    a. Vaginal birth is the preferred mode of delivery.
    b. Cervical ripening agents should be used in the presence of low cervical Bishop score:
        (1) Prostaglandin analogs
        (2) Foley catheter balloon
    c. Cesarean section is reserved for specific indications:
        (1) Failed induction in high-risk pregestational diabetics
        (2) Selected cases of suspected fetal macrosomia
17. Prevention of birth trauma and shoulder dystocia
    a. Selective primary cesarean section
    b. Careful management of arrested and protracted labors
    c. Avoidance of operative vaginal delivery
        (1) In cases of suspected fetal macrosomia
        (2) In cases of dysfunctional labors
    d. Anticipation and expert management of shoulder dystocia
18. Prelabor and labor management
    a. General guidelines
        (1) Patient should take usual dose of intermediate and short-acting insulin the evening before delivery.
        (2) Patient should take dinner and evening snack the evening before delivery.
        (3) No food or subcutaneous insulin the day of delivery.
        (4) Fasting blood sugar should be measured the day of delivery.
        (5) Blood glucose and urine dipstick for ketones every 1 to 2 hours during labor.

(6) Blood glucose should be maintained at 70 to 110, and urine maintained free of ketones.
(7) Rapid glucose infusions for conduction anesthesia should be avoided.
   b. Suggested insulin regimen
      (1) Type I pregestational diabetes
         (a) Type I diabetics have a propensity toward ketosis and hypoglycemia, and labor may predispose toward both conditions.
         (b) Therefore it is prudent in general to begin dextrose and insulin infusions from the onset.
      (2) Five percent dextrose solution is instituted intravenously (IV) at 125 mL/hr.
      (3) Insulin drip at 0.5 U/hr is instituted.
      (4) Insulin and dextrose infusions are adjusted according to glucose and urinary ketone values.
   c. Suggested insulin regimen
      (1) Type II and gestational diabetes:
         (a) Many type II and gestational diabetics may not need any dextrose or insulin infusions during labor.
         (b) Therefore a more conservative approach to these patients is permissible.
      (2) Dextrose-free crystalloid is instituted.
      (3) Dextrose solution is administered IV for persistent glucose less than 70 or for persistent ketonuria.
      (4) Insulin drip is administered starting at 0.5 U/hr for glucose greater than 110.
      (5) Insulin and dextrose infusions are adjusted according to glucose and urinary ketone values.
19. Neonatal management
   a. Delivery of select patients at tertiary facilities
      (1) Diabetics with vascular disease or hypertension
      (2) Diabetics with brittle glucose control
      (3) Diabetes of long standing
      (4) Fetuses suspected of IUGR
      (5) Gestational age less than 37 weeks
      (6) Poorly compliant patients
      (7) Hydramnios
      (8) Suspected or proven fetal anomalies
      (9) Poor maternal glucose control
   b. Anticipation and management of neonatal complications
      (1) Unanticipated congenital anomalies
      (2) Respiratory distress
      (3) Hypoglycemia
      (4) Hypocalcemia
      (5) Birth trauma
      (6) Birth asphyxia
      (7) Polycythemia and hyperviscosity syndrome
      (8) Jaundice
      (9) Diabetic cardiomyopathy and cardiac failure

19.2 Insulin Treatment in Pregnancy

Harold E. Bays and Mary Self

1. Scientifically, studies such as the Diabetes Control and Complication Trial (DCCT) have confirmed that "tight" blood sugar (BS) control can decrease progression of many of the chronic complications of diabetes mellitus (DM). Similarly, studies have demonstrated that normalization of BS control may normalize the risks associated with pregnancy complicated by gestational diabetes or pregestational DM.
2. Practically, the advancement in medical technology, along with the influences of managed health care systems, has increasingly diverted DM medical care toward an outpatient basis.
3. Health care providers recognize the scientific need to maximize BS control and the ability to incorporate technologies and outpatient care systems to implement maximal BS control in the outpatient setting.
   a. Use of new technologies (e.g., home glucose monitors, insulin pumps)
   b. Use of outpatient health systems (e.g., hospital-based, insurance-based, or private educational facilities, or home health care or visiting nurse instruction)

GESTATIONAL DIABETES MELLITUS

Definitions, Etiology, and Diagnosis

1. Gestational diabetes mellitus (GDM) is glucose intolerance with onset during pregnancy.
2. The etiology of hyperglycemia during pregnancy is probably multifactorial and is thought to be significantly caused by placental production of human placental lactogen (HPL) hormone, which results in insulin resistance.
3. Hyperglycemia in GDM is most accentuated after meals.
4. GDM accounts for about 90% of all pregnant women who have DM.
5. Diagnosis
   a. A 50-g oral glucose screening or challenge test is recommended for all women (regardless of risk factors) between 24 and 28 weeks gestation. If subsequent 1-hour BS level is greater than 140 mg/dL, then a glucose tolerance test (GTT) is indicated.
   b. The GTT includes at least an 8-hour fast, followed by a fasting BS. After 100 g of oral glucose, BS levels are obtained at 1, 2, and 3 hours. Interpretation of GTT is described in Box 19-4.
      (1) It should be noted that some authors feel that these guidelines are not sensitive enough. Other, more rigid suggestions have been made.
      (2) Furthermore, other authors suggest that GDM is present if the fasting blood sugar is greater than 105 mg/dL, regardless of other values.

Risks

1. Before delivery, the most common potential fetal complication associated with GDM is macrosomia.

> **BOX 19-4 Interpretation of 100-g Oral GTT**
>
> Gestational diabetes mellitus is diagnosed if two or more subsequent blood sugar values (after 100 g oral glucose) are above:
>
> Fasting 105 mg/dL
> 1 hour 190 mg/dL
> 2 hours 165 mg/dL
> 3 hours 145 mg/dL

  a. Macrosomia can be defined as birth weight greater than 90th percentile, adjusted for sex and gestational age.
  b. Development of macrosomia is related to increased nutrient transport across the placenta (such as "facilitated" glucose transport, and "active" amino acid transport), and subsequent fetal hyperinsulinemia.
2. At delivery, if macrosomia is present, potential fetal complications may include birth trauma such as the following:
  a. Brachial plexus injury
  b. Facial nerve injury
  c. Cephalohematoma
3. After delivery, potential fetal complications associated with GDM may include the following:
  a. Respiratory distress
  b. Hypoglycemia
  c. Electrolyte imbalances
  d. An increased risk of obesity
  e. Type II (adult-onset) DM later in the newborn's life
4. The most common potential maternal complications associated with GDM include the following:
  a. Increased thirst
  b. Increased urination
  c. Increased fetal amniotic fluid
  d. An increased rate of urinary tract infections
  e. Increased rate of yeast infections
  f. Increased rate of spontaneous abortions
  g. Increased rate of hypertension
  h. Increased rate of toxemia
5. If fetal macrosomia occurs, potential maternal complications may include the following:
  a. Difficult delivery
  b. Prolonged labor
  c. Vaginal wall trauma
  d. Need for a cesarean section

Monitoring of Gestational Diabetes Mellitus

1. Once the diagnosis of GDM is made, one monitoring strategy is to recommend that BS be obtained (by home glucose monitoring) fasting and 1 or 2 hours after each meal (four times a day).

2. Monitoring BS levels before meals is not sensitive enough in women with GDM and misses many women with GDM who may benefit from more aggressive treatment.
3. The goal is to maintain fasting BS less than 90 mg/dL, 1-hour postprandial BS less than 140 mg/dL, and 2-hour postprandial BS less than 120 mg/dL.
4. Unless the initial BS is found to be high enough to warrant immediate intervention, glucose monitoring is usually recommended for about a week while on appropriate diet before any decision is made concerning need for insulin therapy.
5. Urinary ketone determination measures starvation states and ketosis, both of which may be harmful to the fetus. Testing is usually recommended fasting, whenever meals are omitted, during periods of nausea or vomiting, or with medical stresses such as during infections.
   a. If the metabolic needs of mother and fetus exceed the carbohydrate consumption and stores of the mother, then a "starvation" state may occur wherein maternal body fat becomes a major source of calories. Fat metabolism may result in the formation of "ketone bodies."
   b. The kidneys are very efficient in clearing ketones so that even if urinary ketones are moderate, it is unlikely that ketone levels in the blood are significantly elevated. However, if urinary ketones become highly positive, this may mean that acidemia is present. Therefore, maintaining urinary ketones less than moderate is a reasonable treatment goal.
   c. Fasting (before breakfast) urinary ketosis can be treated by simple interventions, such as an increase in the bedtime snack or 3 AM glass of milk. Because, for most women, the risk for relative "starvation" is greatest after an overnight fast, a single fasting urinary ketone test each morning may be the most cost-efficient way to detect women at risk for significant ketosis.
6. The total glycated hemoglobin (TGH) or hemoglobin A1C (Hgb A1C) determines the overall BS control for the previous 6 to 8 weeks.
   a. TGH/Hgb A1C may detect patients who had substantial elevations in BS before the glucose tolerance testing.
   b. If the initial blood testing indicates normal TGH/Hgb A1C, and if BS is found to be well controlled by home glucose monitoring, subsequent repeat TGH/Hgb A1C blood testing is usually not necessary.
   c. If the patient develops significant hyperglycemia or requires intensive insulin therapy, or if doubts exist as to the accuracy of home glucose monitoring, then repeat TGH/Hgb A1C blood level testing may be appropriate.
7. Fructosamine and glycated albumin blood levels are of questionable additional clinical benefit in most women with GDM.
8. After diagnosis through glucose tolerance testing, and after obtaining a baseline TGH/Hgb A1C, the best method for determining BS control is home glucose monitoring.

a. Many current home glucose monitoring meters are very user friendly and quite accurate.
b. Some companies may provide "loaner" glucose meters to help reduce cost.

Dietary Treatment

1. Many of the dietary recommendations for women with GDM are similar to the recommendations to any patient with DM. In general, women with GDM should be encouraged to adhere to healthy, low-concentrated sweet diets. If high blood pressure occurs, then reduction in dietary sodium is also important. Some recommendations unique to women with GDM include the following:
   a. To reduce the postprandial glycemic effects of carbohydrates, the recommended diet composition is 40% carbohydrate, 20% protein, and 40% fat.
   b. Women with GDM who are underweight should consume about 40 kcal/kg/day.
   c. Women with GDM at normal weight should consume about 30 kcal/kg/day.
   d. Women with GDM moderately overweight should consume about 25 kcal/kg/day.
   e. Women with GDM massively overweight should consume about 15 kcal/kg/day.
2. However, because the goals of DM control in GDM are often more rigid than for nonpregnant patients with type I or type II DM, dietary compliance and education about the glycemic response to foods is often essential.
   a. The glycemic response to mixed meals is most dependent on the amount (or percentage) of carbohydrates.
   b. The glycemic response to isolated foods may be anticipated by the "glycemic index" (Box 19-5).
   c. Perhaps the best method to educate patients of the glycemic properties of food is through intensive home glucose monitoring. Monitoring postprandial BS 3 times a day, 7 days a week, quickly educates women with GDM as to which foods result in postprandial hyperglycemia.
   d. If the woman with GDM declines to avoid foods with high glycemic potential, then it is recommended that such foods be incorporated into mixed meals. This may blunt glycemic excursions. For example, consumption of cornflakes, potatoes, or bread alone may cause unacceptable elevations in BS, suggesting the need of insulin treatment. However, if these foods are eaten with other foods, insulin treatment may not be needed.
3. To limit postprandial hyperglycemia and limit ketosis, it is often best to recommend spreading the daily caloric consumption to six small meals a day.

Insulin Treatment

1. If initial fasting BS on GTT is greater than 105 mg/dL, then insulin treatment is indicated, along with dietary counseling.

> **BOX 19-5 Glycemic Indexes of Some Foods**
>
> 80% to 90% Cornflakes, carrots, potatoes (instant or mashed), honey
> 70% to 79% Whole wheat or whole meal bread, white rice, potatoes
> 60% to 69% White bread, shredded wheat, brown rice, raisins, beets, bananas, Mars bar
> 50% to 59% Bran, many biscuits, white spaghetti, sweet corn, green peas, potato chips, sucrose, pastry
> 40% to 49% Oatmeal, whole meal spaghetti, sweet potatoes, navy beans, dry peas, grapes, oranges
> 30% to 39% Butter beans, chick and black-eyed peas, ice cream, milk, yogurt, tomatoes, apples, pears
> 20% to 29% Sausage, kidney beans, lentils, fructose, peaches, grapefruit, plums, cherries
> 10% to 19% Soybeans, peanuts
>
> The glycemic index (GI) is defined as the rise in blood sugar (BS) after ingestion of a fixed amount of a certain food, as determined for an individual. For example, if 100 g of glucose ingestion caused a rise in BS by 50 mg/dL, then this is the standard by which other foods are compared. If ingestion of another food caused only a 25 mg/dL rise in BS, then the GI would be 50%. (Please note that sucrose—table sugar—has a GI of about 50%.)

2. If initial fasting BS on GTT is less than 105 mg/dL, but the patient meets the criteria of GDM, then dietary treatment is attempted.
3. If, despite dietary treatment, the fasting BS exceeds 90 mg/dL, or if other goals of BS control are not achieved, then insulin therapy is indicated. In the past, it was commonplace that such women were admitted to the hospital for initiation of such therapy. However, because of the improvement in technology in home glucose monitoring, and the influence of health care systems, outpatient initiation of insulin therapy is becoming the rule.
4. Insulin does not cross the placenta and is not harmful to the fetus. However, insulin treatment of elevated BS in women with GDM has favorable effects on fetal and maternal outcome.
5. The choice of the initial dose of insulin should be based on BS readings. However, different providers may differ with regard to their preferences of insulin dosing, even given the same home glucose monitoring readings.
6. If a woman with GDM is initially found to have marked elevations in BS, and if access to appropriate diabetes education and instruction are not readily accessible, then hospitalization is indicated.
7. If a woman with GDM is initially found to have mild to moderately elevated BS despite diet and is able and willing to receive appropriate DM instruction, then beginning with small doses of insulin may be

the safest and most prudent way to initiate insulin therapy. Further adjustments in dosing can be made every 2 to 3 days afterward, based on the patient's home glucose monitoring.

Follow-Up During Pregnancy

1. Many women who develop GDM are recommended to monitor fasting and 1-hour or 2-hour postprandial BS, as well as fasting urinary ketones, throughout the pregnancy.
2. It is often recommended that women who maintain acceptable BS control with dietary therapy alone reduce their home glucose monitoring and urinary ketone testing to three or four times a week. This recommendation reduces the cost and inconvenience to the patient, yet maintains an acceptable level of monitoring.

Management During Labor and Delivery

1. For most women with diet-controlled GDM who deliver within a few hours of labor, no special treatment or evaluation is usually necessary other than glucose monitoring.
2. If the labor is prolonged, it is the goal that BS readings be maintained between 60 and 100 mg/dL. Furthermore, it is probably best that urinary ketones be kept no higher than moderate.
3. A practical strategy might include glucose monitoring performed every 2 hours until delivery.
   a. If the BS goes below 60 mg/dL and this is not as the result of a hypoglycemic reaction from previously administered insulin, then simply changing the intravenous fluids to something containing dextrose is often sufficient to stabilize the BS.
   b. If the BS exceeds 100 mg/dL, then a low-dose insulin drip (1 to 5 U/hr) is often the safest and easiest way to prevent hyperglycemia.
4. BS should be maintained less than 100 mg/dL during and at delivery to avoid fetal hypoglycemia.
5. Also, the potential for ketosis can be monitored by requesting that urine ketone testing be performed at each void.
   a. If the urinary ketones are found to be greater than moderate, then the patient may be entering into a "starvation state." Intravenous fluids should be changed to something that includes dextrose.
   b. If the BS level subsequently exceeds 100 mg/dL as result of the start of this intravenous dextrose, then an insulin drip should be initiated.
   c. It should be remembered that both glucose and insulin are necessary to prevent ketosis.

After Delivery

1. Once the child has been delivered, insulin therapy is no longer needed for the majority of insulin-treated women with GDM.
2. Some women (particularly if treated with significant amounts of insulin during their pregnancy) may have underlying type I or type II DM. For these women, close follow-up of BS after delivery is indicated.
3. A GTT is recommended 6 weeks postpartum, or when breast-feeding is stopped. At the very least, women with history of GDM should have fasting BS within weeks after delivery. During this postdelivery visit,

the likelihood of developing GDM during future pregnancies and the substantial risk of developing type II DM in the future should be emphasized in patient education.
  a. Women with a history of GDM should be encouraged to adopt and maintain lifestyle habits such as appropriate diet, attaining ideal body weight, and regular physical exercise.
  b. BS monitoring, possibly including GTT, should be performed before any future pregnancy.
  c. Periodic BS monitoring should be recommended to detect potential type II DM later in the mother's lifetime.

Miscellaneous Issues

1. The occasional high BS
   a. Particularly during initial dietary counseling, some women with GDM will experience an occasional high BS after meals as detected by home glucose monitoring.
   b. Little evidence supports that rare, mild, postprandial elevation in BS affords any significant adverse effect to the pregnancy.
   c. Therefore, although it is necessary to counsel women with GDM as to the need for strict BS control, it is also important to reassure them that, if the vast majority of BS levels are well within treatment goals, an occasional mild elevation in BS is unlikely to have any adverse effect on the unborn child.
2. Mixed versus premixed insulin
   a. Insulin administration ameliorates many of the metabolic abnormalities found in patients with DM. Numerous acceptable regimens have proven efficacy, as long as the goals of treatment are met.
   b. Some physicians make extensive use of the premixed insulins.
      (1) These include "70/30" preparations which contain 70% NPH (long acting), and 30% regular insulin (short acting).
      (2) There is a 50/50 premixed insulin preparation as well.
   c. Conversely, other physicians rarely use premixed insulin. They may feel that appropriate BS control can be achieved only through the greater flexibility of dosing achieved through the uncoupled, independent adjustment of moderately long-acting NPH or lente and short-acting regular insulin.
   d. In most cases, adequate achievement of glycemic controls can be achieved with either regimen. In either case, the goal is to reach a fasting BS of less than 90 mg/dL, and 1-hour postprandial BS of less than 140 mg/dL, or 2-hour postprandial BS less than 120 mg/dL.
3. Hypocaloric diets
   a. Pregnancy is not the time to enter into an aggressive, calorie-restricted dietary program for the sole purpose of losing weight.
   b. Most women gain about 25 pounds over the course of pregnancy.
   c. However, some overweight pregnant mothers may not gain or, in fact, may lose weight during pregnancy while adhering to the recommended diet. This is usually acceptable, as long as the weight loss is not excessive, is not the result of an underlying illness, is not caused by uncontrolled BS, and is not associated with positive urinary ketones.

d. Severe hypocaloric diets (such as greater than 50% caloric restriction) may result in significant urinary ketosis.
   e. Some studies suggest that less severe hypocaloric diets (such as a 33% caloric restriction) may prevent the need of insulin treatment and may result in minimal urinary ketosis.
4. Attitudes and realities of GDM and insulin administration
   a. Normalization of BS during pregnancy normalizes the risks of pregnancy complicated by DM.
   b. Most women with GDM are very willing and quite able to learn how to normalize BS with insulin.
   c. Some health care providers are reluctant to recommend insulin treatment to women with GDM for the purpose of normalizing BS.

DIABETES MELLITUS BEFORE PREGNANCY OR PREGESTATIONAL DIABETES MELLITUS

Concerns Before Conception

1. Just as among patients with DM in the general population, the range of BS control, the level of access to quality DM health care, the commitment to self-care, and the severity of the complications of DM vary among women with pregestational diabetes mellitus (PGDM).
2. Some women of childbearing potential may have BS well controlled with diet or oral DM drugs.
3. Some women in the childbearing years have "brittle" DM, with wide swings in BS and, possibly, significant complications of DM, including recurrent diabetes ketoacidosis, hyperosmolar states, retinopathy, neuropathy, nephropathy, cardiomyopathy, and dermopathy.
4. In either event, the risk to the mother and fetus of PGDM is greater than that of GDM. For this reason, one of the most important measures to prevent the complications affiliated with DM and pregnancy is appropriate DM education and treatment before conception.
5. Women with DM treated with diet should be instructed to monitor fasting and 1-hour or 2-hour postprandial BS for months before potential conception.
   a. If the woman's fasting BS exceeds 90 mg/dL, or if postprandial BS consistently exceeds 120 mg/dL, then she may be a candidate for insulin treatment before conception.
6. Women treated with oral DM drugs should be instructed to discontinue these medications months before potential conception and to closely monitor fasting BS and 1-hour or 2-hour postprandial BS for months before potential conception.
   a. If the woman's fasting BS exceeds 90 mg/dL, or if postprandial BS consistently exceeds 120 mg/dL, then she may be a candidate for insulin treatment before conception.
7. It has been suggested that oral DM drugs may cause congenital malformations in humans and in animals.
   a. Sulfonylureas such as glipizide and glyburide have shown no evidence of impaired fertility or harm to the fetus in rats and rabbits given 500 times the human dose.

b. Biguanides such as phenformin have been shown to produce neural tube closure defects, craniofacial hypoplasia, and other congenital malformations in a dose-dependent manner in rats.
c. Other biguanides, such as metformin, may not produce such effects.
d. Prolonged, severe hypoglycemia may occur in newborns whose mothers are treated with oral DM drugs at delivery.
e. Because no well-controlled clinical trials have demonstrated safety in humans with the use of oral DM drugs in pregnancy, such medications should be used only if the benefit is perceived to outweigh the potential risk.

8. For childbearing women with type I DM, "tight" BS control should be initiated before the potential for conception.
   a. In isolated cases, this may be achieved with diet and two shots of insulin per day.
   b. However, in most cases, women with type I DM who wish to become pregnant usually require intensive insulin regimens such as three or four shots of insulin per day, or the use of the insulin pump.

Risks

1. In general, the fetal and maternal risks associated with pregnancy in women with type I DM include those of women with GDM (see Gestational Diabetes Mellitus, Risks).
2. In addition, pregnancies complicated by type I DM have other, often more serious potential complications as well.
   a. Other fetal complications are as follows:
      (1) Fetal malformations or congenital anomalies (with or without spontaneous abortions) are the most common cause of perinatal death of the fetus in diabetic mothers.
      (2) The most common congenital defects include congenital heart disease and neural tube defects with caudal regression syndrome being the most common and most specific. Because these complications will have occurred within the first several weeks of pregnancy, it is crucial that women with type I diabetes inform their doctors for diabetes counseling before considering pregnancy.
      (3) Other potential congenital malformations include anencephalus, anal or rectal atresias, and renal abnormalities.
      (4) Infants of women with DM before pregnancy are also at risk for polycythemia, hypocalcemia, hyperbilirubinemia, respiratory distress syndrome, and hypoglycemia.
      (5) If BS control is good at the time of conception, the risk of fetal malformations is very low—only about 3% to 5%.
      (6) If BS is under very poor control at time of conception, the risks of fetal malformations is about 20% to 25%.
      (7) The percentage risk to the fetus of congenital malformations is roughly equal to the TGH/Hgb A1C. For example, studies have shown that women who conceive with glycated hemoglobin blood levels of 25% have approximately the same percentage risk of congenital malformations.

b. Other maternal complications are as follows:
   (1) For women with type I DM without complications, pregnancy has not been shown to increase the risk or progression of diabetes complications later in life.
   (2) Type I DM kidney or vascular disease increases the risk of spontaneous abortion and low birth weight.
   (3) Type I DM complications such as diabetes retinopathy, neuropathy, and nephropathy may substantially worsen during pregnancy. The risks of worsening diabetes complications should be incorporated in any counseling of diabetic women before conception.

Monitoring of the Woman with Diabetes Mellitus Before Pregnancy

1. If initial BS levels are under good control at conception (as documented by home glucose monitoring and TGH/Hgb A1C), then BS and urinary ketone measurements may be recommended similar to that of women with GDM (see Gestational Diabetes Mellitus). In some cases, BS may also need to be monitored before meals and at bedtime as well.
2. If initial BS levels are not under good control at conception or if the mother has difficulty in controlling BS ("brittle diabetes"), measurements may initially need to be performed before meals and at bedtime until better control is reached. Later during the pregnancy, after significant insulin resistance occurs (which may blunt wide glycemic excursions), BS may become easier to control. Insulin treatment decisions may then more safely be made on fasting BS, 1-hour postprandial BS, and 2-hour postprandial BS.
3. Dietary treatment: Dietary therapy is essentially the same as for women with GDM (described in Gestational Diabetes Mellitus).

Insulin Treatment

1. Hospitalization may be required if close outpatient follow-up and successful outpatient management of BS cannot be achieved.
2. "Tight" BS control is the goal for most pregnant mothers with type I DM. Women with type I DM should try to keep fasting (before breakfast) BS less than 90 mg/dL and 1-hour postprandial BS less than 140 mg/dL or 2-hour postprandial BS less than 120 mg/dL.
3. During the early months of pregnancy, optimal control of BS may not be safely obtainable, particularly among type I DM women with histories of widely unpredictable BS.
   a. If attempts at "tight control" are too aggressive, this may increase the risk of severe hypoglycemic reactions, possibly resulting in coma, seizures, car accidents, falls, etc.
   b. As the pregnancy progresses and insulin resistance develops (blunting glycemic excursions), the ability to control BS may improve.
4. In some cases, women with type I DM can achieve adequate BS control with an insulin regimen of two daily injections. However, in most cases, adequate BS control requires intensive insulin treatment of four daily injections, preferably started months before conception.

5. Insulin pump treatment is indicated if intensive insulin treatment is inadequate in achieving adequate BS control. The use of insulin pumps may not only improve BS control but may also reduce the frequency of hypoglycemic reactions.

Follow-Up During Pregnancy

1. In addition to close monitoring of BS, urinary ketones, and TGH/Hgb A1C, women with PGDM should be monitored for hypertension, which not only is more frequent but may also increase the progression of many of the complications of DM.
2. In women with PGDM, progression of prior DM eye disease may occur. Therefore, it is essential that all women with PGDM have eye examinations before conception and regularly during the pregnancy.
3. In women with PGDM, progression of prior neuropathy may occur. For example, DM gastroparesis or delayed stomach emptying may worsen during pregnancy, requiring hospitalization if feeding is not tolerated.

Management During Labor and Delivery

1. During labor, it is the goal that BS readings be maintained between 60 and 100 mg/dL. Furthermore, it is probably best that urinary ketones should be kept no higher than moderate.
2. A practical strategy might include glucose monitoring performed every 2 hours until delivery.
   a. If the BS goes below 60 mg/dL and this is not as the result of a hypoglycemic reaction from previously administered insulin, then simply changing the intravenous fluids to something containing dextrose is often sufficient to stabilize the BS.
   b. If the BS exceeds 100 mg/dL, then a low-dose insulin drip (1 to 5 U/hr) is often the safest and easiest way to prevent hyperglycemia.
3. BS should be maintained less than 100 mg/dL during and at delivery to avoid fetal hypoglycemia.
4. Also, the potential for ketosis can be monitored by requesting that urine ketone testing be performed every 2 hours, or at least at each void.
   a. If the urinary ketones are found to be greater than moderate, then the patient may be entering into a "starvation state." Intravenous fluids should then be changed to something that includes dextrose.
   b. If the BS level subsequently exceeds 100 mg/dL as result of the start of this intravenous dextrose, then an insulin drip should be initiated.
   c. It should be remembered that both glucose and insulin are necessary to prevent ketosis.

After Delivery

1. During active labor, the need for insulin therapy is markedly decreased. In fact, many women with DM before pregnancy often require little or no insulin for several hours to days after the delivery.

2. Nevertheless, in women with type I DM before pregnancy, the need for insulin treatment will soon return, necessitating close follow-up blood sugar monitoring.

Miscellaneous Issues

1. Breast-feeding
   a. If BS levels remain high after delivery (glucose levels consistently >140 to 180 mg/dL), the glucose may "spill" into breast milk.
   b. Excess sugar in breast milk has been suggested to cause the newborn to be overweight or overactive. It may also cause the baby to prefer sweets in the future.
   c. BS should be well controlled before and during breast-feeding.
2. Need for other testing
   a. Thyroid disease is more common in patients with type I diabetes.
      (1) Because thyroid disease often has few symptoms but can adversely affect the fetus, thyroid testing is recommended for pregnant women with type I diabetes.
      (2) However, thyroid scans should never be obtained during pregnancy.
   b. Women with PGDM with the National Diabetes Data Criteria class A1 and A2 diet may not require antepartum fetal "stress" or "non-stress" testing, if their blood sugars remain under acceptable control.
   c. On an individual basis, women with PGDM with class A2 insulin or class B insulin may benefit from weekly or biweekly NST or BPP around 32 to 34 weeks of pregnancy, especially if there is a suggestion of intrauterine growth restriction, hypertension, poorly controlled BS, or decreased or increased amniotic fluid volumes.
   d. In high-risk pregnant women with PGDM (class R or F), particularly if associated with a growth-retarded fetus, hypertension, poorly controlled BS, or increase or decrease in amniotic fluid, antepartum testing may start as early as 26 to 28 weeks and may be performed more frequently.
3. Drugs that affect BS
   a. Many drugs can increase BS in women with PGDM. For example, terbutaline and betamethasone may substantially increase BS in susceptible women.
   b. Although it has been suggested that some oral diabetes drugs may eventually prove beneficial in women with DM, these drugs have yet to be approved during pregnancy.
4. Glucosuria
   a. Glucosuria may result when BS exceeds 160 to 200 mg/dL.
   b. Because the timing of the onset of action of insulin delivered by subcutaneous insulin administration may not identically match the insulin secretion from a normal pancreas, glucosuria may result.
   c. Even in those patients with otherwise excellent BS control, some asynchrony of the timing of insulin action and insulin need is not uncommon. This may account for the occasional finding of significant glucosuria in a woman with type I DM who has excellent

Practical Guide to the Care of the Gynecologic/Obstetric Patient 395

TGH/Hgb A1C, and excellent BS recorded by home glucose monitoring.
d. One method to improve the match of the hypoglycemic effects of insulin and the hyperglycemic effects of meals is to administer insulin ½ to 1 hour before meals.
e. Shorter-acting insulin may soon be available that may improve the ability to better match the timing of insulin action and insulin need.

PRACTICAL EXAMPLES
See Tables 19-4 through 19-7.

19.3 Intrauterine Growth Retardation

Mark Williams

SIGNIFICANCE

1. Low birth weight (LBW) is a worldwide problem.
    a. Usually defined as birth weight less than 2500 g, irrespective of gestational age
    b. Associated with increased perinatal morbidity and mortality
    c. Widely used as marker of increased neonatal risk
    d. Not an ideal marker of fetal growth and development
        (1) Combines both prematurity and varying degrees of growth retardation
2. Morbidity is associated with LBW and growth retardation.
    a. Twenty-one million LBW babies a year are born internationally, 90% in developing countries.
    b. Proportion of LBWs varies by type of society.
        (1) 3% to 12% rates of LBW in developed countries; 60% premature, 40% growth retarded
        (2) 12% to 40% rates of LBW in developing countries; 20% premature, 80% growth retarded
    c. There are high rates of perinatal morbidity in growth-retarded infants.
        (1) Perinatal depression is three times more likely.
        (2) Hypoglycemia is four to six times more likely.
        (3) Hypothermia is five times more likely.
        (4) Meconium aspiration is 13 times more likely.
        (5) Fetal distress in labor is six times more likely.
3. Components of LBW are as follows:
    a. Proportion of LBW varies by gestational age:
        (1) Of infants at 32 to 33 weeks gestation, 90% are LBW.
        (2) Of infants at 34 to 35 weeks gestation, 50% are LBW.
        (3) Of infants at 37 to 38 weeks gestation, 10% are LBW.
    b. Degree of growth retardation increases as gestational age increases.
4. It is important to distinguish between prematurity and degrees of growth retardation to better understand the etiology of perinatal morbidity and mortality.

Table 19-4 Illustrative Blood Sugar* Level Presentations of Women with Gestational Diabetes Treated with Diet Only

Example 1: Fasting Hyperglycemia

Fasting Urine Ketones[†]	Fasting Blood Sugar (mg/dL)	After-Breakfast Blood Sugar (mg/dL)	After-Lunch Blood Sugar (mg/dL)	After-Supper Blood Sugar (mg/dL)
Large	90-110	110-125	100-120	100-120

Comment and insulin recommendations: This woman with GDM (treated with diet alone) shows a common presentation of morning hyperglycemia with fasting urinary ketosis. A possible insulin regimen may include 6 U of NPH or lente at supper or bedtime. These long-acting insulins, given in the evening, would be expected to lower morning blood sugar (BS) and resolve ketosis. Further adjustments or increases in insulin doses are made based on future BS readings.

Example 2: After-Supper Hyperglycemia

Fasting Urine Ketones[†]	Fasting Blood Sugar (mg/dL)	After-Breakfast Blood Sugar (mg/dL)	After-Lunch Blood Sugar (mg/dL)	After-Supper Blood Sugar (mg/dL)
Mild	80-100	100-120	100-120	120-160

Comment and insulin recommendations: This woman with GDM (treated with diet alone) shows a common presentation of after-supper hyperglycemia, accompanied by mild, occasional increases in morning BS. A possible insulin regimen may include 6 U of regular insulin at supper. This short-acting insulin would be expected to lower after-supper BS. And lowering the evening BS may have residual effect on the morning BS and urinary ketone levels. Alternatively, a combined regimen of 3 NPH or lente and 3 U regular, or 6 U of 50/50 insulin, may also have favorable effects on both the after-supper and before-breakfast BS, and fasting urinary ketone levels. Further adjustments or increases in insulin doses are made based on future BS readings.

*"Blood sugar" represents a range of glucose blood levels as determined by home glucose monitoring for several days, after dietary counseling.
[†]"Fasting urine ketones" represents self-urine ketone testing by urine monitoring strips before breakfast.
GDM, Gestational diabetes mellitus.

Table 19-5. **Illustrative Blood Sugar Level Presentation of a Woman with Pregestational Diabetes Mellitus Before Conception Treated with a Twice-a-Day Insulin Regimen (Before-Breakfast and Before-Supper Split Dose NPH or Lente and Regular Insulin)**

Example 1: Variable Blood Sugar After Supper

Fasting Urine Ketones	FBS (mg/dL)	PPBrkPS (mg/dL)	ACLunBS (mg/dL)	PPLunBS (mg/dL)	ACSupBS (mg/dL)	PPSupBS (mg/dL)	Bedtime BS (mg/dL)
Mild	60-180	80-120	60-100	80-120	60-100	100-180	60-180

Comment and insulin recommendations: This woman, with diabetes before pregnancy (treated with before-breakfast and before-supper insulin) presents with variable blood sugar (BS) levels after supper and before breakfast. Because the BS levels are sometimes low at bedtime, increasing the before-supper regular insulin may increase the risk of bedtime hypoglycemia. Therefore, it may be recommended that supper meals be more consistent in composition, particularly with regard to amount and type of carbohydrates. However, another strategy may be to recommend three or four shots of insulin in a day. Three shots of insulin in a day would likely include (1) before-breakfast NPH or lente mixed with regular, (2) before-supper regular, and (3) bedtime NPH or lente. This would allow greater flexibility in insulin dosing, particularly before supper. Four shots of insulin in a day may include before-meal regular, with nighttime NPH or lente. Before-breakfast NPH is also sometimes mixed with before-breakfast regular in patients treated with four shots of insulin in a day. Afterward, further adjustments or increases in insulin doses are made based on future blood sugar readings.

ACLunBS, Anteciba (before) lunch blood sugar; ACSupBS, before-supper blood sugar; FBS, fasting blood sugar; PPBrkBS, postprandial breakfast blood sugar; PPLunBS, postprandial lunch blood sugar; PPSupBS, postprandial supper blood sugar.

Table 19-6 Illustrative Blood Sugar Level Presentations of Women with Type I Diabetes Mellitus Before Conception Treated with a Four-Times-a-Day Insulin Regimen (Premeal Regular and Nighttime NPH or Lente)

Example 1: Gradually Increasing Blood Sugars

Fasting Urine Ketones	FBS (mg/dL)	PPBrkBS (mg/dL)	ACLunBS (mg/dL)	PPLunBS (mg/dL)	ACSupBS (mg/dL)	PPSupBS (mg/dL)	Bedtime BS (mg/dL)
Negative	60-90	80-120	90-110	90-130	100-140	100-140	80-120

Comment and insulin recommendations: This woman, with diabetes before pregnancy treated with intensive, four-times-a-day insulin (premeal regular—before breakfast, before lunch, and before supper—and bedtime NPH or lente) presents with a gradual increase in before-meal blood sugars and a gradual increase in postprandial blood sugars throughout the day. One option would be to increase the before-lunch and before-supper regular insulin. Another option would be to add NPH or lente to before-breakfast regular insulin.

Example 2: Unpredictable Blood Sugars

Fasting Urine Ketones	FBS (mg/dL)	PPBrkBS (mg/dL)	ACLunBS (mg/dL)	PPLunBS (mg/dL)	ACSupBS (mg/dL)	PPSupBS (mg/dL)	Bedtime BS (mg/dL)
Negative	40-150	80-200	40-150	80-200	40-150	80-200	40-150

Comment and insulin recommendations: This woman, with diabetes before pregnancy treated with intensive, four-times-a-day insulin treatment (premeal regular—before breakfast, before lunch, and before supper—and bedtime NPH or lente) presents with wide fluctuations in blood sugars. Any increase in before-meal insulin may result in hypoglycemia before the next meal or at bedtime. Therefore, recommendations would include improved dietary compliance and better adjustment of regular insulin dosing based on blood sugar, amount and type of carbohydrate consumption, anticipated level of physical activity, anticipated amount of physical or mental stress, etc. If these measures are not successful, then the use of an insulin pump should be considered.

ACLunBS, Anteciba (before) lunch blood sugar; *ACSupBS*, before-supper blood sugar; *FBS*, fasting blood sugar; *PPBrkBS*, postprandial breakfast blood sugar; *PPLunBS*, postprandial lunch blood sugar; *PPSupBS*, postprandial supper blood sugar.

Table 19-7 **Illustrative Blood Sugar Level Presentation of a Woman with Type I Diabetes Mellitus Before Conception, Treated with Insulin Pump**

Example 1: Fasting Hyperglycemia

Fasting Urine Ketones	FBS (mg/dL)	PPBrkBS (mg/dL)	ACLunBS (mg/dL)	PPLunBS (mg/dL)	ACSupBS (mg/dL)	PPSupBS (mg/dL)	Bedtime BS (mg/dL)	2 AM
Mild	90-120	80-120	60-110	80-120	60-110	80-120	60-110	60-110

Comment and insulin recommendations: This woman is treated with an insulin pump. She is receiving basal rate insulin and bolus insulin. Her basal insulin includes 2.0 U of regular insulin per hour between 7 AM and 10 PM, 1.0 U regular insulin per hour between 10 PM and 3 AM, and 2.5 U regular insulin per hour between 3 AM and 7 AM. She also receives bolus insulin based on her blood sugar (BS), amount and composition of meals, anticipated exercise, and anticipated physical and mental stress. Her BS levels demonstrate fasting hyperglycemia with mild ketosis. This suggests a persistent effect of the "dawn phenomenon," despite the increased insulin basal rate of 3 AM to 7 AM. A reasonable approach would be to further increase the 3 AM to 7 AM basal rate.

ACLunBS, Anteciba (before) lunch blood sugar; *ACSupBS*, before-supper blood sugar; *FBS*, fasting blood sugar; *PPBrkBS*, postprandial breakfast blood sugar; *PPLunBS*, postprandial lunch blood sugar; *PPSupBS*, postprandial supper blood sugar.

PATTERNS OF GROWTH

1. General concepts
   a. Two overlapping periods of fetal cellular activity—cellular hyperplasia and cellular hypertrophy—result in three phases of fetal growth and development.
      (1) First phase, occurring from 4 to 20 weeks gestation, is characterized by proportional increases in fetal weight, protein content, and DNA content (cellular hyperplasia).
      (2) Second phase, occurring from 20 to 28 weeks gestation, is characterized by increases in protein and weight and lesser increases in fetal DNA content (hyperplasia and concomitant hypertrophy).
      (3) Third phase, occurring from 28 weeks to term, is characterized by continued increases in fetal protein and weight but no increase in DNA content (hypertrophy).
   b. Population data
      (1) Numerous delivery populations have been described.
         (a) All populations show generally similar growth curves.
         (b) Infants from generally larger (sea level) populations weigh approximately 10% more than infants from smaller (altitude) populations in given racial, gender, gestational age, and birth weight for gestational age centile groups.
      (2) Fetal weight has a sigmoid growth pattern. Linear growth occurs between 24 and 37 weeks gestation.
      (3) Fetuses tend to maintain a given centile range during pregnancy.
      (4) Increased variation in birth weights is noted in postterm infants.
      (5) Absolute birth weights drop in postterm infants.
   c. Timing of the insult to the fetus (predisposes to the type of growth retardation)
      (1) Early insults usually result in symmetric growth retardation, probably by restricting fetal cellular hyperplasia.
      (2) Third-trimester insults restrict cellular hypertrophy; usually result in asymmetric growth retardation.
         (a) Uteroplacental insufficiency and other similar insults result in stresses on the fetus that cause the fetus to redistribute blood flow, maintaining perfusion of the head, heart, and adrenal glands.
         (b) Particularly severe insults to the fetus may cause asymmetric growth retardation to progress to symmetric growth retardation, as redistribution of blood flow fails to maintain growth of the head.
   d. Multiple gestation
      (1) Twins and higher order multiple gestation infants are at increased risk of growth retardation.
         (a) Increased rates of LBW for gestational age
         (b) Increased rates of asymmetric growth restriction (abnormally lean body morphology)

(2) Twins have distinct patterns of growth.
   (a) Growth patterns generally overlap singletons until 32 weeks gestation.
   (b) Twins do not maintain singleton average birth weight growth in the last 6 to 8 weeks of pregnancy.
   (c) The value of separate growth tables for twins is controversial.
   (d) Discordance of more than 20% to 25% in birth weight relative to the larger twin is associated with IUGR and increased perinatal morbidity.

DEFINITIONS OF GROWTH RETARDATION

1. Ideal criteria not well established
   a. Birth weight and length vary by many factors.
      (1) Gestational age (term > preterm)
      (2) Gender (male > female)
      (3) Ethnicity (white > black)
      (4) Multiple gestations (singletons > multiples)
      (5) Altitude (low altitude > high altitude)
      (6) Others (see later text)
   b. Some data are poorly documented.
      (1) Accuracy of gestational age assessment may vary.
      (2) Measures such as crown-to-heel length at term may be inaccurate.
      (3) Some measures of neonatal nutritional status are not always obtained.
         (a) Crown-to-heel length
         (b) Midarm circumference
         (c) Skin fold thickness
2. Gestational age assessment
   a. It is necessary to assign centile rankings of fetal weight properly by gestational age.
   b. Dubowitz scoring of infants often varies 1 or 2 weeks from menstrual dating; unavailable until after delivery of infant.
   c. Obstetric dating is often inaccurate: 15% of patients with proper dating criteria have sonographic dating findings that differ by more than 2 weeks from menstrual dating determinations.
3. Prenatal sonographic estimation of fetal weight
   a. Accuracy limited to ±15%
   b. Should be used with caution
   c. Accuracy less at extremes of estimated weight
   d. Decreased accuracy if fetal positioning precludes accurate measurements or if oligohydramnios is present
4. Types of markers of neonatal growth and development include the following:
   a. Absolute measures
      (1) Example: LBW
      (2) Reproducible
      (3) Tend to "lump" prematurity and growth retardation into the same marker

b. Birth weight relative to gestational age, gender, ethnicity, etc.
   (1) Examples include the following:
      (a) Small for gestational age (LBW centile for gestational age)
      (b) Low fetal growth ratio (observed birth weight/adjusted birth weight)
   (2) Gestational age is not always accurately documented.
c. Body symmetry relative to gestational age
   (1) Examples include the following:
      (a) Ponderal index
      (b) Weight/length ratio
      (c) Body mass index (BMI)
      (d) Midarm circumference/head circumference ratio
   (2) Require gestational age and another body measure, such as length or midarm circumference. Need for other measures increases possibility of erroneous values.
   (3) Identify abnormal growth patterns independent of absolute birth weight.
   (4) Identify groups of infants with otherwise normal birth weights who are at increased risk for perinatal mortality and morbidity; they have sixfold to tenfold increases in rates of hypoglycemia, perinatal depression, meconium aspiration, and prolonged hospitalization.
   (5) Ponderal index may be better correlate of perinatal morbidity than birth weight for gestational age.
5. Correlation between markers and neonatal outcome
   a. Birth weight centile is the most commonly used marker of neonatal status.
   b. Some argue that markers incorporating weight for length, such as the weight/length ratio, may be better correlates of neonatal morbidity than LBW centile for gestational age.
6. Indices of growth retardation
   a. Small for gestational age (low percentile birth weight for gestational age)
      (1) Most commonly used method of neonatal and fetal assessment.
         (a) Birth weight less than 10% for gestational age usually used in the United States
         (b) Birth weight less than 2 SD (birth weight <2.5%) often used in Europe
      (2) Sensitivity and specificity can be adjusted by choice of centile range for population screening versus more specific categorization of growth-retarded infants.
   b. Low birth weight (<2500 g)
      (1) Commonly used criterion to screen for neonatal risk
      (2) Robust, as error in weight determination is minimal
      (3) Confounded by conflicting influences of prematurity and growth retardation
      (4) Does not require accurate knowledge of gestational age
   c. Fetal growth ratio (FGR)

(1) FGR = observed birth weight/adjusted mean birth weight.
(2) Reference mean values for gestational age are relatively easy to determine.
(3) Adjustments for gender and ethnicity are easy to determine.
(4) Correlates well with birth weight centiles.
   (a) FGR less than 0.90 occurs in 18% of patients.
   (b) FGR less than 0.85 occurs in 9.0% of patients.
   (c) FGR less than 0.80 occurs in 4.3% of patients.
   (d) FGR less than 0.75 occurs in 1.7% of patients.

d. Ponderal index
   (1) Ponderal index = 100 (birth weight in g)/(length in cm)^3.
   (2) Ponderal index requires length, as well as other standard data regarding birth weight, gestational age, and occasionally race and gender.
   (3) Use of body length in ratios may decrease sensitivity of marker because of inaccuracy often associated with crown-to-heel measurements. Use of cubed length term may further decrease accuracy of this marker.
   (4) Index varies by gestational age, and by gender and ethnicity to a much smaller degree (Table 19-8).
   (5) Low ponderal index, a marker of asymmetric growth restriction, is associated with increased perinatal morbidity.

e. Weight/length ratio
   (1) Weight/length = birth weight in g/length in cm.
   (2) This requires length, as well as other standard data regarding birth weight, gestational age, and occasionally race and gender.
   (3) Use of body length in ratios may decrease sensitivity of marker because of inaccuracy often associated with crown-to-heel measurements.
   (4) Ratio varies by gestational age, and by gender and ethnicity to a much smaller degree.
   (5) Weight/length ratio less than 5% or 10%, asymmetric growth restriction, is associated with increased perinatal morbidity.

f. BMI
   (1) BMI = birth weight in g/(length in cm)^2.
   (2) BMI requires length as well as other standard data regarding birth weight, gestational age, and occasionally race and gender.
   (3) Use of body length in ratios may decrease sensitivity of marker because of inaccuracy often associated with crown-to-heel measurements.
   (4) BMI varies by gestational age, and by gender and ethnicity to a much smaller degree.
   (5) BMI has not been extensively evaluated as a marker of neonatal status.

g. Midarm circumference/head circumference (MAC/HC).
   (1) HC/MAC = head circumference/midarm circumference.
   (2) Possibly a better marker of neonatal status than ratios of weight to length or birth weight for gestational age.
   (3) Varies by gestational age (Table 19-9).

Table 19-8 Ponderal Index

Weeks	10%	3%
30 weeks	2.05	2.00
32 weeks	2.10	2.05
34 weeks	2.15	2.10
36 weeks	2.23	2.15
≥38 weeks	2.30	2.20

7. Markers for abnormal fetal growth in multiple gestation
   a. Discordance in estimated sonographic fetal weights of 20% to 25% using the larger twin as the index case
   b. Intratwin pair differences in biparietal diameter: greater than 5 mm
   c. Intratwin pair differences in abdominal circumference: greater than 20 mm
   d. Intratwin pair differences in femur length: greater than 4 mm
8. Sonographic (antenatal) markers of abnormal fetal growth
   a. Estimated fetal weight
      (1) Many formulas are available.
      (2) Combinations of biparietal diameter, head circumference, and femur length with the abdominal circumference should be used.
      (3) Estimated fetal weight is generally accurate to ±15% (larger margins of error at extremes of weight range and if oligohydramnios is present).
   b. Head circumference/abdominal circumference ratio
      (1) This ratio is useful to detect asymmetric growth restriction caused by "head sparing effect" active in most cases of growth retardation late.
      (2) Values vary by gestational age.
   c. Femur length/abdomen circumference ratio
      (1) Minimal variation is seen during pregnancy: 0.224 ± 0.015 (mean ±1 SD).
      (2) The ratio is altered if skeletal dysplasia is present.
9. Doppler sonography: Systolic/diastolic flow velocity ratios correlate with placental resistance.

Table 19-9 Midarm Circumference/Head Circumference

Weeks	MAC/HC (±1 SD)
30	0.23 (0.02)
32	0.24 (0.02)
34	0.26 (0.02)
36	0.27 (0.01)
38	0.28 (0.01)
40	0.29 (0.02)
42	0.30 (0.01)

a. Decrease over the course of pregnancy.
  b. Increased values for gestational age indicate increased placental resistance.
  c. Absent or reversed end diastolic flow is often associated with imminent fetal compromise. Reversed flow has occasionally been noted to resolve.
  d. Fetuses with estimated fetal weights in the growth retarded range and normal Doppler flow indices are at increased risk of aneuploidy.

CAUSES OF GROWTH RETARDATION

1. Incorrect dates
   a. Overestimation of gestational age causes centile birth weight to be lower than is actually the case.
   b. Underestimation of gestational age may mask the presence of growth retardation.
2. Aneuploidy
   a. Autosomal trisomies
      (1) Trisomy 13
      (2) Trisomy 18
      (3) Trisomy 21
   b. Triploidy
   c. Turner's syndrome
   d. Extra sex (X) chromosomes (47 XXY, etc.): Average birth weight decreases by 300 g per each additional X chromosome.
   e. Autosomal deletion syndromes
      (1) 5p- (cri du chat)
      (2) 5q-
      (3) 4p-
      (4) 4q-
      (5) 18p-
      (6) 18q-
      (7) Others
3. Open neural tube disorders
4. Renal agenesis
5. Chondrodystrophies
6. Single umbilical artery
7. Maternal factors
   a. Medical conditions
      (1) Advanced stage diabetes (>White class B)
      (2) Collagen vascular disease
         (a) Polymyositis or dermatomyositis
         (b) Systemic lupus erythematosus
      (3) Cyanotic heart disease
      (4) Hypertension
      (5) Renal disease (chronic) without hypertension
      (6) Thyrotoxicosis
   b. Obstetric factors
      (1) Pregnancy-induced hypertension
      (2) Primigravidity

(3) Prior miscarriage, stillborn, or growth-retarded infant
(4) Multiple gestation
c. Medications
  (1) Chemotherapeutic antimetabolites
  (2) Coumadin
  (3) Phenytoin
  (4) Systemic steroid usage
d. Socioeconomic factors
  (1) Poor nutritional status
    (a) Low prepregnancy weight
    (b) Low pregnancy weight gain
    (c) Dietary deficiencies (zinc, others?)
  (2) Substance abuse
    (a) Tobacco
    (b) Ethanol
    (c) Drugs
e. Ethnicity
f. Infection
  (1) Bacterial
    (a) Listeria
    (b) Malaria
    (c) Syphilis
    (d) Toxoplasmosis
    (e) Tuberculosis
  (2) Viral
    (a) Cytomegalovirus
    (b) Rubella

DETECTION OF GROWTH RETARDATION

1. Firm obstetric dates should be established.
   a. Dates are established on the first obstetric visit.
   b. Dating should be modified later in gestation with caution and always with proper documentation.
   c. Menstrual and sonographic dating information must be coordinated.
      (1) Sonograms are generally accurate to within 10% of the composite gestational age.
      (2) Sonography before 22 to 24 weeks gestation is relatively reliable for the purposes of pregnancy dating.
         (a) If a reliable menstrual history of completely regular cycles for the prior 3 months, no hormonal interventions for at least 3 months, and certain dating of the last normal menses is obtained, menstrual dating is accepted if those dates place the gestational age within 10% of the ultrasonographic dates.
         (b) Even if all criteria in 1.c.(2).(a). are met, but the sonographic dating places the gestational age more than 10% earlier or later, the sonographic dating criteria are accepted.

- (c) In the first trimester, trisomy 18 causes significant growth retardation but is sufficiently rare that it does not cause significant problems with pregnancy dating in the first half of pregnancy.
- (3) Sonography after 22 to 24 weeks gestation to establish pregnancy dating can allow cases of early fetal growth disturbances to go undiagnosed.
    - (a) Caution should be used if sonographic dating after 22 to 24 weeks gestation is necessary.
    - (b) If significant disparity is present between sonographic fetal dating information and menstrual dating information, it may be necessary to perform interval fetal surveillance until serial growth measures allow distinctions between incorrect dating and growth retardation to be made. Factors that should heighten concern for significant growth retardation include oligohydramnios, presence of fetal anomalies, and asymmetric growth indices (abnormally small abdominal circumference for gestation or abnormally elevated HC/AC or femur length [FL]/abdominal circumference [AC] ratios)
    - (c) Symmetric growth retardation will be categorized as having a gestational age less than the actual value if no other credible dating information is available, and symmetric growth retardation will escape detection in such circumstances.
    - (d) Early macrosomic fetal growth trends may cause an overestimate of the gestational age.
2. The risk of growth retardation in the pregnancy should be evaluated based on initial history, physical findings, and laboratory evaluations of the patient.
    a. Although commonly employed and inexpensive, fundal height assessment has an unacceptably low negative predictive value for growth retardation in high-risk populations, such as hypertensives, insulin-dependent diabetics, and patients with collagen vascular disorders.
    b. Serial sonographic evaluations during the pregnancy should be considered if a significant risk of growth retardation exists.
3. Methods of serial assessment include the following:
    a. Weight gain: Monitoring the patient's weight gain and ensuring minimum standards are achieved
    b. Fundal height measurements
        (1) The symphyseal to fundal height measurement (in cm) approximates the menstrual gestational age in weeks from 20 weeks to approximately 37 weeks.
            (a) Less reliable if the maternal body habitus is obese
            (b) Not useful in multiple gestations
        (2) Sonography is used to evaluate deviations of more than 3 cm in fundal height from expected values.
        (3) Sonography detects approximately 50% to 60% of cases of growth retardation.

- (a) Suitable for screening of low-risk populations
- (b) Not sufficiently reliable as the only screening modality in patients at high risk of growth retardation
- c. Serial sonographic estimated fetal weights
  - (1) Gestational age should be established, preferably in the first trimester.
  - (2) Estimated fetal weight should be assessed after 24 weeks, at 3-week to 6-week intervals. Intervals of less than 2 weeks may fail to detect ongoing growth.
  - (3) Various parameters are useful to assess fetal growth.
    - (a) Estimated fetal weight for gestational age
    - (b) Abdominal circumference
    - (c) Ratios of head circumference or femur length to abdominal circumference
- d. Doppler sonography
  - (1) Normal Doppler waveforms indicate normal placental resistance.
  - (2) Normal waveforms in growth retardation:
    - (a) May indicate genetic predisposition to small fetal size
    - (b) Indicate increased risk of aneuploidy
  - (3) Doppler sonography is not useful for screening in low-risk populations.

MANAGEMENT OF GROWTH RETARDATION

1. Accuracy of obstetric dating must be determined. Dating should be reassigned with care.
2. Possibility of aneuploidy should be considered.
   a. Symmetric growth retardation is often associated with aneuploidy.
   b. Normal umbilical Doppler flow or normal amniotic fluid volume in fetuses with apparent ultrasonographic growth retardation indicate increased risk for aneuploidy.
   c. Negative targeted sonograms decrease likelihood of syndromes associated with high rates of structural anomalies, such as trisomy 13 or 18.
   d. Negative targeted sonograms in syndromes with low rates of detectable sonographic anomalies, such as trisomy 21, do not appreciably lower the a priori risk of this in a given pregnancy.
   e. Karyotypic evaluation by amniocentesis, placental biopsy, umbilical arterial blood sampling, and occasionally karyotype from the fetal urinary bladder are possible if documentation of the fetal karyotype is judged necessary.
3. Clinical circumstances must be evaluated.
   a. Is the index of suspicion for severe growth retardation and imminent fetal death high?
   b. Do the potential benefits of ongoing fetal assessment and (hopefully) continued growth and development sufficiently balance the perceived risks of continuing the pregnancy?
      (1) Benefits of delaying delivery
         (a) Allows time to reassess interval growth and possibly identify cases of incorrect dating

- (b) Allows time for further growth of the fetus and maturation of critical fetal organ systems
- (c) Decreases subsequent need for neonatal care
- (d) Increases likelihood of subsequent labor induction, if necessary

(2) Risks of delaying delivery
- (a) Ongoing disease processes may put fetus at risk of increased morbidity or mortality.
- (b) Temporization in fetuses near term or at term gestation may not yield any significant gain in growth, development, or maturation of fetal organ systems.
- (c) Cases of falsely diagnosed growth retardation (i.e., incorrectly dated pregnancies) may receive unnecessary interventions, including cesarean delivery after failed induction of labor.
- (d) Increases the need for emergency (cesarean) delivery if fetal status unexpectedly deteriorates.

c. Common clinical presentations
  (1) Size–dates discrepancy noted in the third trimester; no early sonogram
  (a) Presentation
    (i) A patient presents for care in the mid–second trimester and no significant disparity between menstrual dating and physical examination findings (16-cm fundal height at 18 weeks gestation) is noted.
    (ii) Maternal serum alpha-feloprotein (MSAFP) testing shows a low normal value (0.6 multiple of median [MOM]).
    (iii) Menstrual dates are accepted.
    (iv) The pregnancy progresses and a fundal height discrepancy is noted at 32 weeks gestation by dates (28-cm fundal height).
    (v) A sonogram is performed that shows biparietal diameter, head circumference, abdominal circumference, and femur length all approximately 28-week size, and amniotic fluid volume is normal.
    (vi) Doppler flow indices show normal diastolic flow.
  (b) Differential diagnosis
    (i) Symmetric growth retardation (rare)
    (ii) Incorrect dates (very common)
  (c) Plan
    (i) Patient is questioned regarding accuracy of menstrual dating.
    (ii) If history remains consistent with reliable dates, fetal electronic assessment weekly, weekly amniotic fluid assessment, and a follow-up sonogram in 3 weeks to assess for interval growth are considered.
    (iii) Amniocentesis for karyotype may also be a consideration, depending on maternal age and sonographic findings.

(iv) If normal interval growth for a 28-week-gestation fetus occurs, the most likely diagnosis is incorrect dates.
(v) If inadequate growth occurs, growth retardation is more likely.
(vi) If growth retardation appears likely, careful evaluation with serial fetal assessment and delivery when risks to the fetus appear to outweigh perceived benefit of waiting are done.
(vii) Severe degrees of growth retardation may increase the clinical utility of karyotypic evaluation.

(2) Size–dates discrepancy; early sonographic dating
   (a) Presentation
      (i) A patient presents for care in the mid–second trimester and no significant disparity between menstrual dating and physical examination findings (16-cm fundal height at 18 weeks gestation) is noted.
      (ii) MSAFP testing is low (0.4 MOM).
      (iii) Ultrasonography in preparation for genetic amniocentesis reveals biparietal diameter, head circumference, and femur length consistent with 15 weeks gestation at the time of MSAFP testing, when 18 weeks gestation had been assumed.
      (iv) The 3-week disparity is greater than 10% of the menstrual dating gestational age, and sonographic dates are accepted.
      (v) The MSAFP is recomputed based on new dating information, and a new MSAFP value of 0.7 MOM is determined.
      (vi) The pregnancy continues and fundal height discrepancy is noted at 32 weeks gestation by dates (28-cm fundal height).
      (vii) A sonogram is performed that shows biparietal diameter, head circumference, abdominal circumference, and femur length all approximate 28-week size, and amniotic fluid volume is normal.
      (viii) Doppler flow indices show normal diastolic flow.
   (b) Diagnosis: symmetric growth retardation
   (c) Comment: Because of the mid–second trimester sonography, the dating of the pregnancy is firmly established and, in rare cases, adjustment of the dates to a lower value may have temporarily masked the presence of early fetal growth retardation (sometimes associated with aneuploidies such as trisomy 18). The normal Doppler flow pattern indicates that placental (vascular) disease is not likely the cause and increases the risk of aneuploidy.
   (d) Plan
      (i) Targeted sonography is performed; electronic fetal assessment, serial evaluation of amniotic fluid volume, and interval sonography for fetal growth are begun, in 2 to 3 weeks.

- (ii) Amniocentesis should be considered for karyotype.
- (iii) Given the presentation, it is unlikely that growth will normalize.
- (iv) The principal goal of surveillance is to allow adequate time to exclude the presence of semilethal aneuploidies such as trisomy 13, trisomy 18, and triploidy.
- (v) If such aneuploidies are detected, cesarean section for fetal distress is not recommended, after careful explanation of the rationale for avoiding such surgery, where it will provide minimal fetal benefit and much more potential for maternal harm.
- (vi) Delivery should be considered if fetal assessment yields information suggesting imminent fetal compromise before documenting the fetal karyotype.
- (vii) If a normal fetal karyotype is present, timing of delivery will depend on results of ongoing fetal assessment, cervical ripeness for induction, degree of growth retardation (i.e., perceived fetal risk), and gestational age.

(3) Size–dates discrepancy; late access to care
  (a) Presentation
   (i) A patient presents for care in the third trimester and no significant disparity between menstrual dating and physical examination findings (26-cm fundal height at 28 weeks gestation) is noted, although the patient's recollection of her menstrual history is somewhat unclear.
   (ii) No sonographic assessment is performed.
   (iii) The pregnancy continues and, 4 weeks later, a fundal height discrepancy is noted at 32 weeks gestation by dates (28-cm fundal height).
   (iv) A sonogram is performed that shows biparietal diameter, head circumference, abdominal circumference, and femur length all approximately 28-week size, and the amniotic fluid volume is normal.
   (v) Doppler flow indices show normal diastolic flow.
  (b) Differential diagnosis
   (i) Symmetric growth retardation (rare)
   (ii) Incorrect dates (very common)
  (c) Comment
   (i) Because of the lack of any proper dating criteria, accurate pregnancy dating is impossible.
   (ii) Because of the rarity of symmetric growth retardation and the high incidence of incorrect dating in such circumstances, the likelihood of significant fetal pathology is minimal.
   (iii) Because dating is at best uncertain, growth retardation cannot be strongly suspected in such circumstances, and further invasive clinical evaluation with amniocentesis is usually best deferred until the diagnosis is better established.

(d) Plan
   (i) Interval sonography for fetal growth is performed in 3 weeks, and serial electronic fetal assessment on a weekly basis until fetal growth has been reevaluated is considered.
   (ii) Repeat evaluation of the fetal size in such circumstances will usually show normal interval growth for a fetus of the indicated sonographic age.
   (iii) If normal growth is seen, pregnancy dates are changed to sonographic dates, the reasons for the change are documented in the chart, and the pregnancy is allowed to continue.
   (iv) In the rare event of inadequate growth, the plan of evaluation and management would be as noted in 3.c.(2).

METHODS OF FETAL ASSESSMENT

1. General principles
   a. The possibility of false-positive results (i.e., disease indicated when not present) should always be considered.
   b. A positive result in a high-risk patient population has a stronger positive predictive value than a similar result in a low-risk patient.
   c. The minimum interval for many tests is not well established.
      (1) The number of patients necessary to establish distinctions between weekly and twice weekly surveillance precludes the possibility of performing such a study at any individual center.
      (2) Anecdotal reports suggest twice weekly testing is somewhat more sensitive than weekly testing.
   d. Most assessments are valid after 31 weeks gestation (in expert hands, may be applied in range of 24 to 31 weeks gestation).
2. Fetal movement counts
   a. Counts are not proven useful by prospective studies.
   b. Retrospective reports often document decreased fetal movement within 24 to 48 hours before fetal demise.
   c. Time to achieve 10 perceived fetal movements from waking up is noted.
      (1) Lack of 10 movements by noon or 1 pm should be investigated by electronic fetal assessment.
      (2) Significantly increased time required to achieve 10 movements should be investigated by electronic fetal assessment (NST, CST, or BPP).
3. NST
   a. NSTs should be performed weekly or twice weekly, depending on index of suspicion of growth retardation and perceived degree of growth retardation.
   b. Depending on gestational age and cervical ripeness, abnormal testing (nonreactive test) should usually be reevaluated with contraction stress testing or biophysical profiling.

4. CST
   a. CSTs may be administered by controlled nipple stimulation or oxytocin infusion.
   b. Uterine hyperstimulation may occasionally occur.
   c. Once weekly testing is usually adequate.
   d. Depending on gestational age, delivery should be considered for abnormal (positive) test result.
5. BPP
   a. Uses 10-point system (usually)
      (1) Two points are awarded during 30-minute observation for each of the following five criteria:
         (a) Presence of at least one 2 cm × 2 cm amniotic fluid pocket
         (b) Reactive NST
         (c) Presence of 30 seconds of fetal breathing movements
         (d) Presence of one episode of active extension and return to flexion of the fetal limbs, spine, or trunk, or opening and closing of a hand
         (e) Presence of three discrete body or limb movements (Episodes of active continuous movements are considered one movement.)
   b. Biophysical score used to plan obstetric management
      (1) Scores of 8 or 10 indicate low risk for ongoing fetal hypoxia.
      (2) Score of 6 indicates mild suspicion of ongoing fetal hypoxia.
         (a) Testing with BPP repeated in 4 to 6 hours, or with CST.
         (b) If oligohydramnios and gestational age greater than 35 weeks, delivery is considered.
      (3) Score of 4 indicates moderate suspicion of ongoing fetal hypoxia.
         (a) If greater than 35 weeks gestation, delivery is considered.
         (b) If less than 35 weeks gestation, benefits of CST or repeated serial BPP are evaluated versus delivery.
      (4) Score of 0 to 2 indicates high risk for ongoing fetal hypoxia.
         (a) If preterm, testing time is extended to up to 120 minutes.
         (b) Persistent scores of 0 or 2 indicate need for delivery.
         (c) If at term, delivery may be appropriate before completion of 120-minute extended evaluation.
   c. Modified BPP
      (1) Normal amniotic fluid volume in combination with either reactive NST or 30 seconds' fetal breathing movements is strongly predictive of adequate fetal oxygenation.
      (2) If normal modified criteria are present, other components of biophysical profile are unnecessary.
6. Amniotic fluid volume
   a. Two common methods of assessment are as follows:
      (1) Single-pocket technique: Presence of at least one 2 cm × 2 cm (or one 1 cm × 1 cm) pocket of amniotic fluid indicates adequate amniotic fluid volume.
      (2) Amniotic fluid index
         (a) Deepest vertical amniotic fluid pocket in each of four uterine quadrants is measured.

(b) Need for pocket to be completely free of umbilical cord is controversial.
(c) Values vary with gestational age.
(d) Values less than 5-cm to 6-cm quadrants indicate oligohydramnios.
(e) Values in excess of 25-cm quadrants indicate polyhydramnios. If present, evaluation of maternal and fetal correlates of polyhydramnios is indicated.
  b. Weekly evaluations are done for patients at risk for oligohydramnios.
  c. If oligohydramnios is present, the possibility of ruptured membranes should always be considered.
  d. Consider delivery if oligohydramnios is present at term.
7. Sonographic assessment of fetal growth
  a. Many formulas are available to estimate fetal weight.
  b. Physician should use weight derived by the same formula to perform interval comparisons.
  c. An interval of 3 or more weeks is usually necessary for meaningful comparisons of serial growth.

19.4 Genetic Counseling

Beth Buehler
GUIDING PRINCIPLES IN GENETIC COUNSELING

1. Philosophy
  a. Genetic counselors encourage their clients to make informed decisions that reflect the clients' own personal beliefs and values.
  b. Genetic counseling requires knowledge of the specific condition, including the following:
    (1) The clinical presentation
    (2) The natural prognosis
    (3) The diagnosis capabilities, including carrier and prenatal testing if available
  c. A genetic counselor must have communication skills, counseling skills, and time necessary to transmit complex medical information to the family and encourage decision making.
  d. Genetic counselors recognize their own biases but provide nondirective counseling.
  e. They support the informed decisions made by their clients.
2. Goals of genetic counseling in the prenatal setting
  a. Understanding of the medical information: The client is given the most current and accurate information concerning the pregnancy and the fetus, including specifics about diagnosis, appropriate therapies, management of the condition, and etiology of the condition.
  b. Comprehending the recurrence risk:
    (1) The mode of inheritance should be clearly explained (using the client's own pedigree to show inheritance) to the couple or family members.
    (2) Recurrence risks may include empirical data (e.g., nonspecific mental retardation with cause unknown), calculated risks, or

Mendelian genetics risks (25% recurrence risk for cystic fibrosis when a couple are known carriers).
- (3) Clients appreciate risks in many different ways.
  - (a) Numerical risk (Risk for 35-year-old woman to have a child born with chromosomal abnormality is 1 in 192, or 0.5%.)
  - (b) Inverse numerical risk (Risk for 35-year-old woman to have a child without a chromosomal abnormality is 191 in 192, or 99.5%.)
  - (c) Concrete thinking (Either the event will occur or it will not.)
  - (d) Comparison of losses and gains (The condition is analyzed comparing what is the benefit versus what is the risk—positive versus negative aspects of decision.)
- (4) Genetic counselors should encourage clients to evaluate risks in more than one way to understand their implications fully.
- c. Realization of options:
  - (1) When deciding whether or not to have prenatal testing clients understand advantages and disadvantages and may choose from a variety of options including no testing (e.g., chorionic villus sampling [CVS], early amniocentesis, ultrasound alone, or no testing).
  - (2) Options are listed in no particular order to ensure nondirective counseling and examples of different options for different families are emphasized.
- d. Empowering clients to make decisions:
  - (1) The couple is encouraged to choose the best course of action for themselves in light of the medical information, their values and beliefs, the psychological implications (e.g., anxiety over knowing the fetus has Tay-Sachs disease but knowing they would not choose to terminate the pregnancy for religious reasons), and the goals of the family.
  - (2) Encouraging the couple to make their own decisions puts control of the pregnancy back in their hands.
    - (a) Many families feel decisions are made around them or because their doctor told them to do something.
    - (b) These are the clients more likely to blame the doctor if there is a problem or to have unresolved guilt concerning an unhealthy pregnancy.
  - (3) If the client becomes a part of the team deciding what is best for the pregnancy, she will more easily adjust to the outcome.

THE PRENATAL GENETIC SESSION

Individuals are referred for genetic counseling for expert information on specific genetic conditions, possible carrier and prenatal testing, risk evaluation, and guidance in decision making for the family or individual.

1. Indications for genetic counseling referral are as follows:
   a. Advanced maternal age (amniocentesis or CVS is offered to any pregnant woman who will be age 35 years or older at time of delivery) (Table 19-10)

Table 19-10 Chromosome Abnormalities in Liveborn Deliveries

Maternal Age	Risk for Down Syndrome	Any Chromosome Abnormality
35	1/378	1/192
36	1/289	1/156
37	1/224	1/127
38	1/173	1/102
39	1/136	1/83
40	1/106	1/66
41	1/82	1/53
42	1/63	1/42
43	1/44	1/33
44	1/38	1/26
45	1/30	1/21
46	1/23	1/16
47	1/18	1/13
48	1/14	1/10
49	1/11	1/8

  b. Known or suspected hereditary condition in family
  c. Exposure to known or suspected teratogens
  d. A fetus or child with birth defects
  e. Previous multiple miscarriages (three or more) or stillbirth baby
  f. Mental retardation in client or family member
  g. Ethnic population with increased risk for genetic condition (Tay-Sachs in Ashkenazi Jewish population)
  h. Consanguinity
  i. Individual with known genetic condition or birth defect
2. Gathering information
  a. It is important to have all the medical information concerning a client before appropriate genetic counseling can be accomplished.
  b. Analysis of multiple pieces of information is routine in genetics before the most likely diagnosis and recurrence risk can be determined.
  c. Genetic disorders carry with them some stigma, and clients are reluctant to divulge information to individuals they do not trust.
  d. Establishing a good rapport and feelings of trust is imperative to obtaining accurate information from the client.
  e. The pedigree.
     (1) This is the most important tool for establishing the mode of inheritance in a family.
     (2) How to construct a pedigree:
        (a) Specific questions should be asked. (How many pregnancies have you had with Mr. B? versus How many pregnancies have you had?)

(b) Information should never be assumed. (Three pregnancies does not mean three living children.)
(c) Clearly defined symbols should be used, with a key for interpretation.
(d) The informant and the historian should be identified, and the interview dated. (This will make sure the pedigree can be understood and updated in the future by anyone who reviews it.)
(e) Counselor should ask specifically about mental retardation, birth defects, multiple miscarriages, consanguinity, genetic conditions, reasons for death, and age at time of death.
(3) Analysis of pedigree: Careful analysis of the pedigree can establish mode of inheritance (see later section, Mode of Inheritance).
f. Reviewing past medical information:
(1) Autopsy findings
(2) Photography of affected family member
(3) Reports of surgical procedures
(4) Laboratory reports (chromosomes, DNA studies, complete blood count [CBC])
(5) Ultrasound reports
g. Clinical diagnosis.
(1) Visual assessment: Counselor should make eye contact with the client throughout genetic counseling session.
(a) Does the client understand the information?
(b) Does he or she have any unusual physical characteristics, peculiar movements, or obvious medical problems not discussed (e.g., the client has a suspicious scar on lip and nasal speech but has not mentioned having a cleft lip or palate)?
(2) Referral to clinical geneticist: The client or family member has one or more multiple congenital anomalies but no diagnosis.
(a) Counselor should refer client to clinical geneticist for diagnosis.
(b) An incorrect diagnosis can change a client's recurrence risks, prenatal testing, and family planning options.
(c) If after the medical literature is reviewed the diagnosis is suspected to be incorrect, client should be referred to a specialist to make the appropriate diagnosis.
3. Counseling parents
a. Counselor should establish rapport.
(1) The first 1 to 3 minutes of the session should be used to introduce oneself and find out a little about the client.
(2) These 3 minutes will establish a foundation for trust from the client.
b. Counselor should investigate the client's agenda.
(1) The client may be concerned about issues different from those he or she was referred for.

(2) Ascertaining what the client feels is important and alerts the counselor to additional issues for the session and lets the client know he or she is being heard and that his or her concerns will be addressed.
　　c. Counselor should explain personal agenda.
　　　　(1) Counselor should explain what he or she will do during the genetic counseling session and in what order.
　　　　(2) Explaining the counseling agenda before starting helps to keep the genetic counseling session focused and the client aware of its goals.
　　d. Counselor should repeat information.
　　　　(1) Counselor should be prepared to repeat the medical information more than once and in more than one way. (It is desirable to use pictures, diagrams, and visual aids, as well as giving examples.)
　　　　(2) A follow-up letter should be sent to review complex information.
　　e. Counselor should invite questions.
　　　　(1) Counselor should stop several times to invite questions on each subtopic before moving to the next agenda items.
　　　　(2) Counselor should make sure the client understands the information without intimidating him or her. (Am I making myself clear? versus Do you understand?)
4. Giving bad news
　　a. In person:
　　　　(1) Counselor should insist that a client come to the office to get bad news.
　　　　(2) The telephone should be used only as a means to get the client into the office. (Mrs. Jones, the chromosome analysis is finalized, and we would like you and your husband to come in to discuss the information as soon as possible.)
　　b. Counselor should never call client at work.
　　　　(1) Only when a client has specifically asked ahead of time to be called with bad news at work and he or she understands the awkwardness and shock this will cause, or when he or she cannot be reached otherwise, should the client be called at work.
　　　　(2) It is devastating to receive bad news in the workplace.
　　c. Counselor should give news humanely.
　　　　(1) Counselor should always express sympathy for the diagnosis.
　　　　(2) The simple act of saying "I'm sorry" helps the patient in the grieving process.
　　d. The actual news:
　　　　(1) The information discussed during the bad news session varies depending on what type of testing has been done, the accuracy of the testing, and the degree of severity of the problem.
　　　　(2) A specific diagnosis necessitates that clients be given appropriate medical information, be able to review their options and

recurrence risks for themselves and family members, and have support information.
- (3) Nonspecific problems without diagnosis necessitate explanation of follow-up medical procedures or tests and support. The emotional impact of not having a diagnosis is many times far worse for families because they are left with many unanswered questions and unresolved anxiety.
  e. Follow-up: A written letter is sent to the client with the information discussed, recurrence risk, natural prognosis of condition, and the decision to use as a permanent record and to review for the future, or as reference when explaining to the other family members what has happened.
  - (1) A follow-up telephone call after a termination of pregnancy helps the client grieve.
  - (2) Referral to specific specialist (e.g., a neurologist needs to talk with a client who chooses to continue a pregnancy with myelomeningocele).

MODE OF INHERITANCE

Autosomal Dominant Inheritance

One gene on an autosomal chromosome (chromosomes 1 through 22) causes the condition.

1. Criteria
   a. Chromosome affects both male and female equally because the gene is contained on an autosomal chromosome.
   b. Trait appears in every generation.
      (1) The pedigree is vertical (e.g., III-A).
      (2) Exceptions to this rule include new mutations in a family and decreased expressivity.
   c. There is a 50% recurrence risk in any pregnancy of affected individuals.
   d. Unaffected family members do not transmit the trait to their children. If an individual does not have the gene, the risk of having an affected child is no greater than the general population risk.
2. Genetic counseling
   a. Counselor should establish diagnosis.
      (1) Counselor should examine the client and question siblings and other possible relatives for characteristics of the disorder.
      (2) Counselor should rely on a medical geneticist to establish the diagnosis or should obtain medical records with stated diagnostic criteria.
   b. Counselor should explain recurrence risk for individual.
   c. Counselor should explain developmental pathology and how the condition originates from a single dominant gene.
   d. Counselor should outline natural history and management.
3. Examples of autosomal dominant disorders are as follows:
   a. Neurofibromatosis type I

(1) Characterized by café-au-lait spots, axillary freckling, external and internal tumors, and growth abnormalities.
(2) Highly variable expressivity with 50% being new mutations with no family history.
(3) The gene is located on chromosome 17.
b. Achondroplasia
(1) Eighty percent are new mutations.
(2) Mating of two individuals with achondroplasia can cause lethal dwarfism in 25% of offspring.

Autosomal Recessive Inheritance

Condition is caused by two genes inherited from specific autosomal chromosome of each parent or of affected individual.

1. Criteria
   a. Males and females are equally likely to be affected because the gene is on an autosomal chromosome.
   b. Pedigree is typically horizontal, with siblings affected, not parents or offspring (III-B).
   c. There is a 25% recurrence risk when both parents are found to be carriers (having one gene each).
2. Genetic counseling
   a. Individuals with one gene are not affected (heterozygous).
   b. Condition is expressed only when a double dose of the gene is present (homozygous).
   c. Chance to have normal children is 75% when both parents are carriers.
   d. Counselor should explain the nature of the condition, carrier testing or prenatal testing and newborn screening if available, and management.
3. Examples are as follows:
   a. Cystic fibrosis (see Genetic Screening by Ethnic Background, Cystic Fibrosis, later in this section).
   b. Phenylketonuria (PKU)
      (1) PKU is a defect in enzyme phenylalanine hydroxylase.
      (2) Children are normal at birth but cannot digest phenylalanine.
      (3) If children are not put on a specific diet low in phenylalanine, they will become mentally retarded.
      (4) Women of childbearing age should also be on a restrictive diet to prevent having mentally retarded children because of the high maternal plasma phenylalanine.

X-Linked Recessive

The gene is inherited on the X chromosome and expressed in males with one gene and only in homozygous females. Consequently, the condition is usually seen only in males and very rarely in females (pedigree III-C).

1. Criteria
   a. The incidence is much higher in males than in females.
   b. The gene is passed from an affected male to all of his daughters, who in turn pass it to 50% of their sons.
   c. The gene is never passed from father to son.
   d. When the mother is a carrier, there is a 50% recurrence risk for affected males and a 50% chance for carrier daughters.
2. Counseling
   a. Counselor should obtain a pedigree to evaluate the origin of the gene or to determine whether it is a new mutation.
   b. Counselor should explain that the condition is caused by genes from both parents because the mother has given the X chromosome with the gene on it and the father has given the Y chromosome to make the individual male.
   c. Counselor should explain recurrence risk if the mother is a carrier, or the possibility of gonadal dysgenesis.
3. Examples are as follows:
   a. Duchenne muscular dystrophy
      (1) Also known as pseudohypertrophic muscular dystrophy.
      (2) Males have progressive muscle weakness and are usually confined to a wheelchair by early teens.
      (3) Individuals have decreased IQ less than or equal to 75.
      (4) Seventy percent of individuals affected will have a deletion or a duplication of the X chromosome.
      (5) Thirty percent are new mutations; 5% to 15% of cases that appear to be new mutations will actually be germline mosaicism.
      (6) Prenatal and carrier testing is available and should be offered to any women with an affected son.
   b. Hemophilia A
      (1) Blood fails to clot because of lack of factor VIII.
      (2) Internal hemorrhage into joints is the primary clinical characteristic.
      (3) Prenatal testing is available though linkage and direct mutation analysis in some families.
      (4) Fifty percent of severely affected males will have an inversion on the X chromosome.

Multifactorial Inheritance

Multifactorial inheritance is said to occur when a condition is said to be caused by a combination of genetic and nongenetic (environmental) conditions (III-D).

1. Criteria
   a. Condition does not follow any particular single-gene pattern of inheritance but tends to be familial.
   b. Condition tends to occur more frequently in one sex than in the other but is seen in both. (Cleft lip with or without cleft palate is more common in boys. Spina bifida is more common in girls.)

c. The recurrence risk is the same in all relatives who share the same proportion of genes. (Recurrence risk for all first-degree relatives of an individual with a neural tube defect would be the same.)
d. The recurrence risk drops off quickly as the relationship to an affected individual becomes more remote. (The possibility of the condition diminishes in individuals who share fewer genes.)
e. In monozygotic twins the chance that the second twin is also affected is under 100% and usually under 50%.
f. In dizygotic twins the concordance is less than monozygotic twins and usually similar to the recurrence risk in ordinary twins.

2. Counseling
   a. Counselor should explain that parents have not done anything to cause this condition. It is a combination of multiple genetic and nongenetic factors that contribute to making the condition and therefore is unlikely to occur again.
   b. Counselor should explain the treatment, the severity of the condition, and current options.
   c. Counselor should explain future prenatal diagnosis and prevention. (Giving high doses of folic acid before conception and during the first trimester, 4 mg/day, reduces the risk of neural tube defects [NTD] in future pregnancies.)

3. Examples
   a. Pyloric stenosis
   b. Anencephaly

Mitochondrial Inheritance

Mutations involving the mitochondrial DNA are known to cause a limited number of genetic conditions. It is important to remember that only the egg cell contains inheritable mitochondria. The sperm's mitochondria are contained in the tail, which is released during fertilization and therefore not of inheritable significance.

1. Criteria
   a. Pedigree should show both males and females affected; however, inheritance is never through the father.
   b. Specific tissues have different proportions of mitochondria. The more mitochondria, the more severely affected. High areas of mitochondria include cardiac muscles, central nervous system (CNS), and kidney.
   c. Mothers pass mitochondria on to all their offspring.

2. Counseling
   a. It is important that the individual understands that the variability of these conditions is directly caused by the concentration of mitochondria, and this is very difficult to predict.
   b. Currently there is no prenatal diagnosis.
   c. Sons will not transmit the condition to their children.

3. Examples of mitochondrial disorders

a. Leber's optic neuropathy: optic atrophy, occasional movement disorders, electrocardiography abnormalities
b. Kearns-Sayre syndrome: progressive external ophthalmoplegia, retinal pigment abnormalities, heart disease, and cerebellar ataxia; onset usually before age 20

GENETIC SCREENING BY ETHNIC BACKGROUND

Tay-Sachs Disease

Tay-Sachs disease affects 1 in 3600 conceptions and is caused by the lack of an enzyme, hexosaminidase A. Individuals with this condition usually die between the ages of 2 and 5 years from an accumulation of GM_2-ganglioside in the brain and nervous system. Individuals are symptomatic by age 6 to 10 months.

1. Population at risk includes the following:
   a. Ashkenazi Jewish descent (carrier incidence 1 in 25)
   b. French Canadian (carrier incidence 1 in 25)
   c. Cajun (carrier incidence 1 in 12)
2. Carrier testing: When at least one partner is from a population at risk, both partners should be tested to determine whether they are carriers.
3. Inheritance:
   a. Tay-Sachs disease has an autosomal recessive inheritance pattern.
   b. Therefore, if one parent is determined not to be a carrier, the pregnancy is not a risk.
   c. If both parents are carriers, there is a 75% chance for a healthy child and a 25% chance of an affected child.
4. Prenatal diagnosis is available through CVS and amniocentesis by an assay to determine the level of hexosaminidase A activity.

Cystic Fibrosis

Cystic fibrosis affects about 1 in 5000 infants in Northern European populations. Its clinical characteristics include chronic respiratory infection, malabsorption, failure to thrive, and thick secretions of the lung and gut when sodium chloride levels are high. Chronic pulmonary disease begins before 1 year of age and is the cause of death in 90% of individuals. Average life span is 35 years. Treatment includes digestive enzyme replacement therapy, chest physiotherapy, and antibiotics.

1. Population at risk includes the following:
   a. Individuals with a family history
   b. Gamete donors
   c. Individuals with an ultrasound indicative of fetal echogenic bowel, obstructive bowel, or meconium ileus
2. Inheritance is autosomal recessive.
   a. The gene is located on chromosome 7p; however, there are many mutations of the gene that cause it not to work properly.

b. All of the mutations are not known; however, most labs will determine 85% of carriers by analysis of the most common mutations.
c. Specific linkage analysis can be done for families with living affected members.
3. Prenatal diagnosis:
   a. Analysis of six of the common mutations will identify 85% to 90% of carriers.
   b. Family linkage studies can be done for a specific family with a more rare mutation and a living affected family member.
   c. Prenatal diagnosis is possible by CVS and amniocentesis when the mutation in question is known.
      (1) Tests have a 2% to 5% false-positive rate and a 2% to 10% false-negative rate.
      (2) Specific laboratories should be consulted concerning their accuracy.

Sickle Cell Anemia

Sickle cell anemia is a blood disorder involving a structural abnormality in one of the globin chains. Clinical manifestations appear in the first year of life, and repeat episodes may cause organ damage, musculoskeletal infarcts, delay in growth, delay in secondary sex characteristics, increased susceptibility to infections, seizures, ocular abnormalities, pulmonary infarcts, renal abnormalities, skin ulcers, and gallstones. Individuals may have severe pain associated with crisis but variability exists. The only cure is bone marrow transplant, which carries a 15% mortality rate.

1. Populations at risk include the following:
   a. African Americans including Haitians, Jamaicans, and individuals from the Caribbean islands
   b. Hispanics from South America, the Caribbean, Puerto Rico, Cuba, and Southeast Asia
   c. Screening: best done by hemoglobin electrophoresis
2. Prenatal diagnosis is available by CVS or amniocentesis using direct site-specific recombinant DNA analysis.
   a. For prenatal diagnosis of a sickle cell gene in combination with another hemoglobinopathy, family studies or DNA polymorphism by restriction enzyme analysis may be necessary.
   b. Evaluation for these studies should be done by a genetic counselor early in pregnancy.

Beta-Thalassemia

Beta-thalassemia is a blood disorder affecting the globin chain synthesis, resulting in severe anemia with an onset at 2 to 3 months. The disorder is characterized by stunted growth, skull bossing (particularly in frontal and parietal areas), increased susceptibility to infection, bone deformities, fractures, delayed or absent sexual maturation, hepatomegaly, splenomegaly, and shortened life span (second or third decade). Treatment includes blood transfusions, iron chelation, therapy to prevent iron overload, and splenectomy.

1. Population at risk: India, Pakistan, South China, Southeast Asia (Laos, Cambodia, Thailand, Vietnam, Philippines, Malaysia), North Africa.
2. Screening should be done by a CBC, mean corpuscular hemoglobin (MCH), or electrophoresis.
   a. Mean corpuscular volume (MCV) is less than 79.
   b. Mean corpuscular hemoglobin count (MCHC) is normal.
   c. HbA$_2$ is elevated (1% to 6%).
   d. HbF is elevated (2% to 5%).
3. Prenatal diagnosis: Direct DNA analysis by polymerase chain reaction (PCR) can be done following CVS or amniocentesis or through fetal blood samples later in pregnancy.

USING GENETIC RESOURCES

1. Genetic counselors
   a. Genetic counselors are individuals with master's degrees who have been formally trained in genetics.
   b. They are certified by the American Board of Genetic Counseling.
   c. Genetic counselors can be of enormous help to obstetricians.
      (1) They have the expertise and training to decide what type of genetic testing might be necessary for a patient.
      (2) They are usually compassionate individuals who can provide invaluable insight into helping families make decisions because they have extensive experience working with individuals with genetic conditions.
2. Medical geneticists
   a. Medical geneticists are medical specialists with additional training in genetics.
   b. The medical geneticist can establish a genetic diagnosis and review the medical prognosis of the disorder.
   c. Medical geneticists, like genetic counselors, have specific knowledge of genetic disease and how it affects families from firsthand experience.
3. Genetic laboratories
   a. It is important to build up a relationship with the genetic laboratory, whether it is academic or commercial.
   b. A good rapport with a laboratory will provide confidence in results and lead to referrals for research and support groups.
4. Support groups
   a. Counselors should get to know the support groups in their area and those available on a national level.
   b. Directing patients to these valuable organizations can put them in direct contact with others affected by the same condition.
   c. Many of these groups also have newsletters, links to research groups, and local chapters, and some even have yearly conventions.

19.5 Hypertension in Pregnancy

John R. Barton and Baha M. Sibai

1. Hypertensive disorders are the most common medical complication of pregnancy, occurring in approximately 7% to 10% of all pregnancies.
2. Hypertensive disorders are associated with significant maternal and perinatal mortality and present as a wide spectrum of disorders, ranging from minimal elevation of blood pressure to severe hypertension with multiple organ dysfunction.
3. The Committee on Terminology of the American College of Obstetricians and Gynecologists (ACOG) defines hypertension in pregnancy as either:
   a. A systolic pressure of 140 mm Hg or more, or an increment of 30 mm Hg or more from a baseline value established in the first half of pregnancy.
   b. A diastolic blood pressure of 90 mm Hg or more, or an increment of 15 mm Hg or more from a baseline value established in the first half of pregnancy.
   c. The absolute blood pressure levels or threshold increments in pressure must be observed on at least two occasions, 6 hours apart.
   d. If blood pressure in the first half of pregnancy is unknown, readings of 140/90 mm Hg after 20 weeks gestation are considered diagnostic of pregnancy-induced hypertension (PIH).
   e. The committee also regards an increase in mean arterial blood pressure of 20 mm Hg or a mean arterial pressure of 105 mm Hg or more as diagnostic of PIH.
4. Classification guidelines for hypertension disorders of pregnancy by ACOG are as follows:
   a. Pregnancy-induced hypertension
      (1) Preeclampsia
         (a) Mild
         (b) Severe
      (2) Eclampsia
   b. Chronic hypertension preceding pregnancy (any etiology)
   c. Chronic hypertension (any etiology) with superimposed PIH
      (1) Superimposed preeclampsia
      (2) Superimposed eclampsia
   d. Gestational or transient hypertension
5. The following definitions apply to the previously mentioned classifications:
   a. Preeclampsia: hypertension together with abnormal edema, proteinuria, or both
   b. Eclampsia: the development of convulsions or coma in patients with signs and symptoms of preeclampsia in the absence of other causes of convulsions
   c. Chronic hypertension: patients with a persistent elevation of blood pressure to at least 140/90 mm Hg on two occasions before 20 weeks gestation, and patients with hypertension that persists for more than 6 weeks postpartum

d. Superimposed preeclampsia or eclampsia: the development of either preeclampsia or eclampsia in patients with diagnosed chronic hypertension
   e. Gestational hypertension: hypertension appearing in the second half of pregnancy or in the first 24 hours postpartum without edema or proteinuria and with a return to normotension within 10 days after delivery
6. The two most common forms of hypertension are as follows:
   a. PIH, a disorder that appears during pregnancy and is reversed by delivery
   b. Preexisting chronic hypertension, unrelated to but coinciding with pregnancy; may be detected for the first time in pregnancy and is not reversed by delivery

PREECLAMPSIA

Etiology

Preeclampsia is a disorder of unknown etiology that is peculiar to human pregnancy. Many theories regarding its etiology have been suggested and include the following:

1. Abnormal placentation
2. Immunologic phenomena
3. Coagulation abnormalities
4. Abnormal cardiovascular adaptation
5. Dietary factors
6. Genetic factors
7. Vascular endothelial damage
8. Abnormal prostaglandin metabolism

Incidence

1. Preeclampsia is a disorder peculiar to human pregnancy.
2. Reported incidences range from 2% to 35%, depending on the diagnostic criteria and the population studied.
3. It is principally a disease of young primigravidas.
4. The incidence is about 6% to 7% of all pregnancies in the United States.

Risk Factors

Although geographic and racial differences in incidence have been reported, several risk factors have been identified as predisposing to the development of preeclampsia.

1. Nulliparity
2. Multiple gestation
3. Family history of preeclampsia or eclampsia
4. Preexisting hypertension or renal disease
5. Diabetes
6. Nonimmune hydrops fetalis
7. Molar pregnancy
8. Previous preeclampsia, especially if remote from term

Prediction of Preeclampsia

1. The fact that the etiology of preeclampsia remains unknown has made the prediction of preeclampsia very difficult.
2. More than 100 biophysical, clinical, and biochemical tests have been reported in the world's literature to predict the development of preeclampsia, but their overall prediction value remains poor.
3. Examples of clinical tests to predict preeclampsia include the following:
    a. Mean arterial pressure (MAP) at 20 weeks greater than 90 mm Hg
    b. Diastolic blood pressure in the midtrimester greater than 80 mm Hg
    c. Rollover test at 28 to 32 weeks
    d. Angiotensin II infusion test at 26 to 30 weeks
        (1) The angiotensin II test is an invasive procedure that requires infusions of this potent vasopressor at 26 to 30 weeks gestation and subsequent measurement of the diastolic blood pressure.
        (2) Whether the test is positive or negative depends on the amount of angiotensin II required to elicit an increase in diastolic pressure of 20 mm Hg or more.
        (3) Several investigators have studied the value of the angiotensin II test in predicting PIH.
        (4) It has a specificity of 90% to 95%, but the sensitivity is variable, with a high incidence of false-positive results.
        (5) The test is influenced by several factors, including gestational age, with different results obtained on serial testing.
        (6) In addition, it is a very invasive procedure and is not suitable for clinical use.

Diagnosis

1. Preeclampsia traditionally has been described as a triad of hypertension, proteinuria, and edema.
2. However, preeclampsia may present as a spectrum of clinical signs and symptoms, presenting either alone or in combination, often making the diagnosis difficult.
    a. Hypertension: Abnormal blood pressure elevation is the traditional hallmark for the diagnosis of the disease (blood pressure criteria for preeclampsia were presented earlier).
    b. Proteinuria
        (1) Protein excretion in the urine increases in normal pregnancy from approximately 5 mg/100 mL in the first and second trimesters to 15 mg/100 mL in the third trimester.
        (2) Significant proteinuria should be defined as a level greater than 300 mg per 24-hour urine sample.
        (3) When making a diagnosis of severe preeclampsia based on the criterion of proteinuria only, it is recommended that a 24-hour urine excretion of protein of greater than 5 g be documented.
    c. Edema
        (1) Excessive weight gain (more than 2 lb per week in the third trimester) may be the first sign of preeclampsia.

(2) Moderate edema is a feature of 80% of normotensive pregnancies.
(3) In addition, 40% of patients with eclampsia at the University of Tennessee at Memphis had no edema before the onset of convulsions.
(4) Moreover, the assessment of edema is highly subjective.
3. Early recognition of the development of preeclampsia can allow for more timely intervention to improve maternal and perinatal outcome.
4. This reinforces the reason for frequent antenatal visits late in pregnancy to allow early detection.
5. Figure 19-1 is a sample algorithm for the management of a normotensive patient that may be developing subtle signs and symptoms of preeclampsia.

Management of Preeclampsia

1. Once the diagnosis of preeclampsia has been made, definitive therapy in the form of delivery is the desired goal, because it is the only cure for the disease.
2. The ultimate goals of the therapy must always be safety of the mother first, and then the delivery of a mature newborn that will not require intensive and prolonged neonatal care.
3. The decision is between expectant management and immediate delivery and is usually dependent on one or more of the following factors:
   a. Severity of the disease process
   b. Presence of labor
   c. Fetal gestational age

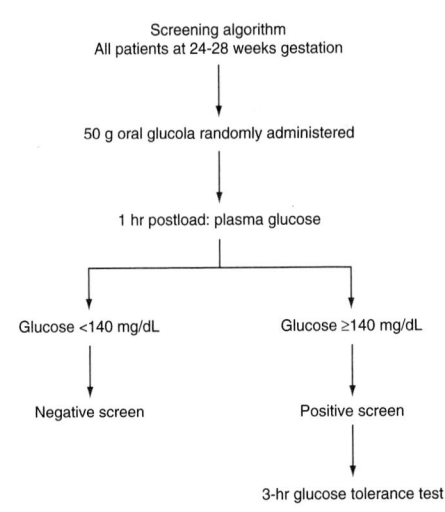

```
Screening algorithm
All patients at 24-28 weeks gestation
              ↓
50 g oral glucola randomly administered
              ↓
1 hr postload: plasma glucose
         ↓              ↓
Glucose <140 mg/dL    Glucose ≥140 mg/dL
         ↓              ↓
  Negative screen     Positive screen
                        ↓
              3-hr glucose tolerance test
```

Figure 19-1 A sample algorithm for the management of a normotensive patient who may be developing subtle signs and symptoms of preeclampsia.

d. Fetal condition
e. Maternal condition
f. Bishop cervical score

Mild Preeclampsia

1. All patients with diagnosed preeclampsia should be hospitalized at the time of diagnosis for evaluation of maternal and fetal conditions.
2. These pregnancies usually are associated with reduced uteroplacental blood flow.
3. Thus, women with mild disease who have a favorable cervix at or near term should undergo induction of labor for delivery.
    a. Even if conditions for induction of labor are unfavorable, the pregnancy should not continue past term (beyond 40 weeks gestation), because uteroplacental blood flow is suboptimal.
    b. The optimal management of mild preeclampsia remote from term is very controversial.
    c. In general, there is considerable disagreement regarding the need for hospitalization versus ambulatory management, the use of antihypertensive drugs, and the use of sedatives and anticonvulsive prophylaxis.
    d. For a patient who has mild preeclampsia with an immature fetus, the goal of therapy should be to do the following:
        (1) Retard the hypertensive process so as not to endanger the mother or the fetus
        (2) Allow time for the fetus to mature and increase the potential for neonatal survival
        (3) Allow the cervix to ripen and therefore increase the probability for a vaginal delivery
    e. Therapy for these patients can be conducted by either ambulatory management or hospitalization.
        (1) Ambulatory management is acceptable for patients who are compliant, who can have frequent office visits including laboratory assessments, and who can perform some form of adequate blood pressure monitoring at home.
        (2) Hospitalization should be required for noncompliant patients and those who show unsatisfactory progress as outpatients.
        (3) In either situation, the regimen given in Box 19-6 is recommended for mild preeclampsia.
4. A patient is considered a candidate for induction of labor if she has reached 37 weeks gestation, the fetus is mature, and the condition of the cervix is favorable. She is also a candidate for induction if her diastolic blood pressure continues to rise despite conservative management.
5. A patient with mild PIH may be followed beyond 37 weeks of gestation if fetal evaluation is normal and the condition of the cervix is unfavorable.
6. Figure 19-2 is a sample algorithm for the management of a patient with mild preeclampsia.

> BOX 19-6 Mild Preeclampsia Regimen
>
> 1. Maternal evaluation
>   a. Physical examination
>   (1) Blood pressure every 4 to 6 hours during the day
>   (2) Urine protein by dipstick daily
>   (3) Assessment of facial or pedal edema daily
>   (4) Weight daily
>   b. Patient history: Symptoms of impending eclampsia or HELLP syndrome (hemolysis, elevated liver, low platelets) include the following:
>   (1) Persistent occipital or frontal headaches
>   (2) Visual disturbances
>   (3) Right upper quadrant or epigastric pain
>   c. Laboratory evaluation
>   (1) Hematocrit and platelet count one or two times a week
>   (2) Liver function tests one or two times a week
>   (3) 24-hour urine collections at diagnosis and every 1 to 2 weeks
> 2. Fetal evaluation
>   a. Daily fetal movement assessment (kick counts)
>   b. NST twice weekly
>   c. BPP if nonreactive NST
>   d. Amniotic fluid volume assessment weekly
>   e. Ultrasound evaluation of fetal growth every 3 weeks

BPP, Biophysical profile assessment; NST, nonstress test.

Severe Preeclampsia

1. The clinical course of severe preeclampsia is usually characterized by progressive deterioration in both maternal and fetal status.
2. These pregnancies are usually associated with increased rates of perinatal mortality and morbidity.
3. Most of the fetal or neonatal complications are related to intrauterine fetal growth retardation and prematurity.
4. The following represent the criteria for the diagnosis of severe preeclampsia (adapted from ACOG Technical Bulletin No. 91):
   a. Blood pressure greater than 160 mm Hg systolic or greater than 110 mm Hg diastolic on two occasions at least 6 hours apart with the patient at bed rest
   b. Proteinuria greater than 5 g in a 24-hour urine collection or greater than 3 g on dipstick in at least two random clean-catch samples at least 4 hours apart
   c. Oliguria (<400 mL in 24 hours)
   d. Cerebral or visual disturbances
   e. Epigastric pain
   f. Pulmonary edema or cyanosis
   g. Thrombocytopenia

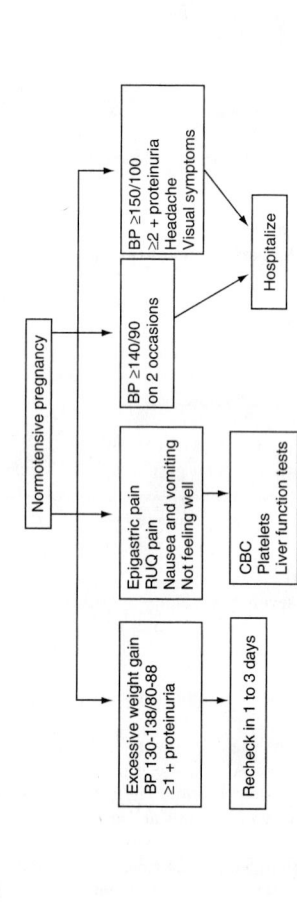

Figure 19-2 A sample algorithm for the management of a patient with mild preeclampsia. *BP,* Blood pressure; *CBC,* complete blood count; *RUQ,* right upper quadrant.

5. Because the only cure for severe preeclampsia is delivery, there is universal agreement to deliver in all patients in which the disease has developed beyond 34 weeks gestation or if there is evidence of fetal lung maturity or fetal jeopardy before that time.
6. In this situation, appropriate management should include the following:
   a. Parenteral medications to prevent convulsions
   b. Control of maternal blood pressure within a safe range
   c. Induction of labor to initiate delivery
7. On the other hand, management of patients with severe disease remote from term (<34 weeks) is highly controversial.
   a. Some institutions consider delivery as the definitive therapy for all cases, regardless of gestational age.
   b. Others recommend prolonging pregnancy in all patients remote from term until one or more of the following is achieved:
      (1) Fetal lung maturity
      (2) Fetal jeopardy
      (3) Maternal jeopardy
      (4) 34 weeks gestation achieved
8. All patients with severe preeclampsia should be admitted to the labor and delivery area for close observation of the maternal and fetal condition.
9. All patients should receive intravenous magnesium sulfate to prevent convulsions.
10. Figure 19-3 is a sample algorithm for the management of a patient with severe preeclampsia.

Severe Preeclampsia in Midtrimester

1. Occasionally, a patient may develop severe preeclampsia at or before 28 weeks gestation.
2. These pregnancies are associated with high maternal and perinatal mortality and pose a difficult management decision for every obstetrician.
3. Immediate delivery will result in extremely high perinatal morbidity and mortality, whereas an aggressive attempt to delay delivery may cause severe maternal morbidity.
4. Figure 19-4 is a sample algorithm for the management of a patient with severe preeclampsia in the midtrimester.

Prevention of Preeclampsia

1. There are numerous reports and clinical trials describing the use of various methods to prevent or reduce the incidence of preeclampsia.
2. Methods used have included the following:
   a. Salt restriction or prophylactic diuretic therapy
   b. Low-dose aspirin
   c. Calcium supplementation
   d. Ingestion of fish or evening primrose oil
3. Because the etiology of the disease is unknown, the reported methods have been used in an attempt to correct the pathophysiologic

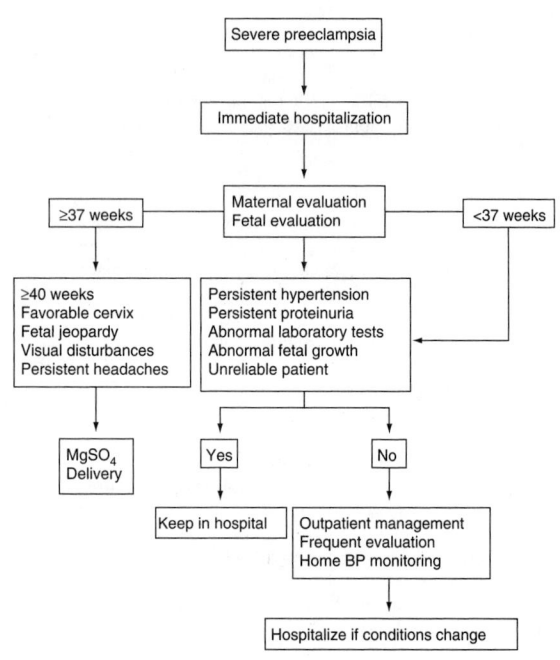

Figure 19-3 A sample algorithm for the management of a patient with severe preeclampsia. *BP,* Blood pressure; *MgSO₄,* magnesium sulfate.

abnormalities of preeclampsia in the hope of preventing the disease or ameliorating its course.
4. Several multicenter studies are currently under way, but there is not yet a consensus on the optimal method for prevention or amelioration of this disease.

ECLAMPSIA

1. Eclampsia is defined as the development of convulsions or coma unrelated to other cerebral conditions during pregnancy and the postpartum period in patients with signs and symptoms of preeclampsia.
2. The hazards of convulsions in pregnancy have been documented for centuries.
3. The reported incidence ranges from 1 in 100 to 1 in 3448 pregnancies.
4. The incidence is increased among nonwhite nulliparous women of low socioeconomic status.
5. At the University of Tennessee at Memphis, a tertiary referral center for several states, the incidence has remained stable at 1 in 300 pregnancies for the past 30 years.

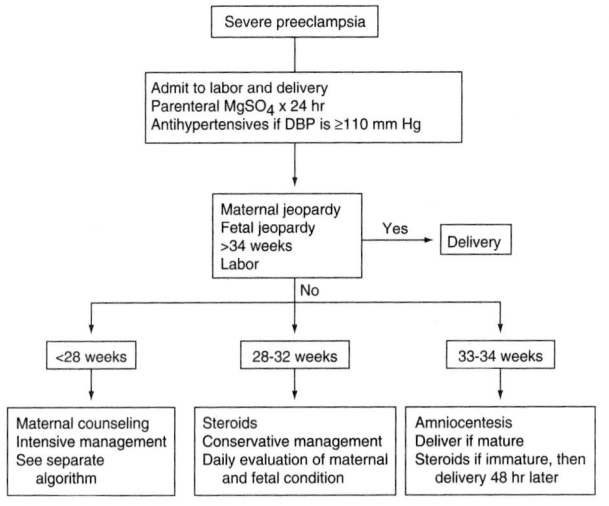

Practical Guide to the Care of the Gynecologic/Obstetric Patient 435

```
                    ┌─────────────────────┐
                    │ Severe preeclampsia │
                    └──────────┬──────────┘
                               ↓
            ┌──────────────────────────────────────┐
            │ Admit to labor and delivery          │
            │ Parenteral MgSO₄ × 24 hr             │
            │ Antihypertensives if DBP is ≥110 mm Hg│
            └──────────────────┬───────────────────┘
                               ↓
                   ┌───────────────────┐    Yes   ┌──────────┐
                   │ Maternal jeopardy │ ────────→│ Delivery │
                   │ Fetal jeopardy    │          └──────────┘
                   │ >34 weeks         │
                   │ Labor             │
                   └─────────┬─────────┘
                             │ No
         ┌───────────────────┼───────────────────┐
         ↓                   ↓                   ↓
    <28 weeks           28-32 weeks          33-34 weeks
```

Figure 19-4 A sample algorithm for the management of a patient with severe preeclampsia in the midtrimester. *DBP*, Diastolic blood pressure; *MgSO₄*, magnesium sulfate.

Below <28 weeks: Maternal counseling, Intensive management, See separate algorithm

Below 28-32 weeks: Steroids, Conservative management, Daily evaluation of maternal and fetal condition

Below 33-34 weeks: Amniocentesis, Deliver if mature, Steroids if immature, then delivery 48 hr later

6. However, considering the number of pregnancies in that area, the incidence actually is about 1 in 1600 pregnancies.
7. For patients obtaining prenatal care, the incidence is about 1 in 800 patients.
8. Eclamptic convulsions constitute a life-threatening emergency.
9. The basic principles in the management of eclampsia involve the following measures:
   a. Support of cardiorespiratory functions
      (1) Airway patency and ensuring maternal oxygenation should be assessed and established.
      (2) Suction should be used as needed and the patient protected from injury by making sure the bed side-rails are elevated and padded.
      (3) Oxygen should be administered to improve maternal oxygen concentration and increase oxygen delivery to the fetus.
   b. Control of convulsions and prevention of recurrent convulsions
      (1) The natural tendency for those caring for an eclamptic patient is to provide therapy to immediately abolish the seizure activity.
      (2) This philosophy is not only unwise, it is potentially dangerous to the patient.
      (3) Parenteral magnesium sulfate is the drug of choice for convulsions resulting from eclampsia in the United States.
         (a) Its major advantages include its relative maternal and fetal safety when used properly.

(b) The mother is awake and alert most of the time and laryngeal reflexes are intact, which helps protect against aspiration problems.
(c) There are several regimens of magnesium sulfate used to prevent convulsions. The two most commonly used are as follows:
  (i) The intravenous (IV) regimen popularized by Sibai at the University of Tennessee at Memphis
  (ii) The intramuscular (IM) regimen preferred by Pritchard used at Parkland Memorial Hospital in Dallas, Texas
(d) The Sibai IV regimen:
  (i) An intravenous loading dose of 6 g of magnesium sulfate prepared as 6 g diluted in 150 mL D5W is administered via infusion pump over 20 to 30 minutes.
  (ii) If the patient develops recurrent convulsions after the initial infusion of magnesium sulfate, a further dose of 2 to 4 g can be infused over 5 to 10 minutes.
  (iii) On completion of the magnesium sulfate loading infusion, a maintenance infusion of 2 to 3 g/hr is used.
  (iv) The infusion rate of magnesium sulfate should be adjusted on the basis of serial serum magnesium levels and physical examination.
(e) Pritchard's IM regimen for severe preeclampsia and eclampsia includes the following:
  (i) Four g of magnesium sulfate IV over 3 to 5 minutes and 10 g IM is administered as a loading dose followed by a maintenance dose of 5 g IM every 4 hours.
  (ii) For mild preeclampsia, 10 g of magnesium sulfate IM is administered as a loading dose followed by a maintenance dose of 5 g IM every 4 hours.
(4) Clinical findings associated with increased maternal plasma levels of magnesium can be found in Table 19-11.
(5) Patients receiving magnesium sulfate therapy require monitoring for evidence of drug toxicity.
(6) Magnesium is excreted by the kidneys, and renal dysfunction may cause toxic accumulation. Magnesium toxicity can be avoided by doing the following:
  (a) Confirming adequate renal function with hourly urinary output assessment
  (b) Doing serial evaluation for presence of patellar deep tendon reflexes
  (c) Making close observation of respiratory rate
  (d) Monitoring serial serum magnesium levels
(7) If magnesium toxicity is suspected the following should be done:
  (a) The magnesium sulfate infusion should be discontinued immediately.
  (b) Supplemental oxygen should be administered.
  (c) A serum magnesium level should be assessed.

Table 19-11 Clinical Findings Associated with Increased Maternal Plasma Magnesium Levels

Serum Magnesium Level (mg/dL)	Clinical Findings
1.5-2.5	Normal pregnancy level
4-8	"Therapeutic range for seizure prophylaxis"
9-12	Loss of patellar reflex
15-17	Muscular paralysis, respiratory arrest
30-35	Cardiac arrest

- (8) If magnesium toxicity is recognized, 10 mL of 10% calcium gluconate is administered (1 g total) intravenously.
    - (a) This medication must be given slowly (i.e., 2 to 5 mL/min) to avoid hypotension and bradycardia.
    - (b) Calcium competitively inhibits magnesium at the neuromuscular junction, but its effect is only transient, because the serum concentration is unchanged.
- (9) Symptoms of magnesium toxicity can recur following calcium gluconate if the magnesium level remains elevated.
- (10) If respiratory arrest is identified, prompt resuscitative measures including intubation and assisted ventilation are indicated.

c. Correction of maternal hypoxemia and acidemia
   - (1) Maternal hypoxemia and acidemia may result from the following:
     - (a) Repeated convulsions
     - (b) Respiratory depression from the use of multiple anticonvulsant agents
     - (c) Aspiration
     - (d) Or a combination of these factors
   - (2) Supplemental oxygen may be administered by face mask or face mask with an oxygen reservoir at 8 to 10 L/min. At 10 L O_2/min, the oxygen concentration delivered approaches 100% using a face mask with an oxygen reservoir.
   - (3) Maternal oxygenation can be monitored noninvasively by transcutaneous pulse oximetry, whereas acid–base status may be assessed by arterial blood gas analysis.

d. Control of severe hypertension
   - (1) The objective of treating severe hypertension is to prevent maternal cerebrovascular accidents and congestive heart failure without compromising cerebral perfusion or jeopardizing uteroplacental blood flow, already reduced in eclampsia.
   - (2) Although the underlying causative factors are not completely delineated, hypertension in preeclampsia is clearly a consequence of a generalized arterial vasoconstriction.

(3) Desirable antihypertensive agent properties for the use in hypertensive emergencies in pregnancy include a rapid onset of action following administration and short duration of action in the event of overtitration.
  (a) Labetalol
     (i) Labetalol is a competitive antagonist at both postsynaptic alpha-1-adrenergic and beta-adrenergic receptors.
     (ii) Labetalol is available in oral and intravenous form.
     (iii) Parenteral labetalol has a rapid onset of action and produces a smooth reduction in blood pressure with rare overshoot hypotension.
     (iv) Labetalol is contraindicated in patients with a greater than first-degree heart block.
     (v) Labetalol is administered in intermittent intravenous boluses of 20 to 80 mg.
  (b) Hydralazine
     (i) Hydralazine is a direct arteriolar vasodilator.
     (ii) Intravenous hydralazine has an onset of action of 10 to 20 minutes with a peak effect in 60 minutes and a duration of action of 4 to 6 hours.
     (iii) Hydralazine is administered in intermittent bolus injections with an initial dose of 5 mg. Blood pressure should then be recorded every 5 minutes.
     (iv) If an adequate reduction in blood pressure is present 20 to 30 minutes after the initial dose, then a repeat dose or one increased to 10 mg in increments of every 20 to 30 minutes should be given.
  (c) Nifedipine
     (i) Nifedipine is a calcium-channel antagonist.
     (ii) Nifedipine improves renal function with a beneficial effect on urine output when treating preeclampsia in the postpartum period.
     (iii) Given sublingually, 10 mg of nifedipine has an onset of action within 3 minutes with a peak effect within 1 hour.
     (iv) Nifedipine is administered 10 to 20 mg orally every 3 to 4 hours.
     (v) Profound reductions in blood pressure with nifedipine can be partially reversed by the slow IV administration of calcium gluconate.
  (d) Sodium nitroprusside
     (i) Sodium nitroprusside relaxes arteriolar and venous smooth muscle equally by interfering with both influx and the intercellular activation of calcium.
     (ii) Onset of action is immediate, and duration of action is very short (1 to 10 minutes).
     (iii) Because preeclamptic patients have a propensity for depleted intravascular volume, they are especially sensitive to its effects. The initial infusion dose

should therefore be 0.2 µg/kg/min, rather than 0.5 µg/kg/min as is standard in nonpregnant patients.

(iv) Cyanide and thiocyanate are products of metabolism of this drug.

e. Initiation of the process for delivery
   (1) Because evacuation of the uterus is the definitive treatment of preeclampsia and eclampsia, patients are evaluated for delivery, once stabilized.
   (2) Vaginal delivery, unless obstetrically contraindicated, is the preferred method of delivery.
      (a) An oxytocin infusion for induction or augmentation of labor may be administered simultaneously with the magnesium sulfate infusion.
      (b) Total fluid intake is limited to 100 mL/hr.
      (c) The protocol for oxytocin infusion for preeclampsia or eclampsia is the same as for routine patients; yet, because of fluid restrictions, oxytocin may need to be more concentrated and dosages per minute adjusted accordingly.
      (d) Continuous fetal monitoring should be employed.
   (3) At delivery, neonatal side effects of maternal administration of magnesium sulfate include the following:
      (a) Hypotension
      (b) Hypotonia
      (c) Respiratory depression
      (d) Lethargy
      (e) Decreased suck reflex
   (4) The pediatrician and newborn nursery should be informed of patients receiving magnesium sulfate.
   (5) Calcium gluconate may also be administered to the newborn if magnesium toxicity is suspected.
   (6) Following delivery, the patient should be monitored in the recovery room under close observation for a minimum of 24 hours.
   (7) During this time, magnesium sulfate should be continued, and maternal vital signs and intake–output should be monitored hourly.
   (8) Some of these patients may require intensive and invasive hemodynamic monitoring, because they are at increased risk of the development of pulmonary edema from fluid overload, fluid mobilization, and compromised renal function.
   (9) Magnesium sulfate administration should continue until improvements in blood pressure, urine output, and sensorium are noted.

Postpartum Eclampsia

1. Approximately 25% of eclampsia cases will occur during the postpartum period, most within the first 48 hours from delivery.
2. Late-onset postpartum eclampsia is defined as convulsions occurring more than 48 hours after delivery in patients with signs and symptoms of preeclampsia.

a. If postpartum eclampsia is confirmed, the management is as previously noted for antepartum convulsions.
b. More vigorous control of blood pressure is possible, however, because there is no longer a concern about compromising the uteroplacental circulation in the postpartum patient.
c. Magnesium sulfate therapy should be continued for 24 to 48 hours from seizure onset.

Complications of Eclampsia

1. There are several maternal complications with eclampsia convulsions, including the following:
   a. Abruptio placentae
   b. Pulmonary edema
   c. Acute renal failure
   d. Aspiration pneumonia
   e. Intracerebral hemorrhage
   f. Retinal detachment
   g. Ruptured subcapsular liver hematoma
2. Abruptio placentae is the most frequent (5% to 10%) complication and intracerebral hemorrhage is the most serious.
3. Fortunately, most of the complications resolve after delivery with proper management.

HELLP SYNDROME

1. Hemolysis, abnormal liver functions tests, and thrombocytopenia have been recognized as complications of preeclampsia and eclampsia for many years.
2. In 1982, Weinstein described 29 cases of severe preeclampsia and eclampsia complicated by these abnormalities.
3. He suggested that this collection of signs and symptoms constituted an entity separate from severe preeclampsia and coined the term HELLP syndrome:
   a. *H* for hemolysis
   b. *EL* for elevated liver enzymes
   c. *LP* for low platelets
4. There are considerable differences regarding the time of onset and the type and degree of laboratory abnormalities used to make the diagnosis of HELLP syndrome.
5. In an attempt to standardize the diagnosis of HELLP syndrome, investigators at the University of Tennessee at Memphis published criteria using cutoff values of more than three standard deviations above the mean to indicate abnormality. Their criteria for the diagnosis of HELLP syndrome are summarized in Box 19-7.
6. The incidence of severe preeclampsia or eclampsia complicated by HELLP syndrome has been reported to range from 2% to 12%.
7. Patients with HELLP syndrome may present with a variety of signs and symptoms, including the following:
   a. Epigastric or right upper quadrant pain
   b. Nausea or vomiting

> **BOX 19-7 Criteria for the Diagnosis of HELLP Syndrome**
>
> **Hemolysis**
> Abnormal peripheral smear
> Total bilirubin >1.2 mg/dL
> Lactic dehydrogenase (LDH) >600 U/L
>
> **Elevated Liver Functions**
> Serum aspartate aminotransferase (AST) >70 U/L
> Lactic dehydrogenase (LDH) >600 U/L
>
> **Low Platelets**
> Platelet count <100,000/mm^3

From Sibai BM: *Am J Obstet Gynecol* 162:311-316, 1990.

    c. Nonspecific viral syndrome–like symptoms
    d. History of malaise for the past few days before presentation
8. It is important to appreciate that severe hypertension (systolic blood pressure > 160 mm Hg, diastolic blood pressure > 100 mm Hg) is not a constant or even a frequent finding in HELLP syndrome. In Weinstein's initial report of 29 patients, less than half (13) had an admission blood pressure greater than 160/100 mm Hg.
9. As a result, these patients are often misdiagnosed as having various medical and surgical disorders, including appendicitis, gastroenteritis, pyelonephritis, or viral hepatitis.

Management of HELLP Syndrome

1. Patients with HELLP syndrome who are remote from term should be referred to a tertiary care center and initial management should be as for any patient with severe preeclampsia.
2. The following is an outline of the management of antepartum HELLP syndrome:
    a. Maternal condition is assessed and stabilized.
        (1) If disseminated intravascular coagulopathy (DIC) is present, coagulopathy is corrected.
        (2) Antiseizure prophylaxis is given with magnesium sulfate.
        (3) Treatment of severe hypertension is begun.
        (4) CT or ultrasound of the abdomen is done if subcapsular hematoma of the liver is suspected.
    b. Fetal well-being is evaluated.
        (1) NST
        (2) BPP
        (3) Ultrasonographic biometry

c. If less than 35 weeks gestation fetal lung maturity is evaluated.
   (1) If mature → delivery
   (2) If immature → steroids → delivery
3. If the syndrome develops at or beyond 34 weeks gestation, or if there is evidence of fetal lung maturity or fetal or maternal jeopardy before that time, then delivery is the definitive therapy.
4. Without laboratory evidence of DIC and absent fetal lung maturity, the patient can be given two doses of steroids to accelerate fetal lung maturity and delivery then should be done 48 hours later.
5. However, maternal and fetal conditions should be assessed continuously during this time period.

CHRONIC HYPERTENSION

1. Management of the woman with chronic hypertension should begin before conception.
   a. If a patient with chronic hypertension is considering pregnancy, she should be advised to have her blood pressure checked several times to establish the cause and severity of her hypertension before pregnancy.
   b. In addition, her response to the antihypertensive drugs should be monitored and drugs with potential adverse effects on the fetus (angiotensin-converting enzyme inhibitors, diuretics) should be replaced by other drugs.
   c. The patient should then be instructed to seek prenatal care once pregnancy is confirmed.
   d. This will ensure accurate determination of the gestational age, as well as the severity of hypertension in the first trimester.
2. For patients who are seen for the first time during pregnancy, the first step in management should include a detailed evaluation and workup to determine the etiology and severity of the hypertension. Attention should be paid to the renal disease, diabetes, thyroid disease, and the outcome in previous pregnancies (superimposed preeclampsia, preterm delivery, abruptio placentae, perinatal outcome).

Causes of Chronic Hypertension in Pregnancy
See Box 19-8.

Management

1. The primary objective in the management of pregnancies in hypertensive women is to reduce maternal risks and achieve optimal perinatal survival.
2. This objective can be achieved by formulating a rational approach that includes the following:
   a. Early antenatal care is provided.
   b. Frequent antepartum evaluations are done.
   c. Delivery is timely.
   d. At the time of initial and subsequent antenatal visits, patients are seen by a dietitian and instructed on nutritional requirements, weight gain, and sodium intake.
   e. Patient should be advised to avoid smoking and caffeine.

> **BOX 19-8 Causes of Chronic Hypertension in Pregnancy**
>
> Essential or idiopathic (90%)
> Secondary (10%)
>   Renal etiology
>   Glomerulonephritis
>   Interstitial nephritis
>   Nephropathy
>   Polycystic disease
>   Renovascular disease
>   Collagen vascular disease
>   Lupus erythematosus
>   Periarteritis nodosa
>   Scleroderma
>   Endocrine etiology
>   Diabetes with vascular involvement
>   Thyroxicosis
>   Hyperaldosteronism
>   Pheochromocytoma
>   Vascular disease
>   Coarctation of the aorta
>   Vasculitis

    f. Patient should be encouraged to have adequate bed rest during the day if possible.

    g. If the patient is well motivated, she can be instructed in self-determination of blood pressure.

3. During the course of pregnancy, the patient is seen once every 2 weeks for the first two trimesters and once weekly thereafter.
4. This schedule of prenatal visits may be adjusted based on maternal and fetal conditions.
   a. Maternal evaluation should include serial hematocrit, uric acid, urine culture, and 24-hour urine testing at least once every trimester.
   b. Fetal evaluation should include serial ultrasonography for growth, and antepartum fetal testing with the use of NST or BPP, or both.
   c. Fetal testing is to be started at 26 weeks gestation and then repeated weekly or more often depending on fetal condition (superimposed preeclampsia, suspected fetal growth retardation).
   d. The biophysical profile needs to be performed only when the NST is nonreactive.
   e. When indicated, amniocentesis is performed to assess fetal pulmonary maturity.
5. The pregnancy may then be continued to term or until onset of superimposed preeclampsia (uric acid >6 mg/dL and proteinuria >1 g/24 hr), or until development of fetal growth retardation or fetal distress.
   a. The development of superimposed preeclampsia is an indication for immediate hospitalization.

b. Subsequent management will depend on severity of the preeclampsia and fetal gestational age.
c. The development of severe superimposed preeclampsia is an indication for delivery in all patients with a gestational age greater than 34 weeks.
d. If superimposed preeclampsia develops before this time, then the pregnancy may be followed conservatively with daily evaluation of maternal and fetal well-being.

Maternal and Fetal Risks

1. Pregnancies complicated by chronic hypertension are at increased risk for the development of superimposed preeclampsia and abruptio placentae.
2. The reported incidence of superimposed preeclampsia ranges from 4.7% to 52% depending on the severity of the hypertension at the onset of pregnancy and on the diagnostic criteria used for superimposed preeclampsia.
3. The reported incidence of abruptio placentae ranges between 0.45% and 1.9% for mild uncomplicated hypertension and between 2.3% and 10% for patients with complicated severe hypertension.
4. The incidence of both of the above complications is not influenced by the use of antihypertensive medications.
5. Despite these risks, more than 85% of women with chronic hypertension have uncomplicated pregnancies.

19.6 HIV in Pregnancy

Stanley A. Gall

Infection with human immunodeficiency virus type 1 (HIV-1) produces a chronic, progressive disease state resulting in acquired immunodeficiency syndrome (AIDS) and subsequent demise. The AIDS epidemic continues to be dynamic, with the first wave of patients being male homosexuals. This was followed by males and females infected because of intravenous drug abuse. During this phase of the epidemic, females were equally involved and 80% were in the reproductive age. The current phase of the epidemic features heterosexual transmission with females up to 20 times more likely to become infected.

EPIDEMIOLOGY

See Box 19-9.

PERINATAL TRANSMISSION

1. Mechanisms of perinatal transmission include the following:
    a. Direct invasion of trophoblast and placental villi by HIV
    b. Passage of infected maternal lymphocyte into the fetal circulation
    c. Infection of cells with CD4 receptors in chorionic villi and villus endothelial cells (Tables 19-12 through 19-14)
2. Role of the placenta in the transmission of HIV is not clear.
    a. In vitro studies have documented that HIV-1 can infect human trophoblast and Hofbauer cells of different gestational ages.

> **BOX 19-9 Changing Epidemiology of AIDS**
>
> 1. 1981-1992: Centers for Disease Control reported 253,448 cases of AIDS
>   a. Male: 87%
>   b. Female: 11%
>   c. Children: 2%
> 2. Women were infected by the following routes during 1981-1992
>   a. Intravenous drug abuse: 50%
>   b. Heterosexual contact: 36%
>   c. Other: 14%
> 3. Women were infected by the following routes 1989-1992
>   a. Intravenous drug abuse: 43%
>   b. Heterosexual contact: 39%
>   c. Other: 18%
> 4. Racial distribution of women with AIDS
>   a. African American: 53%
>   b. Hispanic: 21%
>   c. Other: 26%
> 5. Annual case rate per 100,000 women
>   a. Black: 27.2
>   b. Hispanic: 13.1
>   c. White: 1.8
>   d. Other: 57.9
> 6. Seroprevalence rates (per 1000 women) using neonatal heel stick specimens from 1988 to 1990
>
> | State | Rate |
> |---|---|
> | New York | 5.8 |
> | District of Columbia | 5.5 |
> | New Jersey | 4.9 |
> | Florida | 4.5 |
> | Montana | 0.0 |

From Gwinn M et al: JAMA 265:1701, 1991.

   b. It is unknown whether HIV-1 infection of the placenta can either facilitate fetal HIV-1 infection or inhibit fetal infection by sequestering virus.

RATE OF TRANSMISSION OF HIV-1 FROM MOTHER TO FETUS

Vertical transmission is dependent on a number of factors.

1. Factors that increase transmission
   a. Mother has AIDS
   b. Low CD4 counts, especially less than 200 cell/mm^3

Table 19-12 Evidence for Different Times of Vertical Transmission of HIV

Intrauterine Transmission	Intrapartum Transmission	Postpartum Transmission
Probable	Later onset symptoms (>12 months old) ≈70%	HIV isolation in breast milk
Early onset of symptoms (<12 months old) ≈30%	Delayed viral identification (>4 months old) ≈50%-70%	Cases of transmission via breastfeeding
Neonatal period viral identification (<3 months old) ≈30%-50%	Intrapartum blood and secretion exposure	No evidence of transmission in households
HIV identifiable in fetal tissue (>13 weeks of gestation)	*"Acute Primary Infection"*	
Possible	Viral/immunological pattern	
HIV identified in placentas (≥8 weeks of gestation)	HIV isolated from vaginal/cervical secretion	
In vitro infection of placenta-derived cells	*Discordant twins*	
Unlikely		
Dysmorphic syndrome		

    c. Presence of p24 antigenemia
    d. Presence of histologic chorioamnionitis
    e. Preterm delivery
2. Factors that decrease transmission
    a. Presence of antibody to HIV protein gp 120
    b. Prenatal care
    c. Taking zidovudine (ZDV)
3. European Collaborative Study transmission rate: 25%
4. The AIDS Clinical Trial Group (ACTG) 076 study: showed transmission rate to be 8% in group receiving ZDV antepartum or intrapartum and in the neonate receiving ZDV during the first 6 weeks of life

PATHOGENESIS OF HIV INFECTION: VIRAL REPLICATION AND DISEASE

1. Early studies into viral pathogenesis measured the amount of free culturable virus in peripheral blood and found that viral burden was low in the early stages of HIV infection (e.g., 0 to 10 infective doses per milliliter), rising to 100 to 1000 infective doses per milliliter in later-stage disease.
2. Recent studies have shown a high level of ongoing viral replication during this period of latency.
3. Polymerase chain reaction (PCR) and branched DNA (bDNA) techniques have been used to measure significantly high levels of viral

Practical Guide to the Care of the Gynecologic/Obstetric Patient 447

Table 19-13 **Prevalence of Vertically Acquired HIV Infection and AIDS: 1978-1993**

Birth Year	Vertically Acquired HIV Infection	Vertically Acquired AIDS Cases	Deaths Among Vertically Acquired AIDS Cases
1978	70	50	40
1979	60	40	30
1980	120	70	50
1981	190	110	60
1982	270	150	100
1983	410	220	130
1984	660	290	190
1985	870	370	220
1986	1,100	460	260
1987	1,390	530	280
1988	1,360	610	320
1989	1,590	610	300
1990	1,690	610	270
1991	1,760	590	230
1992	1,750	440	150
1993	1,630	180	50
	14,920	5,330	2,680

From Mofenson LM et al: *Yearbk Obstet Gynecol* xiii-xlii, 1992.

RNA in plasma after initial clearance of virus from peripheral blood. Viral burden is measured at 106 to 107 RNA copies per milliliter during the initial viremia, decreasing to 103 to 104 copies per milliliter during the latent period.
4. Lymph nodes show replicating viruses and intense immunologic reaction in persons with early asymptomatic infection.
5. Antiretroviral treatment with ZDV shows a dramatic fourfold to fivefold decrease in plasma HIV RNA level within 1 week after the drug is initiated.
6. When the drug is withdrawn the plasma level rapidly increases.

CARE OF THE PATIENT WITH HIV

1. Patients seeking prenatal care should be screened for HIV antibodies as a part of routine prenatal care.
2. The Centers for Disease Control and Prevention and the ACOG have recommended antenatal HIV testing be offered to women who admit to a history of risk-associated behavior.
   a. Targeted screening would miss a large segment of the population at risk (40%).
   b. Universal screening is recommended since publication of the ACTG 076 protocol, which showed a 67% reduction in vertical transmission with the use of ZDV.

Table 19-14 Births to Women Who Are HIV Positive and Incidence of HIV Infection in Infants: Estimates Based on Survey of Childbearing Women (SCBW) United States 1988-1993

Year	Number of States in SCBW	Number Tested in SCBW	Percentage Vertically Acquired AIDS Cases	Estimated Number Births to Women Who Are HIV Positive	Estimated Incidence of HIV Infection in Infants*
1988	13	590,128	81.4	5,430	1,360
1989	35	1,747,561	94.1	6,370	1,590
1990	43	2,349,661	96.8	6,770	1,690
1991	44	2,386,430	99.7	7,040	1,760
1992	44	2,711,603	99.7	6,990	1,750
1993	44	2,743,767	99.5	6,530	1,630

From Davis SF et al: *JAMA* 274:952-955, 1995.
*Estimates based on 25% transmission rate.

Table 19-15 1993 Revised Classification System for HIV Infection and Expanded AIDS Surveillance Case Definition for Adolescents and Adults

CD4 count	Asymptomatic or Lymphadenopathy	Symptomatic	AIDS-Indicator Conditions
>500/mm^3	A1	B1	C1
200-499/mm^3	A2	B2	C2
<200/mm^3	A3	B3	C3

From Davis SF et al: *JAMA* 274:952-955, 1995.
*Category A: acute HIV infection, asymptomatic HIV, persistent generalized lymphadenopathy; Category B: persistent vulvovaginal candidiasis, severe cervical dyspasia or carcinoma, pulmonary TBC, pelvic inflammatory disease; Category C: includes conditions previously used as case definitions for AIDS.

    c. Initiation of HIV-1 screening programs in urban obstetric populations has been shown to be both cost effective and medically beneficial.
3. Patients who are HIV-1 positive should be evaluated as follows (Table 19-15):
    a. Physician should determine risk category.
    b. Physician should determine stage of disease.
    c. Sexually transmitted diseases should be detected and treated.

d. Appropriate vaccines and prophylactic medication should be administered.

Evaluations by the Physician

1. Physical examinations
2. Laboratory evaluations
    a. CBC with platelets
    b. CD4 count each trimester
    c. Skin test for tuberculosis
    d. Papanicolaou smear
    e. Liver function tests
    f. p24 antigen levels
    g. Hepatitis B and C antibody levels
    h. Syphilis serology
    i. Cultures for *Neisseria gonorrhoeae* and *Chlamydia trachomatis*

Preventive Care by the Physician

1. Focus on prevention of sexually transmitted diseases (STDs).
2. Hepatitis B vaccine should be given.
3. "Safer sex" measures will reduce exposure to STDs, which may have an adverse effect on the mother and fetus.
4. Zidovudine, 100 mg, five times per day, should be started regardless of CD4 count.
5. Pneumovax vaccine should be given.
6. Trimethoprim-sulfa should be started if the CD4 count is less than 200/mm^3 as prophylaxis against *Pneumocystis carinii* pneumonia.
7. Influenza vaccine should be given (during September-March).

Prenatal Care by the Physician

1. The obstetrician must maintain a high index of suspicion for STDs and opportunistic infections.
2. IUGR is increased in this population; therefore periodic ultrasonic evaluation for growth is indicated.
3. CD4 counts should be performed each trimester.
4. Colposcopy should be performed if Papanicolaou smears are abnormal.
5. Other routine prenatal vitamins should be given, and maternal serum alpha-fetoprotein (MSAFP) triple screen and diabetes screening should be performed.

Intrapartum Care by the Physician

1. Zidovudine intravenously when labor starts: The dosage should be 200 mg IV over 1 hour, then 100 mg/hr until delivery.
2. Intrapartum procedures that expose the fetus to maternal blood and body fluids should be avoided if at all possible (Box 19-10).
3. There is no clear evidence that cesarean delivery reduces the incidence of maternal fetal transmission.
4. Evidence is present that suggests women with CD4 counts less than 200/mm^3 have a greater risk of transmission with longer labors (>12 hours) or prolonged range of motion (ROM) greater than 12.

BOX 19-10 Invasive Obstetric Procedures That May Increase Fetal or Newborn Exposure to Maternal Blood and Secretions

1. Amniocentesis
2. Percutaneous umbilical cord sampling
3. Chorionic villus sampling
4. Fetal scalp sampling
5. Fetal scalp monitoring
6. Amnioinfusion

Postpartum Care by the Physician

1. A private room is desirable to decrease possible exposure of other patients to body secretions.
2. Patient should be fully counseled about contraceptive options and a reliable method advised.
3. Intrauterine devices should not be used because of the patient's immunosuppressive state and increased risk of pelvic inflammatory disease.
4. Forms of successful contraception include sterilization, oral contraceptives, Depo-Provera, Norplant, and barrier methods.
5. A condom should be used with every sexual encounter to reduce transmission of HIV-1 to partner and to reduce the risk of acquiring another sexually transmitted disease.
6. Physician should arrange for follow-up of mother and baby.

PREGNANCY OUTCOME AND FREQUENT COMPLICATIONS

1. Most women who are HIV positive began their prenatal care in the second trimester and 17% have no prenatal care.
2. Women who are HIV positive are more likely to have sexually transmitted diseases and medical complications such as diabetes and chronic hypertension.
3. There is an increased risk of bacterial pneumonia during pregnancy.
4. Women with CD4 counts less than $300/mm^3$ are more likely to develop serious infections in pregnancy.
5. Vaginal candidiasis is a frequent problem and difficult to eradicate; topical antifungals are the treatment of choice.
6. Cervical dysplasia is a common finding and the patient should be managed in the usual manner.
   a. Colposcopy is necessary.
   b. Because abnormal genital cytology is a manifestation of human papillomavirus infection in an immunodepressed patient, therapy should be done.
7. The ACOG has presented statements of physician responsibility in caring for persons with HIV infections. They include the

following:
a. Learning about HIV and its associated conditions
b. Awareness that although it is appropriate to consider physician risk in management decisions, "patient benefit should not be compromised in an effort to protect the physician"
c. Practice of "universal precautions"
d. Respect for the reproductive choices of every woman infected with HIV
e. Not allowing HIV infection to become a barrier to care
f. Providing care regardless of circumstances of infection
g. Providing patient education about the disease, including pretest and posttest counseling
h. Respecting patient confidentiality
i. Becoming familiar with local regulations regarding screening for HIV, reporting and disclosure of results, and confidentiality
j. Avoiding procedures that risk infecting a patient if the care provider is HIV infected

19.7 Group B *Streptococcus* and Bacterial Vaginosis

Michael P. Marcotte and Louis Weinstein

GROUP B *STREPTOCOCCUS* IN PREGNANCY

Epidemiology and Background

1. Synonyms: *Streptococcus agalactiae*, Lancefield group B *Streptococcus*, β-hemolytic *Streptococcus*
2. Not recognized as human pathogen until mid-1960s
3. Asymptomatic colonization present in the genital tract of 15% to 40% of pregnant women in the United States
   a. Highest rates in the lower third of the vagina and the rectum
   b. Lowest rates in the cervix and urinary tract
   c. Asymptomatic urinary tract colonization in 1% to 2% of pregnant women (may represent the highest inoculum size)
4. Presence of colonization dependent on multiple factors (Box 19-11)
   a. Ethnic group: highest in African Americans, then Hispanics (Caribbean descent greater than Mexican), lowest in Caucasians

---

BOX 19-11 **High-Risk Factors for *Streptococcus* Colonization**

Ethnic group: African Americans > Hispanics > Caucasians
Diabetes
Older women
Primigravidas
Medically indigent
Multiple gestations

b. Diabetics
c. Older women
d. Primigravidas
e. Medically indigent
f. Multiple gestations
5. Group B *Streptococcus* (GBS) infections: the most frequent cause of life-threatening infections in the newborn and a significant cause of morbidity in pregnant women in the United States
   a. 10,000 to 15,000 cases of neonatal sepsis annually (compared with 1000 cases of neonatal herpes simplex infections)
   b. Maternal morbidity: chorioamnionitis, endomyometritis, cystitis, and pyelonephritis (50,000 cases annually)
   c. Increased incidence of preterm deliveries with urinary tract colonization
6. Overall cost estimates of GBS-related infections in 1985 in the United States: $726 million

Diagnosis

1. Gold standard: selective culture media (Todd-Hewitt broth), a blood agar media containing gentamycin and nalidixic acid to inhibit gram-negative bacterial overgrowth; increases the pickup rate by 50% over standard aerobic culture media
2. More rapid diagnostic testing (Gram stain, immunofluorescent antibody test, antigen detection with coagglutination, latex particle agglutination, and nucleic acid probes): available but plagued with the problem of low sensitivity in identifying all patients with GBS colonization
3. Serotyping: type I_a, I_b, II, and III shown to be responsible for disease in humans

Clinical Manifestations in the Neonate

1. Early-onset neonatal sepsis (onset before 7 days of life)
   a. Early onset accounts for 66% of neonatal infection with GBS.
   b. Early onset occurs in 1 to 4 per 1000 live births in the United States.
   c. Attack rate is 10 to 40 per 1000 babies born to mothers with positive vaginal rectal colonization.
   d. Early onset neonatal sepsis presents as septicemia, pneumonia, and meningitis, with symptoms present at birth in 50% of neonates (mean age at onset of symptoms is 20 hours).
   e. If infection presents after first few days of life, meningitis predominates.
      (1) This accounts for 30% of early-onset disease.
      (2) Permanent neurodevelopmental deficits occur in 50% with meningitis.
   f. Mortality: Overall is 15%; in preterm infants it is 25% to 30%.
   g. Vertical transmission (colonization of neonates without signs of infection) occurs in greater than 50% of neonates born to mothers with positive antenatal GBS cultures.
      (1) Only 1% of these infants develop early-onset disease.

(2) Forty percent to 75% of GBS are caused by serotype III.
  h. High-risk factors for development of early GBS sepsis include the following:
    (1) Preterm delivery (less than 37 weeks)
    (2) Prolonged rupture of membranes (greater than 18 hours)
    (3) Maternal intrapartum fever or signs of chorioamnionitis
    (4) Preterm premature rupture of membranes
    (5) Previous sibling affected by symptomatic GBS infection
  i. Intrapartum chemoprophylaxis with ampicillin in mothers with GBS colonization and one or more high-risk factors has been shown to decrease occurrence of early-onset infection (see Intrapartum Treatment).
2. Late-onset neonatal infection (onset greater than 7 days of life)
  a. Presenting finding of meningitis is found in 85% of neonates.
  b. Overall attack rate is 0.5 to 1 per 1000 live births.
  c. Infection is not related to intrapartum vertical transmission.
  d. Intrapartum chemoprophylaxis is not effective at reducing the incidence of late-onset disease.
  e. Transmission is postpartum by neonatal contacts: colonized family, friends, and nursing personnel (nursing personnel colonized 15% to 45% of time).
  f. Serotype III is responsible in greater than 90% of late-onset infections.
  g. Mortality is 10%, but 50% of neonates with meningitis have permanent neurodevelopmental abnormalities.
  h. Neonates may also develop other infections from GBS: middle ear, sinuses, conjunctiva, breasts, lungs, bones, joints, and skin.

Clinical Manifestations in the Mother

1. Urinary tract
  a. GBS is found in urine of pregnant women 1% to 2% of the time. Majority are asymptomatic.
  b. Usually associated with heavy colonization of GBS in the genital tract.
  c. The patient should be considered colonized with GBS in the genital tract.
  d. If left untreated, GBS is associated with an increase in the rate of preterm deliveries and premature rupture of membranes.
  e. Also associated with an increase in the rate of neonatal sepsis: 7:100 (whereas genital tract colonization alone is associated with 1:100 cases of sepsis).
  f. If left untreated, GBS is associated with a higher incidence of symptomatic maternal urinary tract infections: cystitis and pyelonephritis.
  g. Treatment: Ampicillin or penicillin (aqueous PCN) is given.
    (1) PCN-allergic patients use erythromycin or clindamycin, for 7 to 14 days, any time GBS is cultured from the urine tract.
    (2) Also plan intrapartum chemoprophylaxis in high-risk patients (see Box 19-11).
2. Chorioamnionitis (intraamniotic infection)

a. Defined as a maternal oral temperature greater than 37.8° C plus maternal tachycardia (>100 beats per minute), fetal tachycardia (>160 beats per minute), uterine tenderness, foul odor of amniotic fluid, or peripheral leukocytosis (>12,000/mm^3).
b. If patient has GBS colonization of the genital tract there is a high rate of colonization (75%) of the intraamniotic cavity after rupture of membranes.
   (1) This amniotic colonization increases with internal monitoring and length of rupture of membranes.
   (2) The amniotic colonization is much higher than the incidence of intraamniotic infection (15%).
c. If chorioamnionitis develops, there is a higher rate of neonatal infection (5 to 7 per 100). Intraamniotic antibiotics may not decrease the rate of sepsis after the mother has signs of chorioamnionitis.
d. Treatment: Immediate initiation of antibiotics is begun: ampicillin (or PCN) and gentamycin along with delivery.
   (1) Chorioamnionitis with GBS is almost always associated with other bacteria.
   (2) For PCN-allergic patients use gentamycin plus clindamycin or a first-generation cephalosporin.
3. Endomyometritis (synonyms: endometritis or endomyoparametritis)
   a. Endomyometritis is defined as a postpartum oral temperature greater than 37.8° C with localized uterine tenderness.
   b. GBS endomyometritis is usually associated with high fever within 12 hours of delivery, tachycardia, and abdominal distension. Some patients are without localizing signs early in the course of the illness.
   c. Bacteremia is present in 35% of cases. Most cases follow cesarean sections.
   d. Treatment: Endomyometritis is usually associated with multiple organisms.
      (1) Broad-spectrum coverage indicated.
      (2) Multiple regimens proposed with activity against GBS.

Prevention of GBS Morbidity and Mortality

1. Antepartum treatment
   a. Strategy
      (1) Ampicillin (or PCN) can be given at the time of positive GBS culture anytime during pregnancy.
      (2) Duration of treatment varies.
      (3) Shortcomings:
         (a) Antepartum treatment is ineffective at preventing GBS infection in mother or neonate as well as preventing premature delivery.
         (b) GBS is transmitted between partners.
         (c) Impossible to eradicate GBS from the rectum because of presence of high concentrations of beta-lactamase producing bacteria, which inhibit the action of ampicillin and PCN.

(d) Large numbers of patients need to be treated with long durations of PCN, which increases the chance of allergic reactions and promotes growth of resistant bacteria.
(e) Only shown to be beneficial if a urine culture is positive for GBS.
(4) Advantages:
(a) Reduces the incidence of preterm delivery, premature rupture of membranes, symptomatic urinary tract infections, and early neonatal GBS sepsis.

2. Intrapartum treatment
   a. Strategy: Ampicillin (or PCN) given to patients with proven GBS colonization and one or more high-risk factors (see Box 19-11).
      (1) Dosage: ampicillin 2 g IV then 1 to 2 g IV every 4 to 6 hours while in labor
      (2) Clindamycin or a first-generation cephalosporin given to PCN-allergic patients
   b. Controversy in determining the patients to be screened, when to screen them in pregnancy, and the diagnostic method to be used.
3. Several proposed methods to implement this strategy
   (1) Method 1
      (a) Patients who present to labor and delivery with a known high-risk factor (preterm premature rupture of the membranes or preterm labor) are cultured.
         (i) Obtain prophylaxis of patients with positive cultures or patients who will deliver before culture results are available.
         (ii) No prophylaxis for patients without risk factors and negative cultures.
      (b) Advantages:
         (i) It has been demonstrated that antibiotics initiated less than 1 hour before delivery are less effective at preventing transmission of GBS to the neonate.
         (ii) This method would allow many patients to receive antibiotics more than 1 hour before delivery (i.e., the neonate would have higher blood levels of the antibiotics).
      (c) Shortcomings:
         (i) A large number of women will be treated unnecessarily.
         (ii) This may increase the incidence of allergic reactions and promote the development of neonatal sepsis from bacteria resistant to ampicillin.
         (iii) This method has never been studied in a large, randomized, double-blind, controlled trial.
   (2) Method 2
      (a) Using a rapid diagnostic technique, patients who present in labor are tested for the presence of GBS. Patients with a positive test and one or more high-risk factors receive prophylaxis.

(b) Advantages:
   (i) GBS has been shown to be transiently present in genital cultures of one third or more of pregnant women throughout their gestation.
   (ii) This strategy would allow for identification of only women with GBS present at the time of delivery (the time when GBS will be vertically transmitted).
(c) Shortcomings:
   (i) Some women presenting will deliver before the results of the rapid diagnostic tests are available.
   (ii) Most importantly, there are currently no tests available that have a high enough sensitivity to be used in clinical practice.

(3) Method 3
   (a) In the mid–second trimester, culture for GBS. When patients present in labor, prophylaxis for all patients with a positive culture and one or more high-risk factors.
   (b) Advantages:
      (i) This method is the only one that has been shown in large, randomized, double-blind, placebo-controlled studies to reduce the incidence of early-onset GBS neonatal sepsis.
      (ii) This method has also been shown to decrease the incidence of maternal postpartum febrile morbidity (endomyometritis).
   (c) Shortcomings:
      (i) Controversy exists in determining which women should have cultures in the second trimester.
      (ii) GBS is transiently present on genital cultures in more than one third of women and, therefore, a number of women who were culture negative earlier in pregnancy will be positive at delivery.
      (iii) Some cases of GBS sepsis occur before screening can be done (delivery before 26 weeks) when the mortality rate if infected may be increased.

(4) Method 4
   (a) Screening with antepartum cultures is not done, and all women who have one or more high-risk factors are treated.
   (b) Advantage: This method will prevent at least the same number of cases of GBS sepsis as method 3, without the cost of GBS screening.
   (c) Shortcomings:
      (i) Many women will be given ampicillin who are not colonized with GBS.
      (ii) This method has not been studied in a randomized, double-blind, placebo-controlled study.

4. Neonatal therapy: prophylactic PCN is administered to all neonates at birth
   a. Advantages

(1) Study has demonstrated a decreased incidence of GBS sepsis in neonates treated with PCN at birth for prevention of gonococcal ophthalmia.
(2) Eliminates the need for GBS screening.
b. Shortcomings
(1) 40% to 50% of neonates who develop sepsis are symptomatic at birth, suggesting that prophylactic PCN after birth may not be adequate treatment and may increase the mortality.
(2) This treatment may select for sepsis from PCN-resistant bacteria.
(3) Also, no randomized, double-blind, placebo-controlled studies have been done.
(4) This strategy will not reduce the incidence of GBS morbidity in the mother.
5. Recommendations
a. The ACOG recommends selective prophylaxis intrapartum of women with GBS colonization who have one or more risk factors (see Box 19-11).
(1) ACOG does not recommend antenatal screening for all women.
(2) ACOG does recommend antepartum screening for women who have threatened or arrested preterm labor or premature rupture of membranes remote from term, and women who undergo cervical surgery in pregnancy.
(3) ACOG does recognize that if GBS colonization status is not known and delivery is imminent it may be beneficial to give intrapartum prophylaxis.
b. The American Academy of Pediatrics (AAP) recommends universal screening of all women at 26 to 28 weeks gestation.
(1) Intrapartum prophylaxis should be given to all patients with positive antepartum cultures and one or more risk factors (see Box 19-11).
(2) AAP states that it may be appropriate to give intrapartum prophylaxis if GBS status is unknown with one of the above risk factors present.
(3) AAP further states that management of neonates of mothers who have received GBS prophylaxis while in labor should be based on clinical findings and gestational age of the neonate.

Summary

1. GBS early neonatal sepsis is the leading cause of mortality by infection in neonates in the United States. GBS is a significant source of maternal morbidity.
2. Controversy still surrounds the ideal way to screen for and prevent GBS morbidity and mortality.
3. Intrapartum chemoprophylaxis with ampicillin has been shown to reduce the incidence of early-onset neonatal GBS sepsis.
4. Selective media (Todd-Hewitt culture media) increases detection of GBS colonization by 50%.

5. Future: Rapid diagnostic tests for GBS that can be used when a patient presents in labor must have a high sensitivity and specificity; intrapartum treatment of those with a positive test and one or more high-risk factors (see Box 19-11).
6. Active immunization of all pregnant women should be performed with a vaccine that stimulates development of protective antibodies of the IgG subtype, crosses the placenta, and protects the neonate in the intrapartum and immediate postpartum period.

BACTERIAL VAGINOSIS

Epidemiology and Background

1. Before 1955, vaginal discharge that was not caused by gonorrhea, trichomonads, or *Candida albicans* was referred to as nonspecific vaginitis.
2. Gardner and Duke, in 1955, isolated a new bacterium from patients with nonspecific vaginitis and called it *Haemophilus vaginalis*.
   a. They concluded that *H. vaginalis* caused nonspecific vaginitis.
   b. They also identified the clue cell as a diagnostic marker.
3. From 1960 to 1980, name changes occurred that reflected changing taxonomy of the bacterium originally identified by Gardner and Duke: The names included *Corynebacterium vaginalis* and *Gardnerella vaginalis*.
4. In the 1980s, it became clear that more than a single organism was responsible for bacterial vaginosis. It again went through several name changes: These included nonspecific vaginitis, anaerobic vaginosis, and finally in 1984 bacterial vaginosis (BV).
5. Data collected throughout this time showed that women with BV had an overgrowth of both aerobic and anaerobic bacteria and a loss of the normal flora of the vagina.
   a. Microbiology
      (1) Normal vaginal flora: Lactobacillus spp. predominate.
         (a) Usual concentration of bacteria less than 10^7 organisms per gram of tissue
         (b) Can find Gardnerella vaginalis in up to 50% of patients without BV
      (2) Flora in bacterial vaginosis: loss of *Lactobacillus* spp. and increased concentration of other bacteria up to 109 organisms per gram of tissue with an increase in anaerobic bacteria. *Gardnerella vaginalis* isolated in 95% of women with BV concomitant with an increase in isolation of *Mycoplasma* spp. and *Mobiluncus* spp. in vaginal secretions of women with BV.
   b. Bacteria found in bacterial vaginosis
      (1) Anaerobes: *Bacteroides* (now known as *Prevotella*) spp., *Peptostreptococcus* spp., *Mobiluncus* spp.
      (2) Aerobes: *Gardnerella vaginalis*, *Mycoplasma* spp.
6. Risk factors: Race, sexually transmitted disease history, hormonal birth control methods, age, and number of lifetime sexual partners are not associated with risk of developing BV.

Practical Guide to the Care of the Gynecologic/Obstetric Patient 459

   a. Current intrauterine device (IUD) use is associated with an increased presence of BV.
   b. Increased rates of BV are seen in women with multiple sexual partners within 1 month of the exam, compared to women in a monogamous relationship.
7. Etiology is unknown.
   a. Some question whether BV is a sexually transmitted disease.
   b. Evidence includes the following:
      (1) Bacteria associated with BV seen in the urine and urethral scrapings of male partners of patients with BV.
      (2) Higher rates of BV in women with multiple sexual partners.
      (3) Decreased rate of BV in monogamous couples.
   c. Evidence against it includes the following:
      (1) Bacteria associated with BV that are found in male partners of women with BV do not persist in these men once they abstain from intercourse.
      (2) No increase in cure rates when partners of women diagnosed with BV are treated.
      (3) BV found in 12% of virginal women.

Diagnosis

1. Symptoms
   a. Malodorous vaginal discharge is the most common presenting complaint.
   b. More than 50% of women diagnosed with BV do not have any complaints.
2. Signs: gold standard: clinical findings
   a. Diagnosis made if three of the four clinical findings are present.
      (1) Vaginal pH greater than 4.5
      (2) Wet preparation showing clue cells (squamous epithelial cells with so many bacteria attached to their surface that the cell borders become obscured)
      (3) A milky homogeneous vaginal discharge
      (4) The release of an amine (fishy) odor after the addition of 10% potassium hydroxide to the vaginal fluid
   b. Advantages:
      (1) Sensitivity, 99.5%; positive predictive value, 98.8%
      (2) Easily and inexpensively performed in the office
   c. Shortcomings:
      (1) Vaginal discharge can appear normal; affected by recent douching and intercourse
      (2) pH of vagina increased by the presence of semen and menstrual blood
   d. Other diagnostic aids: gram stain, cultures for *Gardnerella* and *Mobiluncus*, and rapid diagnostic tests used in research.
      (1) Gram stain:
         (a) In BV the Gram stain will show a loss of normal *Lactobacillus* species and an increase in gram-positive cocci (*Peptostreptococcus*), small gram-negative rods (*Bacteroides*

Table 19-16 **Diagnosis of Bacterial Vaginosis by Gram Stain**

Reading	Normal	Intermediate	Abnormal
Grade	I	II	III
Predominant bacteria	*Lactobacillus*	Mixed	Anaerobes and *Gardnerella*

From *MMWR* 41:1-9, 1992.

and *Gardnerella*), and curved gram-negative rods (*Mobiluncus*).
- (b) Categorizes vaginal flora as normal (*Lactobacillus* predominates), intermediate (mixed flora), or bacterial vaginosis (Table 19-16).
- (2) Advantages:
  - (a) Standard method used in microbiology laboratories to evaluate bacteria
  - (b) Relatively inexpensive
- (3) Shortcomings:
  - (a) Not as sensitive or specific as the clinical criteria
  - (b) Delays the diagnosis if Gram stain equipment not in the office
- (4) Culture for *Gardnerella* and *Mobiluncus:* These are not used in clinical practice because women without symptoms or clinical criteria for BV have positive cultures 50% of the time.
- (5) Rapid diagnostic tests include gas–liquid chromatography, thin-layer chromatography, and enzyme analysis.

Natural History

1. In women who are pregnant, the incidence of BV is 10% to 30%. Approximately 50% of these women will be asymptomatic.
2. Persistent positive diagnosis of BV has been seen in 75% of women not treated.
3. Spontaneous resolution of BV seen in 25% of women. Reasons postulated include the promotion of *Lactobacillus* growth by the hormone milieu and the decreased frequency of intercourse as pregnancy progresses.
4. Treatment with metronidazole (500 mg, twice daily, for 7 days) or clindamycin (300 mg, twice daily, for 7 days) is shown to cure women in pregnancy of BV 85% of the time when cultures are repeated at 4 weeks.
5. BV is associated with preterm labor and delivery, premature rupture of membranes, LBW infants (< 2500 g), chorioamnionitis, and postpartum endomyometritis.

Associated Sequelae from Bacterial Vaginosis in Pregnancy

1. Preterm labor
   a. Evidence suggests that women with BV are at a twofold to threefold increased risk of premature labor and delivery of a preterm low-birth weight infant.
   b. Pathophysiology:
      (1) The bacteria present in BV have been shown to produce phospholipase A_2, an enzyme that liberates arachidonic acid, which may induce prostaglandin synthesis in the amnion, leading to premature labor.
      (2) Another proposed mechanism by which bacteria are thought to induce prostaglandin production is via direct invasion of the amniotic membranes adjacent to the cervix.
      (3) Lastly, the bacteria may stimulate migration of white blood cells that metabolize arachidonic acid leading to labor.
2. Premature rupture of membranes
   a. Studies have consistently demonstrated a twofold to threefold increased incidence of premature rupture of membranes (PROM) in women diagnosed with BV.
   b. Women with BV have been shown to have a much higher incidence of PROM prior to and at term.
   c. Pathophysiology: Bacteria associated with BV have been proved in vitro to produce protease that reduces the strength of the amnion.
   d. Uterine contractions increase intrauterine pressure, which may cause rupture of the already weakened membranes.
3. Chorioamnionitis and subclinical intrauterine infections
   a. Patients in premature labor with BV have a higher incidence of positive amniotic fluid culture for organisms associated with BV (i.e., anaerobic bacteria, *Gardnerella*, and *Mobiluncus*).
   b. These women are at higher risk for developing chorioamnionitis and delivering prematurely.
   c. These women are also less likely to respond to tocolytic therapy.
   d. Although causation has not been conclusively proved for BV and intraamniotic infections, the association is strong.
   e. Pathophysiology:
      (1) The proposed mechanism for the development of chorioamnionitis is through direct ascending invasion of the amnion by vaginal bacteria with proliferation in the amniotic fluid and release of phospholipase A_2.
      (2) These bacteria attract white blood cells, which produce inflammatory mediators, leading to the systemic response.
4. Postpartum endomyometritis
   a. Few prospective reports are available to link the occurrence of intrapartum BV and postpartum endomyometritis.
   b. One study prospectively followed patients with the diagnosis of BV by Gram stain made at the time of labor who subsequently underwent a cesarean section.

c. Those who had BV had a sixfold increase in the rate of postpartum endomyometritis compared with women without BV.
d. All patients received antibiotic prophylaxis at the time of surgery.
e. The authors reported that one third of patients with the diagnosis of BV at the time of labor who had a cesarean section developed endomyometritis despite prophylactic antibiotics.
f. These women grew twice the amount of bacteria on sensitive endometrial cultures than women without BV who developed endomyometritis.
g. Pathophysiology:
   (1) Bacteria gain access to the endometrial cavity by an ascending route.
   (2) Women with BV are shown to have a higher concentration of more virulent bacteria in the vagina than women without BV.
   (3) When a woman in labor undergoes a cesarean section these bacteria not only have access to the endometrial cavity, but also the myometrium, blood vessels, lymphatics, pelvic peritoneum, and the abdominal wound.
   (4) Sutures, which act as foreign bodies, result in a decrease in the bacterial inoculum necessary to establish an infection.

Treatment Strategies

1. Historical perspective:
   a. Gardner and Duke, in 1955, recommended using topical sulfonamides and oral tetracycline.
   b. They believed BV to be caused by a single organism, *Haemophilus vaginalis*, which is sensitive to these antibiotics.
   c. Elimination of this organism was thought to cure the disease.
   d. This was subsequently proved to be incorrect.
   e. Ampicillin was later recommended and has proved to be ineffective.
2. Treatment of the nonpregnant woman:
   a. Standard treatment is oral metronidazole, 500 mg, twice daily for 7 days.
   b. The immediate cure rate is 98%, and long-term cure is expected in 60% to 95% of the cases.
3. Women with BV are encouraged to abstain from douching and some investigators recommend treating partners of patients with recurrent BV.
4. Douching may disrupt the normal *Lactobacillus* predominant microflora of the vagina and promote the overgrowth of organisms responsible for BV.
   a. No studies have conclusively shown a benefit to treating sexual partners.
   b. New regimens shown to be as effective as metronidazole are intravaginal 0.75% metronidazole gel (one applicator full, 5 g, intravaginally, twice daily for 5 days), intravaginal clindamycin 2% cream (one applicator full, 5 g, intravaginally, once daily for 7 days),

short-course oral metronidazole (2 g single dose) and oral clindamycin (300 mg, twice daily for 7 days).
5. Treatment of the pregnant woman:
   a. Multiple studies have examined the role of metronidazole and clindamycin to treat BV in pregnancy.
   b. The hope is that treatment of BV in pregnancy will reduce the incidence of associated morbidity.
      (1) Metronidazole
         (a) Full course: All studies to date have shown a 40% to 50% reduction in the incidence of preterm delivery, PROM, and delivery of a neonate weighing less than 2500 g.
         (b) Short course:
            (i) One study demonstrated that metronidazole, 400 mg, twice daily for 2 days, effectively treated BV in pregnancy with an 85% response rate.
            (ii) Cure was defined as resolution of the woman's symptoms, a negative clinical examination using a wet preparation, and light or no growth of *Gardnerella* on culture.
            (iii) Unfortunately, no information was supplied about the pregnancy outcome.
         (c) Intravaginal: No studies have been published.
         (d) Side effects:
            (i) A recent meta-analysis found no increased risk of fetal malformations of women who used metronidazole in the first trimester of pregnancy.
            (ii) Gastrointestinal side effects are common, occurring in 15% to 20% of nonpregnant patients.
            (iii) No major side effects have been reported in studies published with pregnant patients.
            (iv) Metronidazole does not destroy the normal *Lactobacillus* and it is not associated with an increase in vaginal candidiasis.
      (2) Clindamycin
         (a) Oral therapy
            (i) One study demonstrated that treating women with BV in pregnancy with oral clindamycin, 300 mg, twice daily for 7 days, resulted in a 50% reduction in the incidence of preterm births and PROM.
            (ii) This decrease was observed in both patients with a history of preterm births in preceding pregnancies and in women without such a history.
         (b) Intravaginal therapy
            (i) Two well-designed studies demonstrated that in pregnant women with the diagnosis of BV, intravaginal clindamycin 2% cream was effective at curing BV but did not reduce the incidence of preterm birth or PROM.
            (ii) Cure was defined as both a negative clinical examination and a negative gram stain.

(iii) These authors concluded that intravaginal treatment eliminated the BV-associated bacteria from the vagina but was unable to reach bacteria that had already ascended into the upper genital tract.
(c) Side effects
  (i) Both oral and intravaginal clindamycin are associated with an increase in the rate of subsequent vaginal candidiasis (15% to 20%).
  (ii) Oral clindamycin has been documented to cause pseudomembranous colitis.

Conclusions and Recommendation

1. Bacterial vaginosis is present in 10% to 30% of pregnant women. Half of these women will be asymptomatic.
2. Clinical criteria for the diagnosis of BV have been established, are simple to perform, and are highly sensitive and specific.
3. Studies to date are in agreement that BV in pregnancy is associated with preterm labor, preterm birth, premature rupture of membranes, and LBW neonates. There also appears to be a relationship between BV and chorioamnionitis and postpartum endomyometritis.
4. Oral metronidazole has been shown to be highly effective and safe at eliminating the bacteria responsible for BV from the vagina in the pregnant and nonpregnant patient. There is also evidence demonstrating that metronidazole is effective at reducing the high incidence of preterm birth and PROM.
5. BV is likely to be part of the reason for the high incidence of premature birth and PROM. It is unlikely that treatment of women with BV in pregnancy will prevent all of these events.
6. Current evidence supports screening women in pregnancy for BV and treating infected women with oral metronidazole, 500 mg, twice daily for 7 days.
   a. In women who cannot tolerate oral metronidazole, oral clindamycin, 300 mg, twice daily for 7 days, is an acceptable alternative.
   b. Clindamycin may be associated with a higher incidence of *Candida* vaginitis.
7. In the future, it must be determined whether all women will benefit from screening for BV or only those that are at high risk for premature delivery (specifically, a history of premature birth in the past).
   a. Currently, it seems prudent to screen all pregnant women for BV when they seek prenatal care, and if BV is present, treat them with a full course of oral metronidazole.
   b. The benefit of treatment far outweighs the minimal risk.

19.8 Pulmonary Disease

Michael Parsons

Physiologic changes of the lung during pregnancy were outlined in Chapter 22.6. Pregnancy may also alter underlying pulmonary conditions. Several disease states deserve discussion for management, including appropriate medications.

Practical Guide to the Care of the Gynecologic/Obstetric Patient   465

1. Physiologic changes in normal pregnancy include the following:
   a. Increased
      (1) Vital capacity
      (2) Inspiratory capacity
      (3) Tidal volume
      (4) Minute ventilation
   b. Decreased
      (1) Expiratory reserve volume
      (2) Residual volume
      (3) Functional residual capacity
   c. Unchanged: respiratory rate
2. These changes result in the following:
   a. Increased ventilation with increased basal oxygen consumption
   b. A decrease in arterial PO_2
   c. A slight increase in plasma pH to 7.45
   d. A decrease in bicarbonate

DYSPNEA IN PREGNANCY

Mechanism

More than half of all pregnant women report dyspnea at rest by midpregnancy. Proposed mechanisms include the following:

1. Alveolar hyperventilation, with the patient's subjective awareness
2. A response to decreased PCO_2
3. Consequence of anatomic change in the thorax

Significance

Dyspnea may be a sign of decompensation of an underlying lung or heart disorder.

1. Physiologic dyspnea
   a. Tends to occur early in pregnancy and improves or plateaus in later pregnancy
   b. Is rarely extreme and does not usually interfere with daily activities
   c. Is not associated with specific disease indicators
2. Pathologic dyspnea
   a. May occur at rest or normal levels of activity
   b. May be acute, severe, progressive, intractable
   c. Is associated with signs and symptoms suggestive of pulmonary or cardiac disorders
      (1) Cough
      (2) Orthopnea
      (3) Paroxysmal nocturnal dyspnea
      (4) Syncope during exercise
      (5) Chest pain
      (6) Hemoptysis
      (7) Cyanosis and clubbing
      (8) Grade III or greater systolic murmur
      (9) Diastolic murmur
   d. Pulmonary causes (partial list)

(1) Asthma
(2) Pulmonary thromboembolism
(3) Aspiration
(4) Respiratory infections
(5) Amniotic fluid embolism
(6) Adult respiratory distress syndrome
  e. Cardiac causes (partial list)
(1) Valvular heart disease
(2) Arrhythmias
(3) Ischemic heart disease
(4) Cardiomyopathy

Diagnostic Tests as Appropriate

1. Echocardiogram
2. ECG
3. Exercise stress testing
4. Pulmonary exercise tests

ASTHMA

Asthma is a lung disease that includes the following:

1. Infiltration of the airway with inflammatory cells
2. Increased airway sensitivity and responsiveness
   a. Nonspecific stimuli, including cold air, exercise, strong odors, cigarette smoke
   b. Specific stimuli, including viral infection, F series prostaglandins, ergonovine, aspirin, dust mites, molds
3. Reversible airway obstruction (The reversibility of the obstruction is either spontaneous or as a result of treatment, but in some cases is incomplete.)

Incidence

1. The incidence of asthma during pregnancy is approximately 1%.
2. The incidence of status asthmaticus is about 0.2%.

Morbidity and Mortality

1. Approximately one third of asthmatic women experience worsening of the disease at some time during pregnancy.
   a. Patients with severe asthma experience worsening of the disease more often.
   b. There is an eighteenfold increased risk of exacerbation following cesarean delivery over vaginal delivery.
2. Adverse pregnancy outcomes in patients with severe asthma include the following:
   a. Spontaneous abortions
   b. Preterm labor
   c. LBW infants
   d. Neonatal hypoxia
   e. Maternal morbidity and mortality, including pneumothorax, pneumomediastinum, acute cor pulmonale, cardiac arrhythmias, and muscle fatigue with respiratory arrest

Pathophysiology

The cause of asthma remains unknown. Pathophysiologic causes include the following:

1. Bronchial smooth muscle constriction.
2. Mucus hypersecretion with fluids within the airway lumen.
3. Mucosal edema with thickening of the airway epithelium.
4. Suspected mediators include the following:
   a. Histamine
   b. Leukotrienes
   c. Neuropeptides
   d. Prostaglandins
   e. Thromboxane
   f. Kinins
   g. Others
5. The pathology includes mucosal edema and hyperemia with infiltration of mast cells, eosinophils, and lymphocytes.
   a. Interleukin is produced and IgE synthesized.
   b. The airway wall thickens and fluid within the lumen increases resistance to airflow.
   c. There is obstruction at all airway levels.

Clinical Course

1. Maternal
   a. Acute bronchospasm results in airway obstruction and decreased airflow.
   b. Alterations in oxygenation results from ventilation perfusion mismatching.
   c. Clinical stages of asthma are as follows:
      (1) Hyperventilation compensates hypoxia with normal PO_2 and decreased PCO_2, resultant respiratory alkalosis.
      (2) The airways narrow and hypoxemia results.
      (3) CO_2 retention results from poor ventilation.
      (4) Respiratory failure may follow with hypercapnia and acidemia.
      (5) Pregnant patients are more susceptible to developing hypoxia and hypoxemia because of the smaller functional residual capacity.
2. Fetal
   a. Fetal hypoxemia with decreased umbilical blood flow
   b. Increased systemic and pulmonary vascular resistance
   c. Decreased cardiac output

Diagnosis

1. Clinical evaluation
   a. Cough
   b. Labored breathing
   c. Chest tightness
   d. Anxiety
   e. Breathlessness

f. Prolonged expiration
g. Wheezing unreliable in predicting severity
h. Use of excessory respiratory muscles
i. Tachypnea
j. Tachycardia
k. Pulses paradoxes
l. Central cyanosis
m. Altered level of consciousness

2. Laboratory tests
   a. Forced expiratory volume in 1 second (FEV-1) is the single best measure of pulmonary function for severity.
      (1) Peak expiratory flow rate (PEFR) reflects large airway function to monitor obstruction.
      (2) Of predicted baseline values, 80% or greater are normal for FEV-1 and PEFR.
   b. Arterial blood gas analysis provides objective assessment of moderate to severe asthma.

3. Other tests
   a. Sputum
      (1) Gram stain and Wright stain
      (2) Eosinophils
   b. Chest x-ray
      (1) Chest x-ray is often normal.
      (2) Severe asthma may demonstrate hyperinflation and complications.

Management of Asthma

1. Controlling asthma triggers
   a. Elimination of exposures to irritants
   b. Adjustment for anticipated events, such as pretreatment before exercise
   c. Desensitization

2. Pharmacologic therapy: The two main classes of medications are bronchodilators and antiinflammatories.
   a. Chronic treatment
      (1) Bronchodilator.
         (a) The first-line agents are beta-2-adrenergic agonists.
         (b) They promote cyclic adenosine monophosphate (cAMP) synthesis and facilitate smooth muscle relaxation, mucociliary clearance, and decreased cell mediator release.
         (c) Inhaled beta-2 agonist puffs every 4 hours, as needed, to relax constricted airway smooth muscle (e.g., albuterol, metaproterenol, terbutaline, isoproterenol).
      (2) Inhalational antiinflammatory therapy may be added if treatment with bronchodilators is necessary more than 3 times a week. Choices include corticosteroids, 2 to 5 puffs, bid to qid (e.g., beclomethasone and/or cromolyn sodium), 2 puffs, qid (stabilizes mast cell membranes).
      (3) If asthma is not controlled by the combination in 2.a.2, a tapering dose of oral corticosteroids is indicated (e.g., prednisone,

40 mg PO, qd for 1 week, then taper for 1 week). Daily inhaled corticosteroids may be necessary.
- (4) Additional medications for control of nocturnal asthma may include evening dose of the following:
  - (a) Theophylline
  - (b) Sustained oral beta-2 agonist
- b. Acute exacerbation
  - (1) Lowered threshold for hospitalization during pregnancy
  - (2) Intravenous hydration
  - (3) Supplemental oxygen after a blood gas is obtained
  - (4) Inhaled beta-2 agonists
  - (5) If patient fails to respond, intravenous corticosteroids (e.g., hydrocortisone, 2 mg/kg, or methylprednisolone, 60 mg)
  - (6) Additional treatments: intravenous aminophylline and subcutaneous epinephrine or terbutaline, 0.3 to 0.5 mg of 1:1000 solution

Assessment of Fetus

Evaluate for appropriate fetal growth and fetal well-being during third trimester.

Considerations in Labor

1. Vaginal delivery should be planned for unless there is an obstetric contraindication.
2. Pulmonary status should be assessed by physical exam and expiratory flow measurements or oxygenation as necessary.
3. Fetal monitoring should be performed.
4. Routine inhaled asthma medications should be continued and oral medication transferred to the IV route.
5. Stress dose corticosteroids (e.g., hydrocortisone, 100 mg every 8 hours) if recent systemic steroids.
6. A non–histamine releasing narcotic (e.g., fentanyl) is preferable to meperidine or morphine.
7. PGF-2A uterotonics should be avoided.
8. Regional analgesia should be considered over general.
9. Oxygen to maintain O_2 saturation must be greater than or equal to 95%.

PNEUMONIA

Pneumonia is an acute infection involving inflammation of the lung parenchyma distal to the larger airways.

Incidence

Bacterial and viral pneumonia occur in less than 0.5% of pregnancies.

Morbidity and Mortality

Pneumonia is a major cause of nonobstetric maternal deaths, with a reported mortality of 3% in some series.

1. Increased incidence of preterm labor
2. Perinatal mortality rate: 40 per 1000

Etiology

1. Bacterial:
   a. *Streptococcus pneumoniae (Pneumococcus pneumoniae)* is the most common bacterial pneumonia in pregnancy, causing 30% to 50% of infections.
   b. *Hemophilus influenzae* is more likely in a patient with a smoking history.
   c. *Staphylococcus aureus* is suspected with superimposed pulmonary infections.
   d. *Klebsiella pneumoniae* is seen in chronic alcoholics.
   e. Opportunistic infections include *Acinetobacter, Serratia, Pseudomonas*, increasing in immunocompromised patients.
   f. Overall gram-negative organisms are less common but nosocomial.
2. *Mycoplasma pneumoniae* is most common atypical pneumonia.
3. *Chlamydia pneumoniae*.
4. *Legionella pneumophilae*.
5. Viral:
   a. Influenza A during epidemics should be suspected if respiratory symptoms are present in patient recovering from flulike illness.
   b. *Varicella* is rare but may be life-threatening if a cause of pneumonia in pregnancy.
6. Fungal organisms are uncommon as a cause of pneumonia in pregnancy when compared with other organisms.
   a. Coccidiomycosis is the most common fungal cause in pregnancy (common in southwestern United States)
   b. Other common causes include the following:
      (1) Histoplasmosis
      (2) *Blastomyces dermatitis*
      (3) Cryptococcoses
      (4) *Pneumocystis carinii* pneumonia (PCP) in immunocompromised patients, particularly with AIDS
7. Aspiration:
   a. Pregnant patients are at risk because of delay in gastric emptying and decreased gastroesophogeal sphincter tone.
   b. Aspiration is most associated with general anesthesia but can occur with any condition with decreased consciousness such as seizures, drug overdose, or alcoholism.
   c. Aspiration involves mixes of aerobic–anaerobic organisms and stomach contents.

Pathophysiology

1. The disease process may start by inhalation of organisms from the air or aspiration of organisms from the nasopharynx or oropharynx. Less common mechanisms are hematogenous spread or direct contagious spread.
2. The defense mechanisms of the lung, including ciliated lining epithelium, the cough reflex to expel material, and the immunologic system, are not always successful in preventing infection.

3. Other conditions, such as alteration of consciousness, surgery, or other physical impairments, may predispose to increased infection.
4. Pneumonia can lead to inadequate oxygenation.
5. The viral infections may progress to respiratory failure and acute respiratory distress syndrome.
6. Pregnancy is predisposed to more severe pneumonic infections.
   a. Altered maternal immune status
   b. Increased lung water

Diagnosis

1. Differential diagnosis: The diagnosis of pneumonia is usually evident from the signs, symptoms, physical examination, and laboratory studies. Other causes that should be considered include the following:
   a. Bronchitis
   b. Asthma
   c. Tuberculosis
   d. Tumor
2. History: Symptoms of pneumonia include cough, fever, dyspnea, sputum production, and chest pain; shaking chills may occur. *Mycoplasma pneumoniae* has nonproductive cough.
3. Physical examination: Physical examination reveals fever, tachypnea, and tachycardia. There may be decreased respiratory excursion, and dullness on percussion. If consolidation is present, bronchial breath sounds may be present.
   a. *Mycoplasma pneumoniae* has low-grade fever.
   b. *Varicella pneumoniae* presents 2 to 6 days after cutaneous eruptions.
4. Laboratory examination:
   a. Leukocytosis with a marked left shift is common with bacterial infection. *Mycoplasma pneumoniae* has only mild leukocytosis.
   b. Arterial blood gases may reveal hypoxemia, hypocarbia, and respiratory alkalosis.
   c. Roentgenographic examination is essential.
      (1) If a pregnant woman is suspected of having pneumonia, a chest x-ray film *must* be obtained.
      (2) It may provide a clue to the causative factor.
         (a) Homogeneous, nonsegmental consolidation in a lobe with air bronchogram suggests pneumococcal pneumonia. Pleural effusion may occur.
         (b) A reticular nonhomogeneous pattern suggests *Mycoplasma pneumoniae*.
         (c) *Hemophilus influenzae* pneumonia has air bronchograms in upper lobes.
         (d) Influenza has bilateral lower lobe infiltrates.
   d. Identification of the specific organism is important.
      (1) Gram stain of sputum
      (2) Culture of sputum
      (3) Antigen testing of sputum
      (4) Blood cultures for bacteremia
      (5) Serum testing for *Mycoplasma* IgM

Management

1. Hospitalization
2. Hydration
3. O$_2$ at 3 L/min, nasal cannula, if hypoxia is present
4. Antipyretics
5. Evaluation for fetal well-being and preterm labor if appropriate
6. Antibiotic selection on basis of organism; initial dose empirical
7. Suggested therapy
    a. Penicillin G is given 1.2 to 2.4 million U/day to 1 to 2 million units, IV q4h, in seriously ill patients; ampicillin, vancomycin, erythromycin, or cephalosporins for *Streptococcus pneumoniae*.
    b. Erythromycin is given 500-1000 mg (not estolate), q6h, for *Mycoplasma pneumoniae*, *Streptococcus pneumoniae*, or *Legionella pneumoniae*.
    c. Serious *Hemophilus* infection is treated with third-generation cephalosporins.
    d. Most gram-negative organisms are treated with a third-generation cephalosporin or an aminoglycoside in conjunction with a beta-lactam agent.
    e. Fungal infections may require antifungal agents, such as amphotericin B.
    f. Amantadine hydrochloride is effective for influenza A. Influenza immunization is indicated in susceptible pregnant women and should be given after the first trimester.
    g. Acyclovir is given 5 to 10 mg/kg, IV q8h, as treatment for *Varicella pneumoniae*.
    h. If indicated, initial antibiotic therapy for aspiration pneumonia should include coverage for gram positive, gram negative, and anaerobes such as the following:
        (1) Third-generation cephalosporins
        (2) Penicillin or clindamycin and aminoglycoside

TUBERCULOSIS

Incidence

The incidence of tuberculosis decreased in recent decades until the mid-1980s. Since 1986, there has been an increase in reported cases. In 1990, more than 25,000 cases were reported in the United States, mostly in urban areas.

Pathophysiology

1. Tuberculosis is a systemic disease caused by *Mycobacterium tuberculosis*, a 0.5 × 4 µm aerobic, acid-fast, non–spore forming, nonmotile bacillus.
2. Infection is from the inhalation of droplet nuclei containing the organism.
3. Transmission is most often by close contact with those with cavitary pulmonary disease and productive sputum.
4. Bacteria reach terminal air spaces in the mid and lower air fields.
    a. The apical posterior portions of the lung favor growth.

Practical Guide to the Care of the Gynecologic/Obstetric Patient   473

  b. The infection may spread by lymphohematogenous spread.
  c. A granulomatous tissue reaction then develops, with activated macrophages, lymphocytes, fibroblasts, epithelial cells, and Langhans' giant cells.
  d. Healing usually occurs with calcification.
  e. Tissue necrosis from degenerating macrophages results in caseation necrosis.
5. Two to eight weeks after the infection, cell-mediated hypersensitivity develops and there is a reactive tuberculin test and containment of the infection.
6. Some patients fail to contain the primary infection.

Clinical Presentation

1. Pulmonary disease is the most common manifestation for more than 80% of tuberculosis cases in the United States.
2. The primary pulmonary disease is apical cavitation in later childhood and early adulthood.
3. Chronic pulmonary tuberculosis is its most common disease manifestation in a pregnant woman.
   a. Through activation of bacterial colonies in subapical posterior portion of the upper lobe of the lung, caseous material may liquefy and drain into the bronchial tree, producing a cough.
   b. Early in the infection the patient can have minimal symptoms.
   c. Later she may develop the following symptoms:
      (1) Anorexia
      (2) Fatigue
      (3) Weight loss
      (4) Chills
      (5) Fever
      (6) Night sweats
      (7) Hemoptysis
      (8) Chest pain
      (9) Dullness to percussion (revealed by physical examination)

Diagnosis

1. The Mantoux test is a quantitative use of purified protein derivative (PPD).
   a. This test is a delayed hypersensitivity response to microbacterial antigen.
   b. A 0.1-mg injection of PPD (5 TU [tuberculin unit] strength) is injected intracutaneous, usually in the forearm.
   c. The skin should be read in 48 to 72 hours.
   d. The PPD is safe to give in pregnancy.
   e. Contrary to earlier data, pregnancy does not alter reactivity to the tuberculin skin testing.
      (1) 0 to 4 mm: negative
      (2) To 10 mm: doubtful
      (3) Greater than 10 mm: reactive

2. A positive tuberculin skin test demonstrates that the patient has had a tuberculosis infection.
   a. If there is greater than a 5-mm induration, a chest x-ray with shielding of the fetus should be performed.
   b. The chest x-ray film may show apical or subapical patchy infiltrates with cavitation.
   c. With a positive chest x-ray film, a sputum should be obtained in the early morning for acid fast bacillus (AFB) × 3 days.
   d. Bronchoscopy with endobronchial biopsy could help obtain a culture, which is the definitive diagnosis.
3. If there is a prior history of bacille Calmette-Guérin (BCG), administration guidelines are as follows:
   a. PPD placement is not contraindicated with history of BCG administration.
   b. Ten years after vaccination, a PPD should be interpreted in the usual manner.
   c. If there are concerning symptoms, findings on chest x-ray film, and known exposure history, a prior history of BCG administration should not influence the decision to treat.
4. A chest x-ray examination should be performed in the following:
   a. Tuberculin reactors with known prior negative reactions
   b. Tuberculin reactors in whom the time of conversion is unknown
   c. Patients with suggestive history or physical examination even if the skin test is negative

Tuberculosis and Pregnancy

1. Pregnancy is not associated with the worsening or improvement of tuberculosis.
2. Symptoms are not altered during pregnancy.
3. There is no higher risk of acquiring tuberculosis during pregnancy.
4. Tuberculosis of the fetus is rare.
   a. Means of transmission to the fetus are as follows:
      (1) Hematogenous spread from placenta by umbilical vein.
      (2) Fetal aspiration of infected amniotic fluid in utero or at time of birth.
      (3) The major involvement in the fetus is in the liver and lung, but also dissemination to the CNS, bone, gastrointestinal tract, lymphatics, adrenal, skin, and kidney.
   b. For diagnosing congenital tuberculosis, lesions must be present plus one of the following:
      (1) Lesions in the first week of life
      (2) A primary hepatic complex or caseating granuloma
      (3) Documented primary infection of the placenta or endometrium
      (4) Exclusion of infection by a caretaker in postnatal period
   c. If congenital tuberculosis occurs, perinatal mortality approaches 40%.
5. Infants of mothers with tuberculosis: There is no need for routine separation of the mother if she is undergoing appropriate therapy. A PPD should be placed on the infant at 3 months.

6. Untreated, there is a higher rate of preeclampsia, vaginal hemorrhage, and fetal loss.
7. With chemotherapy, tuberculosis infection does not affect perinatal outcome except for the rare occurrence of congenital tuberculosis.

Less Common Presentations of Tuberculosis

1. Miliary (disseminated)
2. Serofibrinous pleurisy with effusion
3. Female genital tuberculosis endosalpinx, ovaries, and endometrium

Medications for Treatment of Tuberculosis

1. The three medications most frequently used for treatment of tuberculosis during pregnancy are the following:
   a. Isoniazid (INH)
   b. Rifampin (RIF)
   c. Ethambutol (ETH)
2. All of these medications have been successfully used during pregnancy with little risk of teratogenicity.

INH Prophylaxis for Positive PPD

American Thoracic Society (ATS) and CDC recommendations are as follows:

1. For pregnant women less than 35 years old
   a. Greater than 15 mm not previously treated
   b. Greater than 10 mm and from high prevalence area or occupations or recent immigrants
   c. Greater than 5 mm if HIV positive or HIV contact
2. For pregnant women 35 years of age or greater: Less than 15 mm should not receive prophylaxis during pregnancy or immediate postpartum unless they have high-grade risk factors
3. Chemoprophylaxis
   a. INH, 300 mg, every day for 9 months
   b. Pyridoxine, 50 mg a day, for 9 months. Pyridoxine is to decrease the incidence of peripheral neuropathy of INH

Treatment of Active Disease in Pregnancy

Tuberculosis is diagnosed by the culture of the tubercle bacillus from the skin or other bodily fluids. For treatment of active tuberculosis, see Table 19-17.

Medication Risks

1. INH can cause hepatitis, which has an incidence of 20:1000 with a 0.001% risk of death. It causes peripheral neuropathy by competition with pyridoxine.
2. Rifampin also has a risk of hepatitis.
   a. Rare adverse effects, including hydrops, have been reported to the fetus.
   b. Overall, teratogenicity with rifampin has not been shown.
3. Ethambutol side effects have included optic neuritis, with blurred vision and trouble with color discrimination.

Table 19-17 **Treatment of Active Tuberculosis**	
Drug	**Duration**
Isoniazid (INH), 5 mg/kg to a total of 300 mg/day	9 months
Pyridoxine, 50 mg/day	9 months
Rifampin (RIF), 10 mg/kg to a total of 600 mg/day	9 months
Ethambutol (ETH), 5 to 25 mg/kg to a total of 2.5 g/day	8 weeks or until cultures are sensitive to INH/RIF
Pyrazinamide (PZA), 15 to 30 mg/kg to a total of 2 g/day. Start only if resistance to INH is likely or in HIV-infected patients	8 weeks or until cultures are sensitive to INH/RIF
Streptomycin, 15 mg/kg to a total of 1.5 g/day	Generally contraindicated in pregnancy unless no alternative exists

4. Streptomycin can cause fetal defects from mild vestibular damage to bilateral deafness.
5. It is important to monitor for the response to therapy, and also for advanced reaction and drug toxicity.

Tuberculosis and HIV

1. Individuals who are HIV positive develop active tuberculosis by the following means:
   a. More rapid progression of new infections
   b. Reactivation of latent infections
   c. Reinfection with tuberculosis after adequate therapy
2. The diagnosis may be complicated by anergy.
3. Preventive therapy is indicated for the following:
   a. Induration greater than or equal to 5 mm
   b. Anergy and from high-prevalence groups

Public Health Measures

The local health department should be notified of cases of tuberculosis so that contacts may be identified and follow-up provided.

CHRONIC RESPIRATORY DISEASE

Tobacco Smoking

1. Incidence
   a. It is estimated that more than 25% of women are smoking when they become pregnant.
   b. Many will either stop smoking or smoke less frequently during pregnancy, but others will continue to smoke as usual (Box 19-12).

> **BOX 19-12 Surgeon General's Report on Health Benefits of Smoking Cessation in Pregnancy**
>
> 1. Babies born to women who smoke during pregnancy weigh 200 g less on the average than their counterparts born to nonsmoking women.
> 2. There is a dose–response relationship between the amount of maternal smoking and reduced birth weight; the more a woman smokes during pregnancy, the greater the reduction in birth weight.
> 3. If a woman stops smoking by her fourth month of gestation, the risk of delivering a LBW baby approaches that of a nonsmoker.
> 4. Data indicate that maternal smoking during pregnancy may also affect a child's long-term development, intellectual development, and behavioral characteristics.
> 5. The risks of spontaneous abortion, fetal death, and neonatal death increase directly with increasing levels of maternal smoking during pregnancy.
> 6. Maternal smoking significantly increases the incidence of abruptio placentae, placenta previa, bleeding early or late in pregnancy, premature and prolonged rupture of membranes, and preterm delivery.

Data from U.S. Department of Health and Human Services: The health benefits of smoking cessation: a report of the Surgeon General, DHHS Publication No. (CDG) 90-8416, 1990.

2. Morbidity and mortality
   a. The general effects of smoking, including increased risk of lung cancer, emphysema, chronic bronchitis, and cardiovascular disease, are well known.
   b. There are substantial risks to the fetus and neonate, and these are dose related.
   c. Obstetric problems that have been reported from smoking cigarettes include decreased mean birth weight of 200 g, increased incidence of placenta previa and abruptio placentae, prematurity, possible PROM, and possible long-term neurologic abnormalities in the infant.
   d. There is a decreased incidence of PIH.
3. Pathophysiology: The effects on the fetus in smokers have been attributed as follows:
   a. Nicotine causes uterine vasoconstriction and fetal hypertension.
   b. Carbon monoxide reduces fetal oxygen carrying capacity by combining with fetal hemoglobin.
   c. Benzopyrene and other polycyclic hydrocarbons are mutagens and carcinogens.
   d. Smoking is associated with poor nutrition.
   e. Nicotine increases cyanide in the bloodstream.

f. It causes decreased density of fetal vessels in terminal villi of placenta.
4. Management
   a. Management consists of encouraging the pregnant woman to stop or decrease her cigarette smoking. The importance of her infant's health as well as her own should be stressed.
   b. If growth retardation is evident, appropriate monitoring should be performed.
   c. Nicotine transdermal patch use should be individualized. The benefit to heavy smokers (> 20 cigarettes/day) may be greater than the risk.

Kyphoscoliosis

Kyphoscoliosis is a bony deformity of the spine that may have either excessive posterior (kyphosis) or lateral (scoliosis) curvature.

1. Incidence: The incidence is approximately 0.8 to 6 per 10,000 pregnancies.
2. Morbidity and mortality: Kyphoscoliosis has been reported to be associated with increased rates of prematurity and possibly stillbirth.
3. Pathophysiology:
   a. Causes of kyphoscoliosis include idiopathic factors (80%), neuromuscular disease, trauma, tuberculosis, connective tissue disease, and rickets.
   b. Physiologically, the maternal effect of this problem is an alteration of the rib cage configuration, which may lead to compression of the lungs, with emphysema and/or atelectasis.
   c. This can cause decreased vital capacity and cardiopulmonary complications, including cor pulmonale.
4. Diagnosis: Careful physical examination should reveal the spinal deformity.
5. Prognosis:
   a. Successful pregnancies can usually be achieved.
   b. Women with unstable scoliosis or with a curve of greater than 25% are at a greater risk of progressive disease during pregnancy.
   c. There is not an increase in cesarean deliveries.
6. Management:
   a. The maternal status should be monitored for cardiopulmonary compromise, and the fetal status should be monitored for adequate growth and well-being and for preterm labor.
   b. Oxygen should be given if indicated for hypoxia.
   c. Antibiotics should be administered if indicated for pulmonary infection.
   d. Digitalis should be performed if indicated.

Sarcoidosis

1. Sarcoidosis is a systemic granulomatosis disease.
2. The etiology is unknown.
3. It occurs in 0.02% to 0.06% of pregnancies.

4. Morbidity and mortality:
   a. Maternal
      (1) Sarcoidosis itself does not damage the pregnancy, but any disease that has compromised pulmonary or cardiac function may lead to deleterious effects in pregnancy.
      (2) Patients with more severe disease, including dyspnea and skin lesions, often have a worse prognosis.
      (3) Pregnancy does not worsen the clinical course of sarcoidosis, but there is a generalized improvement in disease in most patients, possibly caused by steroids; there is often a relapse postpartum.
   b. Fetal
      (1) Growth retardation and preterm labor have been reported.
      (2) Fetal surveillance may be indicated.
5. Pathophysiology:
   a. A noncaseating granulomatous infiltration occurs in a perivascular pattern.
   b. The most common organs affected are the lungs.
      (1) They may be affected by pulmonary granulomas and alveolitis.
      (2) Progressive fibrosis with loss of volume results in a restrictive ventilatory defect.
   c. Other affected organs include lymph nodes, eyes, skin, bone, nerves, heart, kidneys, and liver.
6. Diagnosis:
   a. Clinical manifestations include dyspnea, nonproductive cough, nonspecific chest pain, fever, fatigue, weakness.
   b. Clinical examination and pulmonary function tests revealing restrictive lung disease are suggestive. Noncaseating granulomas demonstrated by biopsy from the lung, lymph node, skin, conjunctiva, other organs are diagnostic.
   c. Chest x-ray film may demonstrate bilateral hilar adenopathy, interstitial or alveolar infiltrates, or nodular lesions.
   d. Hypercalcemia, hypergammaglobulinemia, elevated liver enzymes in advanced disease.
   e. Angiotensin-converting enzymes have been used as a marker of disease activity but are not consistently helpful.
7. Management:
   a. The goal is preservation of maternal pulmonary function and improvement of symptoms.
   b. Patients with mild, asymptomatic disease do not require treatment because the disease may resolve spontaneously.
   c. Corticosteroids suppress the granulomatous aspect of the disease in more severe cases.
   d. In hypercalcemic patients, prenatal vitamins should not include vitamin D.
   e. Oxygen may be needed during labor and delivery if hypoxia occurs.
8. Prognosis: Pregnancy is well tolerated if the following conditions are not present:
   a. Vital capacity less than 1 L

b. Pulmonary hypertension
c. PaO$_2$ less than 55 mm Hg
d. Dyspnea
e. High doses of steroids required

19.9 Renal Disease

Helen Y. How

RENAL CHANGES DURING NORMAL PREGNANCY

Anatomic Changes

1. Kidney length is increased 1 to 1.5 cm in late pregnancy.
2. Kidney weighs 50 g more in the pregnant state.
3. Dilation of the entire collecting system occurs; right more than left because of dextrorotation of the uterus, because rectosigmoid acts as a cushion for the left ureter, and because of compression of the right ureter by the engorged right renal vein.

Functional Changes

1. Renal hemodynamics
   a. Glomerular filtration rate (GFR) achieves an incremental increase of 30% to 50% by the twelfth week, which is sustained until term.
   b. Renal plasma flow (RPF) increases by 80% between conception and the second trimester and subsequently falls to a level of about 60% greater than the nonpregnant norm.
   c. Creatinine clearance (Cr Cl) of 150 to 170 mL/min/1.73 m^2 occurs by the end of the second trimester.
   d. Blood urea nitrogen (BUN) falls from 13 ± 3 mg/dL to 8.7 ± 1.5 mg/dL.
   e. Creatinine (Cr) falls from 0.67 ± 0.14 mg/dL to 0.46 ± 0.13 mg/dL.
   f. Increased excretion of amino acids, proteins (250 to 300 mg/24 hours), uric acid, glucose, and several water-soluble vitamins.
2. Volume regulation
   a. Total body water increases by 6 to 8 L by term.
   b. The bulk of this is concentrated in the extracellular compartment distributed between the plasma and interstitium.
   c. Plasma volume starts increasing early in the first trimester, accelerates in the second trimester, peaks at around 32 weeks, and stays elevated until term, with average gain of 1.1 to 1.3 L.
3. Sodium (Na$^+$) homeostasis: Net Na$^+$ gain is 950 mEq, the majority of which is stored in the maternal compartment.
   a. Factors increasing urinary Na$^+$ excretion are as follows:
      (1) Increased filtered load
      (2) Antinatriuretic hormone
      (3) Prostaglandins
      (4) Decreased renal vascular resistance
      (5) Progesterone
      (6) Arginine vasopressin

(7) Decreased serum albumin
(8) Increased RPF
b. Factors decreasing urinary Na^+ excretion are as follows:
(1) Aldosterone
(2) Increased filtration flow
(3) Deoxycorticosteroid
(4) Increased ureteral pressure
(5) Exaggerated supine and upright position effects
4. Potassium (K^+) homeostasis:
   a. Net K+ gain is 350 mEq, which is primarily incorporated in the fetus.
   b. Progesterone blocks the effect of mineralocorticosteroids at the level of the renal tubules.
   c. Bartter's syndrome and primary hyperaldosteronism improve.
   d. Body tonicity:
      (1) Plasma osmolality is decreased by 8 to 10 mOsm/kg (270 mOsm/kg H_2O).
      (2) Osmotic threshold is reset for both antidiuretic hormone (ADH) and thirst.
      (3) ADH secretion is increased in pregnancy and, together with increased water intake, results in a decrease of sodium by 5 mEq/L, which effectively decreases serum tonicity.

EFFECTS OF PREGNANCY ON PREEXISTING RENAL DISEASE

Infection

1. Acute pyelonephritis
   a. The most common infectious complication of gestation and is more likely to lead to acute renal failure (ARF) in gravidas than in nonpregnant women.
   b. There are marked decrements of GFR and significant increases in their serum Cr levels.
   c. This can be because the vasculature of the gravidas may be more sensitive to the vasoactive effects of bacterial endotoxins.
   d. Acute pyelonephritis during pregnancy has been associated with hypotension and, on occasion, renal vein thrombosis.
2. Chronic pyelonephritis
   a. The prognosis of pregnancy in women with chronic pyelonephritis is similar to that of gravidas with glomerular disease.
   b. The outcome is favorable in normotensive patients with preserved renal function, but those with hypertension and renal insufficiency at conception do poorly.
   c. Bacteriuria in pregnancy can lead to exacerbation.

Glomerulonephritis

1. Acute glomerulonephritis (GN)
   a. Acute poststreptococcal GN is rare in pregnancy.
   b. It has been mistaken for preeclampsia when it does occur.
2. Chronic GN
   a. Usually no adverse effect if normotensive.

b. Urinary tract infections (UTI) may occur more frequently.

Nephrotic Syndrome

1. Defined by proteinuria, hypoproteinemia, and edema. The most common cause of these is membranous GN or membranous proliferative GN.
2. In the absence of azotemia or hypertension, pregnancy outcome is good and maternal morbidity low.
3. Infant birth weight was related to maternal serum albumin levels.
4. Steroid therapy has been beneficial for patients with nephrotic syndrome and should not be withheld because of pregnancy.
5. Other more common causes of nephrotic syndrome in pregnancy are as follows:
   a. Diabetic nephropathy
      (1) Glomerulosclerosis is part of a widespread angiopathy that involves small blood vessels throughout the body.
      (2) Thus renal involvement is uncommon in the absence of retinal changes.
      (3) The tubules may be affected by diabetes, most often by glycogen deposition in proximal tubules.
      (4) Chronic interstitial nephritis may also be present.
      (5) There is increased predisposition to preeclampsia and infection.
   b. Systemic lupus erythematosus (SLE)
      (1) Some, but not all, studies have demonstrated that lupus patients are more likely to experience a flare during pregnancy if the lupus is active at conception.
      (2) Although controversial, it is suggested that prognosis is most favorable if the disease is in remission 6 months or more before conception.
      (3) Most renal flares are temporary; however, some women will have a permanent decrease in renal function.
      (4) It is difficult to differentiate between lupus renal flare and preeclampsia.
      (5) It is possible that the two conditions can coexist.
      (6) Buyon and colleagues found that a lack of increase in complements C3 and C4 is more characteristic of lupus flare.
   c. Syphilis: Any organ system, including the kidneys, can be affected during the disseminated stage of secondary syphilis.

Polycystic Disease

Functional impairment and hypertension are usually minimal in childbearing years.

Nephrolithiasis

1. Persistent pyelonephritis despite adequate antimicrobial therapy should prompt a search for nephrolithiasis.
2. When calculi are discovered, the possibility of hyperparathyroidism should also be considered.
3. Treatment depends on the symptoms and the duration of pregnancy.
4. In more than half of the cases, the stone passes spontaneously, but about a third of the pregnant women with symptomatic stones will

need cystoscopy, percutaneous nephrostomy, basket extraction, or surgical exploration.

Severity of Renal Impairment and Impact of Pregnancy (Excluding SLE)

1. Mild
   a. Plasma Cr less than or equal to 1.4 mg/dL (124 µmol/L)
   b. Usually a 95% successful obstetric outcome (82% if before 28 weeks)
   c. 20% pregnancy complication and less than 5% long-term sequelae
2. Moderate
   a. Plasma Cr 1.5 to 2.5 mg/dL (133 to 265 µmol/L)
   b. Cr Cl 30 mL/min
   c. Usually a 90% successful obstetric outcome (56% if before 28 weeks)
   d. Accelerated renal deterioration with 44% pregnancy complication and 25% long-term sequelae (77% if before 28 weeks)
3. Severe
   a. Plasma Cr greater than or equal to 3 mg/dL (265 µmol/L)
   b. Amenorrheic and anovulatory
   c. Decreased likelihood of conception
   d. Pregnancy vigorously discouraged with 47% successful obstetric outcome; 84% pregnancy complications (8% if before 28 weeks) and 58% long-term sequelae (92% before 28 weeks)
   e. Pregnancy reconsidered after renal rehabilitation by way of dialysis and a transplant program

Chronic Renal Disease (Antenatal Care)

1. Follow-up every 2 weeks until 32 weeks gestation, then every week thereafter. Recommend induction of labor at 38 weeks.
2. Assess renal function, preferably by 24-hour Cr Cl and protein excretion (monthly). Near term, a 15% decrease in function that affects plasma creatinine minimally is permissible.
3. Early detection of asymptomatic bacteriuria or confirmation of UTI, if possible.
4. Carefully monitor blood pressure (BP) for early detection of hypertension (50%) and assess its severity (20% will develop diastolic pressure of 110 mm Hg). Diastolic pressure should be kept between 80 and 85 mm Hg.
5. Detect preeclampsia early, if possible.
6. Assess fetal size, development, and well-being.

Medical Complications of Renal Insufficiency

1. Neurologic: as a result of water intoxication or electrolyte imbalance, patient seizures
2. Cardiovascular: circulatory congestion secondary to fluid overload, cardiac arrhythmia secondary to electrolyte disturbances, hypertension
3. Gastrointestinal: anorexia, nausea, vomiting, hemorrhage
4. Infections: at operative sites; urinary tract and respiratory system

Renal Biopsy During Pregnancy

1. Packham and Fairley report a series of 111 renal biopsies performed in preterm pregnant women:
   a. Transient gross hematuria: 0.9% (pregnant) vs 3% to 5% (nonpregnant)
   b. Overall complication rate: 4.5%
   c. Conclusion: no increase in morbidity if BP is well controlled, normal coagulation, and an experienced hand
2. Rare indications are as follows:
   a. Sudden deterioration of renal function before 30 to 32 weeks gestation with no obvious cause. Certain forms of rapidly progressive GN may respond to aggressive treatment with steroid, chemotherapy, and perhaps plasma exchange, when diagnosed early.
   b. Symptomatic nephrotic syndrome before 30 to 32 weeks gestation.
   c. When the patient fails to show signs of recovery within 3 weeks; when acute tubular necrosis (ATN) has been suspected clinically.

Chronic Dialysis in Pregnancy

1. GFR less than or equal to 5 mL/min
2. Pregnancies in childbearing age: 0.5% to 0.9% (true frequency unknown)
3. Incidence of abortion: 50% with only 19% to 23% ending in live births
4. Dialysis strategy
   a. All will require a 50% increase in hours and frequency of dialysis.
   b. The aim of this is to do the following:
      (1) Maintain BUN less than 50 mg/dL (8 mmol/L) because intrauterine death is more likely if values exceed this mark.
      (2) Avoid hypotension during dialysis, which could be damaging to the fetus.
         (a) In late pregnancy, the enlarging uterus and supine posture may aggravate this by decreased venous return.
         (b) Continuous external fetal monitoring in the late second and third trimester is recommended.
      (3) Rapid fluctuations in intravascular volume are avoided by limiting interdialysis weight gain to approximately 0.5 to 1 kg.
      (4) Rigid control of BP must be ensured.
         (a) BP must be kept below 140/90.
         (b) First-line treatment is correction of volume overload by dialysis.
         (c) Conventional antihypertensive drugs should be used.
         (d) Phenobarbital or phenytoin should be used for seizure prophylaxis.
         (e) $MgSO_4$ may be given with caution.
         (f) Low-dose aspirin may be beneficial.
      (5) Physician should scrutinize carefully for preterm labor (40%) because dialysis and uterine contractions are associated.
         (a) Postulate progesterone removal.
         (b) This is also a result of increased incidence of abruptio placentae and polyhydramnios.

(6) Plasma calcium should be watched closely to avoid hypercalcemia.
(7) Correcting anemia:
   (a) Hematocrit (Hct) should be kept above 25%, and transfusion with packed red blood cells (RBCs) or erythropoietin therapy (50 to 160 U/g/wk, subcutaneous [SC]) may be necessary.
   (b) If erythropoietin therapy is used, iron and folic acid supplementation should be given simultaneously; Hct values are expected to increase at 0.6% to 2% per week.
   (c) Possible side effects of erythropoietin therapy are hypertension, coagulopathy, fetal polycythemia (passage through the placenta), and polyhydramnios.
   (d) Weekly monitoring of maternal Hct and BP is required, with monthly evaluation of electrolytes, phosphate, Cr Cl, iron, and platelets.
(8) Nutrition: A daily oral intake of 70 g protein, 1.5 g calcium, 50 mmol potassium, 80 mmol sodium, with supplements of dialyzable vitamins is advised.
(9) Pregnant patients are in a state of chronic compensated respiratory alkalosis, and large drops in serum HCO_3 should be prevented. Dialysates containing glucose and HCO_3 are preferred; those containing citrates should be avoided.

Chronic Ambulatory Peritoneal Dialysis (CAPD)

1. Instillation of dialysate (1.5 to 3 L, four or more times daily and left in for 4 to 8 hours) through a permanent indwelling catheter inserted high in the abdomen under direct vision.
2. Advantages over hemodialysis include the following:
   a. No chronic requirement for chronic vascular access or regional heparinization
   b. Lesser degree of fluid and solute shift, more constant chemical and extracellular environment for the fetus
   c. Infrequent episode of hypotension
   d. Higher hematocrit levels
3. There are a total of eight reported cases of pregnancies treated with CAPD. These pregnancies resulted in six live births (one neonatal death) and two spontaneous abortions.

Pregnancy in the Renal Transplant Recipient

1. The following are successful pregnancies:
   a. 1958: donor from twin sister
   b. 1966: living related donor
   c. 1970: cadaveric kidney
   d. 1990: more than 2000 pregnancies
      (1) 1:50 women of childbearing age with a functioning graft becomes pregnant.
      (2) Forty percent had spontaneous abortions and elective termination of pregnancy.

2. Over 90% of pregnancies that do go beyond the first trimester end successfully (40% to 60% preterm delivery).
   a. Ectopic pregnancy: 0.5% of all conceptions
   b. Risk of preeclampsia: 25% to 30%
   c. Permanent decrement in kidney function: 15%
3. Allograft function.
   a. A 30% decline in renal function in the third trimester is normal.
   b. Baseline renal ultrasound at 20 weeks gestation may assist in the evaluation of possible hydronephrosis later in pregnancy.
   c. UTIs are frequent and should be treated energetically as 50% of the transplanted ureters will reflux.
4. Allograft rejection.
   a. Rejection occurs in 9% of patients.
   b. Rejection is difficult, especially in cases of occult chronic rejection with progressive subclinical course.
   c. Clinical hallmarks are present: fever, oliguria, deteriorating renal function, renal enlargement, and tenderness.
   d. Renal biopsy must be performed to distinguish rejection from acute pyelonephritis, recurrent glomerulopathy, possibly severe preeclampsia, and cyclosporine A nephrotoxicity.

Immunosuppressive Therapy

1. Prednisone
   a. Active metabolite is prednisolone.
   b. Cord blood/maternal levels are 1:10.
   c. Two of the 44 live births with adrenal insufficiency.
   d. High dose is necessary to treat documented rejection episode.
2. Cyclosporine A
   a. Possibly less teratogenic potential than azathioprine (limited data)
   b. Adverse effects in nonpregnant patient: renal toxicity, liver dysfunction, tremor, convulsions, diabetogenic effects, hemolytic uremic syndrome, and neoplasia
3. Azathioprine
   a. Liver toxicity
   b. During organogenesis, cannot be activated in the fetus because of its lack of inosinate pyrophosphorylase
   c. May cause chromosomal aberrations in lymphocytes of infants exposed; cleared within 20 to 32 months
   d. Reports of thrombocytopenia and leukopenia in infants
   e. 20% to 50% incidence of intrauterine growth restriction
   f. Infertility, childhood malignancy
   g. Breast-feeding not recommended

Renal Transplant

1. Antenatally, serial ultrasound and antenatal testing starting at 28 weeks is recommended.
2. Delivery and management in labor: Vaginal delivery should be the aim.
3. Obstructive problems and mechanical injury to the transplant are rare.

4. Cesarean section is performed for obstetric reasons or occasionally for cephalopelvic disproportion caused by osteodystrophy related to previous renal failure and dialysis or prolonged steroid therapy.

Maternal Follow-Up After Pregnancy

1. Rejection postpartum may result from a return to a normal immune state (despite immunosuppression) or possibly from a rebound effect from altered gestational immunoresponsiveness.
   a. Five-year survival rate:
      (1) Living related donors: 70% to 80%
      (2) Cadaveric kidneys: 40% to 50%
   b. Threefold increase in cancers of the female genital tracts has been noted.
2. Contraception.
   a. Birth control pills can cause or aggravate hypertension or thromboembolism and can also produce subtle changes in the immune system, but this does not contraindicate their use.
   b. IUD.
      (1) Associated with bacteremia of vaginal origin in 13% of healthy women, so increased risk of pelvic inflammatory disease
      (2) Reduced efficacy in the presence of immunosuppressive and antiinflammatory agents
   c. Bilateral tubal ligation: unwise to offer at the time of transplantation.
   d. Norplant, Depo-Provera: limited data.

IDIOPATHIC POSTPARTUM RENAL FAILURE

Idiopathic condition is characterized by renal failure in association with microangiopathic hemolytic anemia and usually thrombocytopenia occurring within a few days to approximately 10 weeks after an apparently normal pregnancy and delivery.

1. Etiology: unknown
2. Pathophysiology: deposition of platelet thrombi in the microvasculature (platelet aggregating factor)
3. Prognosis: guarded
   a. Most women who have succumbed required chronic dialysis or have survived with severely reduced renal function.
   b. Only a few have recovered.
4. Treatment: supportive, including plasmapheresis, platelet inhibitors

ACUTE OBSTETRIC RENAL FAILURE

1. Incidence: less than 1:10,000 pregnancies: account for 9% of all episodes of ARF in women
2. Site of abnormality
   a. Prerenal
      (1) Renal ischemia is caused by hypoperfusion; it accounts for 75% of the pregnancy-associated ARF.
      (2) Hemorrhage and hypotension are the most common precipitating factors.

b. Intrarenal: renal parenchymal disease
c. Postrenal: obstructive

Workup

To recognize and treat ARF appropriately, the clinician must rapidly identify the precipitating factors and correct them when possible (Table 19-18).

Clinical Course

1. GFR declines rapidly toward a value that approaches zero.
2. Hallmark features include a linear increase in serum creatinine at a rate of 0.5 to 1.5 mg/dL/day; a progressive, rapid rise in serum urea nitrogen (BUN) at a rate of 10 mg/dL/day; and usually a fall in urine flow rate to less than 400 to 500 mL/day.
3. Twenty percent of the ARF cases are nonoliguric; therefore, using urine volume as an index of renal function may be misleading.
4. The next step after a careful history and physical examination is to evaluate urinary sediment.
   a. Prerenal azotemia or obstructive uropathy: normal findings
   b. Glomerular disease or vasculitis: protein or RBC casts
   c. ATN: epithelial or pigmented casts
   d. Interstitial nephritis: eosinophils
5. When ARF results from renal parenchymal injury, the prognosis will depend on the severity of renal ischemia.
   a. Quick recovery is expected with mild ischemia.
   b. Prolonged ischemia leads to reversible ATN.
   c. Severe ischemia leads to an irreversible bilateral renal cortical necrosis (BRCN).
   d. The differences between ATN and BRCN are summarized in Table 19-19.
6. Diagnostic indices (Table 19-20) to differentiate between prerenal and oliguria secondary to intrinsic renal disorder are helpful when there has been no recent administration of diuretics or sodium-containing solutions.
   a. The principle is that the underperfused kidney reabsorbs sodium and water in its glomerular filtrate (GF); thus, the small amount of urine is essentially devoid of sodium and is highly concentrated.
   b. In ARF, secondary to intrinsic renal disorder, the tubular function is lost, the limited GF that may be formed is altered minimally by the tubular system, and the values of the urine excreted closely resemble plasma composition values.

Treatment

1. The main goal of therapy is to eliminate the underlying cause of ARF.
2. Volume and electrolyte and acid–base maintenance are of primary concern.
3. The "rule of 7" is a useful guide in fluid management:
   a. 50 to 200 mL of normal saline or lactated ringers solution can be infused over a 10-minute period.
   b. If the pulmonary capillary wedge pressure (PCWP) increases more than 7 mm Hg over baseline, infusion should be discontinued.

Table 19-18 Causes of Obstetric Acute Renal Failure

Volume depletion	Hemorrhage
	Antepartum
	Postpartum
	Ectopic pregnancy
	Abortion
	Dehydration
	Hyperemesis gravidarum
	Severe diarrhea
Disseminated coagulopathy	Preeclampsia or eclampsia
	Abruptio placentae
	Acute fatty liver of pregnancy
	Postpartum hemolytic uremic syndrome
	Drug or transfusion reactions
Sepsis	Septic abortion
	Acute pyelonephritis
	Puerperal sepsis
	Septicemia
Obstruction	Ureteric damage
	Bilateral pelviureteric obstruction
	Retroperitoneal hematoma
Renal parenchymal disease	Acute glomerulonephritis
	Renal involvement in multisystem disease

From *MMWR* 42(RR-7):1, 1993.

   c. If the PCWP increases less than 3 mm Hg, a second fluid challenge can be given using the same rule.
   d. If central venous pressure is used, the numbers are 5 cm H_2O and 2 cm H_2O.

Table 19-19 Difference Between Bilateral Renal Cortical Necrosis (BRCN) and Acute Tubular Necrosis (ATN)

	BRCN	ATN
Total anuria	2 to 7 days	Rare
Oliguria	Permanent	Oliguria phase: 10 to 14 days
		Polyuria phase (>3 L/day): variable duration
		Recovery phase: 10 to 14 days
Hematuria	Generally at the beginning	Seldom initially
Renal biopsy	Cortical necrosis	Glomeruli are usually normal
Renal scan	↓ Perfusion	Normal perfusion
	↓ Uptake	↑ Cortical retention
	↑ Background activity	

Adapted from Michael J: *Clin Obstet Gynecol* 13:319, 1986.

Table 19-20 **Diagnostic Indices**		
	Prerenal Failure	**ATN**
Urine osmolality (mOsm/kg H_2O)	>500	<350
Urine sodium (mEq/L)	<10-20	>40-60
Urine/plasma ratios		
Osmolality	≥1.5	<1.1
Urea	>8	<3
Creatinine	>40	<20
Fractional Na excretion U/P_{Na} U/P_{Cr}	<1%	>1%
Renal failure index U Na U/P_{Cr}	<1	>1

Adapted from Knuppel RA, Montenegro R, O'Brien WF: *Clin Obstet Gynecol* 28:288, 1985.
ATN, Acute tubular necrosis.

4. Diuretics rarely help or harm the patient.
5. Diuresis after diuretic use in a previously oliguric patient probably indicates that the patient's renal failure is less severe.
6. In the presence of preeclampsia, these drugs are to be avoided because of hemoconcentration unless pulmonary edema is present.
7. In cases of metabolic acidosis, where the blood bicarbonate level is less than 15 mEq/L and the pH is below 7.2, the euvolemic patient may be treated with $NaHCO_3$ (desired increase in HCO_3 × 0.6 × body weight).
8. The decision to dialyze usually depends on the following criteria:
   a. Serum K^+ over 6.5 mEq/L that does not respond to medical treatment (calcium gluconate, $NaHCO_3$ solution with insulin and glucose)
   b. Circulatory congestion secondary to fluid overload
   c. Presence of uremic symptoms such as anorexia and nausea, neuromuscular irritability, confusion, or a pericardial friction rub
   d. A BUN over 120 mg/dL or daily increments of 30 mg/dL in patients with sepsis or tissue necrosis
   e. Metabolic acidosis
   f. The presence of a dialyzable poison or toxic drug
9. ARF secondary to ureteral obstruction by a gravid uterus is a rare occurrence. Treatment consists of positional changes, delivery, and decompressive amniocentesis, because in some cases hydramnios, particularly associated with multiple gestation, is a common complicating factor.

Nutrition

Nutritional recommendations for patients with ARF include a diet low in protein (40 g or 0.6 to 1.5/kg ideal body weight) and a minimum of 100 g of carbohydrates per day.

1. Hyperalimentation is recommended for patients with catabolic ARF.
2. This consists of 25 to 50 kcal/day with 70% as glucose, 20% to 30% as essential amino acids (1 to 1.5 g of protein/kg/day), and fat emulsion (a maximum lipid of 500 mL of a 10% intralipid solution).

Delivery Management

1. Because fetal compromise results primarily from maternal cardiovascular decompensation, improvements in the maternal status will have positive effects on the fetal condition.
2. Furthermore, attempts to deliver the fetus in a hemodynamically compromised mother may lead to increased risks of fetal distress and the need for more aggressive obstetrical management.
3. In a mother who is already partially decompensated, such iatrogenic insults may produce disastrous results.
4. This, of course, assumes that the fetal compartment is not the source of sepsis.
5. Under such circumstances, therapy would include attempts to initiate delivery while stabilizing the mother.

General Guidelines

The guidelines listed below will help prevent ARF in pregnancy:

1. In cases of oliguria secondary to hypovolemia (hemorrhage, vomiting) prompt blood and fluid replacement is essential to avoid hypotension that may lead to renal ischemia, a known trigger mechanism of ATN.
2. Patients at risk to develop postpartum hemorrhage (multiple pregnancies, polyhydramnios, multiparity) should have their blood typed and screened for irregular antibodies.
    a. In addition, the third stage of labor should be actively managed.
    b. The physician should be prepared to manage uterine atony aggressively.
    c. Other conditions such as soft tissue trauma, retained placenta, and blood dyscrasias should be considered and ruled out.
3. In patients with preeclampsia, the pregnancy should be terminated once there is deterioration of renal function, such as oliguria, marked decrease of creatinine clearance, or rarely azotemia.
4. Careful typing and cross-matching for blood transfusion should be done to minimize the risks of a reaction.
5. Patients with septic abortion, puerperal infection, chorioamnionitis, and pyelonephritis should be watched closely for signs of septic shock.
    a. In these cases, antibiotics and removal of the septic focus, when feasible, is the treatment of choice.
    b. The urine output should be monitored.
6. During pregnancy, as well as in gynecologic surgery, the possibility of obstructive uropathy should be considered as the cause of renal failure.
7. Early delivery should be planned in cases of intrauterine fetal death and abruptio placentae to avoid DIC.
8. The use of nephrotoxic drugs should be avoided in the presence of oliguria.
9. Renal function should be monitored when a potentially nephrotoxic drug is being used.

Antenatal Assessment

20.1 Antenatal Assessment

S. J. Carlan

Antepartum fetal surveillance is performed in identified high-risk pregnancies to reduce both perinatal mortality and morbidity. The overall perinatal mortality rate in the United States in 1997 was 7.2 per 1000. These were fetal deaths that occurred from 28 weeks to birth. Up to two thirds of these antenatal deaths may be associated with chronic processes that might be detected with antepartum surveillance. Thus, antenatal fetal assessment is an important component of modern obstetric care.

Although a variety of tests have been proposed, there are six main tests in current use in the United States that are discussed in this chapter:

1. Nonstress test (NST)
2. Contraction stress test (CST)
3. Biophysical profile
4. Modified biophysical profile
5. Umbilical artery Doppler velocimetry
6. Fetal movement

The indications for the tests originally were limited to hypertension and other severe medical complications. However, with the introduction of more sophisticated testing methods, the clinical application has expanded and now includes any pregnancy condition at risk for developing either decreased uteroplacental function or other disorders associated with stillbirth (Box 20-1).

1. Background:
    a. There are variations in technique, timing, frequency, test preference, and interpretation among medical centers.
    b. The time in gestation to initiate surveillance reflects the severity of the condition and the risk of intrauterine fetal death, as well as the likelihood that in utero therapy or delivery would result in a better chance for survival.
    c. The more serious or more unpredictable the condition, the sooner testing should begin.
    d. The frequency of testing depends on the type of test, but typically tests are repeated one or two times per week.

> BOX 20-1 Indications for Antenatal Surveillance

1. Maternal disease
   a. Diabetes mellitus—insulin
   b. Connective tissue disease
   c. Antiphospholipid syndrome
   d. Hypertension—all forms
   e. Hyperthyroidism
   f. Anemia
   g. Preterm premature ruptured membranes
   h. Unexplained vaginal bleeding
   i. Cyanotic heart disease
   j. Advanced maternal age
2. History of poor obstetric outcome
3. Postdate pregnancy
4. Fetal indications
   a. Intrauterine growth retardation
   b. Decreased fetal movement
   c. Nonimmune hydrops fetalis
   d. Irregular or abnormal fetal heart rate tracing
   e. Isoimmunization
   f. Multiple gestation

---

e. Changes in the patient's clinical condition may warrant more frequent studies.

f. Antenatal surveillance cannot prevent most cord accidents, abruptio placentae, or acute fetal compromise.

g. Although most clinicians feel that the use of antepartum surveillance in selected patients provides information that may change obstetric management and lead to improved perinatal outcome, all studies have not demonstrated a uniform improvement in perinatal outcome as a result of antepartum testing.

h. One study concluded that by the time the fetal compromise is diagnosed with antepartum testing, fetal damage may have already occurred.[1]

i. A normal test implies that the fetus is not significantly compromised, and the pregnancy can be extended until either the clinical condition deteriorates or the next scheduled test.

j. Although a normal test accurately predicts a well fetus, an abnormal test does not always mean a sick fetus.

k. Abnormal results, in fact, are seldom reliable and the recommended management of an abnormal test is usually either to repeat the test or to add a backup test rather than to initiate immediate delivery.

l. Antenatal surveillance is more useful in documenting fetal wellness than in determining fetal illness.

NONSTRESS TEST

1. Background:
    a. In 1976, the association of fetal heart rate (FHR) acceleration with fetal movements was reported to signify fetal health.[2]
    b. Although a normal test result can accurately predict a healthy fetus, an abnormal test result is difficult to interpret.
    c. The presence of accelerations is more predictive of health than the absence of accelerations is predictive of compromise.
    d. In late pregnancy, normal, healthy fetuses exhibit 34 accelerations per hour and they average 20 to 25 beats per minute (bpm) in amplitude, lasting 40 seconds.[3]
    e. Between 24 and 28 weeks, about 50% of NSTs are nonreactive.[4]
    f. Between 28 and 32 weeks, 15% of NSTs are nonreactive.[5]
    g. After 32 weeks, the incidence of reactive and nonreactive NSTs is comparable with that seen at term.
    h. At term, fetal movements are associated with accelerations at least 90% of the time.
2. Description: The NST is a noninvasive method of evaluating the immediate condition of the fetus by observing the response of the FHR to fetal movement.
3. Instrumentation: External FHR monitor
4. Contraindications: None
5. Procedure:
    a. The patient should be in a high semi-Fowler's position in a recliner or left lateral decubitus position.
    b. Blood pressures are recorded before the test and every 15 minutes during the test.
    c. Continuous wave Doppler ultrasound is used to record FHR, and the tocodynamometer is placed and adjusted to detect uterine contractions and fetal movement.
    d. The patient or health care provider records fetal movement with an event marker.
    e. The patient is observed up to 120 minutes until the criteria for a reactive test are met, and the patient is rescheduled for follow-up tests if results are normal and tests are clinically indicated.[6]
    f. If the test is read as nonreactive, either plan for additional testing or attempt stimulation with sound (vibroacoustic stimulation [VAS]).
    g. Maintain a permanent record and hard copy of the patient's visit and test.
6. Test modification:
    a. VAS may change a fetus from quiet to active sleep and result in a reactive NST. Most studies have used an artificial larynx to produce the sound stimulus.
    b. A reactive NST after VAS is a reliable indication of fetal well-being.
7. Interpretation:
    a. There are many different definitions of a reactive NST that vary in number, duration, and amplitude of acceleration.[7]

b. Reactive test: The most widely accepted definition of a reactive NST is two or more FHR accelerations of at least 15 bpm and 15 seconds duration in a 20-minute observation period with no decelerations[8] (Fig. 20-1).
c. Nonreactive test is when there is a failure to meet reactive criteria.
d. Unsatisfactory test is when tracing is not satisfactory for interpretation.
e. A test may be reactive with decelerations.
    (1) Mild decelerations, defined as a less than or equal to 15 bpm decrease and a less than or equal to 15-second duration are commonly encountered[9] and are not associated with poor perinatal outcome.[10]
    (2) Prolonged decelerations predict intrapartum fetal distress in 50% of cases and are ominous.[11]
8. Management:
    a. Reactive NST: Repeat the test twice weekly unless clinical condition requires daily or more frequent evaluations. The ideal interval between testing has not been determined.
    b. Nonreactive NST: Perform backup evaluation with biophysical profile, CST, or multiparameter surveillance, or extend test up to 120 minutes.
    c. Unsatisfactory NST: Perform a repeat NST or backup evaluation within 24 hours.
    d. Reactive with variable deceleration: Perform an ultrasound and, if low amniotic fluid, consider delivery based on gestational age and nursery.
9. Predictive value of NST: A reactive NST is associated with a fetal death within 1 week at a rate of 4 to 5 per 1000 patients tested[12] and a tenfold lower risk for intrapartum intervention for fetal distress.

CONTRACTION STRESS TEST

1. Background:
    a. The CST was developed in 1972 by Ray and colleagues[13] and was originally called the oxytocin challenge test (OCT). Historically it was one of the first forms of fetal testing.
    b. The concept of the CST is based on the belief that FHR changes seen intrapartum and associated with a compromised fetus can also be seen antepartum in a fetus evolving into a compromised state when sufficient stress (uterine contractions) is applied.
    c. Studies have shown that this is a sound concept and that the stress of uterine contractions can uncover an evolving uteroplacental insufficiency.
    d. Because the CST could effectively detect diminished fetal oxygen reserve, it became the standard for fetal testing, replacing urinary estriol and human placental lactogen.
    e. The CST is still the only form of antepartum fetal surveillance to use a principle of induced stress to reveal marginal uteroplacental insufficiency.

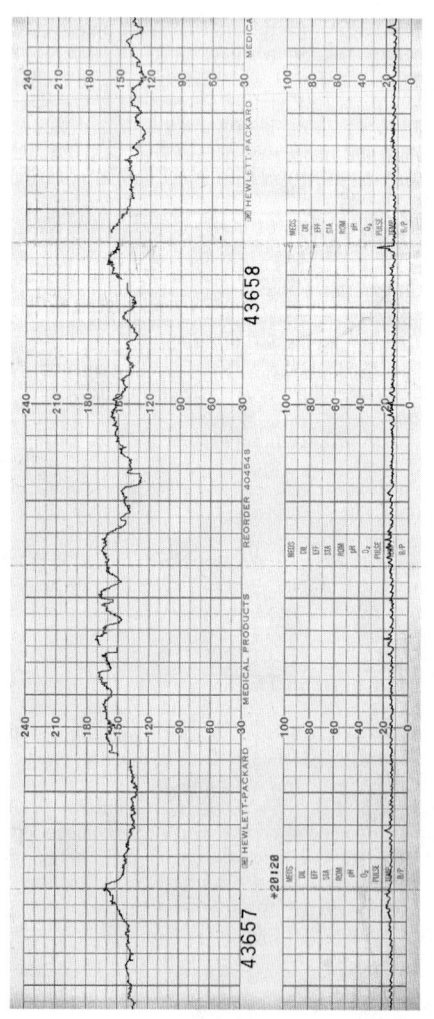

496 Practical Guide to the Care of the Gynecologic/Obstetric Patient

20—Antenatal Assessment

Figure 20-1 Reactive nonstress test.

- f. A negative CST has been consistently associated with good fetal outcome; therefore, a negative CST allows the health care provider to prolong a high-risk pregnancy safely.[14,15]
- g. Fetal death within 1 week of a negative CST is less than 1 per 1000.[16,17]
- h. Therefore, although arbitrary, a negative CST is usually repeated in 1 week. The exceptions to the weekly rule are women with diabetes or a changing clinical condition.
- i. A positive CST has been associated not only with stillbirths, but also with an increased incidence of low 5-minute Apgar scores, intrauterine growth retardation (IUGR), and late decelerations in labor.
- j. The false-positive rate of a positive CST (i.e., calling a healthy fetus sick) is 30%.[18]
- k. The CST can be performed as early as 26 weeks and the results used to manage pregnancy.
2. Instrumentation: Electronic FHR monitor.
3. Description: The CST is a method of assessing the placental respiratory function by observing the response of FHR to uterine contractions.
4. Contraindications: Box 20-2.
5. Procedure:
   a. When the CST is used as a backup for a nonreactive NST, always perform the test in the hospital, preferably in the labor and delivery area.
   b. Place the patient in the semi-Fowler's position or left lateral recumbent position.
   c. Baseline blood pressures are determined at the start of and every 15 minutes during the test.
   d. Attach the monitor belts for both FHR and tocodynamometer in an area on the patient's abdomen where the signals are acceptable.

BOX 20-2 Contraindications to the CST

Absolute Contraindications

Previous classic cesarean delivery
Placenta previa, abruptio, or unexplained vaginal bleeding
Premature ruptured membranes
Funic presentation or vasa previa
Any factor considered to be a contraindication to labor

Relative Contraindications

Preterm labor
Multiple gestation at <36 weeks
Incompetent cervical os

e. Baseline FHR and uterine activity should be reported for 20 minutes before the uterine contractions are initiated with oxytocin.
f. If there are three contractions (each ≥ 40 seconds in duration) in a 10-minute period, the test can be stopped.
g. If baseline uterine activity is insufficient, oxytocin is begun by intravenous (IV) infusion pump at 0.5 mU/min via piggyback into main IV and the rate is increased 1 to 2 mU/min in 15-minute to 20-minute interval until three contractions lasting 40 to 60 seconds over a 10-minute period occur.
h. Discontinue the oxytocin if the following occur:
    (1) The test is positive.
    (2) Hyperstimulation occurs.
    (3) The test is negative.
    (4) Variable decelerations occur.
    (5) Spontaneous rupture of membranes.
i. After the test, observe the patient until uterine activity has returned to baseline.
j. Ninety minutes may be required to perform the CST.

6. Interpretation: Table 20-1.
7. Management:
   a. Positive CST:
      (1) Nonreactive positive CST
         (a) Over 32 weeks: Deliver by cesarean delivery.[19]
         (b) Under 32 weeks: Evaluate the tracing for long-term variability and, if present, manage as though the result were reactive positive.
      (2) Reactive positive CST: individualize
         (a) Over 37 weeks: Induce labor.
         (b) Preterm fetus: Assess fetal maturity.
            (i) Immature: Survey daily.
            (ii) Mature: Induce labor.

Table 20-1 **Interpretation of CST**

CST Result	Definition
Reactive	Two accelerations of 15 sec with maximal increase of 15 bpm above baseline
Nonreactive	Fewer than 2 accelerations of 15 sec with maximal increase of 15 bpm above baseline
Negative	No decelerations noted after any contractions
Suspicious	Under 50% of the contractions have late decelerations, no hyperstimulation
Positive	Over 50% of contractions have an associated late deceleration, no hyperstimulation
Unsatisfactory	Either the quality of the recording is insufficient to assure that no later decelerations are present or the contraction frequency is <3 in 10 minutes

CST, Contraction stress test.

b. Suspicious CST: requires further evaluation with either repeat or backup tests
   (1) Reactive suspicious: Repeat in 24 hours.
   (2) Nonreactive suspicious: Repeat in 24 hours and evaluate for cause of nonreactive tracing, for example, prematurity, medications, and central nervous system (CNS) abnormality.
c. Hyperstimulation:
   (1) If there are no decelerations, the test should be classified as hyperstimulation.
   (2) If hyperstimulation is associated with late decelerations, repeat the test in 24 hours or use a backup test.
d. Unsatisfactory CST: requires further evaluations by using backup test
e. Negative CST (Fig. 20-2):
   (1) Reactive negative: Repeat in 7 days.
   (2) Nonreactive negative: Repeat in 24 hours; evaluate for cause of nonreactive tracing (i.e., prematurity, medication, CNS abnormality).
f. Observable variable deceleration (a decrease in FHR to 90 bpm, or a decrease 40 beats below the baseline for >15 seconds). Perform sonography and, if oligohydramnios, consider immediate delivery

8. Modification of CST:
   a. Nipple stimulation test[20,21]
      (1) Adequate uterine activity can be obtained in 80% to 100% of cases.
      (2) Repeat steps 1 through 6 for the CST.
      (3) Apply warm, moist towel to each breast for 5 minutes.
      (4) If uterine activity is not adequate, massage one nipple for 10 minutes.
      (5) Once contractions begin, the nipples are stimulated only intermittently.
      (6) Note the starting and stopping time of nipple stimulation on the monitor strip.
      (7) Observe carefully for hyperstimulation.
      (8) Interpret CST (see Table 20-1).

BIOPHYSICAL PROFILE

1. Background:
   a. The test was introduced in 1980 and added real-time ultrasound to the NST to evaluate dynamic functions that reflect the integrity of the fetal CNS.[22]
   b. Five biophysical variables are assessed, and the test has a total of 10 points possible, with 0 or 2 points being assigned for the presence or absence of reactivity in the NST, fetal breathing, fetal movement, fetal tone, and amniotic fluid volume (Table 20-2).
   c. Clinical trials report favorable outcomes in a large series using the biophysical profile (BPP) for primary surveillance.[23]
   d. The correlation between abnormal scores and poor outcomes increases as the score decreases from 6 to 0.[24]

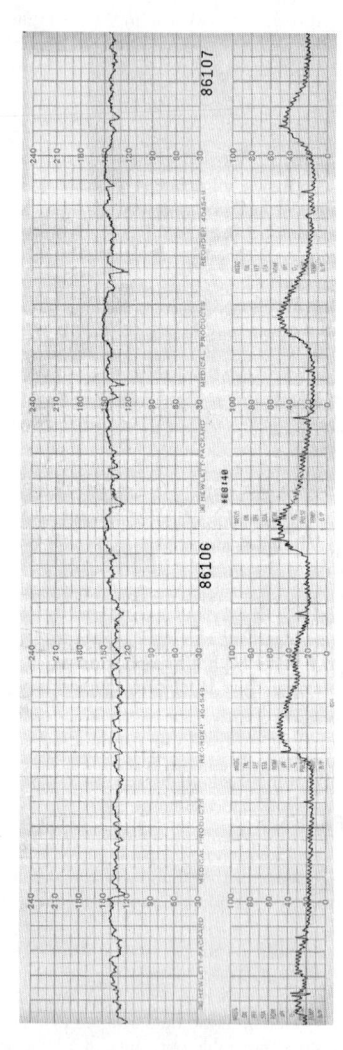

Figure 20-2 Negative contraction stress test.

Table 20-2 Components and Their Scores of the Biophysical Profile

Variable	Score 2	Score 0
Fetal breathing movements	The presence of at least 30 sec of sustained fetal breathing movements in 30 min of observation	Less than 30 sec of fetal breathing movements in 30 min of observation
Fetal movements	Three or more gross body movements in 30 min of observation; simultaneous limb and trunk movements	Less than three gross body movements in 30 min of observation
Fetal tone	At least one episode of motion of a limb from position of flexion to extension and rapid return to flexion	Fetus in position of semi–limb extension or full–limb extension with no return or slow return to flexion with movement; absence of fetal movement counted as absent tone
Fetal reactivity	Two or more fetal heart rate accelerations of at least 15 bpm and lasting at least 15 sec and associated with fetal movement within 20 min	No acceleration or less than two accelerations of fetal heart rate in 20 min of observation
Qualitative amniotic fluid volume	Pocket of amniotic fluid that measures at least 2 cm in two perpendicular planes	Largest pocket of amniotic fluid measures <2 cm in two perpendicular planes

    e. Scores of 8 and 10 are almost always associated with a good outcome, and the false reassuring (negative) rate is comparable to the CST of 1 to 2 per 1000 fetuses dying within 7 days of a reassuring test.

    f. The testing interval is 7 days with all conditions except postdate pregnancies, insulin-dependent diabetes, and IUGR, which are two times per week.

g. In addition to evaluating the fetus for uteroplacental insufficiency, the BPP has also been reported to increase the detection of anomalies and also the probability of diagnosing fetal infection in patients with ruptured membranes if there is absence of fetal breathing.
2. Description: A prenatal physical examination of the fetus using the NST and combination with real-time ultrasound equipment.
3. Contraindications: None
4. Procedure:
    a. An NST is performed as described previously.
    b. Real-time ultrasound is used to assess for four fetal variables (see Table 20-2).
    c. The duration of the ultrasound observation period is extended until normal criteria have been met for each biophysical variable or a maximum 30-minute period has been reached.
5. Interpretation and management: Table 20-3.

MODIFIED BIOPHYSICAL PROFILE (NST AND AMNIOTIC FLUID INDEX)[25-27]

1. Background:
    a. Amniotic fluid volume is a reliable marker of placental perfusion, especially chronic conditions.
    b. When the amniotic fluid index is less than 5 cm, the frequency of nonreactive NST is increased.
    c. This is a noninvasive test designed to assess acute as well as chronic changes in fetal well-being by using the amniotic fluid index and NST.
2. Contraindications: None
3. Procedure:
    a. The NST is performed as previously described with the patient in the semi-Fowler's position.
    b. The amniotic fluid index (AFI)[28,29] is found by first dividing the maternal abdomen into quadrants, with the umbilicus as a reference point and the linea nigra dividing the abdomen into right and left halves.
    c. The ultrasound transducer is held perpendicular to the floor in the longitudinal axis.
    d. The largest vertical diameter without fetal parts or cord in each quadrant is measured.
    e. The total sum of the measurements in centimeters is the amniotic fluid index.
4. Interpretation: Oligohydramnios is defined as an amniotic fluid index either less than the 5th percentile for gestational age (7.0 to 9.8 cm),[30] or less than 5 cm at term.[29]
5. Management:
    a. Patients who have decreased amniotic fluid index, nonreactive NSTs, late decelerations during the NST, or variable decelerations during the nonstress test receive a backup test, either a CST or a biophysical profile.
    b. Depending on gestational age, the patient may be a candidate for obstetric intervention.

Table 20-3 Biophysical Profile Score, Interpretation, and Pregnancy Management

Biophysical Profile Score	Interpretation	Recommended Management
10	Normal nonasphyxiated	No fetal indication for intervention; repeat test weekly except in diabetic patient and postterm pregnancy (twice weekly)
8/10 normal fluid 8/8	Normal nonasphyxiated fetus	No fetal indication for intervention; repeat testing per protocol
8/10 decreased fluid	Chronic fetal asphyxia suspected	Deliver
6	Possible fetal asphyxia	If amniotic fluid volume abnormal, deliver If normal fluid at >36 weeks with favorable cervix, deliver If <36 weeks or lecithin–sphingomyelin <2:1 or cervix unfavorable, repeat test in 24 hr If repeat test ≥4, deliver If repeat test >6, observe
4	Probable fetal asphyxia	Repeat testing same day; if biophysical profile score ≤6, deliver
0 to 2	Almost certain fetal asphyxia	Deliver

DOPPLER VELOCIMETRY

1. Background:
   a. Doppler assessment of the umbilical artery was first reported in 1977, and this vessel remains the most commonly investigated fetal structure in antenatal surveillance schemes using Doppler velocimetry.
   b. The shift in frequency of sound waves between the emitted and returning signals is called the Doppler shift.
   c. The electronics of the Doppler instrument convert the reflected sound into electrical voltage and analyze the shift in frequency between the transmitted and reflected beam.
   d. This is displayed on a screen by a waveform and reflects downstream placental resistance.
   e. Because of the influence of the angle of the sound beam when it strikes the moving column of fetal red blood cells, the diastolic component was added to act as an internal standard, resulting in the commonly used systolic–diastolic (S/D) ratio.

f. Because of the decreasing resistance to flow during fetal diastole in the normal pregnancy, as the gestation advances, the umbilical artery S/D ratio progressively falls.
g. Certain pregnancy disorders are associated with poor placental perfusion, which has been shown to be associated with increased downstream resistance during diastole or decreased flow that results in a progressively higher S/D ratio in these compromised pregnancies.
h. When there is no flow into the placenta during diastole, there is absent end-diastolic velocity (AEDV), a serious clinical condition when it occurs after viability.
i. If there are progressive placental arterial changes, there may even be reversed end-diastolic velocity (REDV), which is almost always associated with other poor surveillance tests and poor perinatal outcome.
j. Umbilical artery Doppler results appear to be most helpful in managing pregnancies complicated by hypertension, IUGR, or both.
k. Clinical action guided by Doppler has been shown to reduce the odds of perinatal mortality by 38%.[31]
l. The beneficial effect of umbilical artery Doppler depends on the incidence of AEDV and not as much on the type of high-risk pregnancy factor.
2. Description: Umbilical artery Doppler velocimetry is a noninvasive method of evaluating placental resistance to flow using sound waves. In most centers, it is not a primary method of fetal surveillance but is used most often to supplement information obtained in pregnancies complicated by IUGR and hypertension.
3. Contraindications: None
4. Instruments: The following two types of Doppler machines are in common use:
    a. Continuous wave Doppler, which uses a continuous wave with a frequency of 2 to 10 MHz
    b. Pulsed wave duplex Doppler, which allows a directed beam to reflect off a specific target
5. Procedure:
    a. Continuous wave Doppler is a "blind" procedure because concurrent real-time images are not performed; therefore, the umbilical artery is identified by its characteristic sound signal.
    b. The pulsed wave duplex Doppler is performed with a real-time ultrasound machine that allows coordinated real-time images and a Doppler signal with a range gate that can be placed over the specific vessel.
    c. Both machines will display the velocity information as waves and the S/D ratios as calculated off the display screen.
6. Pitfalls of Doppler include the following:
    a. *Maternal obesity* hinders ability to obtain waveform.
    b. *Oligohydramnios* hinders ability to obtain waveform.
    c. *Breathing* results in a false abnormal result.
    d. *Doppler angle* can lose lower peak frequency shifts if greater than 60 degrees.

e. *Fetal tachycardia* decreases the S/D ratio.
   f. *Bradycardia* increases the S/D ratio.
7. Interpretation:
   a. The most clinically ominous umbilical artery waveforms that can occur after viability are AEDV and REDV (Fig. 20-3).
   b. Natural history of AEDV and REDV is as follows:
      (1) Once present, AEDV usually persists and may even deteriorate into REDV.
      (2) Without intervention this usually leads to fetal distress or possibly demise.
      (3) The more immature the fetus, the longer the time interval between the appearance of AEDV and fetal distress.
      (4) An improvement in AEDV has occasionally been reported.
8. Management:
   a. The management of patients with umbilical artery AEDV is controversial.
   b. In general, patients are admitted to the hospital for bed rest with treatment of any underlying associated maternal conditions such as hypertension, and intensive fetal monitoring is employed.
   c. Monitoring could be in the form of daily NSTs or even continuous electronic fetal monitoring with biophysical profile testing as often as necessary.
   d. Delivery is indicated when there is acute fetal distress, worsening maternal condition, or severe IUGR with no interval growth over a reasonable time period.
   e. REDV is the most extreme form of increased vascular resistance in the placental bed, and by the time this finding occurs, severe fetal compromise is evident using most of the standard tests of fetal well-being.
   f. It is not clear whether REDV by itself is an indication for early delivery, although this finding practically never occurs in isolation.

FETAL MOVEMENT CHARTING

Assessment of fetal movement in the second half of pregnancy is one of the oldest and simplest methods of monitoring fetal well-being. The "movement alarm signal" was introduced in 1973[32] after the observation that fetal movements decreased before fetal death in pregnancies complicated by placental insufficiency caused by preeclampsia. It is now felt that fetal movement monitoring is especially useful as a surveillance tool for clinical conditions associated with long-standing placental insufficiency. Although several different methods of charting have been proposed, the most commonly used for routine assessment involves a "count to 10" system based on the recognition that most women feel more than 10 movements in a 12-hour period.[33] Of importance, regardless of the method used, the reports of subjective decreases in fetal movement often are inaccurate. Therefore, rigorous methods using graphs with consistent start time and possibly a formal quiet time for counting should be used by the mother to record truly objective fetal movement.

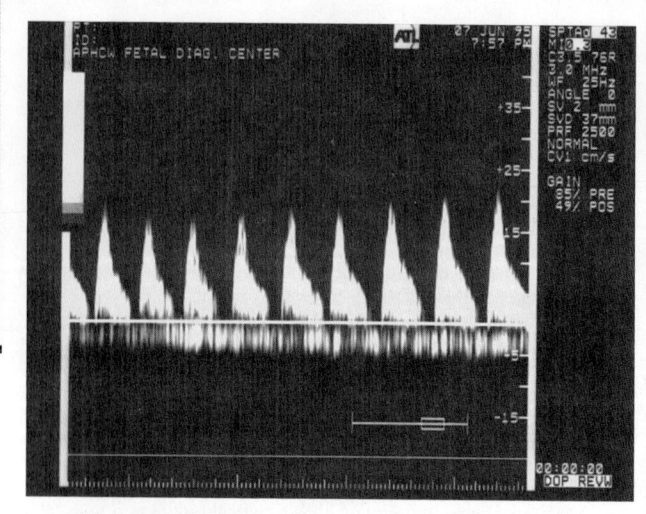

Figure 20-3 Absent end-diastolic velocity of umbilical artery.

1. Background:
   a. The third-trimester fetus makes 30 gross body movements per hour.[34]
   b. The mother perceives 80% of the movements.[35]
   c. Fetal movement peaks between 9 PM and 1 AM and may be related to decreasing maternal glucose levels.[34]
   d. The longest period of inactivity in the normal fetus is 75 minutes.[34]
   e. Factors that influence maternal perception of fetal movement include the following:
      (1) Anterior placental location
      (2) Polyhydramnios
      (3) Maternal activity
      (4) Obesity
      (5) Medications (narcotics and barbiturates)
   f. Decreased fetal movement is shown by 26% of fetuses with major birth defects.[36]
   g. No monitoring method consistently distinguishes between twin fetuses; therefore, fetal movement charting is inadequate to assess the well-being of multiple gestations.
   h. Although the application to low-risk pregnancies has appeal, especially considering that 50% of term stillbirths occur without obvious cause,[37,38] a large study failed to show a reduction of unexplained stillbirths when using routine fetal movement charting.
2. Contraindications: None
3. Method[33,39]:
   a. Fetal movement should be counted beginning in the morning, and they should be recorded.

b. The time of day at which the tenth movement is perceived should be recorded.
4. Interpretation:
   a. If there are greater than 10 movements per 12-hour period, the test is reassuring.
   b. If the mother has fewer than the required movements, further evaluation of fetal condition must be made.

REFERENCES

1. Todd AL: Antenatal tests of fetal welfare and development at age 2 years, *Am J Obstet Gynecol* 167:66-71, 1992.
2. Trierweiler MW, Freeman RK, James J: Baseline fetal heart rate characteristics as an indicator of fetal status during the antepartum period, *Am J Obstet Gynecol* 125:618-623, 1976.
3. Patrick J: Accelerations of the human fetal heart rate at 38 to 40 weeks' gestational age, *Am J Obstet Gynecol* 148:35-41, 1984.
4. Bishop E: Fetal acceleration test, *Am J Obstet Gynecol* 141:905-909, 1981.
5. Druzin ML: The relationship of the nonstress test to gestational age, *Am J Obstet Gynecol* 153:386-389, 1985.
6. Brown R, Patrick J: The nonstress test: how long is enough? *Am J Obstet Gynecol* 141:646-651, 1981.
7. Hage ML: Interpretation of nonstress tests, *Am J Obstet Gynecol* 153:490-495, 1985.
8. Lavery J: Nonstress fetal heart rate testing, *Clin Obstet Gynecol* 25:689-705, 1982.
9. Phelan JP, Lewis PE: Fetal heart rate decelerations during a nonstress test, *Obstet Gynecol* 57:288, 1981.
10. Meis P et al: Variable decelerations during non-stress tests (NST): a sign of fetal compromise? Society of Perinatal Obstetricians, Fourth Annual Meeting, San Antonio, TX, 1984.
11. Druzin ML et al: Antepartum fetal heart rate testing: VII. The significance of fetal bradycardia, *Am J Obstet Gynecol* 139:194-198, 1981.
12. Schneider EP, Hutson JM, Petrie RH: An assessment of the first decade's experience with antepartum fetal heart rate testing, *Am J Perinatol* 5:134-141, 1988.
13. Ray M et al: Clinical experience with the oxytocin challenge test, *Am J Obstet Gynecol* 114:1-9, 1972.
14. Freeman RK et al: The significance of a previous stillbirth, *Am J Obstet Gynecol* 151:7-13, 1985.
15. Freeman R et al: Postdate pregnancy: utilization of contraction stress testing for primary fetal surveillance, *Am J Obstet Gynecol* 140:128-135, 1981.
16. Everston L, Gauthier R, Collea J: Fetal demise following negative contraction stress tests, *Obstet Gynecol* 51:671-673, 1978.
17. Freeman R, Anderson G, Dorchester W: A prospective multiinstitutional study of antepartum fetal heart rate monitoring: I. Risk of perinatal mortality and morbidity according to antepartum fetal heart rate test results, *Am J Obstet Gynecol* 143:771-777, 1982.
18. Collea J, Holls W: The contraction stress test, *Clin Obstet Gynecol* 25:707-717, 1982.
19. Braly P, Freeman RK: The significance of fetal heart rate reactivity with a positive oxytocin challenge test, *Obstet Gynecol* 50:689-693, 1977.
20. Keegan KA et al: A prospective evaluation of nipple stimulation techniques for contraction stress testing, *Am J Obstet Gynecol* 157:121-125, 1987.
21. Oki EY et al: The breast-stimulated contraction stress test, *J Reprod Med* 32:919-923, 1987.
22. Manning FA, Platt LD, Sipos L: Antepartum fetal evaluation: development of a fetal biophysical profile, *Am J Obstet Gynecol* 136:787-795, 1980.

23. Manning FA et al: Fetal assessment based on fetal biophysical profile scoring: experience in 12,620 referred high-risk pregnancies: I. Perinatal mortality by frequency and etiology, *Am J Obstet Gynecol* 151:343-350, 1985.
24. Manning FA et al: Fetal assessment based on fetal biophysical profile scoring: IV. An analysis of perinatal morbidity and mortality, *Am J Obstet Gynecol* 162:703-709, 1990.
25. Eden RD et al: A modified biophysical profile for antenatal surveillance, *Obstet Gynecol* 71:365-369, 1988.
26. Ocak V, Sen C, Madazil R: Is fetal biophysical profile with all parameters needed? *J Matern Fetal Invest* 4:37, 1994.
27. Vintzileos AM et al: The use and misuse of the fetal biophysical profile, *Am J Obstet Gynecol* 156:527-533, 1987.
28. Phelan JP et al: Amniotic fluid index measurements during pregnancy, *J Reprod Med* 32:601-604, 1987.
29. Phelan JP et al: Amniotic fluid volume assessment using the four-quadrant technique in the pregnancy between 36 and 42 weeks' gestation, *J Reprod Med* 32:540-542, 1987.
30. Moore TR: Superiority of the four-quadrant sum over the single-deepest-pocket technique in ultrasonographic identification of abnormal amniotic fluid volumes, *Am J Obstet Gynecol* 163:762-767, 1990.
31. Recent metaanalysis of randomized controlled trials, *Am J Obstet Gynecol* 172:1379–1387, 1995.
32. Sadovsky E, Yaffe H: Daily fetal movement recording and fetal prognosis, *Obstet Gynecol* 41:845, 1973.
33. Pearson JF, Weaver JB: Fetal activity and fetal well-being, *Br Med J* 1:1305-1307, 1976.
34. Patrick J et al: Patterns of gross fetal body movements over 24-hour observation intervals during the last 10 weeks of pregnancy, *Am J Obstet Gynecol* 142:363, 1982.
35. Rayburn WF: Clinical significance of perceptible fetal motion, *Am J Obstet Gynecol* 138:210, 1980.
36. Rayburn W, Barr M: Activity patterns in malformed fetuses, *Am J Obstet Gynecol* 142:1045, 1982.
37. Picquadio K, Moore T: A prospective evaluation of fetal movement screening to reduce the incidence of antepartum fetal death, *Am J Obstet Gynecol* 160:1075-1080, 1989.
38. Rayburn WF: Antepartum fetal assessment: monitoring fetal activity, *Clin Perinatol* 9:1-14, 1982.
39. Sadovsky E et al: The definition and the significance of decreased fetal movements, *Acta Obstet Gynecol Scand* 62:409, 1983.

20.2 Ultrasound and Fetal Aneuploidy

Luanne Lettieri

Obstetric ultrasound is used to assess the well-being of the fetus and the pregnancy. Technologic advances in high-resolution ultrasound have made the ultrasonic detection of fetal chromosomal abnormalities or aneuploidy possible.

1. Frequency of aneuploidy in liveborn infants
   a. Trisomy 21 (Down syndrome): 1:800
   b. Trisomy 18 (Edwards' syndrome): 1:8000
   c. 45X (Turner's syndrome): 1:10,000

d. Trisomy 13 (Patau's syndrome): 1:20,000
   e. Triploidy: very rare
2. Methods of prenatal detection of fetal aneuploidy
   a. Advanced maternal age and history
   b. Maternal serum screening tests (maternal serum alpha-fetoprotein [MSAFP], estriol, human chorionic gonadotropin [HCG]) known as AFP-3
   c. Ultrasound

ULTRASOUND DETECTION OF FETAL ANEUPLOIDY

1. Abnormal biometry
   a. Nuchal fold
      (1) Measurement: Obtain between 15 and 21 weeks gestation (transverse axial scan of fetal head at level of cavum septum pellucidum, cerebral peduncles, cerebellar hemispheres, and cisterna magna); measure from outer skull table to outer skin surface
      (2) Abnormal: greater than or equal to 6 mm (early second trimester)
      (3) Associated with: trisomy 21; 80% of babies with trisomy 21 will have excess nuchal skin
      (4) Sensitivity: 35% to 40%
      (5) False positive rate: 0.5%
   b. Femur length
      (1) Measurement
         (a) Obtain measurement between 15 and 23 weeks gestation.
         (b) Measure only the ossified femoral diaphysis.
         (c) Do not include nonossified cartilage of distal epiphysis or greater tuberosity.
      (2) Abnormal: biparietal diameter/femur length (BPD/FL) ratio greater than 1.5 standard deviation (SD); FL less than 5th percentile for gestational age (GA)
      (3) Associated with: trisomy 21
      (4) Sensitivity: 35%
      (5) False-positive rate: 6%
   c. Humerus length
      (1) Measurement
         (a) Obtain between 15 and 23 weeks gestation.
         (b) Measure only ossified diaphysis.
      (2) Abnormal: BPD/HL greater than 1.5 SD; HL less than 5th percentile for GA
      (3) Associated with: trisomy 21
      (4) Sensitivity: 40%
      (5) False-positive rate: 7%
   d. Ear length
      (1) Measurement
         (a) Measurement can be obtained at any gestational age.
         (b) Nomograms are available only for 14 to 25 weeks gestation.
         (c) Measure from the helix to the end of the lobe.

(2) Abnormal: less than or equal to 10th percentile for GA
(3) Associated with: all types of aneuploidy. (Abnormally short ears are the most sensitive indicators of trisomy 21 in newborn infants.)
(4) Sensitivity: 70%
(5) False positive rate: 8%

e. Hypoplasia of middle phalanx of fifth digit
  (1) Measurement: length of the middle phalanx of the fifth digit as compared with the middle phalanx of the fourth digit
  (2) Abnormal: middle phalanx (MP) 5th/4th less than 0.7 or less than 0.5
  (3) Associated with: trisomy 21; 60% of neonates with trisomy 21 have hypoplasia of middle phalanx of fifth digit
  (4) Sensitivity: 37% for less than 0.7; 75% for less than 0.5
  (5) False-positive rate: 18% less than 0.7; 8% less than 0.5

f. IUGR
  (1) Early onset, second trimester symmetric IUGR—trisomy 18
  (2) Severe asymmetric IUGR—triploidy

STRUCTURAL ABNORMALITIES

Risk of aneuploidy in presence of structural anomalies is detected at the following rates:

Fetus 11% to 35%
Neonate 6% to 7%

1. CNS lesions
   a. Isolated hydrocephaly
      (1) Measurement
         (a) Distance from the lateral wall of the lateral ventricle to the midline compared with the hemispheric width (LV/HW)
         (b) Amount of choroid plexus within the lateral ventricle
         (c) Diameter of lateral ventricular atrium
      (2) Abnormal
         (a) LV/HW: dependent on GA
         (b) Choroid plexus does not fill the lateral ventricle— "dangling choroid plexus sign"
         (c) Ventricular atria greater than 10 mm
      (3) Associated with: trisomy 21, trisomy 18, and triploidy, 3% to 8%
   b. Meningomyelocele
      (1) Sonographic features: separation of the posterior ossification centers on both transverse and longitudinal scans
      (2) "Lemon sign" (lemon-shaped skull)
      (3) Associated with: trisomies 13, 18, and 21, and triploidy, 33% to 50%
   c. Hydrocephaly and meningomyelocele: associated with trisomies 13, 18, and 21, and triploidy, 8% to 15%
   d. Dandy-Walker syndrome
      (1) Definition: range of disorders resulting from abnormal development of cerebellum and fourth ventricle

(2) Sonographic features: separation of cerebellar hemispheres by enlarged fourth ventricle
(3) Associated with: trisomies 18 and 13 and triploidy, 29% to 50%
e. Holoprosencephaly
  (1) Definition: three disorders (lobar, semilobar, alobar) caused by failure of normal forebrain development
  (2) Sonographic features: varying degrees of a monoventricle with fused thalami
  (3) Facial abnormalities frequent: proboscis, cyclopia, cebocephaly, median cleft lip, ethmocephaly
  (4) Associated with: trisomies 13 and 18 and triploidy in 43% to 59% of alobar and semilobar types
f. Agenesis of corpus callosum
  (1) Definition: absence of commissural fibers that radiate to cerebral cortex bilaterally
  (2) Sonographic features:
      (a) Lateral ventricles are displaced laterally and superiorly.
      (b) Frontal horn is indented.
      (c) Third ventricle is elevated, producing an "interhemispheric cyst."
  (3) Associated with: trisomies 13 and 18 and and triploidy, 14% to 20%
g. Choroid plexus cysts
  (1) Sonographic features: cysts within choroid plexus of lateral ventricles; usually seen between 16 and 21 weeks gestation and regresses by 23 to 25 weeks
  (2) Associated with: trisomies 21 and 18
2. Cystic hygroma
  a. Definition: nuchal edema resulting from lymphatic obstruction
  b. Sonographic features: circumferential edema of the head and neck; may contain septation caused by nuchal ligament
  c. Associated with: prenatally diagnosed
    (1) 66% 45X
    (2) 25% normal
    (3) 5% trisomy 21
    (4) 5% trisomy 18
    (5) 1% other
  d. Also associated with parvovirus
3. Facial abnormalities
  a. Cleft lip/palate
    (1) Sonographic features: flattened nose, displaced upper lip, disruption of maxilla; not possible to diagnose cleft in soft palate prenatally
    (2) Associated with: trisomies 13 and 18 and triploidy, 40% to 75%
  b. Common ocular abnormalities
    (1) Holoprosencephaly
    (2) Associated with: trisomies 13 or 18
  c. Micrognathia: Associated with: trisomies 13 and 18
  d. Small, deformed ears: Associated with: trisomies 13, 18, and 21, and triploidy, 23%

4. Hydrothorax
   a. Definition: fluid in pleural cavity
   b. Sonographic features: anechoic fluid collection in fetal chest
      (1) Usually there is return of normal shape and contour of chest; however, with large fluid collections there can be bulging of chest, flattening of diaphragm, and cardiac axis shift.
      (2) Associated with: 45X (most frequent), trisomy 21, and triploidy, 9% to 12%.
5. Diaphragmatic hernia
   a. Definition: failure of fusion of the four structures comprising the muscular diaphragm:
      (1) Septum transversum
      (2) Pleuroperitoneal membranes
      (3) Dorsal mesentery of esophagus
      (4) Body wall
   b. Occurs in 1:2000 to 1:5000 live births.
   c. Sonographic features: visualization of abdominal organs in chest cavity.
      (1) Definitive sign is fluid-filled mass behind left side of heart in a transverse scan.
      (2) Associated features include polyhydramnios, absence of stomach or other abdominal organs in the abdominal cavity, mediastinal shift, and decreased abdominal circumference.
   d. Associated with the following:
      (1) Prenatal studies: trisomies 18 and 21, 4% to 25%
      (2) Neonatal studies: trisomies 18 and 13, 6%
6. Congenital heart disease
   a. Definition: structural abnormality of the heart or valves or cardiac arrhythmia
      (1) Most frequent congenital anomaly (occurs in 8:1000 live births)
      (2) Numerous abnormalities, the most common being septal defects
   b. Sonographic features: depends on type of cardiac anomaly (Recent studies indicate that with prenatal scan, a normal four-chamber view can rule out most cardiac defects.)
   c. Associated with the following:

Chromosome Abnormality	CHD Frequency	Type of Defect*
Trisomy 21	50%	VSD, ECD
Trisomy 18	99%	VSD, ECD, DORV
Trisomy 13	90%	VSD, ASD, dextrocardia
45X	20%	coarc

*ASD, Atrial septal defect; *coarc,* coarctation of aorta; *DORV,* double-outlet right ventricle; *ECD,* endocardial cushion defect; *VSD,* ventricular septal defect.

7. Esophageal malformations
   a. Definition: malformation or absence of esophagus; can range from simple esophageal atresia to tracheoesophageal fistula

(1) Blind proximal esophageal pouch with a tracheoesophageal fistula of the distal esophagus is the most common malformation.
(2) Esophageal atresia occurs in 1:2500 live births.
b. Sonographic features: difficult to diagnose
(1) Nonvisualization of stomach in 50% of fetuses
(2) Polyhydramnios in third trimester
(3) Rarely, visualization of proximal esophageal pouch
c. Associated with the following:
(1) Prenatal detection 20%—aneuploidy, most commonly trisomy 18
(2) Neonatal detection—3% to 4% aneuploidy
8. Duodenal atresia
a. Definition: absence of duodenum, most likely caused by failure of recanalization of duodenum; most common type of small bowel atresia (occurs in 1:10,000 live births)
b. Sonographic features: dilated stomach and proximal duodenum—"double-bubble sign"—two fluid-filled cystic structures in upper abdomen seen on transverse scan; may not be sonographically evident until after 24 weeks gestation
(1) Polyhydramnios—45% of cases
(2) Other anomalies—50%
(3) Cardiac anomalies—20% to 30%
(4) Symmetric growth retardation—50%
c. Associated with: if diagnosed prenatally, 20% to 30% will have trisomy 21
9. Omphalocele
a. Definition:
(1) Extrusion of the abdominal contents through an anterior abdominal wall defect into the amniotic cavity.
(2) The extraabdominal organs are covered by a sac and the umbilical cord inserts into the omphalocele itself, also called exomphalos.
b. Sonographic features:
(1) Midline anterior abdominal mass outside of the abdominal cavity containing abdominal organs—stomach, bowel, liver
(2) Contained within a sac, although sac may rupture, allowing abdominal contents to float freely within the amniotic cavity, resembling gastroschisis
(3) May see ascites
c. Associated with the following:
(1) Risk of aneuploidy dependent on the following:
(a) Associated anomalies (especially cardiac, genitourinary [GU])
(b) Size
(c) Contents (liver vs small bowel)
(2) Prenatal detection: 30% to 40%, trisomies 13, 18, and 21
(3) Neonatal detection: 12%, trisomies 13 and 18
10. Echogenic bowel
a. Definition: most likely represents small bowel that is impacted with meconium
b. Sonographic features: echogenic masses in fetal abdomen

c. Associated with: normal variant, cystic fibrosis, and aneuploidy (trisomies 18 and 21)
11. GU anomalies
    a. Definition: Spectrum of congenital malformations of GU tract can occur.
        (1) Pyelectasis
            (a) Definition: mild dilation of renal pelvis
            (b) Sonographic features: increased diameter of renal pelvis
            (c) Associated with the following:
                (i) 17% to 25% of fetuses with trisomy 21 have pyelectasis.
                (ii) More severe hydronephrosis can be associated with trisomies 13 and 18.
        (2) Multicystic/dysplastic kidneys
            (a) Definition: Renal parenchyma contains numerous cysts of varying sizes.
            (b) Sonographic features: Multiple cysts of different sizes are seen. Cysts may be so small that they cannot be delineated; instead large echogenic parenchyma is seen. Larger cysts may distort shape of the kidney. Oligohydramnios often occurs.
            (c) Associated with trisomies 13 and 18.
        (3) Horseshoe kidney: rarely able to diagnose prenatally; associated with trisomy 18
12. Limb anomalies
    a. Definition: deformities of extremities, particularly hands and feet
        (1) Limb reduction: trisomy 18
        (2) Radial, thumb aplasia: trisomy 18
        (3) Overlapping fingers (clinodactyly): trisomies 13 and 18
        (4) Flexion deformities: trisomy 18
        (5) Polydactyly: all aneuploidies, especially trisomy 13
        (6) Hypoplasia of middle phalanx of fifth digit: trisomy 21
        (7) Wide space between first and second toe: trisomy 21
13. Nonimmune hydrops
    a. Definition: excessive extravascular fluid accumulation
    b. Sonographic features: skin thickening greater than 5 mm, ascites, pleural/pericardial effusions, polyhydramnios, placentamegaly greater than 4 cm
    c. Associated with: trisomies 18 and 21, Turner's syndrome, and triploidy, 14% to 18%
14. Single umbilical artery: This occurs in up to 1% of deliveries. If another anomaly is not present, the fetus is not at an increased risk for aneuploidy.
15. First-trimester ultrasound: Recent studies indicate that an increased nuchal translucency is associated with an increase in the maternal age—related risk for trisomies 13, 18, and 21.

USEFUL ULTRASOUND FINDINGS IN THE DETECTION OF FETAL ANEUPLOIDY

1. Major anomaly: all aneuploidies
2. Combined biometry: all trisomies
3. Early onset severe IUGR: trisomy 18, triploidy

20.3 Nutrition in Pregnancy

Patricia D. Harris and Marcello Pietrantoni

MATERNAL NUTRITION

The goal of nutrition during pregnancy is to nourish the mother while including the additional nutrients necessary to support fetal growth. The need for nutrients increases more than the need for additional calories (Table 20-4).

1. Principles of diet
   a. The mother should be encouraged to eat regularly and to eat a sufficient amount of food to satisfy her appetite. She should avoid skipping meals, especially breakfast, because hypoglycemia and ketonuria can result from an extended fast.
   b. Energy requirements are greatest at gestational weeks 10 to 30, when large amounts of maternal fat are deposited (Fig. 20-4).
   c. An additional 300 calories during the second and third trimesters are needed for optimal weight gain and may be achieved by two additional servings of dairy products and an additional 1 to 2 ounces of meat.

2. Weight gain during pregnancy
   a. A positive linear relationship has been shown between maternal weight gain and newborn weight, and pregnancy outcome (Fig. 20-5).
   b. A positive linear relationship has also been shown between prepregnancy maternal weight and newborn weight (Fig. 20-6).
   c. Low prepregnancy maternal weight and inadequate gestational weight gain have been shown to contribute to decreased intrauterine growth and low birth weight.
   d. Gestational weight gain, especially in the second and third trimesters, is an important determinant of fetal growth (Table 20-5).
   e. The only anthropometric measures of clinical value at this time are prepregnancy weight-for-height, or body mass index (BMI), and serial measurements of gestational weight gain.
   f. Height, without shoes, should be measured at the first prenatal office visit.
   g. BMI = weight (kg) $\div$ height (m^2).
   h. Standard weight-for-height = 100 pounds for the first 5 feet plus 5 pounds for each inch taller than 5 feet or minus 4 pounds for each inch shorter than 5 feet.
   i. Women generally gain 2 to 4 pounds during the first trimester and about 1 pound per week during the second and third trimesters (Fig. 20-7).
   j. The accumulation of some fluid during pregnancy is physiologic as expansion of maternal blood volume may account for 10% of total weight gain. Large shifts of fluid, indicated by sudden large weight gains (8 pounds or more per month), may indicate preeclampsia, especially after 20 weeks gestation.
   k. The components and rate of weight gain are more important than the actual number of pounds gained.

Table 20-4 **Dietary Recommendations for Pregnancy**	
Food Group	**Ideal Number of Daily Servings**
Milk/cheese/dairy	At least 6
Meat/protein	2 to 3
Vegetables/fruits	At least 5
Cereals/breads/starches	At least 6

3. Nutrients of interest during pregnancy
    a. Folic acid is necessary for closure of the neural tube during early fetal development.
        (1) Physiologic needs for folate can be met through a healthy diet that includes dark green, leafy vegetables and enriched cereals.
        (2) Supplementation with low doses (0.8 mg/day) of folic acid is recommended from preconception through the first trimester if there is any question of diet adequacy.
    b. Iron needs greatly increase during pregnancy because of the increased production of blood cells.
        (1) Although iron is found in meats and enriched grain products, the increased requirement is very difficult to obtain through diet, especially during the second and third trimesters.
        (2) Low-dose iron supplements (30 mg/day) are recommended and pose no danger to mother or fetus.
        (3) Higher doses (60 to 120 mg/day, in divided doses bid or tid) are recommended in cases of documented iron deficiency anemia.

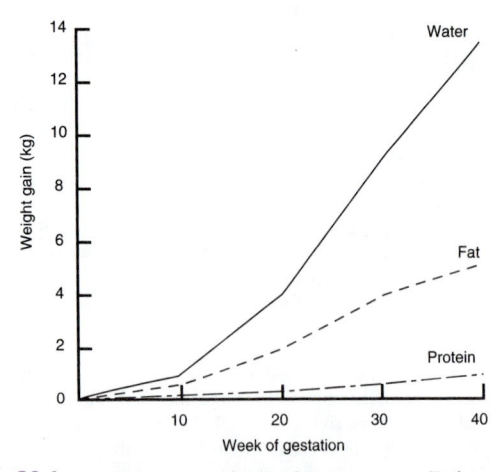

Figure 20-4 Composition of weight gain during pregnancy. (Redrawn from National Academy of Sciences: *Nutrition during pregnancy and lactation: an implementation guide*, Washington, DC, 1992, National Academy Press.)

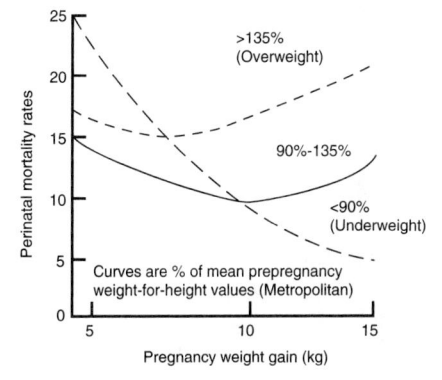

Practical Guide to the Care of the Gynecologic/Obstetric Patient 517

Figure 20-5 Perinatal mortality as a function of maternal weight gain. (Redrawn from National Academy of Sciences: *Nutrition during pregnancy and lactation: an implementation guide*, Washington, DC, 1992, National Academy Press.)

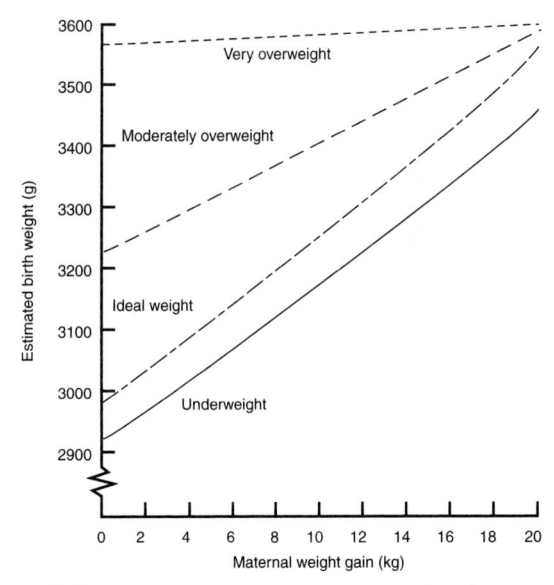

Figure 20-6 Birth weight as a function of maternal weight and prepregnancy weight for height. (Redrawn from National Academy of Sciences: *Nutrition during pregnancy and lactation: an implementation guide*, Washington, DC, 1992, National Academy Press.)

Table 20-5 Weight Gain Recommended for Pregnancy

| Classification | Standard Prepregnancy Body Weight-for-Height (%) | Prepregnancy BMI | Recommended Gestational Weight Gain ||||
| | | | Singleton || Twin ||
			Kg	lb	Kg	lb
Underweight	<90	<19.8	12-18	28-40	18-23	40-50
Normal weight	90-120	19.8-26	11-16	25-35	16-20	35-45
Overweight	120-135	26-29	7-11	15-25	11-16	25-35
Obese	>135	>29	7	15	7-16	15-25

BMI, Body mass index.

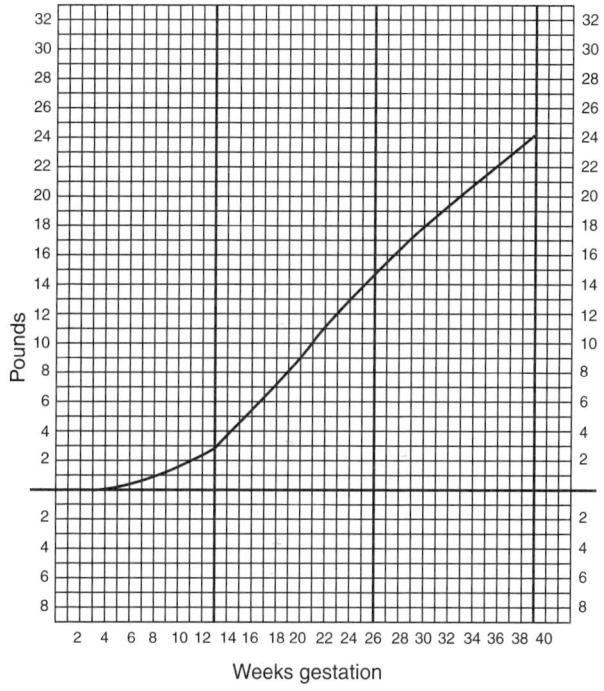

Figure 20-7 Gestational weight gain grid.

- (4) Iron supplements may be better tolerated if taken at bedtime.
- (5) Iron absorption is inhibited if taken with food, prenatal vitamins, or calcium supplements.
 c. Zinc is necessary for protein production, bone building, and DNA and RNA production.
   - (1) The increased requirement for zinc during pregnancy can generally be met through a balanced diet containing meat, fish, and dairy products.
   - (2) Zinc is a component of prenatal vitamins.
 d. Vitamin A is essential to tissues lining the lungs, digestive organs, and GU tract.
   - (1) Birth defects may be caused at much lower doses than previously thought. Research has shown that women who took more than 10,000 IU of preformed vitamin A were five times more likely to have a baby with birth defects than those women who took less than 5000 IU. Therefore, supplementation with preformed vitamin A should be avoided, especially during the first trimester.

(2) Vitamin A requirement is not increased in pregnancy.
(3) Beta carotene, which is found in yellow and dark green leafy vegetables and yellow fruits, need not be restricted.

e. Sodium is needed in increased amounts during pregnancy because of the increased fluid volume in the mother, the requirements of the fetus, and the level of sodium in amniotic fluid. Salt restriction in pregnant women is not recommended.

4. Nutrition-related laboratory values of interest
   a. Generally, it is impractical and expensive to use laboratory or function tests to assess nutrient status in normal prenatal care. However, nutrient status can be assessed using hematocrit (Hct), hemoglobin (Hgb), complete blood count (CBC) and, possibly, serum ferritin.
      (1) Hematocrit (Hct)
         (a) Decreased secondary to bleeding, iron deficiency anemia, or water overload
         (b) Elevated because of dehydration
      (2) Hemoglobin (Hgb)
         (a) Decreased secondary to bleeding, iron deficiency anemia, or protein–calorie malnutrition
         (b) Elevated because of dehydration
      (3) Transferrin
         (a) Decreased secondary to protein malnutrition, pernicious anemia, or iron overload
         (b) Elevated because of iron deficiency, blood loss, or pregnancy
      (4) Albumin
         (a) Decreased secondary to overhydration, decreased protein intake, or impaired digestion or absorption
         (b) Elevated because of dehydration
      (5) Prealbumin
         (a) Decreased secondary to protein malnutrition, stress, or inflammation
      (6) Mean corpuscular volume (MCV)
         (a) Decreased secondary to advanced iron-deficiency anemia, or vitamin B_6 or copper deficiency
         (b) Elevated because of folic acid, vitamin B_{12}, or vitamin C deficiency
      (7) Mean corpuscular Hgb concentration (MCHC)
         (a) Decreased secondary to advanced iron-deficiency anemia
   b. Cholesterol levels in pregnant women may be elevated. This may be secondary to the normal decreased intestinal secretion rate, which allows more circulating exogenous cholesterol for the synthesis of estrogens.

5. Alimentary changes during pregnancy
   a. Increased appetite, usually in the second and third trimesters
   b. Decreased motility because of the increase in progesterone, which may lead to the following:
      (1) Esophageal regurgitation
      (2) Nausea and vomiting
      (3) Delayed emptying of the stomach
      (4) Reverse peristalsis, which may result in heartburn

c. Decreased intestinal secretion for enhanced absorption of nutrients
d. Increased water absorption from the colon, which may lead to constipation
e. An altered sense of taste, which may lead to pica or irregular dietary intake
f. An intensified sense of smell, which may contribute to nausea and vomiting

COMPLICATIONS OF PREGNANCY

1. Multiple fetuses
   a. Ten pounds additional total maternal weight gain is recommended for a twin pregnancy. This recommendation may be adapted for additional fetuses.
   b. As the number of fetuses increases, the duration of pregnancy may decrease. It is therefore essential that nutrition counseling occur early in pregnancy to ensure the most nutrient-dense diet possible.
   c. Additional requirements include the following:
      (1) Folic acid
         (a) 0.4 to 0.8 mg, twins
         (b) 0.8 to 1 mg, triplets, quadruplets, etc.
      (2) Zinc
         (a) 15 mg, twins
         (b) 20 to 25 mg, triplets, quadruplets, etc.
      (3) Iron
         (a) 30 to 60 mg, twins
         (b) 60 mg, triplets, quadruplets, etc.
2. Anemia
   a. Hgb less than or equal to 11.0 g/dL (World Health Organization [WHO] criteria)
   b. Need increased dietary intake of protein, iron-rich foods, and vitamin C–rich foods
   c. Need iron supplementation
3. Diabetes
   a. Preexisting diabetes
      (1) The normal prepregnancy diet should provide the following:
         (a) 30 kcal/kg current weight for active women
         (b) 20 kcal/kg current weight for sedentary and obese women
      (2) The normal nonpregnant woman of average height and stable weight may consume approximately 2200 kcal/day.
      (3) An additional 300 kcal/day in the second and third trimesters are needed for optimal weight gain and prevention of starvation ketosis, indicated by trace or small amounts of urinary ketones.
      (4) Calorie needs should be determined on an individual basis.
   b. Gestational diabetes (GDM)
      (1) GDM is defined as glucose intolerance with onset or first recognition during the current pregnancy.
      (2) Glucose monitoring is important because the criteria for initiating insulin should be based on fasting (fasting blood sugar [FBS]) and postprandial responses to the prescribed diet.

The American Diabetes Association recommends the following guidelines:
- (a) Premeal or fasting: less than or equal to 105 mg/dL
- (b) 1 hour postprandial (pp): less than or equal to 140 mg/dL
- (c) 2 hour pp: less than or equal to 120 mg/dL

(3) Nutrition management is successful if the following occur:
- (a) Necessary nutrients for maternal and fetal health and growth are provided.
- (b) Normoglycemia is maintained.
- (c) Ketonuria is prevented.
- (d) Weight gain is appropriate.

(4) The 1995 American Diabetes Association recommendations for pregnancy include the following:
- (a) If prepregnancy weight was less than 90% ideal body weight (IBW), 36 to 40 kcal/kg current weight per day.
- (b) If prepregnancy weight was 90% to 120% IBW, 30 kcal/kg current weight per day.
- (c) If prepregnancy weight was 120% to 150% IBW, 24 kcal/kg current weight per day.
- (d) If prepregnancy weight was greater than 150% IBW, 12 to 18 kcal/kg current weight per day.
- (e) Keep calories and carbohydrates low at breakfast because of morning insulin resistance.

(5) Elevated fasting triglycerides in GDM are more strongly associated with macrosomia than FBS or pp glucose.

(6) Postpartum women should monitor glucose for 1 week and report any elevations.
- (a) Six to eight weeks postpartum or shortly after breastfeeding cessation, give patient a 75 g 2-hour oral glucose tolerance test (OGTT).
- (b) Check blood glucose at her annual examination.

c. Monitoring
(1) Urinary ketones.
- (a) Trace or small amounts may indicate starvation ketosis.
- (b) Moderate or large amounts may suggest existing or impending diabetic ketoacidosis.

(2) Urine glucose levels imprecisely represent blood glucose concentrations because of varying renal thresholds for glucose excretion resulting from long-standing diabetes or pregnancy.

4. Pregnancy-induced hypertension (PIH)
  a. Increased calcium intake may counteract the effects of sodium in the development of hypertension in salt-sensitive individuals.
  b. The presence of hypocalciuria is a diagnostic aid in differentiating preeclampsia from other forms of gestational hypertension.
  c. There is sufficient recent evidence to support supplementation with large amounts of calcium (2000 mg/day) as a means of preventing PIH/preeclampsia in susceptible women.

d. Calcium competes with copper, iron, zinc, and magnesium for absorption and is best used if obtained from dietary sources or if supplemented in doses of 500 mg qid between meals.
5. "Morning sickness"
   a. Because of varying levels of estrogen, human chorionic gonadotropin (HCG), and progesterone, women may have any or all of the following symptoms, with different intensities, at any time of the day.
      (1) Nausea, vomiting, and retching
      (2) Aversion to odors, bright lights, loud noises, or tight clothes
      (3) Sensitivity to invasion of her personal space
   b. Different things may trigger an episode of "morning sickness" in different women.
      (1) Odors, even those that previously were pleasant
      (2) Abrupt motion
      (3) Bright lights
      (4) Loud noises
   c. Ptyalism, the excessive production of saliva, may alter the sense of taste and increase nausea.
   d. Dietary treatment may include the following:
      (1) Drink liquids 1 hour before or after eating solid foods.
      (2) Avoid water, caffeine, and carbonated beverages.
      (3) Keeping a cut lemon handy to sniff may help to neutralize offensive odors.
      (4) Tart candies, lemonade, etc., may be tolerated.
      (5) Whatever works, eat it.
6. Diarrhea may occur because of iron supplementation or lactose intolerance. Dietary treatment should include the following:
   a. Increase fluids by mouth; restrict caffeine and milk products.
   b. Decrease fiber foods, such as raw fruits (except bananas) and vegetables.
   c. Avoid milk products. Gradually add into diet in small amounts ($1/4$ cup) as tolerated.
7. Constipation may occur because of normal alimentary changes during pregnancy or from iron supplementation. Dietary treatment should include the following:
   a. High-fiber foods such as raw fruits and vegetables, beans, legumes, nuts, and whole-grain breads and cereals
   b. Increased fluids by mouth (excluding caffeine)
8. Pica
   a. Pica is defined as the craving of nonfood items.
   b. Acting on these cravings may limit nutrient intake or absorption and have adverse hematologic and gastrointestinal effects.
   c. Depending on the craving, this can be extremely harmful to the mother and the fetus.
   d. Any unusual cravings should be discussed with a registered dietitian to assess whether they are associated with short-term or long-term nutrition problems.
9. Starvation ketosis
   a. Indicated by ketonuria

b. Causes
   (1) Inadequate carbohydrate intake
   (2) Inadequate calorie intake
   (3) Skipped meals or snacks
   (4) Greater than 10 hours between hour of sleep (hs) snack and breakfast
   (5) Vomiting
10. Vegetarianism
    a. Most vegetarian diets meet or exceed the recommended daily allowance (RDA) for protein.
    b. A lower protein intake than in a nonvegetarian diet may be associated with better calcium retention.
    c. Western vegetarians generally have adequate intakes of iron (because of fortification) and consume greater amounts of ascorbic acid (vitamin C), which enhances the absorption of nonheme (plant) iron.
    d. Vegans (those who eat no animal products) may require vitamin B_{12} supplementation.
    e. Vegans who have limited exposure to the sun may require vitamin D supplementation.
    f. Vegetarian diets tend to be lower in calories and higher in fiber.
    g. For the additional calories needed in the second and third trimesters of pregnancy, add two between-meal snacks rich in calories and nutrients, including nuts, nut butters, and dried fruits.
    h. The vegetarian woman who becomes pregnant should be referred to a registered dietitian to assure that she is informed about a proper diet.
11. Dietary inadequacy
    a. Poor hygiene may be suggestive of life circumstances interfering with adequate nutrient intake.
    b. Untreated dental disease, depression, domestic violence, etc., may interfere with adequate dietary intake.
    c. Signs of eating disorders include the following:
       (1) Dental enamel erosion
       (2) Little subcutaneous fat
       (3) Swollen parotid glands (rare)
       (4) Callouses on the knuckles
    d. Refer to a registered dietitian for assessment and counseling or further referral.
    e. Refer to social services for assistance with housing, food stamps and other federal programs, commodities, etc.
12. Smoking, alcohol, and drugs (SAD)
    a. The use of substances such as tobacco, alcohol, caffeine or coffee, marijuana, and cocaine may affect maternal nutrition as well as have teratogenic effects on the fetus.
    b. Substance abuse may increase the need for one or more nutrients through malabsorption or increased urinary excretion.
    c. Substance abuse may also lead to undesirable changes in food and nutrient intake.

20.4 Assessment of Fetal Pulmonary Maturity

George T. Danakas

1. Lecithin/sphingomylin (L/S) ratio: A ratio of 2 or greater has been generally accepted for pulmonary maturity. Less than 2% chance of neonate having respiratory distress syndrome (RDS). Blood and meconium can affect L/S ratio.
2. Phosphatidylglycerol (PG): The presence of PG is an indicator of pulmonary maturity (even if amniotic fluid is bloody or meconium stained). PG generally does not appear until 35th week of gestation and increases between weeks 37 and 40.
3. TDx test (surfactant/albumin ratio): Assesses surfactant content in amniotic fluid. A value of 55 is the mature cutoff. A value of 70 is needed in a diabetic patient.

20.5 Genetics

Brad Angle, P. Gail Williams, and Joseph Hersh

ABNORMAL TRIPLE MARKER SCREENING

The object of a screening test is to identify, among a large population, a small group that is at sufficiently increased risk for certain disorders to warrant offering specific diagnostic tests. Maternal serum marker screening has become a routine component of modern obstetric management as a noninvasive method of identifying pregnancies at risk for a variety of fetal disorders.

Maternal serum alpha-fetoprotein (MSAFP) testing has been used to identify pregnancies at increased risk for fetal neural tube defects (NTDs) since the 1970s. The use of MSAFP screening expanded in the 1980s to include identification of pregnancies at risk for Down syndrome. More recently, additional serum markers, unconjugated estriol (uE_3) and human chorionic gonadotropin (HCG), have been included in a "triple marker" screening test to improve the detection rate of chromosome abnormalities and possibly to identify other pregnancies at risk for adverse outcomes.

Physiology of Alpha-Fetoprotein

1. Alpha-fetoprotein (AFP) is synthesized in the fetal liver and yolk sac.
2. AFP is the major serum protein early in fetal life.
3. Functional role during fetal development is uncertain.
4. Concentration in fetal serum peaks at the end of the first trimester (Fig. 20-8, A).
   a. Fetal liver continues to produce AFP at a constant rate.
   b. Increasing fetal blood volume results in dilution and decrease in concentration after the first trimester.
5. AFP is filtered by the fetal kidney and appears in amniotic fluid, which is largely composed of fetal urine.
   a. Peak concentration of amniotic fluid AFP (AFAFP) occurs at about 12 weeks gestation.
   b. It decreases by approximately 10% per week during the second trimester (see Fig. 20-8, B).

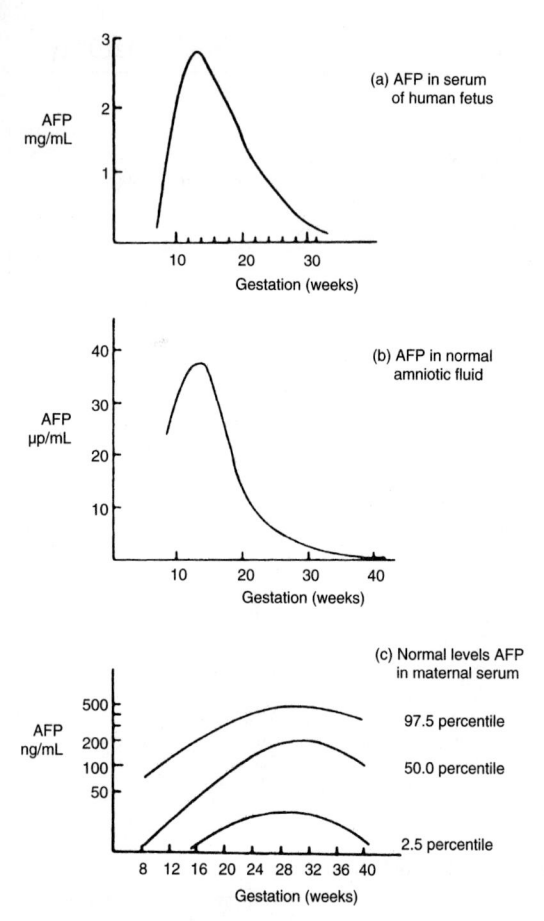

Figure 20-8 The relationship between alpha-fetoprotein levels in fetal serum (a), amniotic fluid (b), and maternal serum (c). AFP, Alpha-fetoprotein. (From Milunsky A, editor: *Genetic disorders of the fetus*, Baltimore, 1992, Johns Hopkins University Press.)

6. Some fetal AFP may reach maternal circulation by the following:
   a. Diffusion across the placenta (70%)
   b. Diffusion across the amnion (30%)
7. MSAFP concentration (0.02 µg/mL) is approximately five orders of magnitude lower than fetal serum (2000 µ/mL).
   a. Placental and amniotic barriers between fetus and mother allow only a small fraction of fetally derived AFP to reach maternal circulation.

b. Greater volume of maternal blood further dilutes the AFP concentration.
8. MSAFP levels increase approximately 15% per week during the second trimester and fall after the 30th week (see Fig. 20-8, C).
9. Paradoxical rise in maternal serum as levels decrease in fetal serum and amniotic fluid results from increased diffusion caused by the following:
   a. Enlarging placental and amniotic surface areas
   b. Increasing placental permeability

Clinical Aspects of MSAFP Measurements

1. Patient sampling.
   a. MSAFP screening may be obtained between 15 and 20 completed weeks of pregnancy.
   b. Optimal time of testing is at 16 to 18 weeks for greatest sensitivity.
   c. MSAFP testing should not be performed after invasive procedures (e.g., amniocentesis), which may give rise to MSAFP elevations.
2. Reporting of measurements.
   a. Results are expressed as a multiple of the unaffected population median.
   b. The absolute concentration of MSAFP is converted to a multiple of median (MoM), which relates it to the median in normal pregnancies at the same gestational age.

   MoM = Measured MSAFP ÷ Median MSAFP for gestational age

   c. The median MSAFP value for each week of gestation is designated as 1.0 MoM (e.g., MSAFP concentration twice that of population median = 2.0 MoM).
   d. Accuracy of gestational dating is critical because MSAFP levels normally rise during the second trimester.
      (1) If actual gestational age is further advanced than estimated, then MSAFP MoM will appear higher than the true value.
      (2) If actual gestational age is less advanced than estimated, then MSAFP MoM will appear lower than the true value.
3. MoM values are adjusted to account for several factors that affect MSAFP levels.
   a. Race
      (1) MSAFP levels in African Americans are approximately 15% higher than in Caucasians.
      (2) Lack of correction results in falsely elevated MSAFP MoM values in the African American population.
   b. Weight
      (1) MSAFP levels decrease with increasing maternal weight as a result of dilutional effects of larger maternal blood volumes.
      (2) Lack of correction results in falsely low MSAFP MoM values in heavier women.
   c. Maternal diabetes
      (1) Insulin-dependent diabetes mellitus is associated with MSAFP levels 20% to 40% lower than nondiabetic women.
      (2) Lack of correction results in falsely low MSAFP MoM values in diabetic women.

MSAFP Screening for Neural Tube Defects

1. Neural tube defects result from the failure of fusion of the neural tube at 20 to 24 days after fertilization.
2. Population incidence of NTDs is 1:1000 to 2:1000 in the United States.
3. The severity of the defects range from anencephaly (absence of forebrain and cranial bones) to spina bifida (myelomeningocele).
4. "Open" neural tube defects are associated with exposed membrane and blood vessels, allowing AFP to leak into amniotic fluid and subsequently diffuse into the maternal circulation.
   a. Anencephaly and 90% of cases of spina bifida are open defects, with complete exposure of neural tissue to amniotic fluid or separation by only a thin membrane.
   b. The larger the exposed surface area, the more AFP diffuses.
      (1) Anencephaly, which has a larger exposed surface, on average, than open spina bifida (OSB), results in higher amniotic fluid AFP and MSAFP levels.
      (2) Median MSAFP approximately 6.5-fold higher than normal with anencephaly and 3.8-fold higher with OSB (Fig. 20-9).
5. Ten percent of spina bifida lesions are "closed" (covered by a thick membrane) and not identifiable by MSAFP screening.
6. There is considerable overlap between MSAFP levels in affected and unaffected pregnancies (see Fig. 20-9).
7. No level of MSAFP can be selected as a screening cutoff that will completely separate unaffected from affected pregnancies.
8. Most screening programs use MSAFP cutoff point of 2.0 or 2.5 MoM (MSAFP level 2 or 2.5 times higher than normal median values). Each cutoff point represents a compromise between maximizing detection rate and minimizing false-positive rate.
   a. Cutoff of 2.0 MoM detects 93% of anencephaly and 85% of OSB with a 4% false-positive rate.
   b. Cutoff of 2.5 MoM detects 89% of anencephaly and 75% of OSB with a 2% false-positive rate.
9. Individual risks based on MSAFP MoM values are commonly reported and used to counsel patients in decision-making process concerning options for further diagnostic evaluation (Table 20-6).
10. MSAFP concentrations are usually higher in multiple gestation pregnancies than in singleton pregnancies, approximately in proportion to the number of fetuses (e.g., median MSAFP MoM in twin pregnancies is approximately 2.0). Data are available to estimate individual risks for women with twin pregnancies.

Other Fetal Anomalies Associated with Elevated MSAFP

1. Ventral wall defects
   a. Elevated MSAFP levels may be associated with open ventral wall defects that allow increased diffusion of fetal AFP into amniotic fluid and maternal serum.

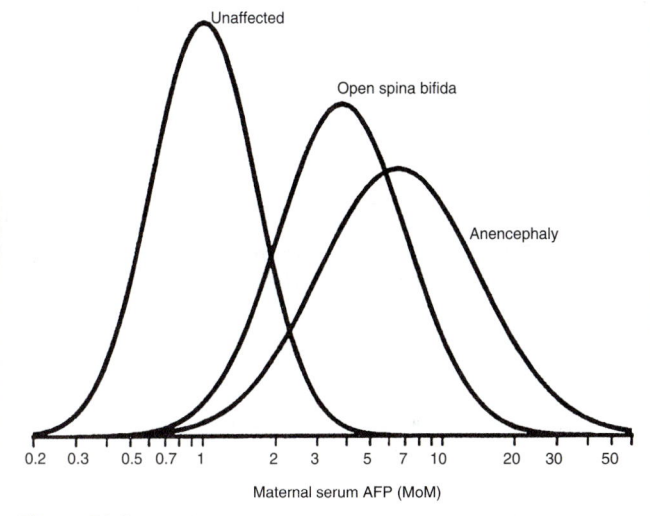

Figure 20-9 Distribution of maternal serum alpha-fetoprotein (AFP) concentrations, expressed as multiple of median (MoM), in normal fetuses, fetuses with open spina bifida, and fetuses with anencephaly.

b. Omphalocele is a midline defect of the abdominal wall with herniation of abdominal organs into a membrane-covered sac from which the umbilical cord arises.
c. Gastroschisis is a defect of the right side of the abdominal wall and is not membrane covered.
d. Because gastroschisis is not membrane covered, higher levels of MSAFP are found, on average, as compared with omphalocele.

Table 20-6 **Individual Odds for Having a Fetus with an Open Neural Tube Defect Based on Specific MSAFP MoM Values**

| Serum AFP (MoM) | Odds at a Given Population Incidence ||
	1 per 1000	2 per 1000
2.0	1:800	1:400
2.5	1:290	1:140
3.0	1:120	1:59
3.5	1:53	1:27
4.0	1:26	1:13
4.5	1:14	1:7
5.0	1:7	1:4

Data from Fourth Report of the O.K. Collaborative Study on Alpha-Fetoprotein in Relation to Neural Tube Defects, *J Epidemiol Community Health* 36:87-95, 1982.
MSAFP, Maternal serum alpha-fetoprotein.

(1) Median MSAFP value with gastroschisis is 7.0 MoM.
(2) Median MSAFP value with omphalocele is 4.0 MoM.
e. MSAFP screening detects almost 100% of cases of gastroschisis and 70% to 80% of omphaloceles at commonly used screening cutoffs.
2. Renal abnormalities
   a. Congenital nephrotic syndrome: Rare autosomal recessive condition in which increased filtration of AFP through fetal kidney into amniotic fluid causes very elevated (>10 MoM) MSAFP levels
   b. Some urinary tract malformations
3. Congenital skin disorders: Epidermolysis bullosa and cutis aplasia are rare conditions in which normal skin barriers are disrupted, resulting in increased diffusion of fetal AFP into maternal circulation.
4. Chromosome abnormalities
   a. Some fetuses with chromosome abnormalities, most commonly trisomies 13 and 18, have an increased MSAFP because of the presence of open fetal defects (e.g., neural tube defects, omphalocele).
   b. Women with elevated MSAFP levels without identified anomalies may be at increased risk for a variety of other chromosome abnormalities, including triploidy, sex chromosome anomalies, and structural anomalies.
   c. The overall risk of a fetal chromosome abnormality in women with elevated MSAFP levels is approximately 1%.
5. Unidentified fetal anomalies: There is a higher incidence of congenital malformations identified at birth in infants whose mothers had elevated MSAFP levels.

Evaluation of the Patient with an Elevated MSAFP Level

Approximately 5% of women who have MSAFP screening have elevated levels. These women should be offered genetic counseling and the option of further diagnostic testing to evaluate for fetal anomalies. With careful follow-up testing, most abnormal MSAFP results can eventually be explained. The following is an example of a protocol for follow-up testing for an elevated MSAFP level (Fig. 20-10).

1. High-resolution ultrasonography is the primary follow-up of elevated MSAFP levels.
2. First priority of ultrasound examination is to confirm estimated gestational age.
   a. Because MSAFP levels vary with gestational age, inaccurate dating used to determine MSAFP MoM may result in a falsely low or high value.
   b. Underestimation of gestational age is the most common reason for an elevated MSAFP level.
   c. If estimated gestational age used for calculating MSAFP MoM differs by greater than 10 days from gestational age determined by ultrasound examination, then the MoM is recalculated using the ultrasound dating.
   d. If ultrasound gestational age is less than 15 weeks, then a repeat MSAFP test must be obtained after 15 weeks.

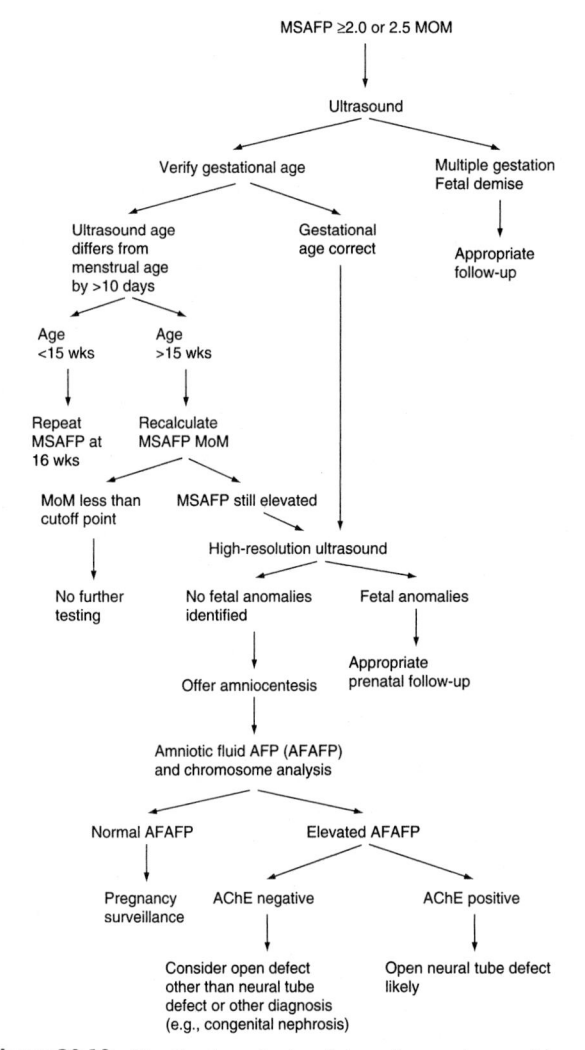

Figure 20-10 Algorithm for evaluation of elevated maternal serum alpha-fetoprotein (MSAFP) levels. *AChE*, Acetylcholinesterase; *AFP*, alpha-fetoprotein; *MoM*, multiple of medium.

3. If gestational dating is correct, then a high-resolution ultrasonogram is performed to evaluate for fetal anomalies.
   a. Detection rate of neural tube defects is 70% to 100%; many centers achieve detection rates of 90% or better.
   b. Detection rate of gastroschisis and omphalocele is 80% to 95%.
4. Some centers provide individual adjusted risks for open neural tube defects based on a normal ultrasound examination.
   a. Prior risk based on the MSAFP test alone may be reduced by 90% to 95%.
   b. Tables for calculating adjusted risks are available.[1]
5. Amniocentesis is an option for further evaluation of an elevated MSAFP that remains unexplained by ultrasonography.
   a. An elevated AFAFP level suggests the presence of an open defect.
   b. Additional test for presence or absence of acetylcholinesterase (AChE) in amniotic fluid is used to differentiate neural tube defects from other fetal defects.
      (1) AChE is an enzyme contained in blood cells and neural tissue.
      (2) Both AFAFP and AChE are elevated in the presence of an open neural tube defect (95% to 98% detection rate).
      (3) Elevated AFAFP and normal AChE suggest the presence of other open defects (gastroschisis, omphalocele).
   c. If a normal AFAFP is obtained after a normal ultrasound examination, the likelihood of an open fetal defect is very low.
   d. Chromosome analysis should be performed on fetal cells obtained by amniocentesis to evaluate for chromosome abnormalities.
6. The detection rate of open neural tube defects using a combination of MSAFP screening and high-resolution ultrasound is comparable with that achieved by amniotic fluid studies.
7. Until more data are available, women with true elevated MSAFP levels and normal ultrasound examinations should continue to be offered the option of amniocentesis for AFAFP, AChE, and chromosome analysis.

Elevated MSAFP in the Absence of Fetal Anomalies

In approximately 50% of pregnancies with elevated MSAFP levels, ultrasonography and amniocentesis do not identify a cause. The majority of patients with unexplained MSAFP elevations have no complications. However, unexplained elevated MSAFP levels are associated with an increased risk (20% to 38%) for adverse pregnancy outcomes. Findings associated with elevated MSAFP levels include the following:

1. Fetal death
   a. Approximately 3% to 5% of all patients with MSAFP elevations and 20% of those with MSAFP levels greater than 5.0 will be found to have experienced fetal demise at the time of ultrasonography.

b. Patients with elevated MSAFP levels who have a viable fetus at ultrasonography are at increased risk for later fetal loss or stillbirth; the higher the MSAFP elevation, the greater the risk.
   (1) A 2.5-fold increased risk for MSAFP MoM in the range of 2.0 to 2.9
   (2) A 10-fold increased risk for MSAFP MoM greater than 3.0
2. Placental anomalies
   a. Transient fetomaternal hemorrhage
   b. Tumor
   c. Infarction
3. Intrauterine viral infections
   a. Cytomegalovirus (CMV)
   b. Parvovirus
   c. Herpes simplex
4. Premature delivery, low birth weight, or intrauterine growth retardation (IUGR): significantly higher risk with MSAFP MoM greater than 5.0
5. Other pregnancy complications
   a. Preeclampsia
   b. Placental abruption

Management of the Patient with Unexplained MSAFP Elevations

It has been suggested that the presence of an unexplained elevated MSAFP level should be considered an indication of a high-risk pregnancy warranting increased surveillance because of the known increased risk of adverse pregnancy outcome. There is currently neither consensus on an appropriate management protocol for such pregnancies nor clear evidence that specific interventions improve pregnancy outcomes. Each pregnancy should be considered on an individual basis.

Individual Serum Markers Used in Screening for Chromosome Abnormalities

1. Low MSAFP levels are associated with an increased risk for fetal Down syndrome.
   a. Reduced MSAFP levels may result from decreased fetal hepatic AFP production.
   b. Detection rate for Down syndrome is 20% to 25% with MSAFP levels less than 0.5 MoM.
   c. Patient-specific risks for Down syndrome are based on a combination of MSAFP MoM values and maternal age.
   d. An assigned risk of greater than or equal to 1:270 (the age-related risk for a 35-year-old woman at midtrimester) is considered abnormal.
   e. Findings other than fetal Down syndrome that may be associated with low MSAFP levels include the following:
      (1) Other chromosome abnormalities (most commonly trisomy 18 and Turner's syndrome)
      (2) Fetal demise
      (3) Hydatidiform mole
      (4) Overestimated gestational age
      (5) Normal variant

2. Elevated maternal serum human chorionic gonadotropin (MSHCG) levels greater than or equal to 2.0 MoM are associated with an increased risk for fetal Down syndrome.
   a. HCG is a placental glycoprotein composed of two nonidentical subunits (alpha and beta).
   b. Intact (total) HCG and free beta-HCG levels peak at 8 to 10 weeks gestation (Fig. 20-11).
   c. As with MSAFP, MSHCG MoM values are adjusted to account for factors that affect MSHCG levels (gestational age, maternal weight, race, diabetes).
   d. Most laboratories measure intact (total) HCG, although it has been suggested that beta-HCG may be a more sensitive marker.
   e. MSHCG is the best single serum marker for the detection of Down syndrome.
   f. Findings other than fetal Down syndrome that may be associated with an elevated MSHCG level include the following:
      (1) Fetal hydrops
      (2) IUGR
      (3) Placental disruption
      (4) Pregnancy-induced hypertension
      (5) Overestimated gestational age
3. Low levels of maternal serum unconjugated estriol (MSuE$_3$) are associated with an increased risk for fetal Down syndrome.
   a. MSuE$_3$ is a steroid derived from dehydroepiandrosterone sulfate (DHEAS) produced in the fetal adrenal glands, converted to alphahydroxy DHEAS in the fetal liver, and metabolized in the placenta.

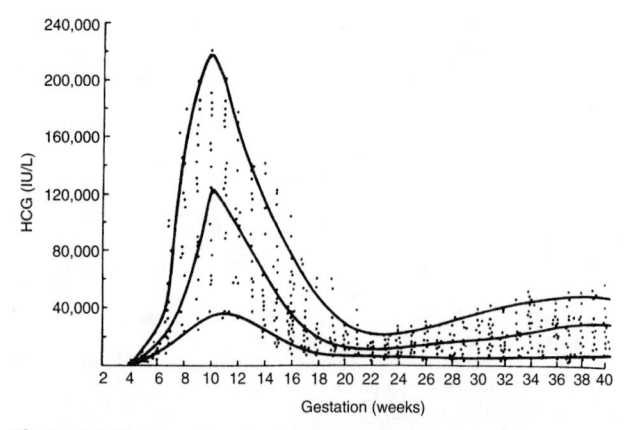

Figure 20-11 The relationship between human chorionic gonadotropin (HCG) levels and gestational age, showing 5th, 50th, and 95th percentiles. (From Hay DL: Br J Obstet Gynecol 95:1270, 1988.)

b. As with MSAFP and MSHCG, MSuE$_3$ MoM values must be adjusted to account for factors that affect levels (gestational age, maternal weight, race, diabetes).
c. The median MSuE$_3$ value for pregnancies affected with Down syndrome is 0.78 MoM.
d. MSuE$_3$ is the second best single indicator for the detection of Down syndrome.
e. Other findings associated with low uE$_3$ values include the following:
    (1) Placental pathology
    (2) Fetal demise
    (3) IUGR
    (4) Maternal chronic hypertension
4. The use of other serum markers for the detection of chromosome abnormalities, including pregnancy-specific beta-glycoprotein and neutrophil alkaline phosphatase, have been considered; however, only the three markers discussed are currently used in clinical settings.

Maternal Serum Triple Marker Screening for Detection of Chromosome Abnormalities

1. A maternal serum triple marker screening test should be offered to all pregnant women under age 35 as a screen for chromosome abnormalities and neural tube defects.
2. The maternal serum triple marker screen consists of the concurrent measurements of MSAFP, MSHCG, and MSuE$_3$.
3. A computerized formula based on Gaussian multivariate analysis is used to derive a specific numerical risk for fetal Down syndrome that is based on the combination of a woman's age-related risk and the three biochemical marker values.
    a. A calculated risk of greater than or equal to 1:270 (midgestational age-related risk for a 35-year-old woman) is considered abnormal.
    b. The detection rate is 60% to 65% in pregnant women under age 35 with a calculated risk of greater than or equal to 1:270.
    c. Detection rate increases to 85% to 90% in women over age 35 because of the effect of maternal age on the calculated risk.
4. In addition to Down syndrome, the maternal serum triple marker test is also useful as a screen for trisomy 18.
    a. Approximately 60% of fetal trisomy 18 will be identified on the basis of combined low levels of MSAFP, MSHCG, and MSuE$_3$.
    b. Although no calculated numerical risk is reported with concurrent low values, it has been estimated that the odds of having an affected fetus given a positive test result are 1 in 15.
5. Other chromosome abnormalities have been identified in pregnancies with abnormal triple marker results.
    a. A pattern of low MSAFP, low uE$_3$, and elevated MSHCG levels may be associated with hydropic Turner's syndrome.
    b. Pregnancies with various other chromosome abnormalities may be identified by subsequent amniocentesis for abnormal triple marker results; however, there have been an insufficient number of cases to confirm a true association with specific chromosome anomalies.

c. Triple marker screening results are currently reported and interpreted only as to the risk for Down syndrome and trisomy 18.
6. Although it has been suggested that inclusion of $MSuE_3$ in the serum marker screen may not add significantly to the detection rate of fetal Down syndrome, it is useful in the detection of trisomy 18 and most laboratories offer the triple marker combination.
7. Triple marker screening cannot be interpreted for multiple-gestation pregnancies because of a lack of normative values for this population.
8. The risk for a neural tube defect is reported as part of the triple marker screen result using the MSAFP MoM value alone (see MSAFP Screening for Neural Tube Defects).
9. Based on the correlation of increased or decreased levels of individual biochemical markers with chromosome abnormalities and neural tube defects, certain patterns of multiple marker values may be associated with increased risks for specific anomalies (Table 20-7).

Evaluation of the Patient with an Abnormal Triple Marker Screening Test for Chromosome Abnormalities

The following is an example of a protocol for follow-up testing for an abnormal triple marker screening test (Fig. 20-12).

1. If the screening test indicates a risk greater than 1:270 for Down syndrome or concurrent low levels indicating an increased risk for trisomy 18, high-resolution ultrasonography is performed to confirm gestational age and evaluate for fetal anomalies.
2. If the estimated gestational age is correct, genetic counseling is provided and the patient is offered the option of amniocentesis.
3. If the estimated gestational age used to calculate triple marker results differs by more than 10 days from that determined by ultrasound, results are recalculated by the laboratory performing the study or the sample is redrawn if the specimen has been obtained before 15 weeks gestation.
4. If the patient elects to proceed with amniocentesis and results are abnormal, the patient receives additional genetic counseling regarding the findings and available options.

Table 20-7 **Patterns of Abnormal Maternal Serum Triple Marker Screen Results**

MSAFP	MSHCG	$MSuE_3$	Differential
Low	High	Low	Down syndrome Hydropic Turner's syndrome
Low	Low	Low	Trisomy 18 (without ventral wall defect)
High	Normal	Normal	Open neural tube defect or ventral wall defect

Practical Guide to the Care of the Gynecologic/Obstetric Patient

```
Abnormal triple marker screen indicating
      increased risk (>1:270) for
         fetal Down syndrome
                │
                ▼
     High-resolution ultrasound
      to verify gestational age
```

- Ultrasound age differs from menstrual age by >10 days
  - Gestational age <15 weeks when sample obtained → Repeat triple marker screen at 16 weeks
    - Triple marker results normal (<1:270 risk) → No further testing
    - Triple marker results abnormal (>1:270 risk) → Genetic counseling; Offer amniocentesis for karyotyping
  - Gestational age >15 weeks when sample obtained → Recalculate risk based on corrected gestational age
- Gestational age correct; No fetal abnormalities on ultrasound
- Gestational age correct; Fetal abnormalities on ultrasound (nuchal fold, choroid plexus cyst, echogenic bowel, etc.) → Genetic counseling; Offer amniocentesis for karyotyping
- Multiple gestation; Fetal demise → Appropriate follow-up

Amniocentesis results:
- Normal chromosomes → No further testing
- Abnormal chromosomes → Further genetic counseling regarding options and implications
- Normal chromosomes → Consider follow-up high-resolution ultrasound

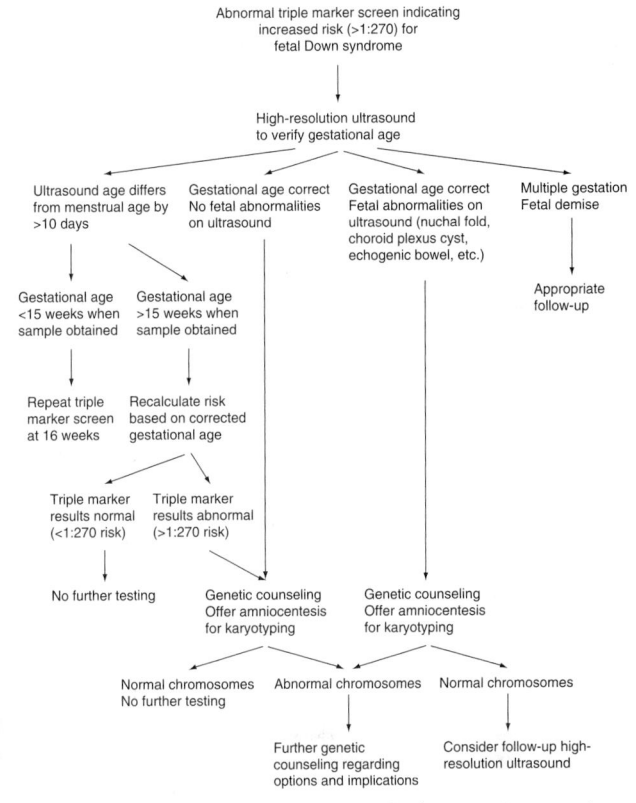

Figure 20-12 Algorithm for evaluation of abnormal maternal serum triple marker screening test indicating an increased risk for Down syndrome.

Issues Regarding the Use of the Triple Marker Screen

1. Benefits include cost effectiveness and potential for identifying fetal chromosome abnormalities and neural tube defects.
   a. Of Down syndrome infants, 80% are born to women under age 35, who are not routinely offered the option of amniocentesis.
   b. Maternal screening is a noninvasive method for identifying pregnancies with an increased risk for fetal anomalies in a low-risk population.
2. Whereas amniocentesis is offered to women 35 years of age or older for diagnosis of chromosome abnormalities, triple marker screening should be offered to these women to provide individual risks for Down

syndrome (which may be higher or lower than their age-related risk alone) and to assist in the decision-making process regarding the options for further testing.
3. Concerns have been raised regarding unnecessary anxiety resulting from false-positive results.
    a. It is estimated that 5% to 10% of screening results will be positive for an increased risk for a chromosome abnormality or neural tube defect.
    b. Of those positive screening tests, only 3% will represent an actual neural tube defect or chromosome abnormality.
4. Screening should be offered with an explanation as to its purposes and limitations.
5. Test results should be provided in a timely fashion to assist in the patient's decision process.
6. It is essential that triple marker screening results be used in conjunction with ultrasound findings and appropriate genetic counseling.

DOWN SYNDROME

In 1866, John Langdon Down described a condition in which affected individuals had mental retardation and a characteristic facial appearance.[2] Although later it was hypothesized that the disorder described by Langdon Down may have resulted from a chromosomal abnormality, convincing evidence that chromosomal abnormalities occurred in humans was lacking. However, in 1959, after techniques were developed to analyze human chromosomes, Lejeune and others[3] identified the presence of 47 rather than 46 chromosomes in affected individuals, and the extra chromosome was designated as human chromosome number 21.

Down syndrome is the most common genetic cause of mental retardation, occurring in approximately 1 in 800 live births. Its incidence increases with advanced maternal age, and especially in pregnant women 35 years of age or older. However, approximately 80% to 90% of cases are born to younger women, because of the significantly greater number of births in this age group.

Although serious and potentially life-threatening medical complications are observed in Down syndrome, in contrast to 25 years ago the infant with this chromosomal abnormality has significantly greater opportunities to live a longer, healthier, and more productive life. These changes reflect greater opportunities in the areas of education, employment, and community living. Although institutionalization was a frequent recommendation after the birth of an affected infant as recently as 15 years ago, institutionalization is no longer considered an option. Even in those infrequent instances when a couple is overwhelmed by the diagnosis and unable to bring an affected infant into their home, adoption of a child with Down syndrome is readily available by other families.

Access to health care has dramatically improved for children with Down syndrome. In 1965, 50% of affected children did not survive beyond 5 years of age, primarily because of the lack of surgical intervention for congenital heart disease. However, with more aggressive medical and surgical intervention for structural abnormalities and medical diseases, especially in the last two decades, survival has improved dramatically and is in excess of 80% at 30 years of age. This figure, in fact, may actually be an underestimate of survival rates now, because a portion of adults did not receive optimum medical care earlier in their lives. Therefore, today, no difference in health care provision exists in the child with Down syndrome when compared with an unaffected population.

Two important federal laws have increased the availability of early developmental and educational programming, beginning in early infancy, after establishment of a diagnosis. Public Law 94-142, legislated in 1977, guaranteed free, equal, and appropriate educational opportunities in the least restrictive environment for all individuals with disabilities from the age of 3 to 22 years. In 1986, Public Law 99-457 enabled an extension of services to include a population of children from birth to 3 years. The recognition of benefits achieved by integrating children with disabilities into regular academic classroom settings has enhanced learning experiences for school-age children with Down syndrome, and in adulthood, greater acceptance of individuals with disabling conditions has led to employment opportunities in the community.

The Neonate with Down Syndrome

Down syndrome is usually diagnosable at, or shortly after, birth, based on a distinctive clinical phenotype, and especially facial characteristics. In fact, the term mongolism, originally used by Langdon Down to describe an affected child, was coined because of the resemblance of the face to Asian individuals; however, this term no longer is regarded as an appropriate one to describe an affected child.

Facially (Figure 20-13 and Box 20-3) the palpebral fissures are upslanting and frequently shortened. The bridge of the nose is flattened, and the ears are small with overfolded helices. Epicanthal folds are present, and Brushfield's spots around the margin of the iris are commonly found. There is facial flattening, with a depressed nasal bridge, and brachycephaly. Tongue protrusions may be observed. Redundant skin over the posterior aspect of the neck is common and, occasionally during pregnancy, can be recognized on ultrasonography in the first and second trimesters. The hands of an infant with Down syndrome tend to be broad and short, and clinodactyly of the fifth fingers is often seen. Frequently, a single palmar crease is identified (i.e., simian crease) and there is evidence of a wide space between the first and second toes with a deep hallucal groove on the plantar surface of the foot, running longitudinally. Muscular hypotonia is a constant feature and may be the first finding identified in the neonate that raises suspicion of the diagnosis. In addition, low muscle tone leads to joint hypermobility and an increased risk for hip dislocation.

Major structural defects are common in Down syndrome and may lead to medical complications shortly after birth or in early infancy if not recognized promptly. The most common structural abnormality is congenital heart disease, which is present in approximately 40% of cases. Although the lesion is frequently asymptomatic at birth and a murmur may not be heard as a result of increased pulmonary vascular resistance, early diagnosis and treatment are critical because of a significant risk for

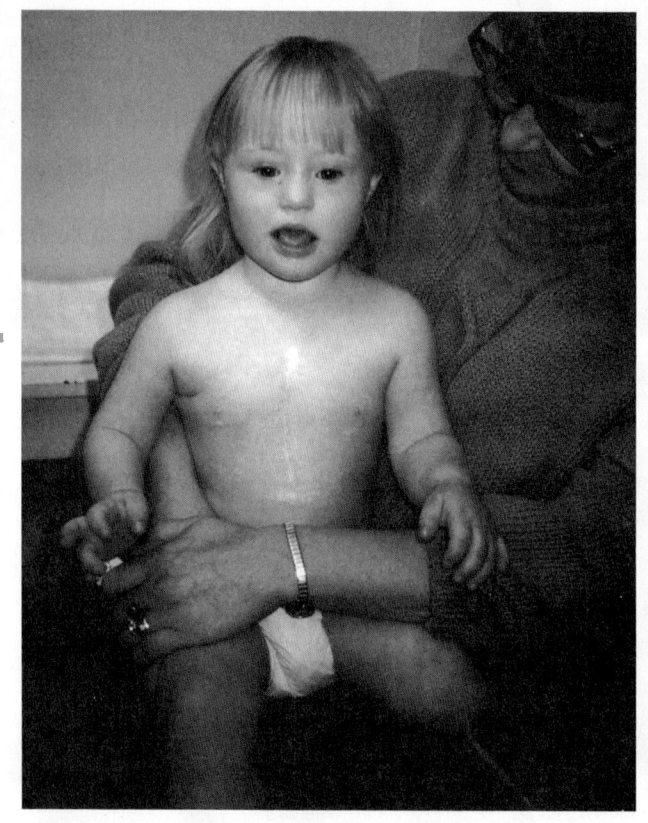

Figure 20-13 Two-year-old female with Down syndrome. Note the incisional scar from a previously repaired heart lesion.

morbidity and mortality resulting from early development of irreversible pulmonary hypertension. In approximately 40% of cases with congenital heart disease, an atrioventricular (AV) canal (i.e., AV communis) is present. Ventricular septal defect is found in about 31% of cases, with approximately 9% of infants having an atrial septal defect, or patent ductus arteriosus, and with teratology of Fallot being present in about 6% of cases. Rarely, a more complex heart lesion is identified. For instance, I have seen a few infants that have had both an AV communis and tetralogy of Fallot. Therefore, in view of the significant risk for morbidity and mortality resulting from congenital heart disease, echocardiography should be performed routinely in all neonates after a diagnosis of Down syndrome is established.

Practical Guide to the Care of the Gynecologic/Obstetric Patient 541

> BOX 20-3 Clinical Features in the Neonate with Down Syndrome
>
> *Craniofacial*
>
> Flat face
> Brachycephaly
> Upslanting and occasionally short palpebral fissures
> Epicanthal folds
> Brushfield's spots
> Flat nasal bridge
> Small ears
> Overfolded ear helices
> Tongue protrusions
> Excessive posterior nuchal skin
>
> *Extremities*
>
> Short, broad hands
> Clinodactyly fifth fingers
> Proximal thumbs
> Single palmar crease
> Gap between first and second toes
> Deep hallucal groove on foot
> Hypermobile joints
>
> *Neurologic*
>
> Hypotonia

Gastrointestinal (GI) anomalies are found in up to 12% of newborns with Down syndrome. Duodenal atresia and stenosis are the most common defects identified, and these obstructive lesions are found in about 2.5% of patients with Down syndrome. In addition, Down syndrome is found in about 25% to 30% of cases of duodenal atresia. Annular pancreas occasionally is present as an associated feature. In utero, diagnosis of duodenal atresia may be suspected on ultrasound in the presence of polyhydramnios, or evidence of a double bubble on examination of the fetal abdomen. Following the infant's birth, bilious vomiting after initiation of feeding should raise suspicion of the diagnosis and the need for further medical intervention. Other GI lesions that occur with increased frequency in Down syndrome include imperforate anus, seen in about 1% of cases; Hirschsprung's disease in 0.56% of cases; and tracheoesophageal fistula in 0.43% of affected infants. Feeding difficulties unrelated to an anatomic GI lesion are not uncommon and result from an inefficient suck resulting from decreased oral muscle tone. The emotional stress of parents dealing with the diagnosis may amplify feeding difficulties, leading to poor weight gain initially. These problems combined with poor growth related to a congenital heart lesion, that may eventually require surgical correction, can result in significant failure to thrive, increasing the risk for postoperative complications in the affected infant. Therefore, intervention from a feeding specialist may be indicated, with patience and support of family members to facilitate adequate growth, especially when surgery to correct a cardiac lesion may be anticipated in infancy.

Congenital cataracts occur in approximately 3% of infants with Down syndrome. Early recognition and surgical extraction are extremely important to retain adequate vision to facilitate growth and development in the future.

In addition, in the neonatal period, an increased risk for developing transient myeloproliferative disorder (i.e., transient acute leukemia) results in a significant elevation of peripheral white blood cells and may include the presence of blast cells. However, unlike leukemia, there are normal numbers of granulocytes and macrophage stem cells in the bone marrow, and ultrastructural differences between leukemoid and leukemic blast cells can be recognized. This disorder is so commonly associated with Down syndrome that its presence, even in the absence of a typical Down syndrome phenotype, should signal the need to search for mosaicism. Although the condition generally is regarded as benign, resolving spontaneously in infancy, an increased risk for developing myeloid leukemia or myelofibrosis later in life exists, warranting closer monitoring of the hematologic status in affected children manifesting this hematologic abnormality.

The Young Child with Down Syndrome

Cognitive deficits represent the greatest long-term disability in Down syndrome. Although development may appear to be normal in early infancy, developmental delay is usually apparent by the latter part of the first year of life. At that time, delays in cognitive and motor development are evident.[4] By school age, most affected children demonstrate a moderate degree of mental retardation on standardized tests of intelligence. Although variability in intellectual abilities exists, including some affected children functioning in an educable range, a progressive decline in IQ is commonly observed. Controversy exists whether there is a relationship between parental educational level or IQ and those observed in affected children, and it has been suggested in one study that a correlation between mothers with 16 or more years of education and higher IQ scores in their affected child exists. Children with Down syndrome have relative delays in the development of language skills, even when compared with children of comparable mental ages. Communication difficulties may be further complicated by significant speech articulation problems. Use of a total communication approach, including both verbal and augmentative therapy, therefore, may facilitate communication abilities in the affected child. An area of strength that is often seen in Down syndrome is the acquisition of social and adaptive skills, and successes in these areas frequently enhance an affected individual's potential to procure some form of meaningful employment in adulthood and to be able to function adequately in a semiindependent living setting. Initiation of early intervention services with motor, cognitive, and speech and language stimulation has had a beneficial effect on development in Down syndrome. Although long-term impact on intellectual functioning may not be great, clear benefits have been seen in the acquisition of social and adaptive skills. Initiation of early services also has provided an important source of support for families dealing with their child's disability.

In addition to surgical correction of anatomic abnormalities, early detection and treatment of several medical problems commonly observed in Down syndrome are critical. Children with Down syndrome have an increased susceptibility to infections, particularly involving the upper respiratory tract. Sinusitis is probably more common than suspected. In my experience, the presence of chronic purulent rhinorrhea frequently is associated with sinusitis that can be demonstrated on computerized tomography. Hearing loss is observed in more than 75% of young children with Down syndrome, and this usually is conductive in nature, resulting from persistent middle ear effusions. Treatment of this problem is necessary to maintain normal hearing to facilitate language development. Audiologic evaluations, therefore, should be initiated in the first year of life and performed, at least, on a yearly basis.

Results of immunologic studies in Down syndrome have been conflicting. Studies have demonstrated both decreased T and B lymphocyte numbers and function. T-cell abnormalities appear to be most consistently present, and in one study, the number of T-helper cells (CD4+) was decreased, resulting in a decreased ratio of T-helper to T-suppressor (CD8+) cells. In addition, an increased risk for autoimmunity is observed in Down syndrome with antithyroid antibodies and alopecia areata being present in about 10% to 15% of cases, and in rare instances there is an association of the latter finding with diabetes mellitus and hypoparathyroidism.

A variety of different ocular abnormalities are common in children with Down syndrome. In addition to congenital cataracts and occasionally glaucoma, congenital nystagmus is observed in about 35% of infants. This finding is not necessarily associated with visual deficits and may resolve spontaneously in childhood. However, refractive errors occur in up to 70% of children with Down syndrome and frequently result from myopia. Strabismus is observed in 60% of cases, and in 20% of affected children, there is evidence of nasolacrimal duct obstruction. The high-frequency association of ocular abnormalities, therefore, necessitates routine ophthalmological evaluation with determination of whether cataracts are present in early infancy, and subsequently followed by ophthalmologic reevaluation in the second year of life, again at about 5 years of age, and in midadolescence.

Thyroid dysfunction, and especially hypothyroidism, is an occasional manifestation of Down syndrome. Congenital hypothyroidism is present in 1.1% of Down syndrome cases. A risk for acquired thyroid disease also exists. In a retrospective study of 49 children with Down syndrome between the age of 4 months and 3 years, in addition to congenital hypothyroidism being present in three cases, two others either had acquired hypothyroidism or hyperthyroidism. In addition, in 13 of the 49 children, there was a mild elevation of thyroid stimulating hormone level in the face of a normal thyroxin level. It has been estimated that thyroid dysfunction may be present in as high as 15% of cases. Because hypothyroidism can further compromise central nervous system function in the child with a developmental disability, prompt recognition and treatment are necessary. However, because early clinical symptoms may be misinterpreted as representing features of Down syndrome, this may not be possible. Therefore, routine screening of thyroid function on a yearly basis until school age is indicated.

In addition to transient myeloproliferative disease that is unique to Down syndrome, an increased incidence of leukemia is also observed and is 10 to 18 times more common than that found in chromosomally normal individuals up to 16 years of age. In addition, in adults with Down syndrome, there is also an increased risk for hematologic malignancies, but not to the same magnitude as that seen in younger individuals. Acute nonlymphoblastic leukemia is the type primarily observed in children who develop this malignancy before a year of age. However, in affected children 3 years of age or older, the distribution of leukemic types is similar to that seen in a chromosomally normal population of children. Survival in children with Down syndrome who have leukemia is lower, in all likelihood, as the result of a lower frequency of remission and increased risk for life-threatening infections. One type of leukemia that is observed up to 200 to 400 times more frequently in Down syndrome is acute megakaryoblastic leukemia. Although not seen frequently, this form of leukemia can be a later manifestation in children who had transient myeloproliferative disorder as a neonate.

Seizures are seen more frequently in Down syndrome, and it has been estimated that the incidence ranges from 2.6% to 8.8%. An increased risk for infantile spasms also exists, and Pueschel reported infantile spasms in 5 of 89 affected children under 1 year of age. Autism also occurs with greater frequency in Down syndrome.

Hypermobility of the joints can result in an increased risk for cervical instability that could lead to spinal cord compression and permanent neurologic sequelae. Radiologically, atlantoaxial instability is observed in approximately 15% of young children with Down syndrome. Although in most instances, the abnormality is asymptomatic, a small percentage have symptoms secondary to spinal cord compression. Risk for neurologic sequelae may be heightened by the presence of bone abnormalities of the cervical spine as well, which are observed on occasion. Therefore, it is generally recommended that radiographs of the cervical spine, including views in flexion and extension, be performed in all affected children between 2½ and 3 years of age, and again before participation in Special Olympics at school age. In the presence of cervical instability, it is generally recommended that participation in competitive sports that could lead to a traumatic neck injury be avoided.[5,6] In addition to the increased risk for atlantoaxial instability, atlantooccipital instability has been found in up to 30% of Down syndrome children as well. Even in the absence of radiographic evidence of cervical instability, the presence of symptoms suggestive of spinal cord compression, such as chronic neck pain, newly developed deficits in motor abilities and bladder and bowel function, pyramidal tract signs, and loss of sensation should necessitate further investigation for the possible presence of this problem. Finally, because a potential risk for spinal cord injury may exist with extreme hyperextension of the neck for intubation, radiographic investigation of the cervical spine before an operative procedure may be indicated.

Problems related to the oral airway and dental development are common in Down syndrome. Upper airway obstruction leading to obstructive apnea may be insidious and potentially life threatening. The presence of a small airway that lacks musculature and connective tissue support, and enlarged tonsils and adenoids, can result in increased airway resistance, leading to hypoxia, pulmonary hypertension, and cor pulmonale. Obesity, a common problem in Down syndrome, may further increase the risk for airway obstruction. Altered sleep habits, such as restlessness, wakefulness with agitation, snoring, daytime fatigue, and apnea should signal the need for further investigation of this potentially serious medical complication. Tonsillectomy and adenoidectomy may be indicated to remedy this problem effectively, but the potential risk must be recognized for vocal resonance problems, with hypernasality developing as a result of velopharangeal incompetence postoperatively. Delayed dental eruption, altered tooth size and morphology, and hypodontia may be observed in up to 50% of Down syndrome cases. Malocclusion is frequent, and although periodontal disease was common in institutionalized patients, the risk for this problem is not felt to be increased in those children reared in a home setting. Macroglossia is observed in Down syndrome, although in some instances, the macroglossia is relative, resulting from a small oral cavity. Both factors plus oral hypotonicity contribute to frequent tongue protrusions. Fissuring of the tongue also is commonly observed. Although tongue protrusions frequently represent a concern of parents, in many instances, they tend to decrease in frequency with age and growth of the oral cavity.

Beginning in early infancy, programming to facilitate neurodevelopmental status should be emphasized. Enrollment in an early intervention program, combined with services provided in the area of occupational, physical, and speech and language therapy are ideal. At 3 years of age, enrollment in a regular preschool with continued provision of ancillary services is important in continuing to optimize an affected child's developmental potential and strengthening social and adaptive skills. Once school age is reached, the child's enrollment in a regular school classroom, for at least part of the day, is mandatory; additional services should be provided by a special educational teacher either by integrating them in the classroom or in a separate setting on an individual basis. Continued efforts at maximizing speech and language development should be pursued on an intensive basis, again incorporating a variety of different modes of communication, if necessary. Occupational and physical therapy, to enhance fine and gross motor development, should be included as part of the academic curriculum. Many children with Down syndrome have demonstrated the ability to learn basic reading, writing, and mathematics skills, and the opportunity to achieve successes in these areas should be readily available.

The Adolescent with Down Syndrome

Adolescence brings its own unique challenges to the person with Down syndrome. In addition to continuing to enhance developmental skills, programming must begin to be directed at developing vocational competency, to enable the person to function in society as an adult. Coping with the desire for independence represents a new challenge for parents and school personnel. In males, pubertal changes occur at an age similar to that of males without Down syndrome. In addition, no differences are noted in the size of external genitalia or gonadotropin levels; however, sterility is present in almost all cases, and there has been only one instance in which reproduction by a male with Down syndrome has been reported. In females, menarche occurs slightly later than an unaffected female, with a mean age at menarche of 12 years 6 months, in contrast to 12 years 1 month in the unaffected female. The development of pubertal changes is not strikingly different, and menstrual periods are similar. The potential for reproduction in a female with Down syndrome is considerably greater than that in an affected male. In a study by Tricomi et al.,[7] it was found that 39% of affected females ovulated, 15% probably ovulated, 15% possibly ovulated, and 30% were not ovulatory. There have been numerous reports of affected females giving birth to offspring and in about 50% of cases the infant was similarly affected.

Adolescence is also a time when most individuals with Down syndrome enjoy good health. However, the risk for obesity increases, necessitating close monitoring of dietary intake, and stressing the importance of participating in a regular exercise program. Dry skin is present in about 90% of cases and skin can become thick and cracked, particularly over the surfaces of the hands, feet, wrists, and elbows. Premature aging from exposure to ultraviolet light is a risk; therefore, protecting skin against excessive sun exposure with sunscreen and protective clothing is important. Beginning in adolescence, follicular skin infections develop in 50% to 60% of affected individuals; these can result in abscess formation if not treated promptly, particularly around the buttocks and thighs. Benign sweat gland tumors (i.e., syringoma) can also develop in the periorbital area, neck, thoracic, and axillary regions and in the periumbilical and pubic areas.

Emotional stresses in the home and at school need to be dealt with in an open, patient, and supportive manner to minimize the risk for abnormal emotional adjustment and behavioral disorders. These problems appear to be seen less frequently in a supportive family setting, where the developmental problems that can adversely impact an individual's self-image can be dealt with promptly in a positive and caring manner.

Growth in Down Syndrome

At birth, a neonate with Down syndrome may be slightly smaller than a chromosomally normal infant, although the difference in size is not significant. Delayed growth velocity occurs in infancy and, even to a greater degree, in the presence of significant congenital heart disease. Adolescent growth spurt is less than that observed in chromosomally normal teenagers, ultimately resulting in a mild degree of short stature. Growth hormone studies in Down syndrome have not revealed growth hormone deficiency. Although growth hormone therapy in this group has been advocated by some, and one study has demonstrated increased mean growth velocity to greater than twice that observed with pretreatment values, the significance of this short-term finding is uncertain and efficacy from growth hormone use has not been proved. Growth charts ranging from 1 month to 18 years of age are available to monitor linear growth after the birth of an infant with Down syndrome.

Survival in Down Syndrome

In the first decade of life, and especially in the first 5 years, the presence or absence of congenital heart disease and surgical correction of the lesion, if one is present, has been a major determinant of survival. Compared with a background population at any point in time, life expectancy in Down syndrome is about 10 to 20 years shorter. Major causes of death in decreasing order of frequency include pneumonia (23% to 41%), congenital heart disease (30% to 35%), other infections (2% to 15%), malignancy (2% to 9%), and senility and stroke (0% to 9%). In a Canadian study, major causes of death up to 30 years of age were complications related to major organ malformations, infection, and leukemia.

More recently, with improved medical and surgical care of individuals with Down syndrome beginning in the neonatal period, life expectancy has increased, and it is anticipated that these figures will continue to improve in the future. Nearly half of Down syndrome patients survive to 50 years of age, with $1/7$ still alive at 68 years of age.

The Adult with Down Syndrome

Because individuals with Down syndrome are surviving well into adulthood, physicians caring for these individuals must become aware of the medical needs of this aging population. Ocular problems are frequent, with cataracts occurring in 30% to 60% of cases, but rarely dense enough to require surgery. Other ocular complications such as glaucoma, blepharitis, and keratoconus occur more frequently and must be monitored for. Hypothyroidism becomes a much more significant problem than in childhood, being present in up to 50% of adults, and yearly monitoring of thyroid function is indicated. Cardiovascular disease is seen more commonly, with an increased risk for mitral valve prolapse and aortic regurgitation. Periodic evaluation of an affected adult's cardiac status appears to be warranted, and in the presence of a cardiac lesion, prophylaxis for subacute bacterial endocarditis should be initiated in the event that instrumentation, such as in the case of dental intervention, is pursued. High-frequency hearing loss is common and may necessitate amplification; therefore periodic audiologic testing is recommended.

The greatest concern associated with the aging process in Down syndrome is the risk for Alzheimer's disease. It has long been recognized that there is a relationship between Down syndrome and dementia, and that the pathologic changes of Alzheimer's disease develop in the brains of middle-age adults with this chromosomal abnormality. Alzheimer changes begin to develop in the fourth decade of life and, by 40 years of age, nearly all Down syndrome adults have evidence of the pathologic hallmarks of Alzheimer's disease, including granulovacuolar changes, senile plaques, neurofibrillary tangles, and neuronal loss. The earliest anatomic change of Alzheimer's disease is the preplaque, which is diffuse deposition of amyloid protein adjacent to cell bodies of morphologically normal neurons. Granular deposition of oligosaccharide is also present. It has been proposed that amyloid progressively accumulates around the cell body until the neuron degenerates with the appearance of tangles and plaques. Therefore, deposition of amyloid protein is presumed to be an early and progressive phenomenon and is possibly a result of overexpression of the amyloid precursor protein gene that is located on the long arm of chromosome 21 at band q21. This gene is also known to be responsible for one familial form of Alzheimer's disease. Although the pathologic changes in the brains of people with Down syndrome are identical to those seen in Alzheimer's disease, a significant portion of adults with Down syndrome do not develop dementia (although dementia is seen in about 25% of cases). It has been proposed that the number of tangles and plaques must exceed a threshold before there is actual evidence of clinical regression in previously acquired cognitive skills, and in Down syndrome it may be higher than in a chromosomally normal adult population, thus lowering the risk for development of dementia.

Regardless of whether or not there is evidence of frank dementia, there is progressive loss of a variety of intellectual functions and receptive language skills that are not simply attributable to mental retardation in the majority of older Down syndrome individuals. Other potentially treatable causes for dementia unrelated to Alzheimer's disease should be searched for, such as depression, which is not an uncommon occurrence, and hypothyroidism.

Allelic variation in apolipoprotein E isoforms has been recognized as being a risk factor for Alzheimer's disease in the general population. The presence of the epsilon 4 isoform has been associated with an increased risk for amyloid deposition in the brain, leading to Alzheimer changes. However, van Gool et al.[8] demonstrated that apolipoprotein E allele frequency was similar in Down syndrome individuals with and without Alzheimer's disease, demonstrating that apolipoprotein E does not play a role in the pathogenesis of Alzheimer changes in this patient population. Schupf et al.[9] have shown that the risk of dementia in mothers that have given birth to a child with Down syndrome before the age of 35 years is increased fivefold, whereas a similar risk is not present when maternal age is greater than 35 years at the time of an affected infant's birth. It has been postulated that the increased risk for Alzheimer's disease in young mothers that have given birth to a child with Down syndrome may be the result of an accelerated aging process that also plays a contributing role in the development of nondysjunction.

Chromosomal Basis of Down Syndrome

Down syndrome results from the presence of an extra chromosome 21. In approximately 95% of cases, the karyotype will reveal trisomy 21 (Fig. 20-14). It has been demonstrated that the extra 21 is maternal in origin in up to 95% of cases of trisomy 21, and the nondysjunctional event occurs in meiosis I in about 77% of cases, and in meiosis II in approximately 23% of cases. A Robertsonian translocation accounts for approximately 3% to 4% of Down syndrome, resulting from fusion of an extra chromosome 21 to another acrocentric chromosome, either in the D group (i.e., chromosomes 13, 14, or 15) or in the G group

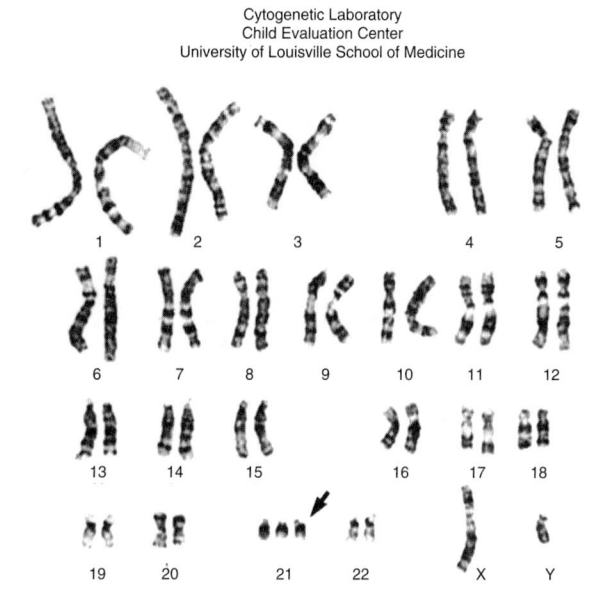

Practical Guide to the Care of the Gynecologic/Obstetric Patient 549

Cytogenetic Laboratory
Child Evaluation Center
University of Louisville School of Medicine

Figure 20-14 Trisomy 21 karyotype.

(i.e., chromosomes 21 or 22). The most commonly observed Robertsonian translocation involves chromosome 14, resulting in a translocated chromosome that contains both a 21 and a 14 chromosome (Fig. 20-15). In contrast to trisomy 21, which is associated with advanced maternal age, age does not appear to play a role in the development of a Robertsonian translocation, and the risk may actually decrease with advancing maternal age. Rarely, Down syndrome can result from a reciprocal translocation, and in one instance, I have seen a child with Down syndrome that was the result of a reciprocal translocation involving one chromosome 6, which was paternally derived. About 1% to 2% of Down syndrome results from mosaicism, in which two populations of cells can be identified, one with a diploid number (i.e., 46 chromosomes) and the other with a trisomic number (i.e., 47 chromosomes). Mosaicism can occur in the presence of either meiotic or mitotic nondysjunction, although the former is probably the more frequent mechanism, with a normal cell line being derived postconceptionally and the monosomic cell line being lost early in embryogenesis. The clinical phenotype in mosaic Down syndrome is somewhat more variable than that seen in classic Down syndrome with the potential for higher cognitive functioning; however, if the child is ascertained because of a suspected clinical

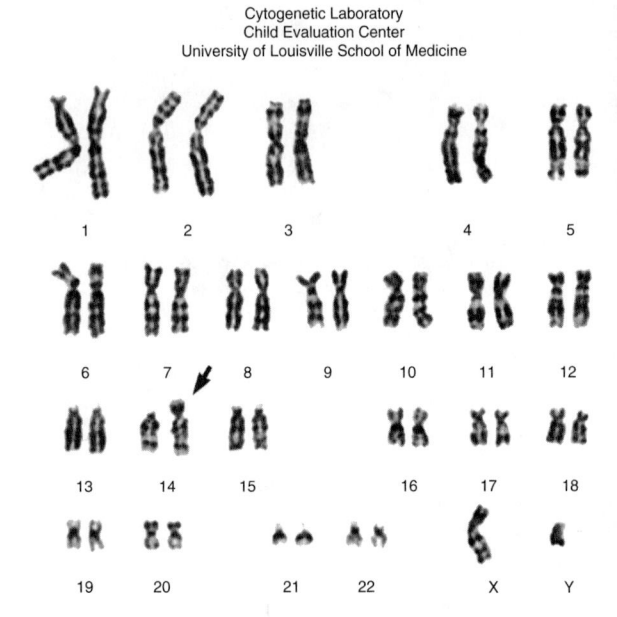

Figure 20-15 14 solids/21 Robertsonian translocation Down syndrome karyotype.

diagnosis of Down syndrome based on physical findings or the presence of mental retardation, little difference in outcome usually is observed, even in the face of mosaicism.

In women under 35 years of age who have given birth to an infant with trisomy 21, an increased risk for recurrence is observed and it is in the range of 1%. There have been rare instances in which multiple family members have had trisomy 21, or a couple has had multiple affected children. This phenomenon may result from two mechanisms: the first is low-grade mosaicism unrecognized in one of the parents, and the second is germ line mosaicism, in which a subpopulation of trisomic germ cells is present only in a reproductive organ.

When Down syndrome results from a Robertsonian translocation, parental karyotyping is important because a balanced Robertsonian translocation can be identified in one of the parents 40% to 45% of the time. In the case of a 14/21 Robertsonian translocation, the presence of a carrier parent increases the risk for recurrence in a subsequent pregnancy, and especially if the mother is identified as the carrier. Risk for recurrence of a maternally derived translocation is 10% to 15%, and in the case of a paternally derived Robertsonian translocation, in the range of 1% to 2%. In the presence of 21/21 translocation Down syndrome, a parent is found to be a carrier in about 4% of cases. In this situation, only two conceptions can be formed (i.e., 21/21 translocation Down syndrome or monosomy 21). All pregnancies surviving to term will have Down syndrome because the latter chromosomal abnormality will result in spontaneous loss. Recurrence risk in the group in which neither parent is identified as being a carrier is approximately 2.6%, probably the result of mosaicism in a germ line in one of the partner's reproductive organs.

Prenatal Diagnosis of Down Syndrome

It has long been recognized that the risk for Down syndrome increases with advanced maternal age. A similar risk has not been demonstrated with advanced paternal age.

Prenatal diagnostic techniques have been established that either can screen a pregnancy for Down syndrome or provide definitive diagnosis of the chromosomal abnormality. The availability of these tests has become extremely valuable for those couples who have an affected child, or who are considering a pregnancy and the woman is 35 years of age, or older, but would not have pursued the option of childbearing without the availability of chromosomal testing in utero. Procedures capable of karyotyping fetal cells include chorionic villus sampling (CVS), amniocentesis, and percutaneous umbilical blood sampling (PUBS). CVS is performed between 10 and 12 weeks gestation. A sample of chorionic villus tissue, which is fetal in origin, is obtained either transcervically, or transabdominally, for the purpose of performing a chromosome analysis. Amniocentesis, on the other hand, is generally offered between 15 and 16 weeks gestation, and fetal cells are cultured from a sample of amniotic fluid that is removed transabdominally. After fetal cells are cultured, chromosome analysis from both procedures is usually available in 8 to 14 days. Risk of miscarriage from the CVS procedure is slightly higher than that of amniocentesis but appears to vary based on experience. Risk of miscarriage from the CVS procedure ranges from approximately 1% to 2%, in contrast to amniocentesis, in which the risk for miscarriage is 0.5%. It has also been suggested that an increased risk for limb reduction defects, and possibly for oromandibular abnormalities as well, may be associated with the CVS procedure. Numerous reports from Europe earlier this decade highlighted this association, although it appears that the greatest risk lies with a procedure that is performed before 10 weeks gestation. Although results of follow-up studies on CVS procedures performed in the United States after 10 weeks gestation are conflicting, it has been suggested that risk for limb reduction defects exceeds that of the background risk in the general population, but is probably somewhere in the range of 1:1000 to 1:3000.

PUBS generally is not offered before 20 weeks gestation because of the technical difficulty of performing the procedure. Late in the second trimester, in instances when a chromosome abnormality is suspected based on ultrasound findings, successful sampling of fetal blood enables more rapid karyotyping, with a result that can be obtained in 3 to 5 days. However, the success rate of the procedure varies from approximately 25% to 75% depending on placental position, and the risk for miscarriage probably is in the range of 1%.

In the early 1970s, in the United Kingdom, measurement of MSAFP was developed as a noninvasive diagnostic tool to screen pregnancies in the second trimester for open NTDs. In 1984, Merkatz et al. demonstrated that approximately 20% to 25% of fetuses with Down syndrome were diagnosable using this screening technique. Low levels of MSAFP were detected. Subsequently, their results were confirmed by other investigators, and in combination with advanced maternal age, measurement of MSAFP also became a method for screening low-risk pregnancies in women under 35 years of age for this chromosomal abnormality. Lower MSAFP levels have been attributed to decreased AFP production or AFP content in the liver of a Down syndrome fetus. More recently, it was discovered that by combining the measurement of AFP with human chorionic gonadotropin and unconjugated estriol levels in maternal serum between 15 and 20 weeks gestation from pregnant women under 35 years of age, 60% to 65% of fetuses with Down syndrome could be detected without increasing the percentage of false-positive results obtained when serum AFP was measured alone, which is in the range of 6% to 8%. It has been suggested that triple marker screening may also represent a valuable tool in a population of pregnant women 35 years of age or older, and particularly in those instances when the couple is uncertain whether they are interested in pursuing invasive prenatal diagnostic testing. It has been demonstrated that close to 90% of Down syndrome fetuses, and close to 50% of a few other forms of aneuploidy, are detectable by triple marker screening, although 25% to 30% of this population will test positive, meaning that the risk for Down syndrome based on the results are equal to or greater than the empiric risk for Down syndrome at midgestation of a 35-year-old woman, which is 1:270.

Approximately 75% of Down syndrome conceptions survive to term. The majority of fetal loss occurs in the first trimester. However, in instances in which a Down syndrome fetus is recognized in the second trimester, there is still a risk for fetal loss during the remainder of the pregnancy, which is approximately 20% to 25%. Although the majority of couples seeking prenatal diagnosis opt to terminate a pregnancy in which the fetus has Down syndrome, couples should be given the option of pursuing invasive prenatal diagnosis if results of the test will provide them with valuable information that will help them prepare for the birth of an affected infant, even if termination is not an option.

Alternative Therapy in Down Syndrome

No definitive treatment is available in Down syndrome. However, because the condition results in a chronic disability and can be associated with significant medical complications, a variety of unconventional therapeutic interventions have been attempted, although typically these have not undergone careful scientific scrutiny before being marketed. The use of a variety of high-dose vitamin and mineral supplements, occasionally in combination with hormones and enzymes, has been advocated as improving both physical characteristics and cognitive functioning in children with Down syndrome. However, several controlled trials in the early

1980s were not able to demonstrate the efficacy of these preparations. More recently, it has been suggested that administration of the drug Piracetam may improve cognitive functioning and physical appearance in Down syndrome, although there have been no scientific studies to corroborate these anecdotal reports.

In Europe, injection of lyophilized or freeze-dried cells from vertebrate animal fetuses has been advocated as a successful intervention in Down syndrome to improve intellectual abilities, and to normalize the physical characteristics of Down syndrome in an affected child. No measurable benefits have been demonstrated from such treatment, and in addition, an increased risk for hypersensitization and the introduction of slow viruses with this procedure also exists. Currently, cell therapy is not available in the United States.

Anecdotal success in improving outcome in Down syndrome has been suggested with the use of patterning and craniosacral manipulation, although outcomes claimed by this form of intervention have been challenged as well.

Finally, reports from both Germany and Israel have suggested that performing plastic surgery on children with Down syndrome to normalize the facial appearance through procedures such as a partial glossectomy; lateral canthoplasty to remove epicanthal folds; nose, cheek, and chin augmentation; and otoplasty could lead to normalization of the affected child's functional abilities. These procedures are occasionally performed in this country, but clearly positive benefits have not been demonstrated with follow-up of children undergoing this surgical intervention.

Molecular Insights into Trisomy 21

With rapid advances in molecular genetics, it is feasible to envision that the genetic structure of chromosome 21 eventually will be completely defined, and that the pathogenetic relationship between the presence of an extra set of genes on chromosome 21 and features of Down syndrome will be understood. To date, the mechanism leading to the phenotype in Down syndrome is not known, although it has been suggested that it may be a nonspecific disturbance of chromosomal balance or a gene dosage effect with an increase in the production of certain proteins encoded by normal genes on the extra number 21 chromosome that alters the delicate balance of several biochemical pathways important in proper development and organ function.[4] Rare instances of translocations involving chromosome 21 leading to a triplication of a portion of the long arm and resulting in a Down syndrome phenotype have helped in narrowing down the region of the chromosome that appears to be critical for developing the phenotype. Currently, band q22 appears to be the candidate for this critical region, and as few as 50 to 100 genes on this portion of the chromosome may be responsible for most of the characteristics typical of Down syndrome. However, identifying a Down syndrome–critical region on chromosome 21 does not provide a complete explanation for the phenotype, because the amyloid precursor protein thought to be involved in Alzheimer changes in the brains of Down syndrome adults lies outside this region, at band q21 (Fig. 20-16).

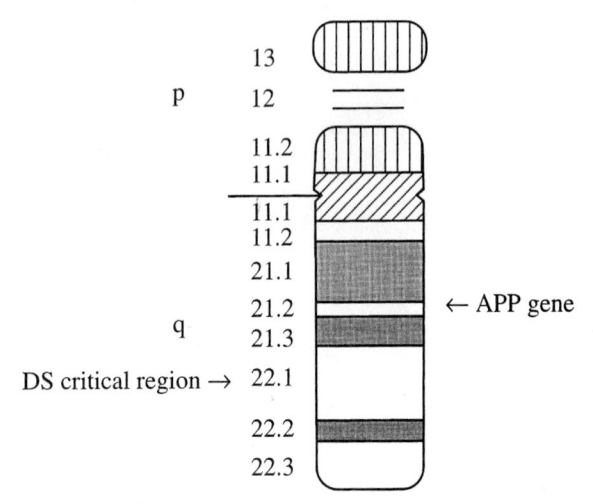

Figure 20-16 Idiogram of chromosome 21 demonstrating presumed Down syndrome (DS) critical region and gene locus for the amyloid precursor protein (APP) gene.

Studying animal models that share biologic similarities with humans also may provide insights into the effects of aneuploidy. Investigations performed on the trisomy 16 mouse, and on other mutant strains homologous to regions of the long arm (q) of human chromosome 21, have helped facilitate a better understanding of the pathogenesis of Down syndrome.

The prognosis for an infant born with Down syndrome in 1996 is considerably brighter than it was previously (Box 20-4). Longer and healthier survival with greater access to successful experiences in the areas of education, employment, and community life are now realistic expectations. Learning of the diagnosis shortly after giving birth to an affected infant is usually overwhelming for a couple and fraught with a great deal of sadness. However, establishing a diagnosis promptly, sharing accurate information in an optimistic and sensitive manner, and being supportive of family members in crisis after learning of the diagnosis can lay down the groundwork for many positive experiences that will occur in the lifetime of the affected individual. The physician can play a critical role in serving as an advocate for the child, to maximize the potential for growth and development. If provided with optimal medical care and developmental intervention, it is anticipated that children with Down syndrome will have an enhanced quality of life and make a substantial contribution to society.

BOX 20-4 Medical and Neurodevelopmental Issues to be Addressed in the Lifecycle of Down Syndrome

Neonate	Child	Adolescent	Adult
Congenital heart disease	Frequent upper respiratory infections	Dry skin and skin infections	Dementia
Gastrointestinal obstructive lesion	Hearing loss	Obesity	Visual deficits
Congenital cataracts	Visual deficits	Pubertal changes	Hypothyroidism
Transient myeloproliferative disorder	Thyroid dysfunction	Mental retardation, behavioral concerns	Cardiovascular disease
Hypothyroidism	Leukemia		Hearing loss
Hypotonia	Cervical instability		Emotional concerns
Feeding difficulties	Upper airway obstruction		
Parental reaction	Dental abnormalities		
	Seizures		
	Growth deficiency		
	Delayed development		

REFERENCES

1. Thornton JG, Lilford RG, Newcombe RG: Tables for estimation of individual risks of fetal neural tube and ventral wall defects, incorporating prior probability, maternal serum alpha-fetoprotein levels, and ultrasonographic examination results, *Am J Obstet Gynecol* 164:154-160, 1991.
2. Down JLH: Observations on an ethnic classification of idiots, London Hospital, *Clinical Lectures and Reports* 3:259-262, 1866.
3. Lejeune J, Gauthier M, Turpin R: Etude des chromosomes somatiques de neuf enfants mongoliens, *CR Acad Sci* 248:1721-1722, 1959.
4. Buckley LP: Congenital heart disease in infants with Down syndrome, *A study of the young child with Down syndrome*, pp. 351-364. New York, 1983, Human Sciences Press.
5. Antonarakis SE: Down syndrome collaborative group: paternal origin of the extra chromosome in trisomy 21 as indicated by analysis of DNA polymorphisms, *N Engl J Med* 324:872-876, 1991.
6. Burton BK, Schulz CJ, Burd LI: Limb anomalies associated with chorionic villus sampling, *Obstet Gynecol* 79:726-730, 1992.
7. Tricomi V, Valenti C, Hall JE: Ovulatory patterns in Down's syndrome, *Am J Obstet Gynecol* 89:651-656, 1964.
8. van Gool, WA Evenhuis, HM van, Duijn CM: A case-control study of apolipoprotein E genotypes in Alzheimer's disease associated with Down's syndrome. Dutch study group on Down's syndrome and aging, *Ann Neurol* 38:225-230, 1995.
9. Schupf N: Increased risk of Alzheimer's disease in mothers of adults with Down's syndrome, *Lancet* 344:353-356, 1994.

20.6 Amniocentesis and Chorionic Villus Sampling

Vernon Cook

AMNIOCENTESIS

History

1. Tissue karyotype technology originated in mid-1960s.
2. Before the ultrasound era (approximately 1980), amniocentesis (amnio) site was selected by palpation.
3. By 1980, amnio site selection was done by ultrasound. Subsequently, needle insertion guidance and observation of needle tip location (relative to fetus and placenta) throughout amniocentesis procedure has become common.
4. Before ultrasound, amnio was not technically feasible before 15 weeks gestation.
    a. The traditional 15-week lower limit for amnio was defined by this limitation.
    b. The 1 in 200 procedure-related pregnancy loss rate data came from the preultrasound era.
5. Since 1990, early amnio (EA), defined by less than 15 weeks gestation, has received additional attention.
    a. EA is associated with a higher, 1% to 4%, pregnancy loss rate and probable increased incidence of inability to retrieve fluid.
    b. Greater than 10,000 EA procedures have been reported in literature.
    c. For each week of gestation (up to 15 weeks), 1 mL of amniotic fluid is removed.

Indications

1. Screening: Karyotype is based on maternal age or other prenatal diagnosis indication.
2. Diagnostic:
    a. Spina bifida
        (1) Amniotic fluid alpha-fetoprotein AFAFP (vs) maternal serum AFP, MSAFP)
        (2) Acetyl cholinesterase
    b. Rh isoimmunization: Liley curve, delta optical density (OD) 450 measurement
        (1) Quantitative evaluation is done for bilirubin.
        (2) Bilirubin is present in proportion to intensity of hemolysis.
        (3) Liley curve zones:
            (a) Zone 1: not affected or mildly affected
            (b) Zone 2: affected; serial observations are required to establish trend; may need fetal transfusion
            (c) Zone 3: intense hemolysis, fetal transfusion required or hydrops will develop
    c. Isoimmunization: fetal antigen status (Rh or irregular antigen) determination by polymerase chain reaction (PCR) (e.g., CDE, Kell antigens)
    d. Single-gene disorders
    e. Ultrasound abnormality
    f. Other (e.g., cytomegalovirus [CMV] culture, PCR viral testing)
    g. Pulmonary maturity: lecithin/sphingomyelin (L/S) ratio, foam stability index (FSI), phosphatidyl glycerol (PG)
3. Therapeutic: reductive amniocentesis.
    a. Removal of up to 5 L has been reported.
    b. Indications include symptomatology (dyspnea, discomfort) and preterm labor complicated by polyhydramnios.
    c. There is little if any association with abruptio placentae; it is not related to volume removed.
    d. It is most frequently performed in twin–twin transfusion syndrome.

Relative and Absolute Contraindications

1. Absence of satisfactory amniotic fluid (AF) pocket away from placenta and fetus; increased risk of fetal hemorrhage
    a. Oligohydramnios or anhydramnios.
    b. Complete anterior placenta in third trimester. Transplacental amnio is relatively contraindicated because of potential fetal hemorrhage from vessel on placental surface.
        (1) Umbilical cord has Wharton's jelly, which stops hemorrhage.
        (2) Placental surface vessels have no jelly and may slowly (or rapidly) hemorrhage until vascular collapse occurs perhaps 2 to 3 hours later.
2. Absence of consent

Patient Counseling

1. Reasonable patient concept: Physician is obligated to explain to patient anything and everything a reasonable person might want to know.

2. Generally all risks and potential complications should be explained before the amniocentesis.
3. Alternatives to amniocentesis include the following:
   a. Explain consequences of not having amniocentesis.
   b. Explain if information be obtained by another method, such as waiting until delivery to determine karyotype, biometry (biparietal diameter, femur length) for pulmonary maturity, maternal serum alpha-fetoprotein triple screening.
4. Benefit to having amniocentesis: Patient should understand rationale for performing amniocentesis.

Risks

1. Second trimester
   a. A 1:200 (0.5%) procedure-related pregnancy loss rate, in excess of gestational age-related loss
   b. Amniotic fluid leakage 1:100 risk (1%)
   c. Controversial increased incidence of neonatal respiratory complications related to gestational age at amnio and amount of fluid withdrawn
   d. Chorioamnionitis: 1:1000 incidence
   e. Inability to retrieve fluid: more than one needle insertion for approximately 5% of amnios
   f. Failure of cell growth: 1:800
2. Third trimester
   a. Fetal hemorrhage and exsanguination: There is a remote possibility.
      (1) Umbilical cord laceration and acute, massive hemorrhage: obvious streaming on ultrasound
      (2) Laceration of placental surface vessel
         (a) Relatively slow hemorrhage; exsanguination is reported though risk is remote; streaming may or may not be observed.
         (b) Wharton's jelly prevents exsanguination from umbilical cord; placental surface vessels lack this protection.
   b. Emergency cesarean section: Incidence is 1:1000 amnios.
   c. Fetal demise has been reported; possibility is remote.
3. Risks not dependent on gestational age
   a. Isoimmunization: Rh immune globulin prophylaxis is indicated for Rh-negative women.
   b. Fetal injury has been reported; possibility is remote.
4. Amnio: not cause of preterm labor, although contractions may be noted after procedure

Complications

1. Isoimmunization: fetal maternal hemorrhage with maternal sensitization to fetal antigen. Rh immune globulin (anti D) prophylaxis is indicated to prevent Rh isoimmunization.
2. Umbilical cord laceration: sudden fetal (or maternal) movement with needle tip laceration of cord vessel. Emergency cesarean section may be warranted in third trimester.

3. Amnion tenting and prevention of fluid retrieval:
   a. Amnion seals to chorion at 13 to 15 weeks. Membrane separation usually can be observed on ultrasound examination.
   b. Amnion is tough; before amnion–chorion fusion, needle penetration of amnion may be difficult because amnion will simply be indented by needle (i.e., tenting) until needle contacts an object (e.g., opposite uterine wall).
   c. Alternatives:
      (1) Persist in present attempt: Stylet replacement and needle repositioning usually will achieve fluid retrieval.
      (2) Reattempt procedure in 1 to 2 weeks when membrane separation cannot be seen on both transabdominal and transvaginal ultrasound.

Procedure Description

1. Informed consent process: Physician explains risks, benefits, and alternatives so that patient understands them.
2. Ultrasound localization of placental and amniotic fluid pocket: Physician selects site away from fetal face (eye injury prevention) and placenta and documents fetal viability.
3. Procedural instructions: Patient is told to minimize body motion during the procedure (no laughing, talking, moving suddenly or unexpectedly).
4. Physician talks to patient during procedure (e.g., play-by-play narrative).
5. Antiseptic precautions are used.
6. Local anesthesia is given if patient desires.
7. Ultrasound guidance and observation occur during (20-gauge or 22-gauge) needle insertion.
8. Aspiration, dye insertion, and needle withdrawal are done.
9. Ultrasound (U/S) transducer is not moved after needle withdrawal to facilitate observation for streaming (blood movement through AF) from needle puncture site.
10. Postprocedural demonstration is given to patient of fetal heart action.
11. Nonstress test × 30 to 60 minutes is performed (if >25 weeks).
12. Explanation and copy of postprocedural instructions (see next section) are given to patient.

Postamniocentesis Patient Instructions

1. For the first 24 hours following the amniocentesis, the patient will need to limit her activities to exclude heavy lifting or strenuous exercise.
2. Patient should refrain from sexual intercourse for the next 48 hours.
3. Patient may eat a regular diet unless restricted by the physician.
4. Patient should report to her physician any of the following:
   a. Moderate to severe cramping or pain continuing for longer than 2 hours following the amniocentesis.
   b. Any unsuspected leakage of amniotic fluid from the vagina.
   c. Any vaginal bleeding.

d. A temperature elevation of greater than or equal to 100.4°F (38°C) within 1 week after the procedure.
5. If not allergic to Tylenol, patient can take two regular Tylenol every 6 hours for mild cramping.
6. If patient has had a genetic amniocentesis, the final results will not be available for approximately 2 to 3 weeks. The results will be given to patient by her private physician.
7. If patient is having amniocentesis to determine fetal lung maturity or delta OD 450, her results will be available later in the day or the next day. The physician will notify patient of the results.
8. If the patient's blood type is A negative, B negative, O negative, or AB negative, she may require Rh immune globulin before leaving the unit.
9. Patient certifies that she has read the above information, she understands her instructions, and has received a copy.

CHORIONIC VILLUS SAMPLING

Chorionic Villus Sampling Overview

The main advantage of chorionic villus sampling (CVS) is the time (10 to 12 weeks gestation) at which it is performed. This first-trimester diagnostic procedure offers couples an opportunity to evaluate the normalcy of the pregnancy during the first trimester. With CVS, those who would not carry an affected pregnancy could have a safer first-trimester termination rather than a mid or late second-trimester procedure.

Indications and Contraindications

1. First trimester
   a. CVS is appropriate for any patient in whom second-trimester amniocentesis would be indicated to exclude aneuploidy, such as the following:
      (1) Maternal age 35 years old or older
      (2) Prior affected child
      (3) Family history of a specific disorder (e.g., hemophilia)
   b. Alternative viewpoint: Because CVS has a higher risk than amniocentesis, CVS may be restricted to conditions with higher risk (e.g., age 40 years old or older).
   c. Postmortem CVS is used for evaluation of recurrent pregnancy loss.
      (1) CVS may be performed at diagnosis of demise.
      (2) Placental tissue remains viable.
      (3) Only 1 in 23 specimens gave normal karyotype.
      (4) 100% of CVS tissue grew in culture; in other tissues (skin, products of conception, amniotic fluid), 36% to 96% failed to grow.
2. Second-trimester CVS
   a. Indications: Amniocentesis or percutaneous umbilical blood sampling (PUBS) is not feasible (e.g., oligohydramnios); rapid karyotype is needed.
   b. Sampling success rate is 91% (200:220).
   c. Complication rate appears similar to PUBS, although data are limited.

3. CVS contraindications
   a. Vaginal bleeding (CVS may exacerbate bleeding)
   b. Cervical infection: gonorrhea, chlamydia, herpes
   c. Vaginal infection
   d. Gestational age less than 10 weeks
   e. Twins
   f. Rh isoimmunization (CVS may exacerbate isoimmunization)
4. CVS limitations
   a. CVS *cannot* check for spina bifida or anencephaly; MSAFP screening is recommended.
   b. CVS does not evaluate for anatomic abnormalities; ultrasound anatomic survey is suggested.

History

1. Initial report for CVS
   a. 4-mm transcervical endoscopic biopsies of chorion were done.
   b. Of 95 patients, all planned elective termination.
   c. Twenty-one patients maintained pregnancy 8 days.
   d. Forty-seven percent of procedures retrieved chorionic villi.
   e. Problems included bleeding and puncture or biopsy of amnion.
2. Subsequent report
   a. Similar endoscopic technique was done with 38 patients.
   b. Nineteen patients were observed 7 to 48 days before termination.
   c. Two patients developed significant infections.
   d. Subsequently there was little further interest in CVS in U.S. or European medicine until the Chinese reported.
3. CVS success in China
   a. A 3-mm transcervical metal cannula aspiration with no optical guidance was done.
   b. Of 100 pregnancies, 99 were successfully sexed with six errors (three male, three female errors).
   c. Four fetal losses occurred.
4. CVS to date
   a. By 1995, 200,000 cases were reported in literature.
   b. Five national trials were completed.
   c. Several series of 10,000 to 20,000 cases were reported from a single center.

Procedure Description

1. Procedural prerequisites
   a. At 10 to 12 weeks gestation: Gestational sac fills uterine cavity (at 12 to 14 weeks, amnion fuses to chorion).
   b. Technically, CVS can be performed earlier but is not because of the increased risk of limb reduction defect (see later section, Complications).
   c. Genetic counseling is provided.
   d. Ultrasound is done for the following:
      (1) Crown rump length (gestational age ± 3 day accuracy)
      (2) Placental site that determines the sampling route

(a) Fundal placenta often requires transabdominal CVS.
(b) Posterior or anterior placentas can often be accessed transcervically.
(c) Lowest complication rates are reported from operators who perform CVS by either approach.
        (3) Placental cord insertion
    2. Transcervical CVS
        a. Bladder filling may facilitate passage of sampling catheter through cervical canal if uterus is anteverted or anteflexed.
        b. Ultrasound guidance: Assistance from technologist is crucial in guiding catheter into placenta.
        c. Cervix and vagina are prepped with betadine. Aseptic technique is observed.
        d. Uterine sound is slowly passed through cervical canal to locate internal os by ultrasound observation.
        e. Uterine sound is removed and replaced by Portex catheter, which should readily advance without force or obstruction.
        f. Catheter is guided into placenta, stylet is removed, and specimen is aspirated. Catheter is removed under suction.
    3. Transabdominal CVS
        a. Fundal placenta or anterior placenta with anteverted uterus
        b. Local anesthesia of skin and uterine serosa for needle insertion site
        c. Ultrasonic guidance of needle into placenta
        d. Several needle passes through placenta during aspiration
        e. From 3% specimens retrieved less than 10 mg tissue, 93% greater than 20 mg (n = 325)
    4. Specimen evaluation
        a. Aspiration syringe contents are inspected; white villi are usually visible.
        b. Petri dish examination is done in cytotechnology laboratory.
        c. Single good aspiration yields 10 to 25 mg of wet tissue.
        d. Some DNA studies require up to 50 mg of wet tissue.
        e. Specimen is reviewed with cytotechnologist to confirm adequacy of specimen before patient leaves.
    5. Specimen processing
        a. Direct method
            (1) Trophoblast cells are analyzed in spontaneous metaphase.
            (2) Karyotype is available in 4 to 12 hours.
            (3) Placental mosaicism and false negatives are about 1% higher than with culture.
        b. Coverslip culture
            (1) Collagenase enzyme releases mesenchymal cells from villi for traditional cell culture in Chang medium.
            (2) Karyotype is available in 10 to 14 days.
    6. CVS registry
        a. All patients are contacted by telephone 2 weeks after procedure.
        b. Karyotype results are explained.
        c. Complications are elicited.

Complications

1. General
   a. Bleeding: 2% is transabdominal, 10% is transcervical.
   b. Cramps: 10% is transabdominal, 2% is transcervical.
   c. Infection: Septic abortion is a remote possibility.
   d. Rupture of the amniotic membrane is a remote possibility.
   e. Rh sensitization: Rh immune globulin prophylaxis is indicated.
   f. Procedure-related pregnancy loss: 1% to 2% above background 2% loss rate.
   g. Limb reduction defect (LRD): See next section.
2. LRDs
   a. Following CVS, LRDs occur at a rate of 1:1000 to 1:3000, "generally increased over background rates."
   b. Background population incidence of LRD is 5 to 6 per 10,000 or approximately 1:2000.
   c. Timing of CVS is related to the rate and severity of LRD; LRD from CVS at 70 days old or older has been limited to fingers or toes.
   d. Proposed LRD mechanism.
      (1) Early gestational age
      (2) Placental trauma and vascular disruption
      (3) Limb ischemia before or after digit formation
      (4) Transient MSAFP elevation post-CVS
   e. LRD model of Quintero et al.
      (1) Before elective abortion, intrauterine fiberscope was placed for observation.
      (2) Placenta was detached or a subchorionic hematoma formed after blunt instrumentation.
      (3) Ecchymotic lesions of scalp, face, head, and thorax were observed.

Patient Counseling

1. Initial counseling session with medical geneticist
   a. Family history
   b. Pregnancy history
   c. Education regarding risks and alternatives
2. Subsequent preprocedural counseling with CVS physician
   a. Indications are reviewed.
   b. Procedural risks are reviewed in detail, including photographs of infants with an LRD.
   c. Alternatives are reviewed.
      (1) Noninvasive screening consisting of ultrasound for nuchal sonolucency (50% sensitivity for trisomy 21) and MSAFP-3 screening (60% sensitivity for trisomy 21)
      (2) Amniocentesis to avoid LRD risk
         (a) Early amnio at 13 to 15 weeks (1% fetal loss rate)
         (b) Traditional amnio at 15 weeks (1:200 fetal loss rate)
3. Postprocedural counseling
   a. Spina bifida MSAFP screening is explained and recommended.

b. Ultrasound anatomic survey at 18 to 20 weeks is recommended with emphasis on digits.
c. Postprocedural instructions are reviewed.

Post-CVS Patient Instructions

1. If patient's blood type is A negative, B negative, O negative, or AB negative, she may need an injection of Rh immune globulin before leaving the unit.
2. Following the CVS procedure, patient may experience spotting or bleeding.
3. Clinician will be concerned if the following occur:
   a. Patient has heavy bleeding like a period.
   b. Patient develops a fever and chills like the flu.
4. If patient has any of these symptoms or any other concerns, she should contact clinician or call her own physician.
5. As a precaution, patient should refrain from sexual intercourse for 3 to 4 days or while bleeding persists. It is also recommended that patient avoid strenuous activity such as jogging, swimming, or tennis during this time.
6. Patient may eat a regular diet unless restricted by her physician.
7. Clinician will call patient as soon as the test results are available.
8. Clinician recommends a follow-up ultrasound and blood test at 17 weeks of pregnancy. The blood test, called AFP, is used to screen for neural tube defects (openings in the baby's brain or spine). CVS does not check for this abnormality. Whereas the AFP test can be scheduled through her physician's office, the clinician suggests the ultrasound be performed at the Reproductive Testing Center to permit an examination targeted on the fetal extremities and face.
9. Patient certifies she has read the above information, understands her instructions, and has received a copy. (Signature copy is kept in patient's chart.)

Postpartum Hemorrhage

John M. O'Brien

21.1 Importance and Perspective

1. Postpartum hemorrhage is a leading cause of maternal death; an obstetric emergency.
   a. Hemorrhage accounts for 16% of all maternal deaths, and postpartum hemorrhage accounts for greater than 50% of these cases.
   b. Significant hemorrhage occurs in 6% of all cesarean deliveries and 3% of all vaginal births. Therefore, this clinical problem likely will be experienced by all practitioners.
2. Recognition and prompt evaluation can reduce the need for transfusion and its associated morbidities.
3. Algorithm for management must be memorized. When a patient is exsanguinating, there is no time to look up treatments or learn steps of proper evaluation.
4. Diagnosis of postpartum hemorrhage is arbitrarily defined as an estimated blood loss of greater than 500 mL. This definition overestimates the population at risk. A more useful estimate may be an estimated blood loss of greater than 1000 mL, which more commonly alters hemodynamics.
5. Hemorrhage may occur either immediately after delivery or be delayed for more than 24 hours. The differential diagnosis differs between immediate and delayed postpartum hemorrhage.

21.2 Etiologies

UTERINE ATONY

1. Uterine atony is the most common etiology for postpartum hemorrhage.
2. Predisposing factors are those factors that either overdistend the uterus, overwork the muscle, or inhibit it from contracting.
   a. Labor arrest or protraction disorder
   b. Prolonged use of higher dose oxytocin
   c. Chorioamnionitis
   d. Multiple gestations
   e. Polyhydramnios
   f. Pharmacologic agents used during labor or delivery

(1) Magnesium sulfate
(2) Betamimetics
(3) General anesthetics
g. Multiple or large uterine leiomyomas
h. Uterine distension by large clot in lower segment or other mass
3. Physical examination notes "boggy" uterus.
4. Other etiologies such as lower genital tract lacerations or retained products of conception must be ruled out, especially if the uterus is firm and continued hemorrhage is noted.

OBSTETRIC TRAUMA

1. Iatrogenic
   a. Forceps or vacuum incorrectly applied or rotation performed
      (1) Vaginal lacerations
      (2) Cervical lacerations
   b. Laceration of pudendal artery at time of pudendal block
   c. Extension of incision during cesarean delivery into uterine vessels
2. Precipitous delivery: may result in cervical or vaginal lacerations
3. Vulvar hematoma
   a. May extend into ischiorectal fossa with potential for extension along the psoas muscle and into retroperitoneum
   b. More common in vaginal deliveries with macrosomic fetus and maternal hematologic or hypertensive disorders

RETAINED PLACENTA

1. Manual extraction attempted before appropriate analgesia, not allowing successful removal, or improper technique used
2. Unrecognized succenturiate lobe or bilobed placenta
3. Abnormal placentation with difficulty creating a plane for removal at time of manual extraction
4. May be cause for either immediate or delayed hemorrhage

PLACENTATION ABNORMALITIES—ACCRETA, INCRETA, OR PERCRETA

1. Do not allow separation of placenta from uterus because of ingrowth of placenta to varying degrees into or through myometrium
2. Most common in patients with placenta previa and a history of cesarean delivery
3. May be recognized antepartum by elevated alpha-fetoprotein or ultrasonography

UTERINE RUPTURE

1. Almost exclusively limited to women with a history of a previous uterine incision (e.g., cesarean delivery, hysterotomy, or myomectomy)
2. Fetal bradycardia most common clinical sign
3. Maternal symptom of persistent rather than intermittent abdominal pain
4. Uterine exploration after successful vaginal birth after cesarean section (VBAC) with postpartum hemorrhage

UTERINE INVERSION
1. Abnormalities in vital signs may be out of proportion to blood loss.
2. Physical examination demonstrates "mass" in vagina or at introitus.

MATERNAL COAGULATION DEFECT OR MEDICAL DISORDERS
1. Uterine bleeding hemostasis is primarily the result of uterine contractions; therefore, it is rarely the result of coagulation defect.
2. Vaginal or vulvar hematoma or excessive bleeding at cesarean delivery may be the result of factor deficiency such as von Willebrand's disease.
3. Other medical conditions such as Marfan's syndrome or Ehlers-Danlos syndrome may not allow sufficient vasoconstriction within the uterus or may result in hemorrhage at other sites involving major vessels because of a defect in connective tissue synthesis.

SUBINVOLUTION OF THE PLACENTAL SITE
1. Cause for delayed postpartum hemorrhage, which is defined as excessive bleeding occurring greater than 24 hours after delivery
2. May be associated with abnormal placental function such as growth restriction or preeclampsia

21.3 Treatments

GENERAL PRINCIPLES
1. Get help.
   a. Anesthesia, nursing, and other physicians experienced in treatment protocols and surgical procedures should be called if they become necessary.
   b. Blood bank should be contacted for type and cross early in evaluation or O negative blood called for if emergency transfusion is necessary.
2. Intravenous (IV) access must be obtained: Two large-bore IV lines are started.
3. Foley catheter is placed to minimize potential trauma to the lower urinary tract and urine output is followed.

MANIPULATIONS
1. Uterine massage for atony
2. Bimanual compression of uterine arteries for temporary control of blood loss
3. Uterine packing for uncontrolled atony
   a. Uterine packing should be considered only after failed pharmacologic therapies.
   b. Patient should desire future fertility or be hemodynamically unstable.
   c. Sterile gauze is packed tightly into the uterus; must be removed within 24 hours of placement.
   d. Prophylactic antibiotics should be considered because of the presence of the internal foreign body.
   e. Packing soaked in thrombin may enhance clot formation.

PHARMACOLOGIC AND MEDICAL THERAPIES

1. Agents for uterine atony
   a. Oxytocin, up to 40 U/L
      (1) Too rapid IV infusion, which can lead to hypotension, is to be avoided
   b. Ergot alkaloids (Methergine), 0.2 mg, given through intramuscular (IM) injection
      (1) Relatively contraindicated in patients with hypertensive disorders
   c. Prostaglandin F2-alpha (Carboprost; Hemabate), 250 µg IM
      (1) Relatively contraindicated in asthmatics, hypertensives, and women with history of cardiac dysfunction
      (2) Dose repeated at 15-minute to 20-minute intervals in refractory cases, but adverse reactions have been reported in patients receiving numerous doses
   d. Dinoprostone (Prostin E2), suppository (vaginal or rectal), 20 mg
      (1) Avoid if patient is hypotensive. Fever is common.
      (2) May repeat every 2 hours.
   e. Misoprostol (Cytotec, PGE1), 800 to 1000 µg rectally
2. Blood products and volume expansion
   a. IV crystalloid
      (1) Ringer's lactate or normal saline at a ratio of 2:1 to 3:1 for each mL of estimated blood loss
   b. Packed red blood cells
      (1) Transfusion if hemodynamically unstable, uncontrolled bleeding with estimated blood loss of 2000 mL, or bleeding controlled and patient symptomatic
   c. Fresh frozen plasma
      (1) Patient should be transfused if consumptive coagulopathy is present or if dilutional coagulopathy is detected.
   d. Calcium gluconate
      (1) Not compatible in IV solution with magnesium sulfate
      (2) Consider if greater than 5 U packed red cells transfused
   e. Platelets
      (1) Transfuse if profound dilutional anemia is present or persistent bleeding occurs with thrombocytopenia
   f. Cryoprecipitate or specific factor replacement
      (1) Cryoprecipitate is necessary for treatment of von Willebrand's disease.
      (2) Other factors may be indicated on diagnosis of preexisting hematologic disorder.
   g. Cell savers
      (1) Have been used in patients with massive blood loss once the risk of collection and transfusion of amniotic fluid is eliminated
   h. For patients who are identified as being at significant risk for obstetric hemorrhage
      (1) Self-donation and directed donation of blood products should be discussed and arranged if applicable.

SURGICAL

1. For retained placenta or subinvolution of placental site
   a. Perform sharp or suction curettage.
   b. Beware of uterine perforation of the gravid uterus.
   c. Consider use of ultrasound for guidance during the procedure.
2. For uterine atony
   a. Bilateral uterine artery ligation: O'Leary stitch
   b. Stepwise devascularization of the uterus with ligation of the vaginal branches of the uterine artery and subsequent ligation of the utero-ovarian pedicles
   c. Bilateral internal iliac artery ligation
      (1) It reduces pulse pressure by 85% to the uterine vasculature but may not be effective in stopping hemorrhage in up to 50% of cases because of extensive pelvic collateral circulation.
      (2) Ligation of posterior branch and superior gluteal artery, which can lead to necrosis of gluteus maximus, is to be avoided.
      (3) Ligation of external iliac by assessing pedal or femoral pulses is to be avoided. Inappropriate ligation may result in loss of lower extremity.
      (4) Ligation is not appropriate if the physician is inexperienced with procedure.
   d. B-Lynch suture
   e. Hysterectomy
      (1) Hysterectomy may be considered earlier in the evaluation of postpartum hemorrhage, depending on family planning desires and amount of active blood loss.
      (2) Most common indications for cesarean hysterectomy are as follows:
         (a) Uterine atony: 43%
         (b) Abnormal placentation: 30%
         (c) Uterine rupture: 13%
         (d) Extension of uterine incision: 12%
         (e) Fibroid uterus: 4%
      (3) Major morbidity is associated ureteral tract injury.
         (a) Obstructed ureter presents as flank pain 2 to 3 days postoperatively.
         (b) Consider intraoperative stenting or other evaluation of ureteral patency.
   f. Abdominal packing
      (1) Abdominal packing may be necessary to perform abdominal mushroom pack with life-threatening bleeding during laparotomy.
      (2) Gauze pads are stuffed inside sterile Mayo stand (plastic bag), which is placed in the abdomen and brought out through the vagina with the end tied to a liter of saline draped off the end of the bed for weight.

3. For abnormal placentation
   a. Accreta
      (1) Oversewing of placental bed (conservative, i.e., retain uterus), or
      (2) Hysterectomy if bleeding persists
   b. Increta
      (1) Hysterectomy, or
      (2) Hysterotomy with placenta left in situ if strong desire for future fertility and placental bleeding not active
      (3) Adjuvant postoperative methotrexate
   c. Percreta (Assistance from an experienced pelvic surgeon or gynecologic oncologist is needed.)
      (1) Hysterectomy with bladder, ureter, or bowel repair, if necessary
      (2) Option of hysterotomy with placenta left in situ if no active bleeding
      (3) Postoperative adjuvant methotrexate
4. For uterine rupture
   a. Repair of uterine defect is primarily with trimming back of incision edges for improved healing.
   b. Hysterectomy may also be required if extensive uterine damage occurs.
5. For uterine inversion
   a. Uterine relaxation is initiated with halogenated anesthetic, IV nitroglycerin, or magnesium sulfate.
   b. Pressure is gently applied circumfrentially to the edge of fundus where the inversion is present.
      (1) Fundus is kneaded back into normal position.
   c. Other maneuvers to replace fundus include the following:
      (1) Hydrostatic pressure: Vagina is filled with saline under pressure, while egress of fluid from the introitus is blocked.
      (2) Laparotomy:
         (a) Traction is placed on the round ligaments from above.
         (b) A figure-eight suture is placed in the fundus and traction is applied.
         (c) Hysterectomy for intractable inversion is performed.
6. For vulvar hematoma
   a. Foley catheter is placed to allow for bladder drainage.
   b. This is followed with serial hematocrit determinations every 6 hours.
   c. Intervention for intractable bleeding or evidence of retroperitoneal extension is considered.
      (1) Angiographic embolization is the treatment of choice.
      (2) Surgical exploration and vulvar packing may allow for identification of bleeding vessel.
   d. Observe closely for infected hematoma, which may require drainage and IV antibiotics.
      (1) Drainage procedure consists of stab incision in vagina and "milking" hematoma.
      (2) Word catheter may be desired if purulent drainage is persistent.

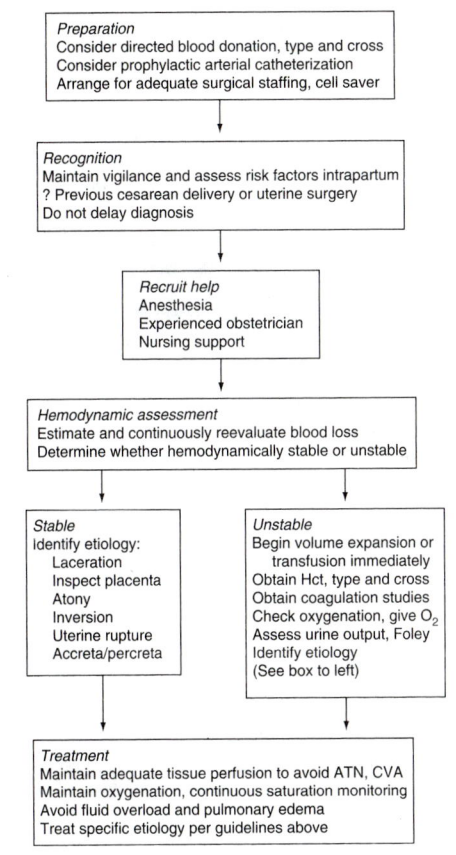

```
Preparation
Consider directed blood donation, type and cross
Consider prophylactic arterial catheterization
Arrange for adequate surgical staffing, cell saver
        ↓
Recognition
Maintain vigilance and assess risk factors intrapartum
? Previous cesarean delivery or uterine surgery
Do not delay diagnosis
        ↓
Recruit help
Anesthesia
Experienced obstetrician
Nursing support
        ↓
Hemodynamic assessment
Estimate and continuously reevaluate blood loss
Determine whether hemodynamically stable or unstable
        ↓                              ↓
Stable                            Unstable
Identify etiology:                Begin volume expansion or
  Laceration                        transfusion immediately
  Inspect placenta                Obtain Hct, type and cross
  Atony                           Obtain coagulation studies
  Inversion                       Check oxygenation, give O₂
  Uterine rupture                 Assess urine output, Foley
  Accreta/percreta                Identify etiology
                                  (See box to left)
        ↓                              ↓
Treatment
Maintain adequate tissue perfusion to avoid ATN, CVA
Maintain oxygenation, continuous saturation monitoring
Avoid fluid overload and pulmonary edema
Treat specific etiology per guidelines above
```

Figure 21-1 Algorithm for management of postpartum hemorrhage. *ATN*, Acute tubular necrosis; *CVA*, cerebral vascular accident; *Hct*, hematocrit.

CATHETERIZATION AND EMBOLIZATION

1. For refractory postoperative hemorrhage
   a. Excellent for bleeding from vessels of the pelvic floor
   b. May not be possible if prior internal iliac artery ligation has been performed
2. Performed under fluoroscopic guidance by interventional radiologist
3. Gelfoam or glue commonly used
4. For patients with anticipated obstetric hemorrhage, such as from a case of placenta percreta diagnosed antepartum
   a. Prophylactic catheterization before delivery may minimize blood loss because embolization can be performed intraoperatively.

21.4 Algorithm for Management

Figure 21-1 shows management for postpartum hemorrhage.

SUGGESTED READINGS

Bobrowski RA, Jones TB: A thrombogenic uterine pack for postpartum hemorrhage, *Obstet Gynecol* 85:836-837, 1995.

Clark SL: Emergency hysterectomy for obstetrical hemorrhage, *Obstet Gynecol* 64:376-380, 1984.

Combs CA, Murphy EL, Laros RK: Factors associated with postpartum hemorrhage with vaginal birth, *Obstet Gynecol* 77:69-76, 1991.

Combs CA, Murphy EL, Laros RK: Factors associated with hemorrhage in cesarean deliveries, *Obstet Gynecol* 77:77-82, 1991.

Gilstrap LC, Ramin SM: Postpartum hemorrhage, *Clin Obstet Gynecol* 37:824-830, 1994.

Hallak M: Transvaginal pack for life threatening pelvic hemorrhage secondary to placenta accreta, *Obstet Gynecol* 78:938-940, 1991.

Herbert W, Zelop C: ACOG Practice Bulletin, no. 76, *Postpartum hemorrhage*, Washington, DC, 2006, ACOG.

Khong TY, Khong TK: Delayed postpartum hemorrhage: a morphological study of causes and their relation to other pregnancy disorders, *Obstet Gynecol* 82:17-22, 1993.

Maier RC: Control of postpartum hemorrhage with uterine packing, *Am J Obstet Gynecol* 169:317-323, 1993.

Mitty HA: Obstetric hemorrhage: prophylactic and emergency arterial catheterization and embolotherapy, *Radiology* 188:183-187, 1993.

Physiology in Pregnancy

Arundathi G. Prasad

The biochemical, physiologic, and anatomic adaptations that occur during the 9 months of pregnancy are profound. Many of these changes begin soon after fertilization and continue throughout gestation. An equally astounding fact is that a pregnant woman returns almost completely to her prepregnancy state following delivery and lactation.

Emotional changes occur early in pregnancy. Starting with the first trimester, the patient experiences easy fatigability and has a desire to spend much of her time sleeping. During the second trimester, the patient frequently experiences a period of euphoria and extreme well-being. Last, in the third trimester, there are again some elements of depression and chronic fatigue, probably a result of the increased weight gain.

22.1 Maternal Nutrition

In the United States the average body mass index (BMI) among women is increasing. BMI is calculated by dividing weight (kg) by height (m^2), using the prepregnancy weight.

The accumulation of body fluid during pregnancy is physiologic; expansion of maternal blood volume may account for 10% of the weight gain.

NUTRITION

1. Adequate nutrition is paramount for optimal fetal growth.
2. Serum markers to measure long-term and short-term protein nutrition in nonpregnant individuals are not valid during pregnancy because of an increased maternal plasma volume.
   a. Prealbumin, albumin, retinol-binding protein.
   b. Decreased serum albumin may also reflect on maternal circulating alpha-fetoprotein.
3. The recommended dietary allowance suggests an additional caloric intake of 300 kcal/day during pregnancy.
4. Increases in caloric intake should be encouraged with teenagers and in women with increased physical activity.

MATERNAL WEIGHT GAIN

1. The relationship between weight gain during pregnancy and birth weight outcome is affected by the prepregnancy weight-for-height status.

a. Patient self-reported weight is reliable within a standard deviation of about 1.5 kg as opposed to actual measurements.
b. An additional 10 lb of maternal weight gain is recommended for multiple gestations.
c. With increased weight gain over what is recommended (24 to 35 lb) during pregnancy, the following may occur:
    (1) Increased incidence of high birth weight (HBW). HBW is defined as greater than 4500 g.
    (2) Decreased incidence of growth restriction. Low birth weight (LBW) is defined as less than 2500 g.
2. HBW infants are 66%, or three times, more likely to die within the first 28 days of life than are normal–birth weight infants.
3. It is recommended that underweight women (BMI <19.8 kg/m^2) gain between 28 and 40 lb.
4. Average weight women (BMI is 19.8 to 26 kg/m^2) should gain between 25 and 35 lb.
5. Overweight women (BMI >26 to 29 kg/m^2) should gain between 15 and 25 lb.
6. For very overweight women (BMI >29 kg/m^2), weight-gain guidelines are set at 15 lb, which accounts for the weight of the fetus, placenta, and amniotic fluid. A gestational weight gain of more than 15 lb in this group is associated with increased perinatal morbidity.
7. The best reproductive outcomes are associated with a weight gain of approximately 20 lb in the last half of pregnancy. A weekly mean rate of gain of 1.0 lb/week from the 20th week of gestation to delivery is recommended.

22.2 Maternal Skin Changes

HAIR AND NAILS

1. The normal ratio of actively growing hair (anagen phase) to resting (telogen) hairs is approximately 9 to 1.
    a. The increased estrogen and progesterone levels during pregnancy stimulate a greater percentage of hairs to enter the anagen phase.
    b. If vellus hairs are also stimulated to become terminal hair, the patient will become aware of increased facial hair and sometimes generalized hirsutism.
    c. After delivery, hair-cycle ratios are reversed and many scalp hairs fall out (telogen effluvium).
    d. The patient should be reassured that this condition is temporary and that hair cycles will return to normal.
    e. Iron and thyroid deficiency should also be considered if scalp hair loss continues for more than a few months.
2. The nails may become more brittle and show signs of dystrophy, including transverse and longitudinal ridging and onycholysis (elevation of the distal nail plate from the nail bed). Changes lasting beyond a few months postpartum should prompt an investigation for thyroid disease and iron deficiency.

SKIN

1. Pruritus itching is the most common skin complaint during pregnancy.
   a. It often originates in the abdominal area and occasionally becomes generalized.
   b. Pruritus without skin lesions is usually attributed to cholestasis of pregnancy.
   c. During pregnancy, the skin has an increased sensitivity, and pruritus may be easily caused by external factors such as body soap, laundry detergent, and radiation.
   d. Relief is obtained by eliminating any irritant and by using mild glycerine cleansing bars, bland lotions with aloe vera, and oils.
2. Vascular skin changes are demonstrated by vessel distension, proliferation, and instability during pregnancy.
   a. Palmer erythema, "spider angiomas" (telangiectasias with a central punctum), and a mottled venous pattern to the skin, particularly on exposure to cold, occur frequently and are usually reversible.
   b. Marginal gingivitis, a condition caused by hyperemia and edema of the gums, occurs in many pregnant women and should be managed by good oral hygiene.
3. Striae (stretch marks) are linear, atrophic, light-red to violaceous lesions and commonly develop over the abdomen, breast, and inguinal areas. Postpartum, the color of the striae will fade; however, they will remain permanently.
4. Melasma is a bilaterally symmetric, lacelike, facial hyperpigmentation often known as chloasma.
   a. Chloasma has a predilection for the malar area, temples, forehead, and the neck region.
   b. Progesterone, estrogen, and melanocyte-stimulating hormone (MSH) play a part in the pigment deposition.
   c. The axillae, pubic skin, and areola show varying degrees of slowly progressing hyperpigmentation.
   d. The linea alba when pigmented is termed the linea nigra.

22.3 Maternal Blood Volume

HEMATOCRIT

1. The hematocrit at the end of pregnancy is usually within the normal range (38% to 45%) in well-nourished women.
2. However, a value less than 34% is highly suspect for true anemia.
3. Maternal red cell mass expansion occurs mostly during the last 8 to 10 weeks of pregnancy.
4. Diluational anemia (first 24 weeks) during pregnancy arises from the increased maternal plasma volume, which occurs before the rise in total erythrocyte mass.
5. Postpartum, the hematocrit will rise approximately 3% to 5% as a result of physiologic diuresis.
6. Changes in hemoglobin and hematocrit values are induced by altitude and smoking.

a. In high-altitude areas (>3300 ft), there is a greater rise in erythrocyte volume to increase oxygen transport.
b. Because of the lower oxygen partial pressure in high-altitude areas, women will have a reduced oxygen saturation with a compensatory increase in red blood cell production.
c. Similarly, this is also seen with smokers; however, this is a result of the increased carboxyhemoglobin, a poor carrier of oxygen.
7. A hemoglobin less than 11 g/100 mL or a hematocrit less than 33% during pregnancy implies anemia.

PLASMA VOLUME

1. There is approximately a 50% increase in maternal plasma volume (equivalent to 2600 mL) over nonpregnant women, and it plateaus at about 30 to 34 weeks.
2. Larger increases are associated with multiple pregnancies and larger fetuses.
3. In tropical climates there is an increase in maternal plasma volume over climates that are cold. This is because of the greater loss in body heat and fluid in tropical climates.

UTERINE BLOOD FLOW

1. As the result of the increase in maternal cardiac output there is also a substantial increase in uterine blood flow.
2. The rate of uterine blood flow is approximately 50 mL/min in early pregnancy, increasing to 500 mL/min at term.
3. The main blood supply to the uterus (approximately 80%) originates from the uterine arteries.
4. Therefore, the progressive increase in uterine arterial blood flow measured by pulsed Doppler ultrasonography is approximately a fourfold increase in flow rate as compared with nonpregnant values.
5. The cardiac output that is distributed to the uterine vessels is approximately 3.5% in early pregnancy and 12% near term.
6. Also, placental perfusion continues to rise until term, when it accounts for 80% to 90% of the total uterine blood flow, which accommodates the exponential growth of the fetus.

22.4 Maternal Vascular Changes

ARTERIAL CIRCULATION

1. The integrity of the maternal vascular arterial circulation is proposed as the primary determinant of body fluid volume regulation.
2. Peripheral arterial vasodilation with relative underfilling of the arterial circulation occurs in early gestation.
    a. This causes a decrease in the systolic and diastolic blood pressures, increased cardiac output secondary to afterload reduction, nonosmotic stimulation of thirst and vasopressin release, stimulation of the renin–angiotensin–aldosterone axis, and renal sodium and water retention.
    b. This results in extracellular fluid and plasma volume expansion.

RENAL BLOOD FLOW

1. In early pregnancy, there is an increase in renal blood flow and glomerular filtration rate of 30% to 50%, secondary to arterial vasodilation, the latter occurring before maternal plasma volume expansion.
2. Also, during pregnancy the sodium-retaining effect of aldosterone is not seen, and similarly in the vascular resistance to angiotensin.
3. Approximately 85% of the total blood volume resides in the venous circulation, because only 15% of the total blood volume circulates in the arterial system.
4. In early pregnancy renal vasodilation with arterial underfilling leads to sodium and water retention.
5. Hence the observed increased renal and glomerular filtration rates during pregnancy of 30% to 50%, respectively.
6. The maternal increase in progesterone may account for the aldosterone escape in pregnancy, because progesterone is known to counteract the tubular sodium transport effects of aldosterone.

22.5 Fetal and Placental Physiology

PLACENTA

1. The placenta regulates maternal–fetal interactions for physiologic exchange and acts as a selective barrier between mother and fetus.
2. It also participates in the immunity of the fetus by actively transporting immunoglobulin G (IgG) antibodies for fetal and neonatal use.
3. The fetus obtains maternal IgG for its in utero immunologic protection, and before 22 weeks gestation the IgG is transported via simple diffusion.
4. After 22 weeks gestation, IgG is transported across the placental membranes by pinocytosis.

FETUS

1. The fetus directs about 50% of its cardiac output through the umbilical arteries.
2. This translates to approximately 500 to 600 mL/min.
3. Therefore, the fetal blood pressure and cardiac output are obvious determinants of umbilical artery flow.
4. Hence, fetal heart failure, arrhythmias, and cord compression could adversely affect umbilical artery blood flow.
5. The fetus contributes to the amniotic fluid volume by urinating approximately 800 mL/day or 5 mL/hour.
6. Also, some of the amniotic fluid is reabsorbed by fetal swallowing and the mechanism of in utero breathing.
7. There is always additional fluid exchange at the chorionic plate between mother and fetus.
8. The fetal skin (keratinized at 24 weeks gestation), chorion–amnion, and umbilical cord contribute little to the amniotic fluid exchange after 24 weeks.

PHYSIOLOGIC FUNCTIONS OF THE PLACENTA

1. Respiratory: exchange of oxygen and carbon dioxide; acts as a lung
2. Nutrition: acts as the gastrointestinal tract with transfer of sugars, amino acids, protein, and lipids
3. Excretion: acts as a kidney in disposing of waste (bilirubin)
4. Protective: acts like the skin by moderating heat transfer; protects against bacterial invasion
5. Endocrine function: produces human chorionic gonadotropin (HCG), luteinizing releasing factor, thyrotropin releasing factor, progesterone, cortisol, estriol, and human placental lactogen (HPL)

PLACENTAL TRANSPORT

Transport of H_2O

1. Transfer of water takes place by what is called "bulk flow."
2. This refers to a process by which small transient changes in hydrostatic and osmotic pressure across the placental membrane result in movement of water.
3. Because water is extremely responsive to such changes, these gradients are transient and difficult to measure.
4. There is a large movement of water in both directions.
5. The net transfer is in favor of the fetus, with an accumulation of water of approximately 0.14 mL/min or 20 mL/day.
6. This large movement of fluid exchange also probably produces a substantial amount of other solutes by "solvent drag."

Transport of Electrolytes

1. The placental membrane is permeable to sodium, potassium, and chloride.
2. So far, no sodium or potassium pump has been discovered in the placental membrane.
3. Transport of these ions occurs by simple diffusion through water-filled "pores" lying between cells.
4. Concentrations of these electrolytes are the same in the fetus as in the mother, and the permeability of the membrane to these electrolytes increases by seventyfold from as early as 9 weeks to 35 weeks, then drops off slightly near term.
5. Calcium, phosphate, iodine, and probably magnesium, as well as many of the trace elements and minerals, are present in higher concentrations in the fetus than in the mother and are transported by active transport mechanisms across the placental membrane.
6. Iron also is present in higher concentrations in the fetus than in the mother and is transported by active transport mechanisms across the placental membrane.
7. Receptors for iron have been found on the placental membrane and its active transport system increases in efficiency as gestation progresses.

Vitamins

1. Water-soluble vitamins such as thiamine (B_1), pyridoxine (B_6), and B_{12}, as well as vitamin C (ascorbic acid) and folic acid, all

have higher concentrations in the fetus and require active transport systems.
2. The concentrations of fat-soluble vitamins (A, D, E, K) are the same or slightly lower in the fetus and these probably traverse the placenta by passive diffusion.

Carbohydrates

1. Glucose is the major metabolic fuel of the fetus and fetal levels are approximately 15% lower in the fetus as compared with the mother's.
2. It is estimated that about two thirds of the glucose uptake is used for placental metabolism, with only the remaining third being transferred for fetal use.
3. Transfer of glucose to the fetus occurs by facilitated diffusion, with glucose being transferred more rapidly than fructose or other sugars of similar molecular weight, which cross by simple diffusion.
4. This transport is not energy dependent but is carrier mediated by a protein carrier in the syncitiotrophoblastic cell membrane.
5. This transport system is very much stereospecific because only d-glucose is facilitated, whereas l-glucose is not.
6. Glycogen storage takes place in the liver, skeletal muscle, and placenta.
7. Near term, the glycogen storage shifts quantitatively from the placenta to the liver.
8. Pyruvate and lactate also cross the placenta by simple diffusion.

Free Fatty Acids

1. Free fatty acids (FFA) are bound to albumin, making them water soluble.
2. FFA traverse the placenta by simple diffusion.
3. FFA are used not for energy but for fetal complex lipid synthesis.
4. Both saturated and unsaturated FFA cross the placenta equally as well, but the rate of transfer is inversely proportional to the fatty acid chain length.
5. As the transplacental supply of FFA falls short of fetal requirements for fat deposition in the third trimester, some of the fetal FFA are probably made de novo by the fetus.

Complex Lipids

1. Complex lipids (triglycerides, cholesterol, and phospholipids) are transported in the mother as lipoproteins and are characterized as low density or high density.
2. Cholesterol, as well as many of these more complex lipids, is probably used by the placenta for its own needs.
3. In addition, transport of these large molecules, if it occurs at all, is probably very small.
4. For these reasons, the fetus synthesizes much of its lipids de novo from precursors.
5. There is a suggestion that the placenta may break down complex lipids for fetal use, but this is unproven.

Amino Acids

1. Amino acids have a fourfold higher concentration in the fetus as compared with the mother.
2. This transport is effected by an active transport mechanism.
3. This mechanism is stereospecific, with the naturally occurring l-forms or isomers crossing more rapidly than the d-isomers.
4. The receptor site, however, is nonspecific, with all of the amino acids competing for the same sites on an equal basis.
5. The fetus synthesizes almost all of its proteins from those amino acids that cross the placenta.
6. In addition, it has been found that the fetus may use these amino acids as a metabolic fuel; some studies show the fetus deriving as much as 25% of its energy requirements from their degradation.

Proteins

1. Most of the fetal protein requirements come from the fetal synthesis of proteins from amino acids that are actively transported across the placenta.
2. Polypeptides and larger proteins cross the placental membrane slowly, if at all.
3. They cross generally by one of two mechanisms:
   a. Simple diffusion: more important earlier in gestation
   b. Pinocytosis: more important later in gestation
4. Plasma proteins, notably albumin, and the beta-globulins such as transferrin and fibrinogen, cross in very small quantities by simple diffusion and the amounts transferred are not significant.
5. Protein hormones such as thyroid-stimulating hormone (TSH), adrenocorticotropic hormone (ACTH), T_4, and T_3 cross the placenta little if at all.
6. Insulin diffuses only in micro amounts, so the fetus must manufacture almost all of its own insulin.
7. The fetus does not manufacture IgG in any appreciable quantities and, indeed, does not attain this ability until well into the newborn period.
   a. The fetus obtains its IgG from the mother.
   b. This sustains the fetus into the newborn period and protects it in utero.
   c. Before 22 weeks, this IgG transfer occurs via simple diffusion.
   d. After 22 weeks, IgG of maternal origin traverses the placental membrane by pinocytosis, an energy-requiring mechanism of "cell drinking."
   e. This transfer is specific only for antibodies of the IgG class. Receptors for the Fc portion of the IgG molecule have been located on the syncitiotrophoblastic cell membrane.
   f. Unfortunately, this transfer is not specific among the IgG antibodies types, and IgG antibodies that may be harmful to the fetus are transferred with the same efficiency as those that are not harmful.
   g. The transfer of harmful IgG antibodies occurs in Rh disease, maternal immune thrombocytopenia (ITP), and myasthenia gravis.

h. In the latter two diseases, the antibodies cross the placenta and induce the same disease in the fetus.

Nucleic Acids

Nucleic acids are synthesized from maternal precursors that cross the placenta by simple diffusion: adenosine triphosphate, adenosine diphosphate, adenosine monophosphate, and purine and pyrimidine bases.

Bilirubin

1. Unconjugated bilirubin rapidly traverses the placenta by simple diffusion; conjugated bilirubin does not.
2. As a result of the ductus venosus through which vena caval and umbilical blood bypass the liver, as well as the immaturity of the liver enzymes, the bilirubin is kept predominantly in the unconjugated form favorable for placental transfer.
3. This explains the absence of jaundice in some neonates who have suffered hemolytic disease in utero.

Nitrogenous Compounds

1. Nitrogenous waste products cross the placenta by simple diffusion and include creatinine, blood urea nitrogen (BUN), and uric acid.
2. If the maternal levels of any of these substances are high, as occurs in maternal renal failure, this will be reflected in the fetus and in the fetal urine.
3. This is important to keep in mind because amniotic fluid creatinine levels (derived from the fetal urine) are often used in lung maturity studies.

Temperature

The placenta functions as a heat exchange unit, with the temperature of the fetus usually 1° C higher than the mother.

22.6 Maternal Respiratory System

Antepartum pulmonary changes begin in the 4th week of gestation. The earliest changes to elicit symptoms are related to mucosal capillary engorgement, resulting in swelling and congestion of the nostrils and throat. The diaphragm becomes elevated because of the enlarging uterus. The subcostal angle is increased from 68 degrees to 103 degrees, causing an increase of approximately 2 cm in the transthoracic diameter. Also, the respiratory rate is usually unchanged.

The increased respiratory effort and concomitant reduction of PCO_2 is caused in large part by progesterone by a central direct stimulatory effect on the respiratory center.

ANATOMIC CHANGES

1. There is a 4-cm rise from the diaphragm.
2. Subcostal angle widens as the transverse thoracic diameter increases by 2 cm.

CHANGES IN PULMONARY FUNCTION

1. Physiologic increase occurs in (not pregnant/pregnant = percentage change) the following:
   a. Tidal volume (487 mL/678 mL = +39% change).
      (1) The tidal volume (TV) lowers PCO_2, causing a mild respiratory alkalosis and a decreased HCO_3.
      (2) Volume increases by about 200 mL.
      (3) This is the volume of air breathed in and out during normal respiration.
   b. Minute O_2 uptake (201/266 = +32% change).
   c. Minute ventilation (7270 mL/10,340 mL = +42%).
   d. Increased airway conductance is caused by a decrease in bronchomotor tone secondary to a progesterone effect.
   e. Inspiratory capacity appears to increase progressively throughout pregnancy, reaching a matrix of approximately 300 mL above nonpregnant levels at term.
2. Physiologic decrease occurs in (not pregnant/pregnant = percentage change) the following:
   a. Functional residual capacity.
   b. Residual volume (965 mL/770 mL = −20% change); decreases by some 300 mL (volume of air remaining in the lung spaces after normal expiration).
   c. Decrease in total pulmonary resistance.
   d. A decrease in the difference between the arterial–venous oxygen content.
   e. Expiratory reserve volume decreases by approximately 200 mL. This is the maximum air volume exhaled after normal resting respiration.
   f. Pulmonary diffusion capacity decreases by approximately 4 mL/min/mm H_2O.
3. No physiologic pulmonary changes occur in the following:
   a. Maximum breathing capacity (102/97 = −5%).
   b. No change in forced vital capacity.
   c. Vital capacity (3260 mL/3310 = +1%).
      (1) May be increased but earlier reports suggest no change.
      (2) This is the maximum total volume of air that can be breathed out after maximal forced inspiration.
   d. No change in lung compliance.
   e. No significant change in the respiratory rate (15/16).
   f. Forced expiratory volume appears to be unaffected.
   g. Peak expiratory flow rate appears not to be affected.
4. Changes in air requirements:
   a. Maternal adaptations to pregnancy in cardiac, renal, and respiratory performance account for approximately two thirds of the extra oxygen need during pregnancy.
   b. The fetus also has an oxygen demand, but its needs are relatively modest because it does not need to regulate its own temperature.
   c. It may be calculated that the extra metabolic activity of pregnancy requires oxygen in the amount of 30 to 40 mL/min or 15% above nonpregnant needs.

d. The developing fetus must off-load its CO_2 into the mother.
   (1) The mother could reduce her basal PCO_2 status.
   (2) The mother "overbreathes" to wash out her PCO_2: This leads to alkalosis, but she compensates by excreting more bicarbonate into the renal system, excreting with it some obligatory sodium.
   (3) Unfortunately, sodium is a major determinant of plasma osmolality, so this decreases.
   (4) Lowering osmolality normally causes a diuresis so that the mother's hypothalamic osmoreceptor centers must be reset to accept and guard this lower value.
   (5) Thus the primary need to lower PCO_2 initiates a series of events that affect the respiratory and renal systems, as well as significantly altering plasma biochemistry.
      (a) Carbon dioxide pressure (PCO_2)
         (i) This is dramatically decreased from the nonpregnant range of 35 to 40 mm Hg to 28 to 30 mm Hg during pregnancy.
         (ii) This pregnancy reduction is almost certainly an effect of progesterone.
      (b) Oxygen pressure (PO_2)
         (i) As would be anticipated from the decrease in PCO_2, there is an increase in PO_2 during gestation.
         (ii) This increase is small, from 85 mm Hg to approximately 92 mm Hg.
      (c) pH
         (i) Maternal arterial pH is unaltered from the normal average of 7.4.
         (ii) The implication is that the decrease in PCO_2, which leads to respiratory alkalosis, is matched by a decrease in the bicarbonate.

22.7 Maternal Urinary System

KIDNEY

1. The mean kidney length was found to increase in size by approximately 1 to 1.5 cm, and the enlargement probably reflects the increase in renal blood flow and renal vascular volume, with perhaps a degree of hypertrophy.
2. Earliest physiologic renal change occurs with dilation of the renal pelvis and ureters (physiologic hydroureter of pregnancy).
   a. These become evident in the first trimester and persist to term and until approximately 6 weeks postpartum.
   b. The proposed mechanisms are as follows:
      (1) External compression of the ureters from the uterus with fetus, iliac arteries, and ovarian veins.
      (2) Hormonal changes are caused by the increases in the levels of progesterone, gonadotropins, and estrogens.

(3) Ureteral hypertrophy is caused by hyperplasia of the connective tissue, hypertrophy of the longitudinal smooth muscles (Waldeyer's sheath), and edema.
c. The hydroureter is more prominent on the right.
d. The maternal renal calyces and ureters dilate and may contain 40 to 100 mL of urine in total.
e. Contrary to popular belief, the ureteral muscular tone is not reduced and may indeed be slightly increased during pregnancy, secondary to the compression and obstruction of the ureter at the pelvic inlet by the pregnant dextrorotated uterus.
f. The dextrorotation is caused by the sigmoid colon.

BLADDER

1. Because of the atonic effects of pregnancy on smooth muscle, the tone of the bladder is progressively decreased and its capacity increased, retaining double its normal volume by term.
2. The trigone area undergoes moderate hyperplasia and muscular hypertrophy, giving a concave appearance to the base of the bladder.
3. As the uterus enlarges hyperemia of the pelvic organs occurs, and the bladder is displaced anteriorly and superiorly, which makes cystoscopy, if necessary, difficult.
4. Near term, the bladder mucosa becomes more edematous and easily traumatized and therefore more susceptible to bacterial infection.
5. Because of the fetal presenting part toward the end of pregnancy, an impairment of the emptying of the venous blood and lymph flow from the base of the bladder often causes edema and more susceptibility for trauma and infection.
6. Urinary tract infections are therefore more common in pregnancy because bacteria can then be transmitted to the ureters via vesicoureteral reflux.
7. The increase in urinary volume in the ureteropelvic system enhances the growth of organisms and hence the observed increase in pyelonephritis in pregnancy.
8. In addition, the maternal bladder vessels tend to increase in size and become tortuous.

RENAL PHYSIOLOGY

1. Renal blood flow increases markedly during pregnancy, with midpregnancy increments attaining 60% to 80% followed by a significant fall in the third trimester from 480 to 890 mL/min.
2. The glomerular filtration rate (GFR) is increased by approximately 50% throughout pregnancy.
   a. This is increased from the nonpregnant state average of 97 mL/min to 128 mL/min by the 10th week of gestation; also, there may be a small decrease between 36 weeks of gestation and term.
   b. Urinary flow and sodium excretion decrease by half in the supine position, and the BUN and creatinine decrease because of the increased GFR.
   c. However, the creatinine clearance is not affected by pregnancy.

d. As a test of renal function, dye excretion urinary tests may be misleading because during daylight pregnant women tend to accumulate water in the form of dependent edema and at night, while the patients are recumbent, they mobilize and excrete fluid (nocturia).
3. Homeostatic control during pregnancy causes women to retain some 2 L of water, 290 mEq sodium, 155 mEq of potassium, and the corresponding anions. The normal kidney has an almost unlimited ability to control water and electrolytes; during pregnancy the kidney resets to achieve a new balance.
   a. Acid–base physiology
      (1) During pregnancy, the mean arterial PCO_2 decreases from approximately 39 to 30 mm Hg.
      (2) The blood levels of hydrogen ions are also slightly decreased, as is the bicarbonate (HCO_3) by some 4 mEq/L.
      (3) The effect of these changes is that the arterial pH averages 7.44 during pregnancy versus 7.40 in nonpregnant women.
   b. Potassium
      (1) Approximately 350 mEq is retained in the course of pregnancy.
      (2) This resistance for choleresis has been ascribed to the action of progesterone.
   c. Sodium
      (1) Renal sodium is the prime determinant for the maintenance of volume homeostasis.
      (2) Despite an increase of about 47% in the amount of sodium presented to the renal tubules every 24 hours, their reabsorption efficiency is maintained at better than 99%.
      (3) Approximately 950 mEq of sodium is accumulated throughout pregnancy.
   d. Urinary output
      (1) The 24-hour urine volume is largely unchanged.
      (2) The increased filtered load of water is reabsorbed with equal efficiency when required.
   e. Posture: Changes in maternal posture cause only a short-term effect on the kidneys' ability to handle water and sodium.
   f. Excretion of nutrients
      (1) Glucose
         (a) Glucose is excreted in increasing amounts; but the pattern of glycosuria and amount excreted per 24 hours appear to be random.
         (b) Therefore it is apparent that testing or screening for glycosuria during the antenatal period for diabetes mellitus is not appropriate.
         (c) Other sugars are also excreted in increased amounts, except arabinose.
      (2) Amino acids: The total amount of amino acids excreted is increased, but there is a variation among individual amino acids.
      (3) Vitamins: Water-soluble vitamins are excreted in greater amounts.

Table 22-1 **Creatinine Clearance**

	Plasma	
	Creatinine	**BUN**
First trimester	0.73/100 mL	11
Second trimester	0.58/100 mL	9
Third trimester	0.53/100 mL	10

  (4) Proteins: Proteins are unchanged over a 24-hour period and up to 200 mg/dL is considered normal.
  (5) Creatinine clearance
    (a) The creatinine clearance is taken as an index of the GFR.
    (b) By the eighth week of pregnancy, a mean increment of 45% has occurred in a 24-hour creatinine clearance.
    (c) Throughout the second trimester, it remains elevated, but during the weeks preceding delivery there is a consistent decrease down to the nonpregnant levels (Table 22-1).
    (d) Values of 0.8 mg/100 mL and 14 mg/100 mL should alert the clinician to investigate renal function.
  (6) Uric acid
    (a) During normal pregnancy, there is a relative hypouricemia.
    (b) Plasma uric acid concentrations decrease by 25% as early as the eighth week of pregnancy and begin to increase once more during the third trimester, reaching a concentration equivalent to the nonpregnant mean.
    (c) Uric acid concentration and renal reabsorption are significantly higher in pregnancies complicated by preeclampsia or intrauterine growth restriction.
    (d) Above a critical level of 580 mg/100 mL, there is a significant perinatal mortality in hypertensive patients.
  (7) Renin–angiotensin system
    (a) During normal pregnancy, the level of the circulating renin begins to increase during the early first trimester and continues to increase progressively until term, achieving values 5 to 10 times greater than nonpregnant concentrations.
    (b) Like most globulin fractions, angiotensin also increases, and it rises from a mean nonpregnancy value of 0.7/L to a mean peak of 3.6 mg/L.
    (c) As might be anticipated, the concentrations of angiotensin I and II also increase, but the anticipated effects, vasoconstriction and consequent rise in blood pressure, do not occur.
    (d) Indeed, pregnant women are remarkably resistant to the pressor effects of the infused angiotensin from as early as 10 weeks gestation.

22.8 Maternal Gastrointestinal System

APPETITE
1. Pregnant women appear to have a significant increase in appetite.
2. In some cases, this tends to take bizarre forms.
3. These few peculiar habits in themselves are unlikely to cause any adverse effects.
4. Such things as coal and clay have a significant absorption and buffering capacity and could, if taken in excess, reduce the absorption of minerals and vitamins from the gastrointestinal system.
5. In a few women, appetite may be decreased secondary to nausea or reflux esophagitis, and attention to these symptoms usually improves appetite.

GASTRIC REFLUX
1. Gastric reflux is probably caused by a combination of the esophageal (cardiac) sphincter laxity and the anatomic displacement of the lower esophageal sphincter, increased intraabdominal pressure, and even a hiatal hernia.
2. Management with an antacid preparation is usually effective in improving appetite.

GASTRIC SECRETION
1. Gastric secretion decreases in terms of acidity during early and midpregnancy.
2. However, it increases late in pregnancy, although the amount of mucus production may also be increased.

GASTRIC MOTILITY
1. Gastric motility almost certainly decreases, and with a delay in complete emptying time, this is probably further reduced during labor.
2. Gastric emptying is double in time in pregnant women compared with nonpregnant women.

INTESTINAL ABSORPTION
Efficiency of gastric absorption may be increased, either by specific mechanisms or by a delay in transit time that allows more time for digestion and absorption.

LARGE INTESTINE
Absorption efficiency appears to be greater (more water absorption) during pregnancy, and intestinal transit time is probably slower, which may also explain constipation.

LIVER
1. In functional terms, liver function tests are probably unchanged, with normal levels of serum bilirubin.
2. Also, nonspecific alkaline phosphatase increases in pregnancy are attributable to the alkaline phosphatase isoenzymes from the placenta.

GALLBLADDER

1. Gallbladder may be passively dilated and hence larger in size; however, the composition of the bile itself appears to be unchanged.
2. There is anecdotal evidence that gallstones are more frequent during pregnancy with the decreased motility of the gallbladder and incomplete emptying; this causes the large residual volume of bile, which causes cholesterol crystals to be formed and retained.

22.9 Maternal Reproductive System

Most of these changes result from an increase in the hormones estrogen and progesterone.

BREASTS

1. Size and nodularity are increased (soon after missed period).
2. Superficial veins are more prominent because of increased blood supply and blood vessels. This causes the feelings of fullness and tingling (end of second month).
3. Striae (stretch marks) may appear.
4. Pigmentation usually increases.
5. There is an increase in sebaceous glands in areola (Montgomery's tubercles), which lubricate the nipple.
6. Precolostrum starts the 16th week; colostrum is noted in the third trimester.

OVARIES

1. No ovulation occurs during pregnancy because necessary hormones are suppressed.
2. Blood vessels to ovaries enlarge.

FALLOPIAN TUBES

1. Fallopian tubes elongate but otherwise experience few changes.
2. Blood vessels to fallopian tubes enlarge.

UTERUS

1. The uterus enlarges from a solid organ (approximately 2 oz) to a thin-walled muscular sac (2.2 lb) for gestation as a result of hormones that do the following:
   a. Provide new muscle fibers
   b. Increase blood supply and enlarge blood vessels
   c. Enlarge preexisting fibers
   d. Develop the lining of the uterus
2. Braxton Hicks contractions
   a. Begin at fourth month
   b. Painless; stimulate blood flow through placenta
3. Blood flow
   a. One sixth of maternal blood flow in the uterine system
   b. Affected by hemorrhage, malnutrition, maternal position, uterine contractions

Table 22-2 **Bishop Prelabor Cervical Score**

	0	1	2	3
Dilation (cm)	Closed	1-2	3-4	5 or greater
Effacement (%)	0-30	40-50	60-70	80 or greater
Station	−3	−2	−1, 0	1+ or greater
Consistency	Firm	Medium	Soft	—
Position	Posterior	Midposition	Anterior	—

VAGINA AND VULVA

1. Increase in size and number of cells
2. Increase in secretions: acidic to prevent growth of microorganisms (except yeast)
3. Increase in blood vessels and blood supply
   a. Increased sensitivity
   b. Increased sexual interest

CERVIX

1. Endocervical glands enlarge.
2. Glandular activity increases: secretion of thick, tenacious mucus (mucus plug).
   a. Seals the cervix, preventing bacteria and other organisms from entering the uterus
   b. Leads to much vaginal discharge
3. Table 22-2 shows the Bishop scores for evaluating changes in the cervix.

22.10 Common Discomforts of Pregnancy: Causes and Relief

See Box 22-1.

ACHE IN BACK, HIPS, OR THIGHS

1. Cause: Pressure of baby on small nerves on inside of vertebrae and pelvis
2. Relief: Pelvic rock on all fours or creeping on all fours; this may encourage fetus to readjust its position

BACKACHE

1. Causes
   a. Poor posture
      (1) This is more common in multiparous women whose muscle tone is poor.
      (2) Lax abdominal muscles let uterus fall forward; this leads to lordotic posture for maintenance of balance.
   b. Softening effect of hormone action on spinal discs and sacroiliac joints
   c. Obesity

BOX 22-1 The Discomforts of Pregnancy

First Trimester	Second Trimester	Third Trimester
Ambivalence	Ankle edema	Anxiety
Backache	Backache	Backache or hip pain
Breast tenderness	Changing body image	Changing body image
Changing body image	Constipation	Constipation
Depression	Depression	Depression
Emotional lability	Emotional lability	Emotional lability
Fatigue	Fainting or dizziness	Fatigue
Fearfulness	Fearfulness	Fearfulness
Gingival hyperplasia	Gingival hyperplasia	Fetal movements
Headache	Headache	Gingival hyperplasia
Increased urinary frequency	Heartburn	Headache
Increased or decreased libido	Increased or decreased libido	Heartburn
Increased sensitivity	Increased fetal movements	Hemorrhoids
Indecisiveness	Increased sensitivity	Increased sensitivity
Irritability	Increased vaginal discharge	Increased or decreased libido
Morning sickness	Indecisiveness	Increased urinary frequency
Nasal congestion	Irritability	Increased vaginal discharge
Skin changes	Leg cramps	Indecisiveness
	Ligament pain	Insomnia
	Nasal congestion	Irritability
	Shortness of breath	Leg cramps
	Skin changes	Ligament pain
	Varicose veins	Nasal congestion
	Weight gain	Shortness of breath
		Skin changes
		Slight nausea
		Varicose veins
		Weight gain

2. Relief
    a. Careful attention to correct posture and body mechanics
    b. Pelvic rock, especially on all fours
    c. Kneeling in a crawling position several times a day
    d. When standing, lifting one foot and placing it on an object so it is higher than the other foot; or standing with one foot in front of the other and rocking back and forth slightly
    e. Firm mattress on bed
    f. Cautions
        (1) Not all backaches can be classified as to the same cause.
        (2) Each patient must be dealt with privately to find the exact location and type of pain.
        (3) Backache high and to one side may indicate kidney problems.
        (4) Ache in the middle of a buttock with muscle cramping may be caused by a sacroiliac problem.
        (5) Manipulative exercises can help but must be done by an operant with expertise in this area.

BREAST TENDERNESS

1. Causes
    a. Exaggerated sebaceous glands (Montgomery's glands)
    b. Hyperplasia of the breast
2. Relief: Wearing a good support bra (during sleep as well)

CONSTIPATION

1. Causes
    a. Diminished peristalsis caused by pressure of the enlarged uterus and the relaxing effect on muscle coat of intestines
    b. Decreased physical activity
    c. Impaired tone of stretched abdominal muscles
2. Relief
    a. Drinking three glasses of cool water at 5-minute intervals on rising, then a glass of fruit juice with breakfast
    b. Making sure diet includes plenty of vitamin B, found in wheat germ, liver, whole grains, and brewer's yeast
    c. When sitting on toilet, assuming a semisquatting position by putting feet up on a stool; relaxes pelvic floor

DIAPHRAGM PRESSURE (CRAMP OR STITCH UNDER RIBS)

1. Cause: When baby is high in abdomen, diaphragm is compressed against the base of the lungs
2. Relief: Lifting rib cage by raising arms sideways and upward above head, then stretching

DIZZINESS, FAINTING, AND LIGHT-HEADEDNESS

1. Causes
    a. Vasomotor changes
    b. Pressure of gravid uterus on greater abdominal vessels

c. Anemia
d. Decreased blood sugar
2. Relief
   a. Avoiding sudden changes in posture, especially after practice of conscious release
   b. After lying down, getting up slowly, rolling to side, then pushing up to sitting position (using arms)
   c. Avoiding standing or lying flat on back for long periods
   d. Following physician's advice for treatment of anemia
   e. Not skipping meals; eating properly
   f. Avoiding hot, stuffy rooms

DYSPNEA (SHORTNESS OF BREATH)

1. Causes
   a. When baby is high in abdomen, diaphragm is compressed against the base of the lungs.
   b. Dyspnea may indicate anemia.
2. Relief
   a. Sleeping propped up with pillows or spending first 10 minutes in bed lying on back with arms extended above head and resting on the bed
   b. Lightening during late pregnancy

EDEMA

1. Causes
   a. Peripheral arterial vasodilation with a resultant decreased filling of arterial circulation
   b. Sodium and water retention
   c. Pressure on the iliac vein and inferior vena cava caused by an enlarging uterus increases capillary pressure in the lower extremities, with a resulting filtration of fluid into the interstitial spaces
2. Relief
   a. Lying on left side for 30 minutes three to four times daily
   b. Getting regular exercise
   c. Increasing fluid intake
   d. Eating three servings of protein daily

EMOTIONAL DISCOMFORTS (ANXIETY, DEPRESSION, AND EMOTIONAL LABILITY)

1. Causes
   a. Perceived lack of control during childbirth experience
   b. Fear of the "unknown" (labor, etc.)
   c. Physical discomforts (nausea, vomiting, backache, fatigue)
   d. Changing body image
   e. Unresolved conflicts, ambivalence about pregnancy and its subsequent changes, emotional turmoil, poor coping skills, and genetic predisposition
   f. External pressures, such as finances
   g. Physical and hormonal changes of pregnancy

2. Relief
   a. Maintenance of physical health
   b. Encouragement, positive reinforcement, and communication therapy
   c. Pharmacologic treatment with sustained serotonin reuptake inhibitors (SSRIs) such as Prozac or Paxil

FATIGUE

1. Causes
   a. Significant hormonal increases
   b. Poor nutrition, anemia, and slowed circulation
   c. Sleep disturbances caused by urinary frequency, leg cramps, respiratory difficulties, vomiting, or other problems
2. Relief
   a. Daily exercise to improve circulation
   b. Toward term, lying down at least once daily

FINGERS (TINGLING, NUMBNESS, AND A FEELING OF SWELLING)

1. Causes
   a. Enlargement of breast tissue high in armpit, resulting in pressure on nerves and blood vessels
   b. May indicate need for more iron
2. Relief: Placing hands on shoulders and rotating elbows in a circle

FLATULENCE

1. Cause: Decreased motility of intestinal tract
2. Relief
   a. Avoiding gas-forming foods: parsnips, beans, cabbage, corn, fried foods, pastry, very sweet desserts, and any food known by patient to cause problems
   b. Encouraging regular bowel habits (see constipation relief)
   c. Eating bulky foods; drinking plenty of liquids

FOOT PAIN

1. Cause: Excessive weight gain (40 to 60 lb) and lordotic curvature of the spine may affect stability of foot, causing a breakdown of the arch
2. Relief
   a. Inverting foot (i.e., turning it in when walking barefoot to hold arch up)
   b. Wearing shoes with arch supports

GROIN ACHE OR PAIN

1. Causes
   a. Poor posture
   b. Standing too long
   c. Pressure of baby
   d. Spasm of round ligaments
2. Relief

a. Doing light effleurage (small circular massage) in groin area, giving a slight lift as hands come upward gives relief. Pressure should not be used on the down stroke.
b. Pulling up leg on same side as spasm, as if tying a shoe; or lying down on affected side with leg drawn up will provide relief for a sudden spasm.

HEARTBURN

1. Causes
    a. Enlarged uterus displaces stomach upward.
    b. Progesterone relaxes cardiac sphincter of stomach.
    c. Nervous tension, worry, and fatigue intensify problem.
2. Relief
    a. Eating several small meals a day instead of three large ones
    b. Avoiding greasy or highly spiced foods and coffee
    c. Chewing gum
    d. Breathing slowly and deeply
    e. Taking a tablespoon of cream one-half hour before meals (This will not help if heartburn is already present.)
    f. Avoiding over-the-counter remedies, especially baking soda and Alka-Seltzer, because of their high sodium content
    g. If problem is especially bad at night, sleeping propped up with pillows

HEMORRHOIDS (VARICOSE VEINS OF THE LOWER BOWEL AND RECTUM)

1. Causes
    a. Relaxing effect of progesterone and pressure of heavy uterus on lower part of large bowel
    b. Obesity
    c. Lack of exercise, excessive sitting
    d. Constipation
    e. Failure to empty bowel when urge is felt
    f. Straining to move bowels
2. Relief
    a. As for constipation
    b. Doing Kegel exercise regularly to stimulate circulation in the pelvic area
    c. Applying cold compresses (e.g., ice, witch hazel, Epsom salts)

INCREASED VAGINAL DISCHARGE

1. Causes
    a. Prevention of the growth of microorganisms (except yeast)
    b. Irritations or allergic reactions
2. Relief
    a. Bathing vaginal area frequently with cool water and unperfumed soap
    b. Wearing cotton underwear
    c. Avoiding pantyhose and tight-fitting pants

d. Avoiding vaginal sprays, powders, feminine hygiene products, and colored or scented toilet tissues

LEG CRAMPS

1. Causes
   a. Pressure of gravid uterus on blood vessels, lessening the flow of blood to legs
   b. Overextension of the foot: this occurs with pointing of the toes (e.g., when bedcovers are too heavy, with tightly made beds, or when exercises are improperly done)
   c. Sudden stretching
   d. Fatigue or chilling
   e. Lack of calcium in diet
   f. Excessive amounts of phosphorus absorbed from milk and milk products
2. Relief
   a. The object is to stretch the cramped muscle, thus improving circulation.
   b. For a foot cramp, standing on affected foot will provide relief.
   c. For cramp in calf, straightening knee, pulling foot toward head, holding, then relaxing and repeating if necessary gives relief.
   d. For cramp in front of thigh, stretching leg backward helps.
   e. For cramp in buttock, stretching leg forward helps.
   f. A cramped muscle should never be massaged. Massage enhances rather than relieves the cramp and may cause tenderness that can last for days.
      (1) Because phlebitis could be present, the leg should be examined before massage is used for any reason.
      (2) If the physician feels inadequate calcium or excessive phosphorus intake is the cause, he or she will probably suggest various dietary adjustments.
      (3) An instructor may be in a good position to help a woman replan her dietary habits.
      (4) For this, some background information on nutrition and foods containing calcium and phosphorus is needed.

NAUSEA

1. Causes
   a. Increased estrogen or HCG levels
   b. Combination of hormonal, psychologic, and neurologic factors
2. Relief
   a. Consuming dry crackers, toast, or cereal before getting out of bed or whenever nausea begins
   b. Eating five or six small meals each day so that the stomach does not get empty
   c. Avoiding greasy or spicy foods
   d. Limiting fluid intake during meals but drinking water freely between meals
   e. Avoiding strong food smells

VARICOSE VEINS OF VULVA

1. Cause: Same as varicose veins of legs
2. Relief
   a. Lying with hips elevated several times a day, either on back or in Sims' lateral position
   b. Putting entire body in slant position by lying on a slant board
   c. Wearing firmly applied perineal pad for support (special pads are available from surgical supply companies)

VARICOSE VEINS OR LEG ACHE

1. Causes
   a. Hereditary predisposition
   b. Relaxing effect of progesterone on walls of veins
   c. Pressure of enlarged uterus on abdominal veins (slows blood return from lower limbs)
   d. Fatigue
   e. Standing with knees locked, causing a muscular constriction, preventing proper venous return
2. Relief
   a. Avoiding round garters, thigh highs, or any clothing that causes pressure on any part of the body.
   b. Changing positions frequently; avoiding long standing or sitting.
   c. Doing Kegel exercises regularly.
   d. Taking long walks; the massaging action of muscles close to veins is good for stimulating circulation.
   e. Crawling on hands and knees several times a day; doing pelvic rock.
   f. Elevating legs and hips several times a day; keeping knees flexed and supported by pillows.
   g. Wearing support hose or stockings made of elastic. (These should be put on while lying down, ideally before getting up in the morning.)
   h. Cautions: Patients should never stand "at attention" with knees locked. Knees should always be slightly flexed.

22.11 Endocrinology and Physiologic Changes

THYROID

Thyroid disorders are much more common in women than in men.

Normal Adult Thyroid Function

1. Thyrotropin-releasing hormone (TRH) is synthesized in the supraoptic and paraventricular nuclei of the hypothalamus and is stored in the median eminence.
2. TRH stimulates the anterior pituitary to both release and synthesize TSH.
3. TSH stimulates both synthesis and release of thyroid hormones: thyroxine (T_4) and triiodothyronine (T_3).
4. T_4 and T_3 have feedback control of TSH at the pituitary level and, possibly, at the hypothalamus level.

5. Thyroid hormone synthesis and release:
   a. Trapping
      (1) Iodide accumulates within the thyroid gland from plasma by active transport via iodide pump.
      (2) Pump is stimulated by TSH and iodide deficiency within thyroid.
      (3) Pump is inhibited by perchlorate and thiocyanate.
   b. Iodination
      (1) Glandular iodide reacts with a peroxidase and the thiouracil groups of thyroglobulin to create monoiodotyrosine (MIT) and diiodotyrosine (DIT).
      (2) This step is inhibited by propylthiouracil (PTU) and methimazole (TAP).
   c. Coupling: Previously formed iodotyrosines oxidatively couple to create thyroxine (T_4 by DIT + DIT) and triiodothyronine (T_3 by DIT + MIT).
   d. Release
      (1) Thyroglobulin-bound T_4 and T_3 are released into the circulation by the action of a protease.
      (2) This step is stimulated by TSH.
      (3) This step is inhibited by iodine and lithium.
   e. Peripheral conversion
      (1) Circulating T_4 is converted to T_3 (active) and rT_3 (reverse T_3; inactive).
      (2) This step is inhibited by PTU and is decreased by propranolol.
6. Pregnancy normally results in certain physiologic alterations that influence clinical and laboratory evaluation of thyroid function.
   a. Increased iodine renal clearance
   b. Increased thyroid clearance of iodine
   c. Possible role of placental thyrotropins (HCT, HCG)
   d. Increased synthesis of thyroxine-binding globulin (TBG): TBG doubles by 8 to 12 weeks gestation.
   e. Decreased thyroxine-binding prealbumin (TBPA)
7. Laboratory evaluation of thyroid function during pregnancy (Table 22-3) should be done.
8. Normal ranges for laboratory tests of thyroid function are listed in Table 22-4.
9. The free thyroid index (FTI) is a mathematic expression without units used to compensate for pregnancy-related changes in total T_4 and rT_3U.
   a. Its normal range approximates that of total T_4 in nonpregnant patients.
   b. It is calculated by the following equation:

   $$FTI = T_4\ total \times rT_3U / Mean\ NL\ rT_3U = 30$$

Normal Fetal Thyroid Function
1. Like other fetal tissues, the fetal thyroid gland shows progressive maturational changes as gestation advances.

Table 22-3 **Alterations in Thyroid Function During Pregnancy**

Measure of Function	Status
Protein-bound iodine	Increased
T_4 (total)	Increased
T_3 (total)	Increased
TBG	Doubled
Reverse T_3 uptake (rT_3U)	Decreased
T_4 (free)	No change
T_3 (free)	No change
Free thyroid index (FTI)	No change
TSH	No change

TBG, Thyroxine-binding globulin; *TSH*, thyroid-stimulating hormone.

    a. By 11 to 12 weeks, fetal thyroid can produce iodotyrosines and iodothyronines.
    b. Fetal thyroid concentrates iodine by 12 to 14 weeks.
    c. TSH appears at 10 weeks, increases between weeks 20 and 30, and then declines.
    d. Total T_4 and free T_4 rise in response to an increase in TSH.
    e. Amniotic fluid T_4 increases to peak at 25 to 30 weeks gestation and then declines.
    f. Amniotic fluid T_3 increases progressively.
    g. Amniotic fluid T_3 increases to peak at 17 to 20 weeks and then declines.
2. The role, if any, of maternal thyroid hormones in fetal development, especially in the first 12 weeks, remains unclear and is highly disputed. Placental passage from mother to fetus is shown in Table 22-5.

Table 22-4 **Normal Ranges for Laboratory Tests of Thyroid Function**

Test	Nonpregnant	Pregnant
T_4 (total)	5-12.5 µg/dL	6-15 µg/dL
T_3 (total)	50-175 ng/dL	125-275 ng/dL
T_4 (free)	2.5 ng/dL	2.5 ng/dL
T_3 (free)	0.3 ng/dL	0.3 ng/dL
TSH	1.9-5.9 µU/mL	1.9-5.9 µU/mL
FTI	4.5-12	4.5-12
rT_3U	25%-35%	15%-25%

FTI, Free thyroid index; *rT_3U*, reverse T_3 uptake; *TSH*, thyroid-stimulating hormone.

Table 22-5 Placental Passage of Maternal Thyroid Hormones

Hormone	Passage
TSH	Negligible
T_4	Very poor
T_3	Poor
TRH	Good
Thyronine analogues (Dimit)	Good
Thyroid-stimulating immunoglobulins (TSIg)	Good
Iodine	Rapid

TRH, Thyrotropin-releasing hormone; *TSH*, thyroid-stimulating hormone.

Normal Neonatal Thyroid Function

Following birth, very rapid changes in thyroid function occur.

1. Thyroid iodine uptake increases at birth to peak at about 48 hours of life.
2. Uptake normalizes by the fifth day of life.
3. Cord serum T_3 values are low at birth.
4. Cord serum rT_3 values are elevated at birth.
5. TSH rises sharply minutes after birth and peaks within 3 hours.
6. Following the rise in TSH is an increase in total T_4 and free T_4.
7. Serum T_3 rises and rT_3 decreases as a result of alterations in peripheral conversion of T_4.

PITUITARY

The pituitary gland is not essential after 12 weeks gestation; however, pituitary mass increases by 50%, primarily because of increased prolactin from the anterior pituitary.

1. Prolactin levels increase from 10.5 to 250 ng/mL.
   a. Function is uncertain.
   b. Lactation requires the basal metabolic level.
   c. Episodic nature of release continues.
   d. Present in amniotic fluid: not under the influence of dopamine.
   e. Questionable role in Na^+/H_2O homeostasis.
2. Follicle-stimulating hormone (FSH) is suppressed.
   a. Suppression is primarily secondary to increased estrogen levels.
   b. Increased HCG also suppresses FSH.
3. Luteinizing hormone (LH) is suppressed.
4. Growth hormone (GH) is suppressed. Paradoxical because E_2 normally increases GH.
5. ACTH is increased. Paradoxical because elevated cortisol seen with pregnancy is not associated with negative feedback.
6. TSH level is unchanged.
7. MSH is increased. Function = hyperpigmentation (linea nigra, chloasma, areola, etc.).

8. Vasopressin level is unchanged.
   a. This is paradoxical because the hypoosmolality associated with pregnancy causes no change.
   b. Osmoreceptors are reset at lower level.
9. Oxytocin level is increased. Function is equal to milk letdown; has no correlation with strength of contractions.

ADRENAL

The adrenal glands are not significantly altered during pregnancy; however, there is an expansion of the zona fasciculata (glucocorticoid production).

1. Corticosteroid-binding globulin (CBG) increases from 33 mg/dL in nonpregnant women up to 70 mg/dL during pregnancy.
   a. This increase results from increased hepatic synthesis, which is secondary to elevated maternal estrogen levels.
   b. The estrogen-mediated increase in CBG elevates plasma cortisol levels.
2. Free cortisol is also elevated during pregnancy and progressively increases from the first trimester until term. The increase in free cortisol results from its increased production and delayed clearance.
3. Desoxycorticosterone (DOC) is elevated; however, plasma levels of DOC during pregnancy do not respond to ACTH stimulation or to dexamethasone suppression.
   a. The increase is secondary to a possible second site of production, which is fetoplacental.
   b. Mineralocorticoid activity is weak.
4. Dehydroepiandrosterone sulfate levels are decreased during pregnancy because of the increased metabolical clearance.
5. Aldosterone levels are increased because of increased production.
6. Androstenedione levels are increased.
7. Testosterone levels are increased. However, because of increased sex hormone–binding globulin (SHBG), free testosterone decreases.
8. Dehydroepiandrosterone/dehydroepiandrosterone sulfate (DHEA/DHEAS) are decreased.

PANCREAS

Pancreatic hypertrophy and hyperplasia of the pancreatic beta cells occur during pregnancy.

1. Insulin (beta cells)
   a. Fasting: small increase by change 3
   b. Fed: slower response to rise/peak; higher peak; longer duration
2. Glucagon (alpha cells): basal levels are increased

OVARY/PLACENTA

1. Source of progesterone
   a. Corpus luteum until 8 to 12 weeks
   b. Placenta after 8 to 12 weeks
2. Source of estradiol: placenta from DHEA (maternal and fetal origin)

3. 17-hydroxyprogesterone (OHP)
   a. Source is corpus luteum.
   b. Graph peaks at 12 weeks, then declines.
4. Estriol
   a. Source is placenta 16-hydroxy DHEAS.
   b. Graph is increased.
5. HPL
   a. Source is placenta.
   b. Function is unknown but it has a metabolic role.
6. HCG
   a. Structure
      (1) Alpha subunit: greater than LH, TSH, FSH
      (2) Beta subunit: greater than LH
   b. Graph
      (1) Initial peak at 8 to 10 weeks
      (2) Second peak at 32 to 38 weeks
   c. Function: to maintain corpus luteum

SUGGESTED READINGS

American Academy of Pediatrics and American College of Obstetricians and Gynecologists: *Guidelines for perinatal care,* Washington, DC, and Elk Grove Village, IL, 1983, ACOG and AAP, p.166.

Brown MA et al: Measuring blood pressure in pregnant women: a comparison of direct and indirect methods, *Am J Obstet Gynecol* 171:661-667, 1994.

Clark SL et al: Position change and central hemodynamic profile during normal third-trimester pregnancy and post partum, *Am J Obstet Gynecol* 164:883-887, 1991.

Cogswell ME et al: Gestational weight gain among average-weight and overweight women—what is excessive, *Am J Obstet Gynecol* 172:705-712, 1995.

Institute of Medicine (United States): *Nutrition during pregnancy,* Report of the Committee on Nutritional Status During Pregnancy and Lactation, Food and Nutrition Board, Washington, DC, 1990, National Academy Press.

Joffe GM et al: Diagnosis of cervical change in pregnancy by means of transvaginal ultrasonography, *Am J Obstet Gynecol* 166:896-900, 1992.

Kimura M et al: Physiologic thyroid activation in normal early pregnancy is induced by circulating hCG, *Obstet Gynecol* 75:775-778, 1990.

Lopez MC et al: The measurement of diastolic blood pressure during pregnancy: which Korotkoff phase should be used, *Am J Obstet Gynecol* 170:574-578, 1994.

Maher JE et al: Indicators of maternal nutritional status and birth weight in term deliveries, *Obstet Gynecol* 81:165-169, 1993.

Schrier RW, Briner VA: Peripheral arterial vasodilation hypothesis of sodium and water retention in pregnancy: implications for pathogenesis of preeclampsia-eclampsia, *Obstet Gynecol* 77:632-639, 1991.

Thaler I et al: Changes in uterine blood flow during human pregnancy, *Am J Obstet Gynecol* 162:121-125, 1990.

Index

Page numbers followed by f refer to figures; those followed by t refer to tables; and those followed by b refer to boxed material.

A

Abdomen
  Langer's lines of, 46, 47f, 50-61
  physical examination of, 3, 235
Abdominal incisions, 50, 52f
  Cherney, 56, 59-61, 60f
  Maylard, 52f, 56-59, 57f, 59-61, 66
  median, 62-65, 62f
  midline, 50, 52f
  paramedian, 65, 66f
  Pfannenstiel, 52f, 53f, 52-56
  selection of, 50, 51f
  transverse, 50, 65
  vertical, 61, 68, 74-75
Abdominal pain
  adhesions, 253
  adnexal origins of, 244
  anatomy of, 233
  assessment of, 234
  description of, 233
  differential diagnosis, 237b
  dysmenorrhea, 251
  early pregnancy complications as cause of, 238
  history-taking, 234-235
  intestinal causes of, 246
  laparoscopy evaluations, 236-238
  ovarian hyperstimulation syndrome, 245
  physical examination for, 235-236
  physiology of, 233
  systemic causes of, 251

Abdominal pain (Continued)
  "trigger point," 255
  ultrasound evaluations, 236
  urinary tract sources of, 249
  vascular sources of, 250
Abdominal pressure, 90
Abdominal wall muscles, 9, 13
Abdominal–pelvic diagnostic laparoscopy, 72
  bipolar forceps test, 75
  examination procedure, 74
  general anesthesia for, 74
  Hasson cannula, 74-75
  hemostasis during, 77
  instruments for, 73
  operating room preparation for, 73
  operative report, 77
  preadmission preparation for, 72
  three-step, 75-77
  trocar placement, 75
Abdominal-Valsalva leak point pressures, 94-95
Abnormal uterine bleeding
  amenorrhea. *See* Amenorrhea
  anatomic causes of, 181b
  definition of, 179
  definitions, 179
  diagnosis of, 180
  dilation and curettage for, 183
  endometrial ablation for, 183
  estrogen-progestin contraceptives for, 183
  etiology of, 179, 180b, 181b

603

Abnormal uterine bleeding (*Continued*)
  hypermenorrhea, 179
  hypomenorrhea, 179
  hysterectomy for, 183
  management of, 182
  medical therapy for, 183
  menometrorrhagia, 180
  menorrhagia, 179
  metrorrhea, 180
  oligomenorrhea, 180
  organic causes of, 179
  polymenorrhea, 180
  progestin contraceptives for, 183
  surgical therapy for, 183
  systemic diseases that cause, 180b
Abortion, 239
Absent end-diastolic velocity, 504, 506f
Abstinence, 123, 134t
Acetic acid, 70
Achondroplasia, 420
Acrosin assay, 165
Acute cystitis, 249
Acute pyelonephritis, 481
Acute renal failure, 487, 489t, 490t
Acute tubular necrosis, 488, 489t
Acute urethral syndrome, 198
Acyclovir, 206, 207
Adenomyosis, 145, 253
Adhesions, 253
Admission orders, 4
Adnexal pain, 244
Adrenal glands, 600
Albumin, 520
Alcohol, 524
Allen stirrups, 73
Alpha-fetoprotein, maternal serum, 370, 410, 525
  chromosomal abnormalities, 530
  Down syndrome and, 533
  elevated levels of
    amniocentesis evaluations, 532
    evaluation of patient with, 530, 531f

Alpha-fetoprotein, maternal serum (*Continued*)
    fetal anomalies associated with, 528
    fetal death and, 532-533
    management of, 533
    nonfetal anomaly causes of, 532
  factors that affect, 527
  fetal levels of, 526, 526f
  measurement of, 527
  neural tube defect screening using, 528, 529t
  physiology of, 525
  renal abnormalities, 530
Alprazolam, 317t, 318t
Alspingostomy, 242-243
Alzheimer's disease, 547-548
Amenorrhea
  central nervous system lesions that cause, 176
  classification of, 167, 168b
  clinical assessments of, 171
  definition of, 179
  Depo-Provera and, 112, 176
  diagnostic procedures for, 171, 172f
  differential diagnosis, 261
  drug-induced, 176
  estrogen therapy for, 178
  eugonadotropic, 174-176
  exercise-induced, 175
  extragonadal anomalies that cause, 169-170
  galactorrhea and, 176
  gonadal abnormalities associated with, 167-169
  hypergonadotropic, 173-174
  lactation-related, 123
  ovulation induction for, 178
  physiologic, 167
  polycystic ovarian disease and, 176-177
  postpill, 175
  primary, 167-170, 261
  pseudocyesis, 175
  psychogenic, 174-175
  secondary, 173, 174b
    classification of, 173, 174b

Amenorrhea (*Continued*)
    definition of, 173
    diagnostic workup for, 177
    treatment of, 178
treatment of, 178
weight loss–induced, 175
Amino acids, 580, 585
Amniocentesis, 208, 537-538, 556
    complications of, 558
    contraindications, 557
    fetal hemorrhage risks, 558
    history of, 556
    indications for, 557
    maternal serum alpha-fetoprotein evaluations, 532
    patient counseling, 557
    postprocedural instructions, 559
    procedure, 559
    reductive, 557
    risks associated with, 558
    in second trimester, 558
    in third trimester, 557, 558
    umbilical cord laceration risks, 558
Amnion tenting, 559
Amniotic fluid index, 502
Anabolic agents, 325
Anafranil. *See* Clomipramine
Anal canal, 21f
Anal triangle, 13, 15f, 16
Analgesia, 348
    comparison of, 349t
    considerations for, 360
    continuous techniques, 354
    inhalation, 351
    intravenous adjuvants, 351
    ketamine, 350-351, 352t
    ketorolac, 351
    neuraxial, 349, 353, 349t
    nonpharmacologic techniques, 350
    opioids, 350, 356-357
    psychoprophylactic, 349t, 350
    single-injection techniques, 356
    subarachnoid, 353, 354t, 356
    systemic intravenous, 349t
Androgen
    binding of, 305
    exogenous ingestion of, 305

Androgen (*Continued*)
    metabolism alterations, 305
    production of, 305, 306
Androgen insensitivity syndrome, 170
Androgen-producing tumors, 306-307
Android pelvis, 330f
Anemia, 485, 521
Anencephaly, 528
Anesthesia, 5
    combined spinal and epidural, 357
    epidural, 353, 354t
    general, 357
    nonobstetric surgery during pregnancy, 359
Aneuploidy, 508
    choroid plexus cysts and, 511
    cleft lip/palate and, 511
    congenital heart disease and, 512
    corpus callosum agenesis and, 511
    cystic hygroma and, 511
    Dandy-Walker syndrome and, 510-511
    diaphragmatic hernia and, 512
    duodenal atresia and, 513
    echogenic bowel and, 513-514
    esophageal malformations and, 512-513
    frequency of, 508-509
    genitourinary anomalies and, 514
    holoprosencephaly and, 511
    hydrocephaly and, 510
    hydrothorax and, 512
    limb anomalies and, 514
    meningomyelocele and, 510
    nonimmune hydrops and, 514
    omphalocele and, 513
    prenatal detection of, 509
    pyelectasis and, 514
    structural abnormalities associated with, 510
    ultrasound detection of, 509, 514
Angiotensin II infusion test, 428

Angiotensin-converting enzyme inhibitors, 368-369
Anococcygeal raphe, 14f, 15f, 18f, 21f, 29f
Antenatal assessment, 492
 indications for, 492, 498t
 tests used in, 492
  amniotic fluid index, 502
  biophysical profile.
   See Biophysical profile
  contraction stress. *See*
   Contraction stress test
  Doppler velocimetry, 506f, 503
  fetal movement charting, 505
  nonstress, 496f, 494
Anterior abdominal wall
 anatomy of, 50
 blood supply to, 50
 fascial layers of, 47
 Langer's lines, 46, 47f, 50-61
 lateral. *See* Anterior lateral abdominal wall
 muscles of, 47, 49f
 nerve supply to, 50, 51f
 skin of, 46
 subdivisions of, 9f
 transverse sectional image of, 48f
Anterior gluteal line, 22f
Anterior lateral abdominal wall, 8, 9f
 deep layer of, 8, 10f
 fascia of, 8, 10f
  deep, 9
  subcutaneous, 8, 10f
  superficial, 8, 10f
  thoracolumbar, 11
  transversalis, 11, 47
 muscles of, 13
Anterior superior iliac spine, 15f
Anthropoid pelvis, 330f
Antibiotics
 oral contraceptives and, 102b, 102
 prophylactic use of
  description of, 6
  hysterosalpingogram, 142
  during intrauterine device insertion, 117

Antibody-agglutination testing, 162-163, 163b
Antidiuretic hormone, 481
Antihypertensive agents, 438-439
Antiinflammatories, 468
Antiresorptive agents, 325
Anus, 14f
Aponeuroses, 12f
Appendices epiploicae, 249
Appendicitis, 246-247
Arcuate line, 12f, 46, 49f
Arcus tendineus, 21f, 22f
Ascites, 263
Asherman's syndrome, 173
Aspermia, 158
Aspiration pneumonia, 470
Asthenozoospermia, 158
Asthma, 466
 clinical course of, 467
 diagnosis of, 467
 fetal assessment, 469
 incidence of, 466
 labor considerations, 469
 management of, 468
 morbidity and mortality, 466
 pathophysiology of, 467
Atrophic vaginitis, 321-322
Atypical squamous cells of undetermined significance, 69, 70t
Autonomic nervous system, 40, 41f, 43f, 44f
 parasympathetic division, 40
 sympathetic division, 40
Autosomal dominant inheritance, 419
Autosomal recessive inheritance, 420
Azathioprine, 486
Azithromycin
 chancroid treated with, 204
 chlamydia treated with, 199
 donovanosis treated with, 205
 gonorrhea treated with, 196
Azoospermia, 155, 156b, 158

B
Bacteremia, 195

Bacterial vaginosis, 213, 214t, 458
  background, 458
  clindamycin for, 463-464
  diagnosis of, 459-460, 460t
  epidemiology of, 458
  etiology of, 459
  metronidazole for, 215, 462-464
  natural history of, 460
  pathophysiology of, 462
  in pregnancy, 461
  risk factors for, 458-459
  sequelae associated with, 461
  signs and symptoms of, 459-460
  treatment of, 462
Basal body temperature, 125, 126f
Benign breast disease, 103
Betamethasone, 370
Beta-thalassemia, 424
Bethanechol supersensitivity test, 95-96
Biguanides, 391
Bilateral renal cortical necrosis, 488, 489t
Bilirubin, 581
Billings method, 125
Bimanual examination, 4
Biophysical profile, 413, 499
  background, 499-502
  components of, 501t
  interpretation of, 503t
  modified, 502
  procedure, 502
  scores, 503t
Biopsy
  endometrial, 143
  renal, 484
Bipolar forceps test, 75
Bisphosphonates, 325
Bladder
  anatomy of, 30
  autonomic innervation of, 43f
  innervation of, 31f
  maternal, pregnancy-related changes in, 584
Bladder compliance, 90-91
Bladder distention, 249
Bladder filling, 90-92, 91f
Blood urea nitrogen, 480
Blood volume, 575
Body mass index, 403

Bowel preparation, 5
Bowel sounds, 3
Brandt-Andrews maneuver, 339
Braxton-Hicks contractions, 333
Breast(s)
  inflammatory lesions of, 263
  physical examination of, 1, 3
  pregnancy-related changes in, 588
Breast cancer, 104-132, 328
Breast mass, 264
Breast-feeding, 394
Breech presentation, 331-332, 342-344, 343f, 344b
Brenner tumor, 307
Broad ligament, 23-24, 25f
Bronchodilators, 468
Brow presentation, 345
Bulbospongiosus muscles, 19
Bupropion, 317t
Butoconazole, 217
Butorphanol, 352t

C

CA 125, 301-302
Calcitonin nasal spray, 325
Calcium gluconate, 568
Calymmatobacterium granulomatis, 204
Camper's fascia, 9, 46
Cancer
  cervical. *See* Cervical cancer
  oral contraceptives and, 108-111
  ovarian. *See* Ovarian cancer
  uterine. *See* Uterine cancer
  vaginal, 295, 296t
  vulvar, 297, 299t
Candida spp., 215, 216
Carbohydrates, 579
Carbon dioxide, 583
Cardinal ligaments, 28
Cardiovascular disease, 105b, 104, 325
Cardiovascular system, 2, 3
Caudal epidural anesthesia, 355-356

Cefixime, 196
Cefotaxime, 196
Cefoxitin, 211, 212t
Ceftizoxime, 196
Ceftriaxone
  chancroid treated with, 204
  gonorrhea treated with, 196
  pelvic inflammatory disease treated with, 211
Celexa. See Citalopram
Central nervous system
  lesions of, 176
  physical examination of, 1
Cervical canal, 23-24, 26f
Cervical cancer, 290
  clinical presentation of, 290
  diagnosis of, 291
  epidemiology of, 290
  etiology of, 290
  oral contraceptives and, 104
  prognosis for, 291
  risk factors for, 290
  staging of, 291, 292t
  treatment of, 291
Cervical cap, 118, 119f, 120
Cervical dysplasia, 450
Cervical mass, 274
Cervical mucus
  description of, 143
  sperm penetration testing, 165
Cervical neoplasia, 227-228
Cervix
  anatomy of, 23-24, 26f
  digital examination of, 334
  pregnancy-related changes in, 589, 589t
Cesarean section, 347, 360, 373
Chancroid, 203, 226
Charting
  history-taking, 1
  physical examination, 1
Chasteberry, 316t, 319
Cherney incision, 56, 59-61, 60f
Chest, 3
Chief complaint, 1
Childbirth. See Labor and delivery
Chlamydia, 197
  diagnosis of, 198
  epidemiology of, 197

Chlamydia (Continued)
  etiology of, 197
  follow-up for, 199
  lower genital tract infection, 198
  in pregnancy, 199
  risk factors for, 197
  screening criteria for, 197b
  treatment of, 199
  upper genital tract infection, 198
Chlamydia sp.
  C. trachomatis, 196-197, 209
  cervicitis, 104
Chloasma, 575
Cholesterol, 520
Chorioamnionitis, 453-454, 461
Chorionic villus sampling, 551, 560
  complications of, 563
  contraindications, 561
  first-trimester, 560
  history, 561
  indications for, 560
  limb reduction defects, 563
  overview of, 560
  patient counseling, 563
  postmortem, 560
  postprocedure instructions, 564
  procedure, 561-562
  registry, 562
  second-trimester, 560
  transabdominal, 562
  transcervical, 562
Choroid plexus cysts, 511
Chromosome abnormalities
  alpha-fetoprotein screening. See Alpha-fetoprotein
  Down syndrome. See Down syndrome
  maternal age and, 415, 416t
  serum markers used to screen for, 533
  triple marker screening for, 535-536
Chronic ambulatory peritoneal dialysis, 485
Chronic hypertension, 442
  causes of, 443b
  definition of, 426

Chronic hypertension (Continued)
  fetal risks, 444
  management of, 442
  maternal risks, 444
Chronic pelvic pain, 233
Chronic pyelonephritis, 481
Chronic renal disease, 483
Chronic respiratory disease, 476
  kyphoscoliosis, 478
  sarcoidosis, 478
  tobacco smoking, 476, 477b
Cimetidine, 309
Ciprofloxacin
  chancroid treated with, 204
  donovanosis treated with, 204
  gonorrhea treated with, 196, 196
Citalopram, 317t, 318t
Cleft lip/palate, 511
Clindamycin, 215, 463-464
Clitoris, 13, 14f, 18f
Clomid, 145-146
Clomiphene citrate, 178
Clomipramine, 317t, 318t
Clotrimazole, 217
Coccidiomycosis, 470
Coccygeal joint, 34
Coccygeal plexus, 36
Coccygeus muscle, 21f, 22f, 23
Coccyx, 15f, 29f
Collateral circulation, 34
Colon
  abdominal–pelvic diagnostic laparoscopy of, 76
  injuries to, during diagnostic studies, 79
Colon tumors, 249
Colposcope, 70
Colposcopy, 70, 71b
Common iliac arteries, 30, 32f
Complete abortion, 239
Complex lipids, 579
Condoms
  effectiveness rates, 134t
  female, 121f, 121-122
  male, 121, 122f
Condylomata acuminata, 226-227
Congenital adrenal hyperplasia, 170, 177, 306
Congenital heart disease, 512

Congenital hypothyroidism, 543-544
Congenital nephrotic syndrome, 530
Constipation, 523
Continuous lumbar epidural analgesia, 354-355
Contraception
  abstinence, 123, 134t
  barrier methods, 118
  basal body temperature monitoring, 125, 126f
  cervical cap, 118, 119f, 120
  complications, 132, 134t
  condoms. See Condoms
  Depo-Provera. See Depo-Provera
  diaphragm, 118, 119f, 120
  effectiveness rates, 134t
  history-taking, 102
  hormonal implants, 107-112, 114t, 134t
  intrauterine device. See Intrauterine device
  lactation amenorrhea method, 123
  Minipill, 113
  natural family planning, 124
  oral, 101. See also Oral contraceptives
  in patients with HIV, 231
  postcoital, 113
  progestin-only contraceptives, 107, 114t, 134t
  in renal transplantation patients, 487
  rhythm method, 124, 134t
  spermicides, 123
  sterilization, 125. See also Sterilization
  vaginal sponge, 120
  withdrawal method, 124
Contraceptive patch, 101
Contraction stress test, 495
  background, 495-497
  contraindications, 497b
  interpretation of, 498t
  management of, 498-499
  modification of, 499

Contraction stress test (*Continued*)
  negative, 500f
  nipple stimulation test, 499
  positive, 498
  procedure for, 497-498
  reactive positive, 498
Corpus callosum agenesis, 511
Corpus cavernosum, 18f
Corpus luteum cyst rupture, 245
Corticosteroid-binding globulin, 600
Craniopharyngiomas, 170
Creatinine, 480
Creatinine clearance, 480, 586, 586t
Credé maneuver, 339
Crohn's disease, 247
Culdocentesis, 236, 241
Cushing's syndrome, 306
Cyclosporine A, 486
Cyproterone acetate, 309
Cystic fibrosis, 423
Cystic hygroma, 511
Cystic teratoma, 245
Cystitis, 249
Cystometrogram, 88-90, 90f

D

Danazol, 144, 317-318
Dandy-Walker syndrome, 510-511
Dapsone, 230
Deep circumflex iliac artery, 32f
Deep perineal nerve, 19-20
Dehydroepiandrosterone sulfate, 305-306, 308, 600
Delayed puberty, 267
Delivery. *See* Labor and delivery
Dentition, 1
Depo-Provera, 112, 114t, 176
Desoxycorticosterone, 600
Detrusor instability, 286
Detrusor leak point pressure, 95
Detrusor pressure, 90
Dexamethasone, 309, 370
Diabetes Control and Complication Trial, 383

Diabetes mellitus
  birth trauma prevention, 381, 373
  breast-feeding, 394
  cardiovascular disease and, 327
  classification of, 362-363, 364t
  congenital anomalies, 370, 379
  dietary considerations, 375, 376b, 386, 521-522
  fetal complications, 391-392
  fetal growth abnormalities in, 371
  fetal well-being surveillance, 380
  gestational. *See* Gestational diabetes mellitus
  gestational age, 369
  glucose monitoring and control in, 371, 372t, 375-376
  insulin therapy for, 376-377
  intrapartum asphyxia prevention, 373
  intrauterine fetal death prevention, 372
  intrauterine growth retardation, 371
  labor and delivery, 381
  management of, 375
  maternal disease, 368
  neonatal complications, 374
  neonatal management, 382
  preconception counseling, 367
  pregestational. *See* Pregestational diabetes mellitus
  pregnancy viability, 369
  preterm labor prevention and treatment, 370
  type I, 362
  type II, 362
  ultrasound surveillance in, 378
Diabetic fetopathy, 379
Diabetic nephropathy, 482
Diagnostic studies
  abdominal–pelvic diagnostic laparoscopy. *See* Abdominal–pelvic diagnostic laparoscopy
  colon injuries during, 79
  colposcopy, 70, 71b

Diagnostic studies *(Continued)*
  Papanicolaou smear.
    See Papanicolaou smear
  rectal injuries during, 79
  small bowel injuries during, 77
  ureteral dissection.
    See Ureteral dissection
Dialysis
  chronic ambulatory peritoneal, 485
  during pregnancy, 484
Diaphragm (anatomy)
  pelvic, 20, 21f, 22f
  urogenital, 18f, 20f, 22f
Diaphragm (contraception), 118, 119f, 120, 134t
Diaphragmatic hernia, 512
Diarrhea, 523
Diazepam, 352t
Diet. *See* Nutrition
Dihydrotestosterone, 305
Dilation and curettage
  abnormal uterine bleeding treated with, 183
  ectopic pregnancy diagnosis using, 241
Diltiazem, 369
Diphenhydramine, 352t
Discharge summary, 7
Diverticulitis, 248-249
Donovanosis, 204
Doppler velocimetry, 503, 506f
Down syndrome, 508, 538
  in adolescent, 545, 555b
  in adult, 547, 555b
  alternative therapies in, 552
  Alzheimer's disease risks, 547-548
  cataracts associated with, 542
  cervical spine instability in, 544-545
  in child, 542, 555b
  chorionic villus sampling diagnosis of, 551
  chromosomal basis of, 548, 549f, 550f
  clinical features of, 539, 540f, 541b
  cognitive deficits associated with, 542-543

Down syndrome *(Continued)*
  dental problems in, 545
  discovery of, 538, 539
  epidemiology of, 538
  fetal loss in, 552
  gastrointestinal anomalies in, 541-542
  growth in, 546
  health care access for, 538-539
  joint hypermobility in, 544-545
  life expectancy in, 547
  maternal serum alpha-fetoprotein levels and, 533, 552
  medical issues, 555b
  molecular insights into, 553
  myeloproliferative disorders and, 542, 544
  natural history of, 538
  neonate with, 539, 555b
  neurodevelopmental interventions in, 545
  ocular abnormalities in, 542-543
  percutaneous umbilical blood sampling diagnosis of, 551
  prenatal diagnosis of, 551
  prognosis for, 554-556
  recurrence risks in subsequent pregnancies, 550-551
  Robertsonian translocation as cause of, 550f, 550-551
  seizures in, 544
  serum markers associated with
    maternal serum human chorionic gonadotropin, 534
    maternal serum unconjugated estriol, 534-535
  structural defects in, 539-540
  survival in, 547
  thyroid dysfunction in, 543-544
  triple marker screening for, 26f, 536
  upper airway obstruction in, 545
  ventricular septal defects in, 539-540

Doxycycline
  chlamydia treated with, 199
  donovanosis treated with, 204
  gonorrhea treated with, 196
  lymphogranuloma venereum treated with, 200
  pelvic inflammatory disease treated with, 211, 212t
  syphilis treated with, 202
Duchenne muscular dystrophy, 421
Duodenal atresia, 513, 541-542
Dysfunctional uterine bleeding, 179
Dysmenorrhea, 2, 138, 251
Dyspareunia, 284
Dysplastic kidneys, 514
Dyspnea, 465, 592
Dystocias, 331-332
  classification of, 341-347
  definition of, 340-341
  inlet, 346
  midpelvic, 346-347
  passage, 346-347
  shoulder, 345-346, 374, 381

E

Ears, 1, 3
Echogenic bowel, 513-514
Eclampsia, 434
  complications of, 440
  convulsion control and prevention, 435-437
  definition of, 426, 434
  incidence of, 434
  magnesium sulfate for, 435-436, 437t
  management of, 435-439
  maternal hypoxemia and acidemia associated with, 437
  postpartum, 439
  severe hypertension associated with, 437-439
Ectopic pregnancy, 239
  definition of, 239
  Depo-Provera and, 112
  diagnostic tests and modalities, 240, 242f

Ectopic pregnancy (Continued)
  differential diagnosis, 240
  epidemiology of, 239
  etiology of, 239
  incidence of, 239
  laparoscopy applications, 241-242
  oral contraceptives and, 111t, 103
  persistent, 243
  risk factors for, 240
  signs and symptoms of, 240
  surgical treatment of, 242-243
  treatment of, 241
Edema, 592
Edwards' syndrome, 508, 535
Effexor. See Venlafaxine
Electrolytes, 578
Electromyography, 93f, 92-93
Endocervicitis, 198
Endocrine system, 2
Endometrial ablation, 183
Endometrial biopsy, 143
Endometrial cancer, 107
Endometriosis
  acute, 188
  assessments, 187
  bowel, 191
  chronic, 188
  clinical manifestations of, 185
  definition of, 184, 252
  description of, 184
  diagnosis of, 146
  disease patterns, 189
  epidemiology of, 184
  excision of, 81-82
  follow-up for, 192
  histogenesis, 185
  host responses to, 188
  infertility caused by, 139-140, 186, 190
  laparoscopy for, 147, 187
  laparotomy for, 147
  malignant, 192
  management of, 192
  pain associated with, 185, 190, 252
  peritoneal pockets with, 188
  physical examination for, 186, 252

Endometriosis (*Continued*)
  risk factors for, 184, 185
  surgical therapy for, 146-147
  symptomatic bowel, 191
  treatment of, 144-145
    complications of, 189
    options for, 189
  ureteral, 192
  in vesicouterine pouch, 188
Endometriotic plaque, 81, 82
Endomyometritis, 454, 461-462
Epidural analgesia, 353, 354t
Episiotomy, 339
Ergot alkaloids, 568
Erythromycin
  chancroid treated with, 204
  chlamydia treated with, 199
  donovanosis treated with, 205
  lymphogranuloma venereum treated with, 200
Escitalopram, 317t
Esophageal malformations, 512-513
Estradiol, 328, 600
Estriol, 601
Estrogen therapy
  amenorrhea treated with, 178
  contraindications for, 327
  indications for, 327
  oral estrogens, 328
  osteoporosis treated with, 325
Ethambutol, 475, 476t
Ethinyl estradiol, 101
Eugonadotropic amenorrhea, 174-176
Evening primrose oil, 316t, 319
Exercise-induced amenorrhea, 175
Exophthalmos, 138
Expressed prostatic secretions, 163-164
External genitalia
  anatomy of, 13, 14f
  physical examination of, 3
External iliac artery, 31
External iliac lymph nodes, 34
External oblique muscle, 10f, 11, 12f, 48
Extremities, 3
Eyes, 1, 3

F

Face presentation, 345
Falciform ligament, 10f
Fallopian tubes. *See* Uterine tubes
Famciclovir, 206-207
Family history, 1
Fascia
  anterior lateral abdominal wall, 8-9, 10f, 11
  of Camper, 9, 46
  of Colles, 8, 16
  Gallaudet's, 9
  rectovaginal, 28
  rectovesical, 27
  rectus, 47, 67
  Scarpa's, 8, 16, 46
  superficial, 67
  superficial perineal, 16
  thoracolumbar, 11
  transversalis, 11, 47, 49f
Fasting hyperglycemia, 396t
Fat necrosis, 264
Female infertility
  causes of, 139
  cervical factor, 140, 145, 147
  diagnostic studies for, 141
  differential diagnosis, 271
  endometriosis as cause of, 139-140
  evaluation, 137-139
  gamete intrafallopian transfer for, 149
  history-taking, 137
  hysterosalpingogram evaluations, 141-142
  laparoscopic evaluations, 143
  medical management of, 144
  oocyte donation for, 149
  surgical therapy for, 146
  tubal embryo transfer for, 149
  unexplained, 141, 146
  uterine factor, 145, 147-148
  zygote intrafallopian transfer for, 149
Female pseudohermaphroditism, 170
Female sterilization, 129
  bipolar coagulation, 130-131
  clip application technique, 130, 131f

Female sterilization (Continued)
  complications, 132, 134t
  effectiveness rates, 134t
  failure rates, 132, 132t, 133t
  Falope Ring, 131-132
  fimbriectomy, 129, 131f
  interval, 130-132
  Irving technique, 129, 131f
  minilaparotomy tubal, 132
  Pomeroy technique, 129, 131f
  postpartum tubal, 130
  spring clip, 132
  Uchida technique, 130-132, 131f
  unipolar coagulation, 130
Femoral artery, 32f
Femoral nerve, 33, 37f
Femur length/abdomen circumference ratio, 404
Fentanyl, 352t
Fetal death, 532-533
Fetal growth ratio, 402-403
Fetal hemorrhage, 558
Fetal movement counts/charting, 412, 505
Fetal position, 331-332, 335f
Fetal presentation
  abnormalities of, 342-346
  breech, 331-332, 342-344, 343f, 344b
  brow, 345
  description of, 331-332, 334
  face, 345
  occiput posterior, 344
  occiput transverse, 344-345
Fetal weight, 332-333, 401, 404
Fetus, 577
  amino acids for, 580
  carbohydrates for, 579
  carbon dioxide production, 583
  complex lipids for, 579
  free fatty acids for, 579
  heart rate of, 334
  hyperinsulinemia in, 379
  lung maturity assessments, 381, 525
  macrosomia in
    description of, 332-333, 342, 371

Fetus (Continued)
    ultrasound predictors of, 378
  proteins for, 580
  pulmonary maturity assessments, 381, 525
  thyroid function in, 597
  vitamins for, 578
  well-being assessments, in diabetes mellitus, 380
Fimbriectomy, 129, 131f
Finasteride, 309
Flatulence, 593
Fluconazole, 217, 218
Fluoxetine, 317t, 318t
Flutamide, 309
Fluvoxamine, 317t
Folic acid, 516-520
Follicle, 143
Follicle-stimulating hormone, 599
Forced expiratory volume in 1 second, 468
Forceps delivery, 347
Foreign body mastitis, 264
Fossa ovalis, 8
Free fatty acids, 579
Free thyroid index, 597
Fresh frozen plasma, 568
Fructosamine, 385
Functional bowel disorders, 255
Fundi, 3

G

Galactorrhea, 176
Gallaudet's fascia, 9
Gallbladder, 588
Gamete intrafallopian transfer, 149
Gardnerella vaginalis, 458
Gas cystometry, 92
Gastric motility, 587
Gastric reflux, 587
Gastric secretion, 587
Gastroenteritis, 248
Gastrointestinal system
  physical examination of, 2
  pregnancy-related changes in, 587
Gastroschisis, 529

General anesthesia, 357
   for abdominal–pelvic diagnostic laparoscopy, 74
Genetic counseling, 414
   chromosomal abnormalities, 415, 416t
   client decision making, 415
   goals of, 414-415
   indications for, 415-416
   information gathering, 416-417
   inheritance modes
      autosomal dominant, 419
      autosomal recessive, 420
      mitochondrial, 422
      multifactorial, 421
      X-linked recessive, 420
   parents, 417-418
   prenatal, 415
   principles of, 414
Genetic counselors, 425
Genetic screening, 423, 525
   beta-thalassemia, 424
   cystic fibrosis, 423
   sickle cell anemia, 424
   Tay-Sachs disease, 423
   triple marker, 525, 535
Geneticists, 425
Genital discharge, 269
Genital tract
   bleeding of, 258
   congenital anatomic defects of, 169
   fistulae of, 269
   upper, infection of, 285
Genitofemoral nerve, 37f, 39, 39t
Genitoreproductive system, 2-4
Genuine stress incontinence, 286
Germ cell tumors, 307-308
Gestational age, 329, 369
   assessments, 401
   body symmetry relative to, 402
   low birth weight correlated with, 395
   ultrasound determinations, 530, 532
Gestational diabetes mellitus, 363, 365b, 383
   blood sugar monitoring, 384, 389, 396-399t
   definition of, 383

Gestational diabetes mellitus (Continued)
   diagnosis of, 383
   dietary treatment of, 386, 521-522
   etiology of, 383
   follow-up, 388
   glycemic index of foods, 386, 387b
   hyperglycemia in, 383
   hypocaloric diets, 389-390
   insulin therapy for, 377, 382, 386, 389
   ketone evaluations, 385
   labor and delivery management, 388
   maternal complications associated with, 384
   monitoring of, 384
   nutritional considerations, 386, 521-522
   postpartum monitoring, 388
   risks associated with, 383
   screening algorithm for, 366t
Gestational trophoblastic disease, 243
Gestational weight gain, 515, 516-517f, 518t, 519f
Glomerular filtration rate, 480, 584-585
Glomerulonephritis, 481
Glucose, 579, 585-586
Glucose control, 371, 372t
Glucose tolerance test, 383, 388-389
Glucosuria, 394-395
Gluteal line, 22f
Glyburide, 377
Glycemic index, 386, 387b
Glycopyrrolate test, 96-97
Glycosylated hemoglobin, 375-376, 385
Gonadal dysgenesis, 167-169
Gonadal genesis, 169
Gonadotropin-releasing analogs, 144-145
Gonadotropin-releasing hormone agonists, 309, 317t, 318

Gonorrhea, 194
  bacteremia associated with, 195
  diagnosis of, 196
  etiology of, 194
  incidence of, 194
  pelvic inflammatory disease associated with, 195
  in pregnancy, 195
  prevalence of, 194
  risk factors for, 194
  septic arthritis associated with, 195
  signs and symptoms of, 195
  transmission of, 194
  treatment of, 196
Granuloma, 264
Granuloma inguinale, 204
Granulosa-theca cell tumors, 308
Graves' disease, 138
Group B *Streptococcus*, 451
  antepartum treatment, 454-455
  background, 451
  colonization risk factors, 451b
  diagnosis of, 452
  epidemiology of, 451
  intrapartum treatment, 455, 457
  maternal manifestations of, 453
  morbidity and mortality prevention, 454
  neonatal manifestations of, 452, 456-457
  screening for, 457
  sepsis, 452, 453
  urinary tract manifestations of, 453
Growth retardation. *See* Intrauterine growth retardation
Gynecoid pelvis, 330f
Gynecologic history, 2

H

Haemophilus ducreyi, 203
Haemophilus influenzae, 470
Haemophilus vaginalis, 458
Hair growth
  description of, 304
  pregnancy-related changes, 574

HAIR-AN syndrome, 307
Hasson cannula, 74-75
Head circumference/abdominal circumference ratio, 404
Headaches, 104
Heartburn, 594
HELLP syndrome, 440, 441b
Hematocrit, 520, 575
Hematopoietic system, 1
Hematospermia, 155-166
Hemizona assay, 165
Hemoglobin, 520
Hemophilia A, 421
Hemorrhage. *See* Postpartum hemorrhage
Hemorrhagic corpus luteum of pregnancy, 243
Hemorrhoids, 594
Hepatocellular carcinoma, 107
Hereditary nonpolyposis colorectal cancer, 292-293
Herpes simplex virus, 205
  diagnosis of, 206
  epidemiology of, 205
  HIV infection and, 225
  laboratory tests for, 206
  neonatal infection, 207, 207-208
  in pregnancy, 207
  recurrent, 205-206
  signs and symptoms of, 205-206
  treatment of, 206-207
Hip fractures, 323
Hirsutism
  definition of, 304
  differential diagnosis, 265
  etiology of, 305
  evaluation of, 308
  hair growth, 304
  ovarian causes of, 307-308
  treatment of, 308
History-taking, 1
  chief complaint, 1
  family history, 1
  past surgical history, 1
  preoperative evaluation, 5
  present illness, 1
  systems review, 1-3

HIV
  background, 222
  care of, 447
  chancroid and, 226
  clinical manifestations of, 224
    gynecologic, 224
    initial, 224
  counseling for, 224, 229
  diagnosis of, 224
  epidemiology of, 222
  evaluations, 449
  herpes simplex virus and, 225
  opportunistic infections caused by, 230
  pathophysiology of, 223, 446
  pelvic inflammatory disease and, 226
  in pregnancy, 228, 444
    cervical dysplasia, 450
    complications of, 450
    contraceptive counseling, 231
    counseling, 229
    epidemiology of, 445b
    intrapartum care, 449
    intrapartum management of, 230-231
    obstetric management of, 229
    outcomes, 450
    perinatal transmission, 444, 447t
    postpartum care, 450
    postpartum management of, 231
    prenatal care, 447, 449
    tests for, 228
    transmission, 228, 444, 445
    zidovudine for, 229-230, 449
  preventive care, 449
  risk factors for, 224
  syphilis and, 225-226
  testing for, 223, 228
  transmission of, 222, 228, 444, 445
  tuberculosis and, 476
Holoprosencephaly, 511
Hormonal implants, 107-112, 114t, 134t

Hormone replacement therapy, 327
Hot flashes, 320-321
Human chorionic gonadotropin, 601
  Down syndrome and, 534
  pregnancy verification using, 146, 210, 236, 240
Human immunodeficiency virus. *See* HIV
Human papillomavirus, 104, 290
Human placental lactogen, 601
Humegon, 146
Hydralazine, 438
Hydramnios, 379-380
Hydrocephaly, 510
Hydrothorax, 512
17-Hydroxyprogesterone (17-OHP), 306, 308
  deficiency of, 169
  production of, 601
Hydroxyzine, 352t
Hypercortisolism, 324
Hyperglycemia, 396t
Hypergonadotropic amenorrhea, 173-174
Hypergonadotropic hypogonadism, 152
Hyperkeratosis, 71b
Hypermenorrhea, 179
Hyperparathyroidism, 324
Hyperprolactinemia, 176, 266
Hypertension, 426
  antihypertensive agents for, 438-439
  chronic. *See* Chronic hypertension
  definition of, 426
  eclampsia. *See* Eclampsia
  epidemiology of, 426
  gestational, 427
  HELLP syndrome, 441b, 440
  preeclampsia. *See* Preeclampsia
  pregnancy-induced, 427, 522-523
Hyperthyroidism, 324
Hypertrichosis, 304
Hyperviscous semen, 157
Hypocaloric diets, 389-390

Index

Hypoglycemia, 368, 372
Hypogonadotropic hypogonadism, 152
Hypomenorrhea, 179
Hypoosmotic swelling test, 165
Hypothalamic-pituitary-gonadal axis, 150-152
Hypothyroidism, 543-544
Hysterectomy
  abnormal uterine bleeding treated with, 183
  cervical cancer treated with, 291
  total abdominal, 294
  uterine atony treated with, 569
Hysterosalpingogram, 141-142
Hysteroscopy, 71, 144

I

Idiopathic postpartum renal failure, 487
IgG, 580-581
Iliococcygeus muscle, 21f, 22f, 23t
Iliohypogastric nerve, 36, 37f, 39t, 51f
Ilioinguinal nerve, 39, 39t, 51f
Iliolumbar artery, 32f, 34
Iliopectineal line, 80-81
Immunosuppressive therapy, 486
Incisions, 50, 52f
  Cherney, 56, 59-61, 60f
  Hasson cannula placement, 74-75
  Maylard, 52f, 56-61, 57f, 66
  median, 62f, 62-65
  midline, 50, 52f
  paramedian, 65, 66f
  Pfannenstiel, 52f, 53f, 52-56
  selection of, 50, 51f
  transverse, 50, 65
  vertical, 61, 68, 74-75
Incomplete abortion, 239
Incontinence
  genuine stress, 286
  menopause-related, 322
Inevitable abortion, 239

Infections
  bacterial, 272
  fungal, 273
  male genital tract, 163
  opportunistic, 230
  parasitic, 273
  pelvic, 244
  protozoal, 273
  upper genital tract, 285
  urinary tract, 584
  viral, 273
Inferior epigastric artery, 32f, 48
Inferior gluteal artery, 32f, 33
Inferior gluteal line, 22f
Inferior hypogastric plexus, 43
Inferior vesical artery, 32f
Infertility
  differential diagnosis, 270
  female
    causes of, 139
    cervical factor, 140, 145, 147
    diagnostic studies for, 141
    differential diagnosis, 271
    endometriosis as cause of, 139-140, 186, 190
    evaluation, 137-139
    gamete intrafallopian transfer for, 149
    history-taking, 137
    hysterosalpingogram evaluations, 141-142
    laparoscopic evaluations, 143
    medical management of, 144
    oocyte donation for, 149
    pelvic inflammatory disease as cause of, 212
    surgical therapy for, 146
    tubal embryo transfer for, 149
    unexplained, 141, 146
    uterine factor, 145, 147-148
    zygote intrafallopian transfer for, 149
  male, 150
    causes of, 140-141
    diagnostic tests, 150-165
    differential diagnosis, 270
    endocrine system evaluations, 150-152
    evaluation, 150

Infertility (*Continued*)
    history-taking, 150, 152b
    incidence of, 150
    physical examination for, 150, 153t
Inflammatory bowel disease, 247
Informed consent, 5
Inhalation analgesia, 351
Inheritance
    autosomal dominant, 419
    autosomal recessive, 420
    mitochondrial, 422
    multifactorial, 421
    X-linked recessive, 420
Inlet dystocia, 346
Insulin therapy
    gestational diabetes mellitus treated with, 377, 382, 386, 389
    pregestational diabetes mellitus treated with, 382, 392
    in pregnancy, 383
Integument, 1, 3
Intercostal nerves, 51f
Internal genitalia
    anatomy of, 23-24, 25f
    physical examination of, 3
Internal iliac artery, 31, 32f
    anterior trunk, 31
    posterior trunk, 34
Internal iliac lymph nodes, 34
Internal oblique muscle, 10f, 11, 48-49
Internal pudendal artery, 19, 32f, 33
Interstitial cystitis, 250
Intestinal obstruction, 247
Intrauterine adhesions, 148
Intrauterine catheters, 342
Intrauterine device, 115-116
    antibiotic prophylaxis, 117
    composition of, 115-116
    considerations before using, 116
    effectiveness rates, 134t
    insertion of, 117
    mechanism of action, 115
    patient education about, 116
    in patients with HIV, 231
    perforation caused by, 118
    pregnancy while using, 118-120

Intrauterine device (*Continued*)
    removal of, 117, 117f
Intrauterine growth patterns, 396-397
    in multiple gestations, 400-401
Intrauterine growth retardation, 395
    amniotic fluid volume assessments, 413-414
    aneuploidy and, 510
    assessments, 407-408
    causes of, 405
    clinical presentations, 409-412
    definitions, 401
    delivery delays, 408-409
    detection of, 406
    diabetes mellitus and, 371, 378
    fetal assessments, 412
    indices of, 402-403
    karyotyping, 408
    management of, 408
    obstetric dates, 406-407
    risk evaluations, 407
    significance of, 395
    size—dates discrepancies, 409-412
    ultrasound detection of, 404, 406-407
Intravenous pyelogram, 84-85
Intravesical pressure, 90
Involuntary detrusor contraction, 92
Iron, 516-519
Irritable bowel syndrome, 255-256
Irving technique, 129, 131f
Ischial tuberosity, 15f
Ischiocavernosus muscle, 18f, 19
Isoniazid, 475, 476t
Itraconazole, 218

J
Joints
    pelvic, 34
    physical examination of, 2, 4

K
Kallmann's syndrome, 170
Karyotyping, 171, 408

Kearns-Sayre syndrome, 423
Ketamine, 350-351, 352t
Ketorolac, 351
Ketosis, 385, 388, 393
Kidneys
  biopsy of, 484
  blood flow changes during pregnancy, 584, 577
  diseases of. See Renal disease
  failure of. See Renal failure
  pregnancy-related changes, 480, 583
  transplantation of. See Renal transplantation
Klebsiella pneumoniae, 470
Krukenberg tumor, 307
Kyphoscoliosis, 478

L

Labetalol, 438
Labia majora, 13, 14f
Labia minora, 13, 14f, 29f
Labor and delivery, 335. See also Pregnancy
  abdominal examination, 333-334
  abnormalities of, 340
    arrest disorders, 342
    breech presentation, 331-332, 342-344, 343f, 344b,
    description of, 340-341
    passage dystocias, 346-347
    passenger, 342-346
    power, 341-342
    prolonged latent phase, 341
    protraction disorders, 341
    shoulder dystocia, 345-346, 374, 381
  asthma considerations, 469
  Cesarean section, 347, 360
  in diabetes mellitus patients, 388, 393
  digital examination, 334
  engagement, 337
  episiotomy, 339
  evaluations, 333
  factors involved in, 329
  fetal descent, 337

Labor and delivery (Continued)
  fetal presentation, 331-332, 334
  first stage of, 337-338
  forceps, 347
  fourth stage of, 339
  gestational age, 329
  in gestational diabetes mellitus patients, 388
  history-taking, 333
  initiation of, 329
  lacerations during, 339
  mechanism of, 337
  normal, 329
  operative, 347, 358
  oxytocics used in, 340
  pelvic examination, 334-335
  pelvic types, 329-331, 330f
  physical examination, 333-334
  placental separation, 338-339
  in preeclamptic patients, 430
  in pregestational diabetes mellitus patients, 393
  preterm, 370
  second stage of, 338
  stages of, 335-339, 336f
  term, 329
  third stage of, 338-339
Labor pain
  analgesic or anesthetic interventions for, 348
  combined spinal and epidural, 357
  comparison of, 349t
  considerations for, 360
  continuous techniques, 354
  epidural, 353, 354t
  general anesthesia, 357
  inhalation, 351
  intravenous adjuvants, 351
  ketamine, 350-351, 352t
  ketorolac, 351
  neuraxial, 349, 349t, 353
  nonpharmacologic techniques, 350
  opioids, 350, 356-357
  psychoprophylactic, 350, 349t
  single-injection techniques, 356
  subarachnoid, 353, 354t, 356

Labor pain (Continued)
    systemic intravenous, 349t
    characteristics of, 347
    physiologic effects of, 348
Lacerations
    small bowel, 78
    umbilical cord, 558
Lactation amenorrhea method, 123
Lamivudine, 230
Langer's lines, 46, 47f, 50-61
Laparoscopy
    abdominal pain evaluations, 236-238
    abdominal–pelvic diagnostic. See Abdominal–pelvic diagnostic laparoscopy
    ectopic pregnancy indications, 242, 241
    endometriosis uses, 147, 187
    female infertility evaluations, 143
    pelvic pain evaluations, 236-238
Laparotomy, 147
Lateral femoral cutaneous nerve, 37f, 39, 39t
Lateral sacral artery, 34
Leber's optic neuropathy, 423
Left-frozen-pelvis, 82-83
Leg cramps, 595
Leiomyomas, 246
Leiomyomata, 147-148
Leopold maneuvers, 331-332, 332f, 334
Leuprolide, 318t
Levator ani muscle, 18f, 20, 23t
Levofloxacin
    chlamydia treated with, 199
    gonorrhea treated with, 196-197
    pelvic inflammatory disease treated with, 211
Lexapro. See Escitalopram
Ligaments, 35
    broad, 23-24, 25f
    cardinal, 28
    falciform, 10f
    ovarian, 23-24, 25f, 26f
    round, 26f

Ligaments (Continued)
    sacrospinous, 15f, 35, 36f
    sacrotuberous, 15f, 18f, 35, 36f
    suspensory ligament of the ovary, 23-24
    uterosacral, 28
Ligamentum flavum, 353
Ligamentum teres, 10f
Limb reduction defects, after chorionic villus sampling, 563
Linea alba, 9-11, 10f, 12f, 47
Linea arcuata, 11
Linea semilunares, 11
Lipids, 579
Lipoid cell tumors, 308
Liver, 587
Lorazepam, 352t
Low birth weight, 395, 402
Lower motor neuron lesions, 93
Lumbar plexus, 36, 37f
    anatomy of, 36
    branches of, 36, 39, 39t
    femoral nerve, 33, 37f
    genitofemoral nerve, 39, 39t
    iliohypogastric nerve, 36, 37f, 39t, 51f
    ilioinguinal nerve, 39, 39t
    lateral femoral cutaneous nerve, 37f, 39, 39t
    obturator nerve, 39, 39t
Lumbosacral joint, 34
Lumbosacral trunk, 35
Lung maturity assessments in fetus, 381, 525
Luteal phase defect, 141, 143
Luvox. See Fluvoxamine
Lymph nodes
    external iliac, 34
    internal iliac, 34
    paraaortic, 34
    physical examination of, 3
    sacral, 34
Lymphatic system
    of pelvis, 34
    of perineum, 20
Lymphogranuloma venereum, 199

Lymphoproliferative disease, 146

M
Macroglossia, 545
Macrosomia, 332-333, 342, 371
 definition of, 384
 ultrasound predictors of, 378
Magnesium, 316
Magnesium sulfate, 435-436, 437t
Male infertility, 150
 causes of, 140-141
 diagnostic tests, 150-165
 differential diagnosis, 270
 endocrine system evaluations, 150-152
 evaluation, 150
 history-taking, 150, 152b
 incidence of, 150
 physical examination for, 150, 153t
Male pseudohermaphroditism, 169-170
Mannitol, 246
Mantoux test, 473
Marginal artery, 23-24
Marshall-Marchetti-Bonney stress test, 97
Mastitis, 263-264
Maternal changes during pregnancy. *See* Pregnancy, maternal changes during
Maternal nutrition. *See* Nutrition
Maternal serum alpha-fetoprotein, 370, 410, 525
 chromosomal abnormalities, 530
 Down syndrome and, 533
 elevated levels of
  amniocentesis evaluations, 532
  evaluation of patient with, 530, 531f
  fetal anomalies associated with, 528
  fetal death and, 532-533
  management of, 533

Maternal serum alpha-fetoprotein (*Continued*)
  nonfetal anomaly causes of, 532
 factors that affect, 527
 fetal levels of, 526, 526f
 measurement of, 527
 neural tube defect screening using, 528, 529t
 physiology of, 525
 renal abnormalities, 530
Maternal serum unconjugated estriol, 534-535
Mayer-Rokitansky-Kuster-Hauser syndrome, 169
Maylard incision, 52f, 56-61, 57f, 66
McBurney's point, 247
McRoberts maneuver, 346
Mean corpuscular hemoglobin concentration, 520
Mean corpuscular volume, 520
Meckel's diverticulitis, 248-249
Median incision, 62f, 62-65
Medical geneticists, 425
Mefenamic acid, 319
Melasma, 575
Meningomyelocele, 510
Menometrorrhagia, 180
Menopause, 320
 atrophic vaginitis associated with, 321-322
 definition of, 320
 epidemiology of, 320
 hot flashes associated with, 320-321
 incontinence associated with, 322
 mood changes associated with, 322
 pathophysiology of, 320
 sexual changes secondary to, 322-323
 sleep disturbances associated with, 322
 symptoms of, 320
Menorrhagia, 179

Menstrual cycle
  abdominal pain and, 234
  follicular phase of, 142
  luteal phase of, 141-143
  menstrual phase of, 143
  phases of, 142-143
Menstrual history, 138
Menstruation
  body fat levels for, 175
  endometriosis risks, 185
  oral contraceptives effect on, 103
Mentum, 345
Meperidine, 352t
Mesentery
  avulsion injury to, 78-79
Mesometrium, 25f
Mesosalpinx, 25f, 26f
Mesovarium, 25f
Mestranol, 101
Metformin, 377-378
Methylergonovine, 340
Metrodin, 146
Metronidazole
  bacterial vaginosis treated with, 215, 462-464
  pelvic inflammatory disease treated with, 211
Metrorrhea, 180
Miconazole, 217
Micrognathia, 511
Micturition, 83
Midarm circumference/head circumference, 403, 404t
Midazolam, 352t
Middle rectal artery, 32f, 33
Middle sacral artery, 30
Midpelvic dystocia, 346-347
Midpelvis, 331
Minipill, 113
Minute ventilation, 582
Mitochondrial inheritance, 422
Mittelschmerz, 254
Mixed neuron lesions, 93
Mons pubis, 13, 14f
Montevideo unit, 341
Morning after pill, 113-115
"Morning sickness," 523
Morphine, 352t
Mouth, 3

Müllerianosis, 189
Multicystic kidneys, 514
Multifactorial inheritance, 421
Multiple gestations, 400-401, 521, 574
Multiple myeloma, 324
Muscles, 2
Musculoskeletal system, 2
Mycobacterium tuberculosis, 209
Myomas, 145, 147
Myometrium, 26f

N
Nails, 574
Nalbuphine, 352t
Naloxone, 352t
Natural family planning, 124
Nausea, 595
Neck, 3
Necrospermia, 158
Neisseria gonorrhoeae, 194, 209
Neonate
  with Down syndrome, 539
  growth of, 401-402
  sepsis in, 452-453
  thyroid function in, 599
Nephrolithiasis, 482
Nephrotic syndrome, 482, 530
Neural tube defects, 528, 529t
Neuraxial analgesia, 349, 349t, 353
Neurofibromatosis type I, 419-420
Neurologic system
  physical examination of, 4
Neurosyphilis, 201-202
Nevirapine, 230
Nifedipine, 438
Nipple stimulation test, 499
Nitrogenous compounds, 581
Nonimmune hydrops, 514
Nonstress test, 412, 494, 496f
Norplant. *See* Hormonal implants
No-scalpel vasectomy, 128f, 127
Nose, 1, 3
Nuchal fold, 509
Nutrition
  in diabetes mellitus, 375, 376b, 386, 521-522
  maternal, 515, 573

Nutrition (Continued)
  in pregnancy, 515
    anemia, 521
    complications-related considerations, 521
    folic acid, 516-520
    goals, 515-521
    inadequacies, 524
    iron, 516-519
    "morning sickness," 523
    multiple fetuses, 521
    pregnancy-induced hypertension, 522-523
    recommendations, 516t
    sodium, 520
    vitamin A, 519-520
    zinc, 519
  premenstrual syndrome and, 312-316
  vegetarianism, 524
Nystatin, 217

O

Obstetric history, 2
Obstetric trauma, 566
Obturator artery, 32f, 33
Obturator externus muscle, 18f
Obturator internus muscle, 18f, 21f, 23
Obturator nerve, 39, 39t
Occiput posterior presentation, 344
Occiput transverse presentation, 344-345
Ofloxacin
  chlamydia treated with, 199
  gonorrhea treated with, 196, 196, 197
  pelvic inflammatory disease treated with, 211
17-OHP. *See* 17-Hydroxyprogesterone
Oligoasthenoteratozoospermia, 158
Oligohydramnios, 414, 504
Oligomenorrhea, 180
Oligospermia, 155-166, 156b
Oligozoospermia, 158
Omphalocele, 513, 529

Oocyte donation, 149
Opioids, 350, 356-357
Opportunistic infections, 230
Oral contraceptives, 101
  abnormal uterine bleeding treated with, 183
  administration of, 103, 114t
  amenorrhea and, 175, 178
  antibiotics and, 102, 102b
  benefits of, 103-104
  cancer risks, 108-111
  cardiovascular disease and, 104, 105b
  cervical cancer and, 104
  contraindications, 107b, 108t
  disadvantages of, 103-104
  ectopic pregnancy and, 103, 111t
  effectiveness rates, 101-102, 134t
  endometriosis treated with, 145
  estrogen, 101
  headaches caused by, 104
  hirsutism treated with, 308
  mechanism of action, 101
  patch, 101
  premenstrual disorder treated with, 316-317, 317t
  progestins, 101
  selection of, 109t
  side effects of, 103-104, 105b
  types of, 101
Oral glucose tolerance test, 364, 366t, 384b
Oral hypoglycemic agents, 377-378
Organomegaly, 3
Orgasm dysfunction, 284
Osteomalacia, 324
Osteopenia, 324
Osteoporosis, 323
  definition of, 323-324
  diagnosis of, 324
  differential diagnosis, 324
  endometriosis and, 186, 192
  epidemiology of, 323

Osteoporosis (Continued)
  hip fractures associated with, 323
  pathophysiology of, 323
  risk factors for, 323
  treatment of, 192, 325
Ovarian artery, 23-24, 25f, 30
Ovarian cancer, 299
  clinical presentation of, 301
  description of, 299
  diagnosis of, 301
  epidemiology of, 299
  epithelial, 103
  etiology of, 300
  histological classification of, 300, 300t
  oral contraceptives and, 103, 107
  prevention of, 301
  prognosis for, 303
  staging of, 302t, 303
  treatment of, 303
Ovarian cyst rupture, 245
Ovarian failure, 141, 146, 273
Ovarian hyperstimulation syndrome, 245
Ovarian insensitivity syndrome, 169
Ovarian ligament, 23-24, 25f, 26f
Ovarian mass, 277
Ovarian neoplasms, 307-308
Ovarian remnant syndrome, 254
Ovarian torsion, 245
Ovaries
  abdominal–pelvic diagnostic laparoscopy of, 77
  anatomy of, 23-24, 25f
  pregnancy-related changes in, 588
Ovulation disorders
  female infertility caused by, 141
  treatment of, 145-146
Ovulation method, 125
Ovulatory pain, 254
Ovum, 124-125
Oxytocics, 340
Oxytocin, 340, 568

P
Packed red blood cells, 568
Pain
  abdominal. See Abdominal pain
  adnexal, 244
  endometriosis-associated, 185, 190, 252
  labor. See Labor pain
  ovulatory, 254
  pelvic. See Pelvic pain
  "trigger point," 255
  urinary tract sources of, 249
  vascular sources of, 250
Pancreas, 600
Papanicolaou smear, 3-4, 69
  classification of, 70t
  grading of, 70t
  HIV testing, 227
  liquid-based screening systems, 69
  patient preparation for, 69
  sampling of, 69
Paraaortic lymph nodes, 34
Paramedian incision, 65, 66f
Pararectal space, 24
Parasympathetic nervous system, 40, 44f
Paravesical space, 24, 27f
Parlodel, 176
Paroxetine (Paxil), 317t, 318t
Parturition, 329
Past surgical history, 1
Patau's syndrome, 509
PCT. See Postcoital text
Peak expiratory flow rate, 468
Pelvic adhesions, 141, 146, 148-149
Pelvic congestion syndrome, 254
Pelvic diaphragm, 20, 21f, 22f
Pelvic examination, 235-236, 334-335
Pelvic floor, 28, 29f
Pelvic infections, 244
Pelvic inflammatory disease, 208
  cervical neoplasia and, 227-228
  chlamydia, 198
  definition of, 208
  diagnosis of, 210
  differential diagnosis, 285
  epidemiology of, 209
  etiology of, 209
  follow-up for, 212

Pelvic inflammatory disease (Continued)
  gonorrhea, 195
  HIV infection and, 226
  incidence of, 209
  infertility caused by, 212
  laboratory findings, 210
  long-term sequelae of, 212
  management of, 211, 212t
  microbial causes of, 209
  prevalence of, 209
  risk factors for, 209
  signs and symptoms of, 210
Pelvic inlet, 329-331
Pelvic joints, 34
Pelvic kidney, 250
Pelvic lymphadenectomy, 291
Pelvic mass
  gynecologic causes of, 274
  nongynecologic causes of, 280
Pelvic outlet, 331
Pelvic pain, 281
  acute, 281
  adenomyosis, 253
  adhesions, 253
  adnexal origins of, 244
  anatomy of, 233
  assessment of, 234
  chronic, 233, 256, 282
  differential diagnosis, 237b
  dysmenorrhea, 251
  early pregnancy complications as cause of, 238
  history-taking, 234-235
  laparoscopy evaluations, 236-238
  leiomyomas, 246
  physical examination for, 235-236
  physiology of, 233
  ultrasound evaluations, 236
  urinary tract sources of, 249
  vascular sources of, 250
Pelvic peritoneum, 28
Pelvic thrombophlebitis, 250
Pelvis
  abdominal–pelvic diagnostic laparoscopy of, 72-77
  android, 330f
  anthropoid, 330f
Pelvis (Continued)
  blood supply of, 30, 32f, 33f
  collateral circulation, 34
  fetal positions in, 331-332, 335f
  gynecoid, 330f
  ligaments of, 35
  lymphatic drainage of, 34
  measurements of, 331f
  midpelvis, 331
  nerves of, 35
  platypelloid, 330f
  types of, 329-331, 330f
  viscera of, 23
Penicillin, 202
Pentazocine, 352t
Pentobarbital, 352t
Percutaneous umbilical blood sampling, 551
Perforation, small bowel, 78
Pergonal, 146
Perimenopause, 320
Perimetrium, 26f
Perineal body, 14f, 15f, 18f, 21f
Perineal lacerations, 339
Perineal muscles, 19
Perineal pouch
  deep, 19
  superficial, 16
Perineum, 13
  anal triangle, 13, 15f, 16
  anatomy of, 8, 15f, 17f, 18f
  boundaries of, 13
  floor of, 13
  lymphatic drainage of, 20
  urogenital triangle. *See* Urogenital triangle
Peripheral arterial vasodilation, 576
Peripheral pulses, 3
Peritoneum, 10f
  closure of, 65
  pelvic, 28
Pessary test, 98
Pfannenstiel incision, 52-56, 52f, 53f
Phentolamine testing, 96
Phenylketonuria, 420
Physical examination, 1, 3-5
Pica, 523
Pinocytosis, 580

Piriformis muscle, 20, 21f, 22f, 23
Pituitary gland, 599
Placenta, 577
  amino acids transport via, 580
  bilirubin transport via, 581
  carbohydrate transport via, 579
  complex lipids transport via, 579
  electrolytes transport via, 578
  free fatty acids transport via, 579
  hormones produced, 600
  nitrogenous compounds transport via, 581
  nucleic acids transport via, 581
  physiologic functions of, 578
  protein transport via, 580
  temperature regulation by, 581
  thyroid hormone transport via, 599t
  vitamin transport via, 578
  water transport via, 578
Placenta accreta, 566, 570
Placenta increta, 566, 570
Placenta percreta, 566, 570
Plasma volume, 576
Platypelloid pelvis, 330f
Plexus
  coccygeal, 36
  inferior hypogastric, 43
  lumbar. *See* Lumbar plexus
  sacral, 35
  superior hypogastric, 40-43
Pneumonia, 469
  aspiration, 470
  diagnosis of, 471
  etiology of, 470
  incidence of, 469
  management of, 472
  morbidity and mortality, 469
  pathophysiology of, 470
Podofilox, 227
Podophyllin, 227
Polycystic ovarian syndrome, 141
  amenorrhea and, 176-177
  androgen production and, 307
Polymenorrhea, 180
Polyps, 147
Polyzoospermia, 158
Pomeroy technique, 129, 131f

Ponderal index, 403, 404t
Postcoital test (PCT), 143, 165
Posterior gluteal line, 22f
Posterior labial artery, 16
Posterior labial nerve, 16
Postoperative orders, 6
Postpartum endomyometritis, 461-462
Postpartum hemorrhage
  algorithm for, 571f
  diagnosis of, 565
  etiologies of, 565
    maternal coagulation defect, 567
    obstetric trauma, 566
    placental abnormalities, 566, 570
    placental site involution, 567
    retained placenta, 566
    uterine atony, 565, 567-569
    uterine inversion, 567, 570
    uterine rupture, 566, 570
    vulvar hematoma, 570
  importance of, 565
  maternal deaths caused by, 565
  treatment of, 567
    abdominal packing, 569
    algorithm for managing, 571f
    blood products, 568
    catheterization and embolization, 571
    manipulations, 567
    pharmacologic and medical, 568
    principles, 567
    surgical, 569
Postpill amenorrhea, 175
Potassium homeostasis, 481
Pouch of Douglas, 28
Prealbumin, 520
Precocious puberty, 266
Prednisone, 486
Preeclampsia
  angiotensin II infusion test for, 428
  definition of, 426
  diagnosis of, 428
  etiology of, 427
  incidence of, 427

Preeclampsia *(Continued)*
  labor and delivery induction in, 430
  management of, 429, 429f
  mild, 430, 431b, 432f
  prediction of, 428
  prevention of, 433
  risk factors for, 427
  severe, 431, 433, 434f
Preganglionic sympathetic fibers, 40
Pregestational diabetes mellitus, 367, 390
  discontinuation of medications, 390
  follow-up, 393
  insulin regimen for, 382, 392
  labor and delivery management, 393
  monitoring of, 392
  postpartum monitoring, 393
  preconception concerns, 390
  risks, 391
Pregnancy. *See also* Labor and delivery
  adrenal glands during, 600
  alimentary changes during, 520-521
  bacterial vaginosis in, 215, 461
  chlamydia infection in, 199
  complications of, 521
  creatinine clearance during, 586, 586t
  dialysis during, 484
  diarrhea during, 523
  discomforts during, 589, 590b
    aches, 589
    backache, 589
    breast tenderness, 591
    constipation, 523, 591
    diaphragm pressure, 591
    dizziness, 591
    dyspnea, 592
    edema, 592
    emotional, 592
    fainting, 591
    fatigue, 593
    finger tingling, numbness or swelling, 593

Pregnancy *(Continued)*
    flatulence, 593
    foot pain, 593
    groin pain, 593
    heartburn, 594
    hemorrhoids, 594
    leg cramps, 595
    light-headedness, 591
    nausea, 595
    vaginal discharge, 594
    varicose veins, 596
    vulvar varicose veins, 596
  ectopic. *See* Ectopic pregnancy
  gonococcal infection in, 195
  hemorrhagic corpus luteum of, 243
  herpes simplex virus in, 207
  history-taking, 2
  HIV in. *See* HIV, in pregnancy
  insulin treatment in, 383
  maternal changes during
    acid-base physiology, 585
    appetite, 587
    arterial circulation, 576
    bladder, 584
    blood volume, 575
    breasts, 588
    cervix, 589, 589t
    fallopian tubes, 588
    gallbladder, 588
    gastric motility, 587
    gastric reflux, 587
    gastric secretion, 587
    gastrointestinal system, 587
    glomerular filtration rate, 584-585
    hair, 574
    intestinal absorption, 587
    kidneys, 583
    large intestine, 587
    liver, 587
    nails, 574
    ovaries, 588
    plasma volume, 576
    potassium levels, 585
    pulmonary function, 582
    renal blood flow, 577, 584
    reproductive system, 588
    respiratory system, 581
    skin, 575

Pregnancy (*Continued*)
   sodium levels, 585
   urinary output, 585
   urinary system, 583
   uterine blood flow, 576
   uterus, 588
   vagina, 589
   vulva, 589
  nonobstetric surgery during, 359
  nutrition during. *See* Nutrition, in pregnancy
  pancreatic function during, 600
  renal changes during, 480
  in renal transplantation patient, 485
  renin–angiotensin system during, 586
  smoking cessation during, 477b
  syphilis in, 202-203
  thyroid function during, 596, 598t
  uric acid levels in, 586
  uterine incarceration, 243
  weight gain during, 515, 516-517f, 518t, 519f, 573
Pregnancy-induced hypertension, 427, 522-523
Premature ovarian failure, 320
Premature rupture of membranes, 461
Premenstrual dysphoric disorder
  definition of, 310
  diagnosis of, 311, 313b
  epidemiology of, 310
  treatment of, 317, 318t
Premenstrual syndrome, 105b, 283
  alternative therapies for, 316t
  definition of, 310
  diagnostic criteria for, 312b, 310, 311
  epidemiology of, 310
  etiology of, 310
  management of, 311, 316t
  nutritional considerations, 312-316
  pharmacologic treatment of, 316-319, 317t

Premenstrual syndrome (*Continued*)
  symptoms of, 311
Preoperative evaluation, 5
Preoperative note, 6
Present illness, 1
Preterm labor, 370
Primary amenorrhea, 167-170, 261
Primary dysmenorrhea, 251-252
Progestagens, 328
Progesterone, 328
  amenorrhea treated with, 178
  withdrawal test, 171
Progestins
  contraceptives, 107, 114t, 134t
  endometriosis treated with, 145
Progress notes, 4
Prolactin, 599
Promethazine, 352t
Propiomazine, 352t
Prostaglandin F2, 340, 568
Proteins, 580
Proteinuria, 428, 431
Prozac. *See* Fluoxetine
Pruritus, 575
Pseudocyesis, 175
Pseudohermaphroditism
  female, 170
  male, 169-170
Psychogenic amenorrhea, 174-175
Puberty
  delayed, 267
  precocious, 266
Pubic symphysis, 15f, 29f, 34
Public Law 94-142, 539
Pubococcygeus muscle, 21f, 23t
Puborectalis muscle, 21f, 23t
Pubovaginalis muscle, 21f, 23t
Pudendal cleft, 13
Pudendal nerve, 19-20, 36
Pulmonary capillary wedge pressure, 488
Pulmonary disease, 464
  asthma. *See* Asthma

Pulmonary disease (Continued)
  chronic respiratory disease, 476
  dyspnea, 465
  pneumonia. See Pneumonia
  tobacco smoking, 476, 477b
  tuberculosis. See Tuberculosis
Pulmonary maturity assessments in fetus, 381, 525
Pyelectasis, 514
Pyelonephritis, 481
Pyospermia, 155-166, 164
Pyramidalis muscle, 11-13, 12f
Pyrazinamide, 476t
Pyridoxine, 316, 476t

Q
Q-tip test, 97-98

R
Rapid fill cystometry, 95
Rectal injuries, 79
Rectouterine fossa, 28, 29f
Rectovaginal examination, 4, 235
Rectovaginal fascia, 28
Rectovaginal pouch, 76
Rectovesical fascia, 27
Rectus abdominis, 10f, 47-48, 49f
Rectus fascia, 47, 67
Rectus sheath, 11, 46
Renal biopsy, 484
Renal blood flow, 584, 577
Renal disease, 480
  chronic, 483
  glomerulonephritis, 481
  nephrolithiasis, 482
  nephrotic syndrome, 482
  polycystic disease, 482
  preexisting, pregnancy effects on, 481
  pyelonephritis, 481
  severity of, 483
Renal failure
  acute obstetric, 487, 489t, 490t, 490-491
  delivery management in, 491
  idiopathic postpartum, 487
  nutritional considerations for, 490

Renal insufficiency, 483
Renal plasma flow, 480
Renal transplantation, 486
  immunosuppressive therapy, 486
  maternal follow-up, 487
  pregnancy in recipient of, 485
Renin—angiotensin system, 586
Reproductive tract
  abnormalities of, 268
  bacterial infections of, 272
  fungal infections of, 273
  infections of, 272
  parasitic infections of, 273
  protozoal infections of, 273
  viral infections of, 273
Residual urine measurements, 85
Respiratory system
  physical examination of, 2
  pregnancy-related changes, 581
Retropubic space, 27
Reversed end-diastolic velocity, 504, 505
Rhythm method of contraception, 124, 135t
Rifampin, 475, 476t
Round ligament, 26f

S
Sacral evoked responses, 94
Sacral plexus, 35
Sacrococcygeal joint, 34
Sacroiliac joint, 34
Sacrospinous ligament, 15f, 36f, 35
Sacrotuberous ligament, 15f, 18f, 35, 36f
Sacrum, 21f, 24-27
Saddle block, 356
Salpingectomy, 243
Salpingiocentesis, 242
Salpingitis, 240
Sarcoidosis, 478
Scarpa's fascia, 8, 16, 46
Sciatic nerve, 35
Secobarbital, 352t
Secondary dysmenorrhea, 252
Selective estrogen receptor modulators, 325

Semen
  cellular components of, 163-164
  definition of, 152-164
  hyperviscous, 157
  liquefaction of, 155-166
  white blood cells in, 163-164
Semen analysis
  agglutination, 160-162
  antibody-agglutination testing, 162-163, 163b
  definition of, 152-164
  differential diagnoses based on, 156b
  macroscopic examination, 155
  morphology evaluations, 160, 161f, 162f
  motility evaluations, 158-160
  normal parameters, 140
  requirements for, 152-155
  semen collection, 155
  sperm count, 157-158, 159t
  viscosity, 157
Septic abortion, 239
Septic arthritis, 195
Sertoli-Leydig cell tumors, 307
Sertraline, 317t, 318t
Sex hormone-binding globulin, 305
Sexual dysfunctions, 284
Sexual history, 2, 137-138
Sexuality disorders, 285
Shoulder dystocia, 345-346, 374, 381
Sickle cell anemia, 424
Single umbilical artery, 514
Sinuses, 1
Skin, 575
Skull, 3
Small bowel
  abdominal-pelvic diagnostic laparoscopy of, 76
  injuries to, during diagnostic studies, 77
  laceration of, 78
  perforation of, 78
  thermal injury to, 78
Small bowel mesenteric occlusion, 250-251
Small for gestational age, 402

Smoking, 104, 476, 477b, 524
SOAP format, 4
Sodium
  homeostasis of, 480-481
  during pregnancy, 520, 585
Sodium nitroprusside, 438-439
Spaces
  pararectal, 24
  paravesical, 24, 27f
  retropubic, 27
Spectinomycin, 196
Speculum examination, 3-4
Sperm, 124-125
  agglutination of, 160-162
  morphology of, 160, 161f, 162f
  motility of, 158-160
Sperm count, 157-158, 159t
Sperm function tests, 164-165
  acrosin assay, 165
  cervical mucus penetration, 165
  hemizona assay, 165
  hypoosmotic swelling test, 165
  sperm penetration assay, 164-165
Spermicides, 123
Sphincter urethrae muscle, 19
Spina bifida, 528, 557
Spironolactone, 308-309, 317t, 318-319
Splanchnic nerves, 44f
Spontaneous abortion, 239
Squamous intraepithelial lesion, 70t
Staphylococcus aureus, 470
Starvation ketosis, 523-524
Sterilization
  effectiveness rates, 134t
  female. *See* Female sterilization
  vasectomy, 125, 127f, 128f
Streptococcus pneumoniae, 470
Streptomycin, 476, 476t
Stress incontinence, 286
Subarachnoid anesthesia, 353, 354t
Subarachnoid block, 356
Subcostal nerves, 51f
Sulfonylureas, 390
Superficial perineal pouch, 16
Superior gluteal artery, 32f, 34
Superior hypogastric plexus, 40-43

Index

Superior rectal artery, 30
Superior vesical artery, 32f
Suspensory ligament of the ovary, 23-24
Swyer's syndrome, 169
Sympathetic nervous system, 40
Symptothermal method, 124-125
Syphilis, 200
  congenital, 201
  diagnosis of, 201
  etiology of, 200
  HIV infection and, 225-226
  latent, 201
  neurosyphilis, 201, 202
  in pregnancy, 202-203
  primary, 201
  secondary, 201
  tertiary, 201
  treatment of, 202
  treponemal tests for, 202
Systemic lupus erythematosus, 482
Systems review, 1-3

T

Tamoxifen, 178
Tay-Sachs disease, 423
Teeth, 1
Terconazole, 217
Teriparatide, 325
Term labor, 329
Testosterone, 305
Tetracycline, 202
Thoracolumbar fascia, 11
Threatened abortion, 239
Throat, 1, 3
Thromboembolic prophylaxis, 6
Thrombophlebitis, 250
Thyroid function, 596, 598t
Thyronine, 596
Thyrotropin-releasing hormone, 596
Tidal volume, 582
Tioconazole, 217
Tobacco smoking, 476, 477b
Total abdominal hysterectomy, 294
Transferrin, 520
Transvaginal ultrasound, 293

Transversalis fascia, 11, 47, 49f
Transverse abdominis muscle, 10f, 11, 49
Transverse ducts of epoophoron, 26f
Transversus abdominus, 46
Treponema pallidum, 200
Trichloroacetic acid, 227
Trichomonal vaginitis, 214t
Trichomonas vaginalis, 218, 219
Trichomoniasis, 218
"Trigger point" pain, 255
Triiodothyronine, 596
Trimethoprim-sulfamethoxazole, 204
Triple marker screening, 525, 535
  abnormal results, 536t
  benefits of, 537
  chromosome abnormality detection using, 535, 536
  Down syndrome, 26, 536
  issues regarding, 537
Trisomy 13. *See* Patau's syndrome
Trisomy 18. *See* Edwards' syndrome
Trisomy 21. *See* Down syndrome
Trocars, 75
Tubal embryo transfer, 149
Tuberculin skin test, 474
Tuberculosis, 472
  clinical presentation of, 473, 475
  diagnosis of, 473
  HIV and, 476
  incidence of, 472
  isoniazid prophylaxis for, 475, 476t
  Mantoux test for, 473
  pathophysiology of, 472
  in pregnancy, 474
  treatment of, 475, 476t
  tuberculin skin test for, 474
Turner's syndrome, 167-168, 508
Tzanck smear, 206

U

Uchida technique, 130-132, 131f
Ulcerative colitis, 247

Index

Ultrasound
  abdominal pain evaluations, 236
  aneuploidy detection using, 509, 514
  ectopic pregnancy diagnosis using, 241
  fetal growth assessments, 414
  fetal macrosomia determinations, 378
  gestational age determinations, 369
  intrauterine growth retardation detection using, 406-407
  intrauterine growth retardation determinations, 378
  ovarian cancer evaluations, 302-303
  pelvic pain evaluations, 236
  primary amenorrhea evaluations, 171
  transvaginal, 293
  umbilical artery Doppler, 381
  uterine cancer evaluations, 293
Umbilical artery, 31
Upper motor neuron lesions, 93
Ureter
  abdominal, 28-30
  congenital anomalies of, 81
  injuries to, 83
  pelvic, 31f, 30
Ureteral calculi, 249-250
Ureteral catheters, 83
Ureteral dissection, 80
  endometriosis, 81-82
  indications for, 80
  left-frozen-pelvis, 82-83
  operative procedures for, 81
  topographical anatomy, 80
Urethra, 18f
Urethral denervation sensitivity testing, 97
Urethral pressure profile, 87-88, 89f, 89t
Urethral sphincter, 15f
Urethral syndrome, 250
Urethroscopy, 85, 86t
Uric acid, 586
Urinalysis, 84
Urinary incontinence, 286
Urinary tract
  anatomy of, 28
  Group B *Streptococcus* manifestations, 453
  physical examination of, 2
Urinary tract infections, 584
Urine flow rates, 87b, 87f, 88t
Urodynamic studies, 83
  abdominal-Valsalva leak point pressures, 94-95
  bethanechol supersensitivity test, 95-96
  bladder filling, 90-92, 91f
  cystometrogram, 88-90, 90f
  definition of, 83
  detrusor leak point pressure, 95
  electromyography, 92-93, 93f
  evaluative process, 84
  frequency/volume voiding diary, 84
  glycopyrrolate test, 96-97
  Marshall-Marchetti-Bonney stress test, 97
  micturition, 83
  pessary test, 98
  phentolamine testing, 96
  physical examination, 84
  Q-tip test, 97-98
  radiographic evaluations, 84-85
  rapid fill cystometry, 95
  residual urine, 85
  sacral evoked responses, 94
  urethral denervation sensitivity testing, 97
  urethral pressure profile, 87-88, 89t, 89f
  urethroscopy, 85, 86t
  urinalysis, 84
  uroflow studies, 87
  video cystourethrography, 85
  videourodynamics, 94, 94f
Uroflow studies, 87
Urogenital diaphragm, 18f, 20f, 22f
Urogenital triangle
  anatomy of, 14f, 15f, 16
  deep perineal pouch, 19
  description of, 13
  superficial perineal pouch, 16

Uterine artery, 25f, 32f, 33
Uterine bleeding. *See* Abnormal uterine bleeding
Uterine blood flow, 576
Uterine cancer, 291
  clinical presentation of, 293
  diagnosis of, 293
  epidemiology of, 291
  etiology of, 292
  prevention of, 293
  prognosis for, 295
  staging of, 293, 294t
  treatment of, 294
Uterine contractions, 341
Uterine mass, 275
Uterine tubes
  anatomy of, 23-24, 26f
  mass, 276
  pregnancy-related changes in, 588
  sterilization techniques, 131f, 129
Uterosacral ligaments, 82
Uterus
  abnormalities of, 182b
  anatomy of, 23-24, 25f, 26f
  atony of, 565, 567-569
  bicornuate, 148
  congenital anomalies of, 148
  incarceration during pregnancy, 243
  innervation of, 31f
  inversion of, 570, 567
  pregnancy-related changes in, 588
  rupture of, 570, 566
  unicornuate, 148

V

Vagina
  anatomy of, 26f, 28, 29f
  digital examination of, 334
  innervation of, 31f
  pregnancy-related changes in, 589
Vaginal artery, 33
Vaginal cancer, 295, 296t
Vaginal discharge, 2
Vaginal intraepithelial neoplasia, 295-296
Vaginal mass, 274
Vaginal orifice, 14f
Vaginal sponge, 120
Vaginosis, 213, 214t. *See also* Bacterial vaginosis
Valacyclovir, 206-207
Varicose veins, 596
Vasectomy, 125, 127f, 128f
Vasopressin, 600
Vegetarianism, 524
Venlafaxine, 317t
Ventricular septal defects, 539-540
Vesicouterine fossa, 29f
Vesicouterine pouch, 188
Vestibular bulbs, 19
Vestibule, 13, 14f, 18f
Video cystourethrography, 85
Videourodynamics, 94, 94f
Virilization, 304
Vitamin A, 519-520
Vitamin E, 316
Vitamins, 578, 585
Voiding diary, 84
Vulva
  cancer of, 297, 299t
  lesions of, 287
  pregnancy-related changes in, 589
  varicose veins of, 596
Vulvar hematoma, 570
Vulvar intraepithelial neoplasia, 297
Vulvovaginal candidiasis, 215
  diagnosis of, 217
  etiology of, 215
  recurrent, 218
  signs and symptoms of, 216
  treatment of, 217
Vulvovaginitis, 214t

W

Water-soluble vitamins, 578-579
Weight gain during pregnancy, 515, 516-517f, 518t, 519f, 573

Weight loss–induced amenorrhea, 175
Wellbutrin. *See* Bupropion
Wharton's jelly, 557
White blood cells, 163-164
Withdrawal method of contraception, 124
Wood's screw maneuver, 346

X
Xanax. *See* Alprazolam
X-linked recessive inheritance, 420

Z
Zidovudine, 229-230, 449
Zinc, 519
Zoloft. *See* Sertraline
Zygote intrafallopian transfer, 149

Key Telephone Numbers

This is a listing of the phone numbers of departments and individuals in the hospital who might be needed for immediate consultation.

Department

Admitting _____

Anesthesia _____

CCU _____

ECG _____

EEG _____

ER _____

ICU _____

Information _____

IV Team _____

Laboratory _____

    Chemistry _____

    Hematology _____

    Microbiology _____

    Other _____

Medical Records _____

Nuclear Medicine _____

Paging _____

Pathology _____

Pharmacy _____

Physical Therapy _____

Pulmonary Function _____

Radiology _____

Recovery Room _____

Respiratory Therapy _____

Security _____

Social Service _____

Sonography _____

Other _____

Nursing Stations

House Staff

Attending Staff

